PSYCHOTHERAPY IN CORRECTIONS

A Supportive Approach

PSYCHOTHERAPY IN CORRECTIONS

A Supportive Approach

Peter N. Novalis, M.D., Ph.D.
Virginia Singer, D.N.P., PMHNP-BC, CARN-AP
Carol M. Novalis, M.A.

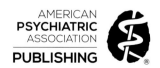

AMERICAN
PSYCHIATRIC
ASSOCIATION
PUBLISHING

If you wish to buy 50 or more copies of the same title, please go to www.appi.org/specialdiscounts for more information.

Copyright © 2023 American Psychiatric Association Publishing

ALL RIGHTS RESERVED

First Edition

Manufactured in the United States of America on acid-free paper
26 25 24 23 22   5 4 3 2 1

American Psychiatric Association Publishing
800 Maine Avenue SW, Suite 900
Washington, DC 20024-2812
www.appi.org

Library of Congress Cataloging-in-Publication Data
A CIP record is available from the Library of Congress.

British Library Cataloguing in Publication Data
A CIP record is available from the British Library.

Dedicated to the courageous people fighting the
pandemics of the world—of disease, violence,
crime, poverty, incarceration, and social injustice;
and to the survivors of these pandemics, who
deserve a better life

Contents

PART I

Introduction to Psychotherapy in Corrections and Supportive Techniques

PART II
Core Issues

PART III

Key Disorders

PART IV
Important Considerations

About the Authors

Peter N. Novalis, M.D., Ph.D., is a psychiatrist in Las Vegas, Nevada. He has more than 30 years of clinical experience, most of it in public psychiatric institutions, including state and federal psychiatric hospitals and correctional facilities. Early in his career he developed an interest in supportive psychotherapy and was the primary author of the first major textbook on the subject, *Clinical Manual of Supportive Psychotherapy*. Recognizing a need for the application of supportive psychotherapy in correctional facilities, he has developed the current project along with his coauthors.

Virginia Singer, D.N.P., is a nurse practitioner, board certified in psychiatric mental health and addictions. She has more than 25 years of experience in mental health and has worked in jails, state prisons, inpatient psychiatric hospitals, and inpatient and outpatient drug and alcohol treatment centers.

Carol M. Novalis, M.A., is an adult educator and researcher with 30 years of experience in both private and public institutions. She has a special interest in improving the education of socially disadvantaged adults.

Introduction

2020 and the years that followed were difficult ones, and it seems like we're still counting. The world had to deal with a biological injustice called COVID-19, and at the same time in the United States there broke into flames some issues of social injustice that had been smoldering for hundreds of years. Ironically, scientists encouraged the public to aim for "herd immunity" to the virus, while legal scholars urged the abolition of "qualified immunity" for police officers. Attention was called to the unequal treatments of minority groups and increased harassment of persons of color, women, Asian American–Pacific Islanders, LGBTQ individuals, immigrants, the poor, the disabled, and others as well. There was moderate success in addressing the biological injustice of the disease (which itself was inflicted disproportionately on certain groups such as elderly, Hispanic, and Black persons and economically disempowered groups such as immigrants and women) and its social and economic effects. There was perhaps partial success followed by ongoing efforts to deal with the multiple social injustices especially in American society.

These issues may not seem germane to psychotherapy in prisons and jails, but they are perhaps central to it. Social consciousness of the problems created by confining people has increased and become more important to policy-making. The term "carceral" is increasingly used to emphasize the fact that persons are held against their will within walls and that the term "criminal justice system" is self-contradictory in its meaning. The specter of COVID-19 caused fear, infection, and death within prisons over and above the usual numbers. It drew attention to the existing injustices throughout the American criminal justice system, not just the carceral component and the predominantly American propensity to arrest and lock people up. And persons with enlightened social consciousness were called "woke," a term (and its variants) that actually goes back to the antebellum era and its use by antislavery proponents.

In January 2021, the American Psychiatric Association apologized for its institutional history of racism and devoted its May annual meeting to (among many) issues of properly diagnosing Black persons and recruiting Blacks to a profession where they have been conspicuously absent (Warner 2021). It is also of note that historical racism includes the attributions of mental illness, violence, and criminality to minority groups. This apology did not exactly come on the heels of the one made by the American Medical Association (Associated Press 2008). However, there had been a history of efforts to address the racial disparities and injustices, including the attention drawn to the issue by APA's first Black president, Altha Stewart (Richmond 2018).

Cultural sensitivity is not a new concept in psychotherapy, although the upheaval in social consciousness of these years drew attention to the need for sensitivity in working with persons of diverse cultures in the criminal justice system. But even cultural sensitivity can be a double-edged sword. As therapists are exhorted to eschew damaging stereotypes, such as reading emotion as anger in Black men, they can also risk losing their sensitivity to knowing their patients completely as individuals (e.g., approaching a Latino man with the expectation that he will have only macho attitudes rather than getting to know him as a unique person).

In this really challenging year—or two, or three—we have tried to be cognizant enough of the above-mentioned issues to write usefully about psychotherapy that, in the circumstances we practice, is highly focused on treating the poor, minorities, and traditionally disadvantaged persons. There is still a tremendous variability in criminological theories, some of which might well attribute all criminal behavior to social injustice, and theorists who think that the American system should become completely "uncarceral" (i.e., prison-free). Your personal attitudes toward these issues will definitely affect your style and the content of therapy, but we hope we have produced a book that works for most people who are willing to deal with the stresses and challenges of doing psychotherapy in prison and jails.

While this book is not overtly political, we are concerned primarily with the individuals we treat. We are informed by and hope we reflect the need to "do right" by our patients in the light of the problems that are present in, and in many cases caused by, the system itself. In addition to the cultural issues that reflect various ethnic, class, gender, and physical subgroups of the prison population, we also need to address the culture of the prison, the staff and justice system that underlie the circumstances of our patients, the criminal backgrounds of the group as well as of the persons we are treating, and the circumstances of their interactions with the system. Understanding our patients' experience within this system may start with recognizing their distrust of us and of anything to do with their current situation and anyone who has not been in that situation, not just people who work for the system.

The humanity of the person we treat must always be the first consideration. Our patients are not defined as people sentenced to incarceration: what they did to get into prison is not the only measure of who they are. In reading such works as *The New Jim Crow* (Alexander 2020), *Caste* (Wilkerson 2020), or *Social (In)justice and Mental Health* (Shim and Vinson 2021), one learns how policy, assumptions, and history have led to injustice and suffering. One need only look at the rates of incarceration, arrests, and even killings by police of unarmed persons of color to see the effects of slavery, persistence of poverty, and bigotry and to get an indication of the pervasive nature of social injustice. Robert T. Carter and his colleagues have identified and defined race-based trauma as a factor in the emotional well-being of oppressed people, especially African Americans, exacerbating social adjustment and mental health issues in oppressed populations (Levine 2020). While we can only do so much in our individual roles within this system, understanding the history and its current consequences can help us understand the individuals we treat. As El-Amin and Sufrin (2020) comment, this is hard work and everyone, including staff and patients, may be affected by racism in prison environments. To the extent that this engenders outrage and, perhaps, fear response, it affects therapy and therapeutic alliances in complex ways. We must individually commit to speak up, and not be bystanders but upstanders (p. 14). There is something to be said about an advocacy role as discussed further in Chapter 1.

Correctional institutions may lack funding, but they have a wealth of data and research about themselves. Throughout the United States, legislators at all levels are intensely interested in issues such as trauma, drugs, suicide, and opportunities for education and rehabilitation within jails and prisons. Most research has as its goal the reduction of recidivism, the rate at which released prisoners return in 1, 3, 5, or 7 or more years. We have had to set our own "funding" limits on what we could cover in one volume, and our emphasis is on treating individuals.

This book is about doing psychotherapy, in particular a type of psychotherapy known as *supportive psychotherapy*, in correctional institutions. We have limited the scope to individual psychotherapy with adults. Mostly, we concentrate on psychotherapy with individuals who are involuntarily confined, although there is nothing terribly different when doing psychotherapy with those who are not incarcerated. However, one issue that is uniquely relevant to working with confined populations is what can be said to them to prevent them from coming back after they are released.

Stepping into a jail or prison might be likened to entering an alien space vessel. The denizens dress oddly and speak a strange lingo. It is a challenge to learn the customs by which they behave, and you are certainly concerned that you will not fit in or belong, or perhaps stir up some hostility you did not intend to create. In science fiction terms, such a meeting is called a Close Encounter of the Fourth Kind. Although it is used to describe the experience of entering an alien spaceship, it is typically invoked when someone has abducted and experimented upon you. Such might be your impression when you enter a prison for the first time, thinking you are the subject and they are working their experiments upon *you*. And you would be right.

Is there any kind of travel book or Fodor's guide that can ameliorate this culture shock of entering a place that is so alien to normal society? Mark Twain's *Innocents Abroad* is highly critical of the travelogues that have gone before him, as noted in the Wikipedia entry for the book: "If all the poetry and nonsense that have been discharged upon the fountains and the bland scenery of this region were collected in a book, it would make a most valuable volume to burn" (Wikipedia 2020b).[1] Books about prisons and prisoners do run the range from poetry to nonsense, and if put together they would make quite a pile to burn. (Ironically, some of Mark Twain's own books, such as *Huckleberry Finn*, were banned, and probably some were also burned.) Where do you find the truth? How much do you have to read? How many years do you need to work?

Is what matters here "the truth" or "the truth, the whole truth, and nothing but the truth"? Popular mystery writer (and Amazon Prime executive producer) Michael Connelly writes of his protagonist detective Harry Bosch that there are two kinds of truth. One is an immutable kind upon which you can base your whole life mission, but the other is malleable and belongs to such folks as corrupt lawyers and politicians because it can be molded to any purpose (Connelly 2017, p. 132). We mention this because we think the field of corrections abounds with these two kinds of truth, and it takes a lot of digging, and sometimes a modicum of courage, to distinguish the two and be willing to work for the truth. Which truth is it that you believe about prisons and prisoners? And FYI, there may be two kinds of truth, but Harry Bosch says there are NO coincidences (TV Tropes 2021)!

---

[1]Speaking of Wikipedia, we have utilized it as a universally accessible reference to read about publicly posted or generally relevant information. However, it should be kept in mind that Wikipedia says that "Wikipedia itself is not considered a reliable source" (Wikipedia 2020a). There are numerous articles of disputed accuracy even on such topics as basketball or Chicago.

Psychotherapy is done by psychologists; social workers; physicians, including psychiatrists; psychiatric nurse practitioners; and physician assistants. Licensed nurses, including registered nurses and licensed vocational or practical nurses, are involved in counseling inmates. There is also a group of correctional counselors for whom there are specialized textbooks. We have greatly benefited from reviewing the knowledge base in that area, and we do hope this book will be of value to most people who counsel inmates, provided that they do not undertake anything that is beyond the scope of their licensure. Prisons are also able to cost-effectively use trained personnel for therapy who might not have licenses in the outside world. (For an example, see the use of master's-level therapists for the psychotherapy of depression in Chapter 9.)

Our experience in these areas has been in state and federal men's and women's jails, prisons, forensic units, and mental health units. We have also had years of experience in private hospital and office practices, so we know the differences in standards and practice between these worlds. The experts, of course, say that the standards and practices should be the same, but the world has not caught up with that ideal.

Occasionally, we have put in brief case vignettes. Unlike the lengthy and detailed studies of individuals you might find in some texts, we like short stories that make a point, although we based these vignettes on our actual experiences or those of our colleagues, with the usual alterations to avoid HIPAA concerns.

We have tried to reference many of the things that we consider important, interesting, or both. But this is not a scholarly book, which would have hundreds or even a thousand more references. However, you can easily find "everything else." It just requires judicious use of the prefix "www" and in our country the suffix ".gov." As you can see from the individual bibliographical entries, many can be found, read, and printed for free.

Here is the arrangement we thought best. Part I is an introduction to psychotherapy in corrections and supportive techniques. In Chapter 1 we introduce the subject and talk about the relationship of supportive psychotherapy and corrections. Chapter 2 is a minihandbook of supportive therapy techniques. Chapter 3 carries the knowledge base into the prison itself, dealing with issues that affect new or returning prisoners. Finally, we expand on the issues of managing therapy in Chapter 4. Part II addresses core issues in helping prisoners: self-harm and suicidal behavior in Chapter 5, trauma in Chapter 6, and substance use in Chapter 7. Part III covers key disorders encountered in corrections, including serious mental illness, or SMI (Chapter 8), and mood disorders (Chapter 9). Then, in Chapter 10, we cover personality disorders, including psychopathy, addressing related issues of violence and anger. Part IV addresses important considerations that will be relevant to many readers. We discuss women in prison in Chapter 11. Chapter 12 is about behaviors and problems that tend to disrupt or impair good care, such as hunger strikes and malingering. Chapter 13 covers a variety of special topics, such as cultural issues, that could probably fill a bookshelf each if they were covered in depth but can here only be touched on. Chapter 14 covers the issues about going home and reducing the recidivism we mentioned above. Then there are a few concluding remarks.

Out there are also many books ranging from the textbooks you might have used in your course work and scholarly treatises to individual memoirs, often poignant or heartbreaking. We hope to impress upon our readers that there is more to a person than their crime, and to try to humanize the subject and our patients as much as possible. There are many persons caught up in criminal justice systems from whom we have learned much—of what it is to be an imperfect, fallible, or just unfortunate human being born in the wrong place or the wrong time in the wrong family, dominated by a different culture or caught up in circumstances beyond their control. Yet, there are those who are somewhat beyond the reach of well-meaning helpers. Good or evil, or the usual mixture of both—we have learned a little or a lot from each of our patients. Likewise, we hope that here you will learn through us from them.[2]

Peter N. Novalis, M.D., Ph.D.
Virginia Singer, D.N.P.
Carol M. Novalis, M.A.
Las Vegas, Nevada
2022

References

Alexander M: The New Jim Crow: Mass Incarceration in the Age of Colorblindness, Tenth Anniversary Edition. New York, The New Press, 2020

American Psychiatric Association: APA's apology to Black, Indigenous and People of Color for its support of structural racism in psychiatry. January 18, 2021. Available at: www.psychiatry.org/newsroom/apa-apology-for-its-support-of-structural-racism-in-psychiatry. Accessed July 4, 2021.

Associated Press: Group apologizes for its racial bias. New York Times, July 11, 2008 Available at: www.nytimes.com/2008/07/11/health/11ama.html. Accessed July 4, 2021.

Connelly M: Two Kinds of Truth. New York, Grand Central Publishing, 2017

El-Amin WW, Sufrin C: Addressing racism in correctional health care. CorrectCare: The Magazine of the National Commission on Correctional Health Care 34(3):5, 14, Summer 2020

Levine J: "Changing the outcomes, not just the symbols." Teacher's College Newsroom (Columbia University), July 23, 2020

Richmond LM: Mental health needs of blacks not being met, says APA president. Psychiatric News 55(19):1, 21, October 5, 2018

Shim RS, Vinson SY (eds): Social (In)justice and Mental Health. Washington, DC, American Psychiatric Association Publishing, 2021

TV Tropes: The Black Echo. Available at: https://tvtropes.org/pmwiki/pmwiki.php/Literature/TheBlackEcho. Accessed January 1, 2021.

Warner J: Psychiatry confronts its racist past, and tries to make amends: but there is a lot to apologize for—from Reconstruction to today. New York Times, April 30, 2021. Updated May 21, 2021. Available at: www.nytimes.com/2021/04/30/health/psychiatry-racism-black-americans.html. Accessed July 4, 2021.

Wikipedia: Accuracy dispute. Available at: https://en.wikipedia.org/wiki/Wikipedia:Accuracy_dispute. Accessed September 8, 2020a.

Wikipedia: Innocents Abroad. Available at: https://en.wikipedia.org/wiki/The_Innocents_Abroad. Accessed September 8, 2020b.

Wilkerson I: Caste: The Origins of Our Discontents. New York, Random House, 2020

---

[2]There are those who say that the belief in absolute good and evil should be relegated to the scrap heap of ideas along with the hardware in our prisons, the argument being that such a belief results in hardline correctional philosophies with cruel and unusual punishments (the hardware in our prisons being a not much enlightened evolution of the instruments of the Inquisition). Ask yourself where you stand on this age-old debate. Does it depend on your religion, or whether you are religious at all? Does it depend on your political affiliations? Is everyone and everything forgivable, or are there still unforgivable evils and persons? Finally, and this might help you to answer the preceding questions: Have you ever worked with a psychopath?

Notes on Usage

We try to vary pronouns for males and females except when the context makes it desirable to refer to one rather than the other. We have decided to usually use "Black" and "white" and similar terms, but sometimes we will use "African American," usually to reflect the preference of a source being discussed. (The designation "Black" is now capitalized, reflecting the change in the editorial practices of the major news organizations in the summer of 2020.) We strive to use correctly the terms "Hispanic" and "Latino," which are not synonymous. Some writers are now using the term "Latinx" to avoid the gendered terms "Latino" and "Latina," but that has not become general usage, so we have continued to use the present terminology.

But let's consider who is the person being treated. Is he or she a client, patient, resident, inmate, criminal, prisoner, detainee, incarceree (a newer term that was originally used to refer to those in Japanese interment camps during World War II), or offender? The term *client* does not seem right because of the involuntary settings, but for anyone receiving direct treatment it seems appropriate to use the term *patient*. Many persons in jails or prisons have not have actually broken any law if they are in a pretrial setting or innocent of the crimes of which they are accused. *Detainee* does appropriately apply to many persons awaiting trial or in immigrant detention centers. During the preparation and publication of this book, there has been a concern among advocates of better care to eliminate what is felt to be dehumanizing language regarding persons who have been incarcerated. This includes the elimination of the terms *prisoner* and *inmate* in lieu of person-first descriptions such as an "incarcerated person" or a "person with a substance use disorder" (National Commission on Correctional Health Care 2021). We recognize the importance of person-centered terminology, but as a descriptive rule it is not yet seen in recent publications, in the media such as *The New York Times*, or among the professionals with whom we work. We have adopted the practice of the advocacy group The Marshall Project of continuing to use the word *prisoner* but attempting to eliminate the term *inmate* (Solomon 2021); the latter may be still found in articles and books (e.g., Batastini et al. 2020) and in references to the research using such terms. We shall also comment on the use of the term *criminal* in a later chapter.

We also have made a concerted effort to avoid objectifying diseases, so, therefore, we do not call a person who has schizophrenia a "schizophrenic" or a person who has borderline personality disorder a "borderline." Some practices, such as not applying diagnoses to women because traditional oppression has created their symptoms, are worth understanding, but we have considered them "a bridge too far" for this work. At the end of our introduction above, however, we did refer to a "psychopath." In that case, our justification is that psychopathy is not a mental illness.

The Substance Abuse and Mental Health Services Administration of the U.S. National Institutes of Health is usually referred to as "SAMHSA."

There are two major diagnostic resources. One is the *International Classification of Diseases*, Tenth Revision, which is referenced worldwide in multiple versions (www.cdc.gov/nchs/icd/icd10.htm). This will be referred to as ICD-10. Some authors are making references to ICD-11, and there are some diagnostic differences that will affect researchers, but we will continue with ICD-10 until it has been effectively replaced.

Our most used diagnostic reference manual is, of course, usually called "DSM-5," which refers to the American Psychiatric Association's *Diagnostic and Statistical Manual of Mental Disorders*, 5th Edition (Arlington, VA, American Psychiatric Association, 2013). A text revision, DSM-5-TR, was published in March 2022 and is also discussed where relevant. There are also a few other revisions and text revision editions, but we do not refer to them in a substantial way in this book. A list of the editions we refer to is as follows:

- DSM-5-TR: American Psychiatric Association: *Diagnostic and Statistical Manual of Mental Disorders*, 5th Edition, Text Revision. Washington, DC, American Psychiatric Association, 2022
- DSM-5: American Psychiatric Association: *Diagnostic and Statistical Manual of Mental Disorders*, 5th Edition. Arlington, VA, American Psychiatric Association, 2013
- DSM-IV: American Psychiatric Association: *Diagnostic and Statistical Manual of Mental Disorders*, 4th Edition. Washington, DC, American Psychiatric Association, 1994
- DSM-III: American Psychiatric Association: *Diagnostic and Statistical Manual of Mental Disorders*, 3rd Edition. Washington, DC, American Psychiatric Association, 1980
- DSM-II: American Psychiatric Association: *Diagnostic and Statistical Manual of Mental Disorders*, 2nd Edition. Washington, DC, American Psychiatric Association, 1968
- DSM: American Psychiatric Association: *Diagnostic and Statistical Manual: Mental Disorders*. Washington, DC, American Psychiatric Association, 1952

References

Batastini AB, Morgan RD, Kroner DG, Mills JF: A Mental Health Treatment Program for Inmates in Restrictive Housing: Stepping Up, Stepping Out. New York, Routledge, 2020

National Commission on Correctional Health Care: Position Statement on Use of Humanizing Language in Correctional Health Care. 2021. Available at: www.ncchc.org/filebin/Positions/Use-of-Humanizing-Language-in-Correctional-Health-Care-2021.pdf. Accessed March 2, 2022.

Solomon A: What words we use—and avoid—when covering people and incarceration. The Marshall Project. 2021. Available at: www.themarshallproject.org/2021/04/12/what-words-we-use-and-avoid-when-covering-people-and-incarceration. Accessed March 2, 2022.

PART I

Introduction to Psychotherapy in Corrections and Supportive Techniques

1

Supportive Psychotherapy in the Correctional Environment

Have you been to jail lately? No, we don't mean to work there, but to live. If you have, you would be one of 10.6 million people. That's not the number of people who live in jail, but it reflects what is called the enormous *churn* of people who come in and out of jails in the United States every year. As for those who live there: in early 2020, there were 631,000 people in jail; 1,291,000 in state prisons; 226,000 in federal prisons and jails, including 66,000 being held by federal marshals; 44,000 in youth facilities; and 42,000 in immigration detention centers (Bronson and Berzofsky 2017). Because of COVID-19, the numbers in immigration detention centers dropped precipitously to under 20,000 (Solis 2020). Smaller numbers of people are held in territorial prisons (11,000), facilities operated by tribal authorities or the Bureau of Indian Affairs (2,500), and military facilities (1,500). There are also 22,000 involuntarily committed in mental hospitals, including some forensic facilities (Sawyer and Wagner 2020). Another 4,537,300 people are under community supervision of some sort (parole or probation) (Kaeble and Cowhig 2018).

Generally speaking, do those numbers sound high? Yes, they are. (For a slight diversion and learning experience of how high, see the dialogue box "The *Lakh*-up Monster.") More than half of state prisoners are serving sentences for violent offenses, while nearly half of federal prisoners are there for drug-related offenses. There are also tremendous racial and cultural differences in the U.S. criminal justice system. For example, the imprisonment rate for sentenced Black males is six times that for sentenced white males; the ratio is less but still elevated for persons of Hispanic affiliation (Bronson and Carson 2019). Women are the fastest growing group of incarcerated people, and they have unique needs arising from the traditionally unequal position they have held in society because of structural inequalities and life trajectories leading to prison.

The *Lakh*-up Monster

JACK: I'm working on our book about prisons, and I'm reading this really cool monograph about the prisons in India, but I don't understand this sentence. It says, "At any given time, over 3.5 *lakh* people are imprisoned in correctional institutions in India" (Math et al. 2011, p. 3). Who are these *lakh* people? Are they a special type of prisoner?

JILL: Really, are you quite stupid or what?

JACK: Okay, okay, I assume a *lakh* is a number, but how much is it?

JILL: Why don't you just look it up on Google?

JACK: Because you're a general fount of all knowledge, and you probably know the answer already.

JILL: Yes, I do, but I want you to work for it. *Lakh* is a Sanskrit word and is commonly known in Asia. So do the math. The population of India is a bit more than four times the population of the United States, and as you know, the United States incarcerates about 2.1 million people. So how many people do you think they incarcerate in India?

JACK: That sounds like a trick question. I know that the United States has the highest incarceration rate in the world. So if India incarcerated people at the same rate as we do, it would incarcerate about 8.4 million people, since it has four times the population. But accounting for the fact that the rate is much higher in the United States, I would assume that they incarcerate only 3.5 million people, which would mean that a *lakh* is a million.

JILL: How wrong you are! A *lakh* is 100,000, and at the time that monograph was written in 2011, India incarcerated only 3.5 *lakh*, or 350,000 people.

JACK (*excited*): Well, knock me down and break my crown! That's unbelievable.

JILL: Yes, because the incarceration rate in the United States is *24* times the incarceration rate in India!

JACK: Why is that?

JILL: There are a lot of reasons. But a good analogy would be to use another Sanskrit word, *juggernaut*, which was used to refer to a huge processional wagon bearing an image of a Hindu god. The U.S. correctional system is like a *juggernaut*, a relentless wagon (I'd call it a paddy wagon but that would probably be politically incorrect) that rolls down the streets of our cities arresting people in its path for minor reasons that we call "misdemeanors." Then we put them in jail and make it impossible for them to pay bond and get out. And since they can't get out, they lose their jobs and it destroys their families. And prison doesn't do much to help them. And when they get out, the system doesn't give them the resources and opportunities to stay out. And so it goes. Can you tumble to that?

JACK: Cute phrase, coming from you. But that's a great analogy. I think I'll use it in our book.

Trestman (2018) has reviewed the statistics of nondominant populations in prison and points out that the system is biased against such individuals in many ways, starting with the likelihood of arrest (on the basis of appearance or community rather than behavior that might be overlooked or discounted) and extending to bail money (which is not affordable and leads to longer detention) and sentencing (which is statistically longer for nondominant populations). In his article, Trestman acknowledges the cumulative disadvantages faced by individuals who are Black, Hispanic, or Native American, or from other disadvantaged groups, and suggests that the justice system needs to address how such cumulative disadvantages impact both these individuals' experiences at first contact with police and the beliefs and attitudes of professionals (police, courts, mental health providers) with the goal of diverting individuals away from incarceration and toward personal goals that are more likely to keep them out of the system altogether.

To sum up what is going on here, and alluding to what we said in the Introduction, the United States has been accused of running a "carceral state" that is not only obsessed with incarceration but historically biased against minority populations, and especially Blacks, because of a national history of slavery and racism. An accessible collection of essays will elucidate that point (Hernández and Muhammad 2015).

So, in the United States we are rather good at putting people in jails and prisons and detention centers. But we are not so good at keeping people out after they are released. For example, five out of six state prisoners released in 2005 were rearrested within 9 years of their release, and on average, there were five arrests per prisoner (Alper et al. 2018).

The take-home point (or take-to-jail point, if you are reading this at work) is this: Although correctional settings are not likely anyone's favorite place to spend a Saturday night, they are places where many people *do* spend a Saturday night—if not yourself, then perhaps a family member or friend, especially if your heritage is African American or Hispanic. In a widely reported study, it was found that nearly one-half of respondents had had a family member incarcerated (Renner 2019). The figure is 60% for families of African Americans and families with low education levels and only 15% for families of college-educated whites.

Why do people commit crimes, and why does the United States in particular arrest and incarcerate so many people with a predilection for people of color? There are numerous theories of crime, and the field is not shrinking (somewhat like the field of psychotherapy), since criminal behavior is after all a form of human behavior. We have briefly mentioned some of the leading theories in Table 1–1. As for the United States being an "incarceration nation," there are numerous reasons for that as well but a lot less controversy. The inequalities start in disadvantaged communities that are oppressed by the rest of the society and also mistreat and marginalize women (Miller 2008). The incarceration starts with a massive misdemeanor system and a monetary bail system that entraps people from disadvantaged backgrounds.

As a mental health professional, you probably want to understand why and how people are incarcerated and how to help them once they get there. This does not mean that everyone in jail has a mental illness or even close. But mental health professionals have always had an interest in the causes of criminal behavior and ways to prevent people from coming back (i.e., reducing recidivism). Correctional institutions have numerous programs, some with more or less of what we would call "psychological content." In the two tables that follow, we present a brief survey of the programs or characteristics that affect prisoners psychologically (Table 1–2) or have planned-for psychological content (Table 1–3). Focusing on the person rather than the activity, Table 1–4 lists many activities—be they therapeutic, quasi-therapeutic, or totally nontherapeutic (e.g., quelling a riot)—that may be assigned to psychotherapists. The point of these tables is to emphasize that you are but one of many persons in a great enterprise that influences your patients' physical and mental health. You must know something about the other things in your patients' lives, minimally, so that you don't contradict or undo the effects of their other programming. You may also want to refer patients to such programs or convince them to enroll.

TABLE 1–1.   Leading theories of crime

Theory or group of theories	Proponents	Basic assertions	Comments
Classical and Rational Choice and Deterrence; Routine Activity (see the last two names under "Proponents")	John Locke (1632–1704) Thomas Hobbes (1588–1679) Jeremy Bentham (1748–1832) Cesare Beccaria (1738–1794) Lawrence E. Cohen Marcus Felson	Criminal behavior reflects the rational choice of criminals; therefore, it can be deterred by punishment.	Has some empirical support, but it is definitely not the whole story; yet, it is the dominant paradigm of many persons and especially correctional facilities in terms of management.
Neoclassical, Positivism, Hard Determinism	Oscar Newman Robert Martinson (1927–1979) James Q. Wilson (1931–2012)	Associated with the (outmoded) doctrine that "nothing works."	Not accepted by researchers now because it is believed that programs and therapy can lessen recidivism.
Conflict, Marxist, Radical Critical (includes Peacemaking, Convict Criminology, Green Criminology)	Karl Marx (1818–1883) Willem Bonger (1876–1940) Otto Kirchheimer (1905–1965) William J. Chambliss (1933–2014) Harold Pepinsky and Richard Quinney (Restorative and Participatory Justice) George Rusche (1900–1950) William Graham Sumner (1840–1910) Austin Turk George B. Vold (1896–1967) Max Weber (1864–1920)	The criminal justice system reflects interest of powerful groups.	Feminist theory is an outgrowth of the power imbalance recognized in Marxist theories; many of the others represent smaller interest groups based on political ideologies.

TABLE 1–1. Leading theories of crime *(continued)*

Theory or group of theories	Proponents	Basic assertions	Comments
Feminist and Female Pathways	Freda Adler Rita Simon Anne Campbell (1951–2017) ("Staying Alive") Kathleen Daly Meda Chesney-Lind and Lisa Pasko (Female Pathways) James W. Messerschmidt John Hagan (Power-Control Theory)	Recognized androcentricity in previous theories of criminology and the historical and current position of women as nondominant and suppressed; women's pathways follow trajectories of escape from abuse and victimization.	Has major implications in understanding criminality in women, the nature and labeling of mental problems in women, and appropriate treatment in corrections.
Biological, Developmental	Franz Joseph Gall (1758–1828) Ernst Kretschmer (1888–1964) Robert Agnew Cesare Lombroso (1835–1909) Hans Eysenck (1916–1997) William Ferrero (1871–1942) Charles Goring (1870–1919) E. A. Hooton (1887–1954) William Sheldon (1898–1977) Otto Pollak (1908–1998) Sarnoff Mednick (1928–2015) Terrie Moffitt	Kretschmer and Sheldon described three body types; criminality results from biological/genetic defects; role of punishment may be limited.	Applied to so-called psychopaths who were previously considered relatively untreatable.
Psychological	Sigmund Freud (1856–1939) Kate Friedlander (1902–1949) Hervey Cleckley (1903–1984) Robert M. Hare	Mental conflicts or personality defects result in aggression and hence crime; Cleckley and Hare developed the modern concept of psychopathy.	Still useful in understanding how psychological processes are responsible for criminal behavior; also applied to psychopaths and individuals with severe personality disorders, but generally not the source of most crime.

TABLE 1–1.   Leading theories of crime (continued)

Theory or group of theories	Proponents	Basic assertions	Comments
Social Process, Social Learning, Differential Association	Ronald Akers Albert Bandura (1925–2021) Robert Burgess Delbert Elliot Edwin Sutherland (1883–1950) (Differential Association) Daniel Glaser (Differential Identification) Erving Goffman (1922–1982) (Dramaturgy)	People learn to become criminals from their social environment; crime is a social illness or deviance.	Fairly widely accepted as accounting for various forms of delinquency and also the way individuals can learn to become prosocial, such as by learning to model the therapist's behavior.
Social Bonding and Control, Containment	Michael Gottfredson and Travis Hirschi (1935–2017) (General Theory of Crime) David Matza (1930–2018) F. Ivan Nye (1918–2014) Walter Reckless (1899–1988) (Containment), Gresham Sykes (1922–2010)	Addresses the effect of or lack of social bonds.	Also a theory of delinquency; shows that low self-control is a remediable factor in criminals.
Labeling and Reintegrative Shaming, Restorative Justice	Howard Becker John Braithwaite Charles Horton Cooley (1864–1929) Edwin M. Lemert (1912–1996) Frank Tannenbaum (1893–1969)	Labeling and stigmatization create a vicious circle that results in increased criminality.	Attractive and also relevant to our comments on labeling of women, but the empirical support is weak.
Social Disorganization	Lloyd Ohlin (1918–2008) Robert Ezra Park (1864–1944) Clifford R. Shaw (1895–1957)	Explains the development of crime in disadvantaged areas.	Applicable to understanding the development of many prisoners we treat.

TABLE 1–1. **Leading theories of crime** *(continued)*

Theory or group of theories	Proponents	Basic assertions	Comments
Anomie and strain	Emile Durkheim (1858–1917) Robert Agnew Ernest Burgess (1886–1966) Richard Cloward (1926–2001) Henry D. McKay (1899–1980) Robert K. Merton (1910–2003) Steven F. Messner Walter B. Miller (1920–2004) Richard Rosenfeld	Absence of social norms is one factor; the tension between social goals and blocked opportunities leads individuals to commit crimes.	Explains why many people see crime as an attractive option or at least one that has no negative implications for them.
Integrative and Pathways	Ronald L. Akers Thomas Bernard Mark Colvin Francis T. Cullen Delbert S. Elliott Howard B. Kaplan (1932–2011) Marvin D. Krohn Robert Sampson and John H. Laub (Pathways and Age-Graded Life-Course Theory) Terence P. Thornberry Charles R. Tittle	Represents the attempts of theorists to develop overarching integrative theories that explain crime.	Social learning and social bonding and strain theories seem to have been the main "winners" in this multitheory competition.
General Personality and Cognitive Social Learning (GPCSL)	Donald A. Andrews (1941–2010) and James Bonta (Andrews and Bonta 1994; and later editions)	Role of biological factors (genetic, temperament, traumatic brain injury), psychological and family factors, and social-environmental factors in causation.	Encompassing elements of several previous theories, this theory is related to the risk-need-responsivity (RNR) model of treatment (see text).

Source. Based on Pittaro 2010; Schram and Tibbetts 2014; See and Kieser 2013; Walsh and Jorgensen 2020.

TABLE 1–2.	Examples of prison programming that affect prisoners psychologically

Incarceration itself

Location of the prison (often far from family and reentry resources)

Housing assignment based on classification, security, racial and gang affiliations, a special need, and other reasons

Special Management Units ("SMUs")[a]

Protective custody[b]

Medical department services other than psychological or psychiatric (e.g., medication group, exercise group, occupational therapy)

On-site recreational therapy

Off-site specialists

Camp and/or forestry programs, or boot camp

High-security units (all levels may exist in some prisons, especially women's prisons)

Detox unit

Mother and baby units

Low-security community residences (work and go to school during the day)

Work-in unit (porter)

Other work onsite (prison wages, minimum wages, market wages)

Work programs run by outside contractors

Vocational training (e.g., sheet metal, furniture, highway flagger)

Dog pod or other animal-involved units

Victim recovery

Other restorative justice programs

Education (GED, high school, vocational or trade school, college)

Literacy or English as a second language

Library or law library

Recreation therapy and recreational yards

Commissary, food service, or chow hall

Chorus

[a]SMUs may variously be called "Special Housing Units" and may include Disciplinary Housing (Restrictive Housing Unit, versions called solitary confinement, segregation, closed cell restrictions, and, by prisoners, "the hole"). Disciplinary housing may lock down detainees for 23 out of 24 hours, and these detainees may be denied access to television, commissary, face-to-face visitation, or even phones other than to make calls to legal counsel and services.
[b]Protective custody, or "PC," may be self-selected or involuntary for protection of others in the institution and ordered by the disciplinary committee; the typical PC unit may allow individuals out for 4–6 hours a day for exercise and socialization, and they may access television, video games, and commissary.

Correctional environments are physically and psychologically dangerous. Except in the highest security institutions, when you enter one you will be surrounded by prisoners much of the day. Although you go home at the end of that day, you may still feel a little bit of what it is like to be confined there, and after you go home you may still feel oppressed by your encounters of the day. This includes a common experience of feeling abused or harangued in the therapy session but not quite badly enough to call for assistance or send the patient out the door. Outside of the therapy sessions, prisoners (even those who are pleasant and cooperative during therapy sessions) can be

TABLE 1–3.	Examples of prison programming with significant psychological content

Psychology and mental health counseling services including groups (see Table 1–4)

Psychiatry or similar mental health medication services

Medication groups (often led by nurses)

Mental health unit (temporary or permanent housing assignment)

Therapeutic Community (usually for mental health or substance abuse treatment)

Alcoholics Anonymous, Narcotics Anonymous, Rational Recovery

Mental illness peer groups

Yoga

Exercise groups

Religious services

Outside volunteers

Outside halfway house programs

Transitional programs

Reentry pod and groups

Art

Music

Bibliotherapy

Drama therapy

Crafts and crafts programs

Family (systemic) therapy

bullying, threatening, and physically assaultive and frequently make unjustified complaints of abuse against staff members.

Plucking a volume from our shelf, we encounter the renowned galactic chef Gurronsevas, traveling incognito as a dietitian, sneaking into Sector General, a 384-level (levels, not beds) hospital that serves all sentient species at the edge of the galaxy. He is discovered and receives a quick course in First Contact Procedures from his captain. *Don't show a strong reaction to anything you see or hear even if it is personally repugnant. Show an interest in everything and try to praise rather than criticize. Most of all, be agreeable and diplomatic* (White 1996, p. 192).

Admittedly it is an analogy, but as the preceding indicates, it is important to pay attention to your personal responses and reactions when entering a correctional environment, and as we said in the Introduction, you may have the disquieting feeling that you are being scrutinized closely or examined for personal flaws. When we talk about doing psychotherapy (particularly supportive psychotherapy) with people in correctional settings, we will not in general talk about how to do highly specialized (usually forensic) evaluations. Evaluations of this type would include the formal reports listed in Table 1–3. Such reports are the responsibility of specialists in forensic psychology, psychiatry, and court social workers.

Therapists are frequently asked or required to make recommendations based on information acquired from interviewing patients. Examples would be the decision to move a person in or out of an infirmary suicide watch, the decision to seek outside hospitalization, or the determination of mental suitability for discipline (sometimes

TABLE 1–4.   Activities of psychotherapists in correctional settings

Various institutional functions related to employment and safety

Specialized forensic evaluations (generally not covered in this book) for NGRI (not guilty by reason of insanity), parole (often done as a committee)

Individual psychotherapy (just a few examples; some are related to group modalities)

   Supportive

   Psychodynamic

   Psychoanalytic

   Cognitive-behavioral therapy (CBT)

   Motivational interviewing

   Interpersonal psychotherapy (IPT)

   Acceptance and commitment therapy (ACT)

General group psychotherapy

Specialized groups (overlap with specialized offender and victim programming)

   CBT and/or sleep hygiene for insomnia or nightmares

   Moral reconation therapy

   Meditation/Mindfulness

   Guided imagery

   Progressive relaxation

   Thinking for a Change

   InsideOut Dad

   Social work

   Parenting

   Seeking Safety

   STOP (Sexual Treatment of Offenders in Prison)

   STEPPS (Systems Training for Emotional Predictability and Problem Solving)

   SOAR (Survivors of Abuse and Rape)

   Reoffense prevention groups

   Offense-related groups (Good Lives Model or other programming for sex offending, domestic violence/intimate partner violence, DUI, child neglect, elder neglect, drug-related crimes)

   Anger management (e.g., Cage Your Rage)

   Trauma

   Drug-related crimes group

   Victim awareness group

   Anger management

   Aggression Replacement Training

   Addiction treatment or relapse prevention

   Newcomers group

   Lifers group

   Short-timers group

TABLE 1–4.　　**Activities of psychotherapists in correctional settings *(continued)***

Evaluations related to psychotherapy (but not specialized forensic) functions

　Suicide and self-harm related (placement on levels of suicide watch and observation, develop Crisis Response Safety Plans (described in Chapter 5 and elaborated on in Chapters 6, 7, 13, and 14)

　Level of care determinations (including hospitalizations)

　Safety determinations (e.g., for travel outside institution)

　Placement determinations (e.g., for single cell, certain classes, lay-in from work)

　PREA (Prison Rape Elimination Act)–related assessment (many possible capacities)

　Other evaluative functions

　　Determine culpability for discipline (e.g., so-called baseline stable evaluations)

　　Do individual or group interventions for hunger strikes

　　Authorize permissions for lower bunk, lower tier, or single cell

　　Determine if patient is malingering illness

　　Serve as gatekeeper to prescribers

　　Evaluate referrals from others

　　Talk down or defuse violence

　　Report misconduct (dealing with confidentiality issues)

called a "baseline stable" evaluation). When it's appropriate to do so, we will advise you about some of those issues. However, the primary subject of this book is psychotherapy, and particularly supportive psychotherapy. To give an example of what we may minimize or exclude, there is abundant literature on assessing suicidality in corrections, and it's not our intention to introduce a new system or method for you to make such decisions in your own institution. So as far as the various duties of Table 1–4 go, use what you are given, but we *will* give you guidance on doing psychotherapy with suicidal patients in a separate chapter.

Given the great number of persons in carceral settings, an important question is "Who needs treatment?" That is, "Who needs psychological treatment?" Or, without begging the question, "Is it just mentally ill people who need treatment?" Of course not. People in situational crises need treatment, and not all of them have what is traditionally considered a mental illness. DSM-5-TR and ICD-10 have a range of codes to cover various life circumstances, many of which fall short of what clinicians call mental illness. For example, there are codes for psychosocial circumstances, a history of trauma or mental illness, and legal problems, and a specific code for incarceration. The Bureau of Justice Statistics of the U.S. Department of Justice uses a number of methods to measure various mental illness and illness-like conditions that occur in incarcerated persons. Their methods of collection vary and so, too, do the numbers. For example, some numbers come from what the Bureau of Justice Statistics calls "SPD," or Serious Psychological Distress. About one in seven state and federal prisoners and one in four of those in jail reported SPD in a survey ending May 2012. Also, 37% of prisoners and 44% of the jailed population said they had been told by a mental health professional that they had a mental disorder (Bronson and Berzofsky 2017). A third statistic is that of symptoms of mental disorder as determined by a structured clinical interview for DSM (in this case, DSM-IV) disorders. The 2004 data showed that the rate of DSM-IV disorders, based on structured interview, was 64% among people in jail, 56% among state prisoners, and 46% among federal prisoners. In the same Bureau of Justice Statistics report are some comorbidity numbers that you frequently hear about in discussions of substance use disorders in prison: About 74% of state prisoners and 76% of the local jail population who have a mental health problem also have a substance use problem. Prisoners with mental health problems are slightly more likely (49% vs. 46%) to have committed a violent offense, A violent criminal record is also more prevalent among mentally ill prisoners (61% vs. 56% in state prisons), as is a history of violent recidivism (47% vs. 39% in that group). These findings contradict the common belief that mentally ill persons are sentenced for minor offenses. Such a belief is more likely true of subpopulations of mentally ill persons such as homeless persons (Bronson and Berzofsky 2017).

What about serious mental illness? A frequently cited estimate is that about 16% of people in jail or prison have serious mental illness. We will discuss this in Chapter 8.

Where Do They Live? A Prison Primer

Some fairly small places where persons are held briefly prior to a disposition are called *lockups*. Mental health services are still important in such facilities because of the catastrophic reactions of newly arrested persons and their high suicide rate. In the United States, jails and detention centers may house presentence detainees or sentenced persons, often in separate locations so that the populations do not mingle.

Felony is the most serious type of crime, and punishment is typically a year or more. A *misdemeanor* is a lower level of crime for which punishment is up to a year. You will also hear about "aggravated felonies" and other classes of crimes such as sex offenses. In most states, persons convicted of misdemeanors are housed in jails, and persons convicted of felonies are sent to state prisons. But in some states, persons convicted of low-level felonies are housed for several years in jails. Once assigned to a prison, prisoners do not usually return to jail unless they incur some other charge. But because of a program called realignment in California, a prison-to-jail reassignment of prisoners began in 2011, and although community safety did not seem to worsen, there was a tremendous increase in prisoner-on-prisoner murders in the jails outside of Los Angeles. The number of such murders is not huge, but it went from 12 to 30 in the 7 years before to the 7 years after realignment (Pohl and Gabrielson 2019). There were similar concerns about the lowering of the total prison population by court order because of the inhumane overpopulation of the prison system as a whole.

While politicians of all stripes continued to argue about the proper and humane treatment of prisoners, in March 2020 along came an international mass/serial killer known as coronavirus, aka COVID-19, and a few other aliases that were politically inflammatory. Within weeks, judges were diverting people from jail and prison, sheriffs were releasing low-level nonviolent jail residents charged or convicted of low-level offenses both pre- and postsentence, and state and federal authorities were releasing thousands of prisoners.

Did the world descend into postapocalyptic anarchy? Apparently not, as we discuss in Chapter 14. However, prison is thought to serve several purposes, and it may be argued (see below) that some of these purposes, such as punishment, retribution, and general deterrence, may not be served by early release, even if there is no effect on recidivism.

Presentence institutions in the United Kingdom are called *remand prisons*. Most countries have multilevel prison systems, from high to minimum security. In minimum security (some countries call them "open" prisons), a person, who is usually in transition to leave the prison system, may be allowed to work on the grounds with minimal supervision or may spend the day in the community going to school or work. Many of these people may receive their mental health services in community facilities. All systems provide penalties (e.g., a 5-year sentence) for leaving minimum security, so escapes, or "elopements," are rare, and such persons are not considered dangerous.

At the periphery of the mainline institutions are transitional living facilities and halfway houses, some private but many state-run, where a resident is legally speaking still a prisoner of the state. There are many mental health services in parole and probation clinics for those completing sentences or avoiding sentencing. There are also facilities that house prisoners whose sentences have expired but who are being held indefinitely on civil commitment.

Stays in jails may range from a few hours (until a newly arrested person posts bond and is released) to several years (for complicated pretrial cases). The majority of persons who do not post bond fairly rapidly will stay several months until trial. Highprofile cases will take longer as parties mutually agree upon delays in coming to trial, or a person convicted of several misdemeanors may serve sentences for all of them in jail.

At the heart of it, however, you find out that 470,000 out of those 631,000 people in jail (or 74%) have not even been convicted yet. Also, many of the people you see in jail are innocent. Many of them are there because they cannot afford the typical bond of $10,000, which represents more than half of a year's salary for them (Sawyer and Wagner 2020). Fortunately, this situation now appears to be changing rapidly as many jurisdictions are abolishing cash bond. Some sentenced prisoners are also innocent. Some may have plea-bargained based on poor advice or pressure from others, including police, family, or attorneys. Of course, there are other sentenced prisoners who falsely protest their innocence. Some patients do have a constant hope of getting up enough bond to be released or of finally winning their case. At the end, hope may be dashed upon conviction, a dangerous period of time because of the stress it creates. Depending on the level of offense, this may be followed shortly by a transfer to prison.

What Do I Need to Know About Working With Corrections Staff?

Correctional culture is paramilitary in approach and reflects a male-dominated "macho" culture. It is a culture in which people do not complain of pain and all aberrant behavior tends to be treated as criminal (i.e., ascribing criminal motives rather than seeing the signs of mental or behavioral disorders), and sensitivity or "softness" is viewed as a weakness. Correctional officers (COs) often believe that therapists "coddle" their patients, whereas they believe that they see the "real" patient where he or she lives and works in the dormitory and kitchen. (In general, you should never call COs "guards," although you will frequently hear them called that by prisoners and on television, and even in some of the articles that you read. Similarly, television shows typically call prisons "jails," as in "You'll go to jail for the rest of your life.")

Therapists who work successfully with COs get to know them. You can visit a CO where he or she works in the dormitory and the control "bubble." You need not make a pest of yourself, but there are many occasions when stopping by to deal with an issue is useful. Good mental health departments also invite custody to provide input into their meetings. This does sometimes create concerns in prisoners who see the officers going into the mental health office. HIPAA compliance is not usually the issue, since HIPAA allows the sharing of information on a need-to-know basis even to COs and all the way up to the warden. For example, if a person should be observed for suicidal behavior, then the CO needs to know what to look for. However, the CO would not be allowed to read the mental health chart.

What Do I Need to Know About Supportive Psychotherapy to Work With Prisoners?

Whether you are a beginning or an experienced psychotherapist, you probably already know a lot about supportive psychotherapy and have been using some of its techniques from your first day on the job. In training and subsequent professional readings, you have frequently encountered and learned about so-called supportive techniques and interventions, even though you may have heard that they are to be saved for the most impaired or seriously ill of your patients.

Supportive therapy does have a collection of techniques, and supportive interventions were described over 2,000 years ago by the Ancient Greeks, who wrote about rhetoric, or the art of persuading people with words (as opposed to the use of force such as in war). As one historian notes: "This art or technique [of the Ancient Greek philosophers] favorably compares with several of the methods called supportive psychotherapy" (Kourkouta 2002, p. 39).

Sigmund Freud, who had himself elaborated and then abandoned the use of direct suggestion and hypnosis in lieu of associative psychoanalytic technique, predicted that "the large-scale application of our theory will compel us to alloy the pure gold of analysis freely with the copper of direct suggestion" (Freud 1919 [1918]/1955, p. 168). We (Novalis et al. 1993, 2020) and many others portray supportive psychotherapy as a type of psychotherapy, as are cognitive-behavioral therapy (CBT), psychoanalytic therapy, psychodynamic therapy, humanistic therapy, and many others.

Supportive therapy has been conceived of as being on a spectrum of techniques ranging from supportive at one end to expressive at the other. A particular kind of therapy encompassing the spectrum and the Core Conflictual Relationship Model was developed by Luborsky (1984). An update of such studies may be found elsewhere (Leichsenring and Leibing 2007). Other presentations may be found in books by Winston et al. (2020), Battaglia (2019), and Sharpless (2019). Some practitioners say that they hold a "Y-theory" of psychotherapy, with supportive techniques being the stem for cognitive or psychodynamic techniques (Plakun et al. 2009). Given the numerous available "psychotherapies" that are used in corrections, our view of supportive psychotherapy does not place it on a two-dimensional spectrum of supportive-expressive treatments; rather, we view it as the root of all successful psychotherapeutic methods. Supportive psychotherapy involves three components:

1. Supportive goals
2. Supportive techniques
3. A supportive therapist-patient relationship

The relationship between therapist and patient will be discussed in Chapter 3, where we will address the issues that patients in corrections have in their interpersonal relationships, including their relationship with therapists. We discuss the first two elements in this chapter and the next.

Supportive psychotherapy has also been described as *eclectic* and *integrative*. An eclectic therapy is one that draws from multiple sources of techniques that have been found to work. Typically, this is how most therapists enhance their skills. "The truth is that most therapists practice the eclectic approach, even if they identify as a specialist in one type of therapy" (Dean 2021, p. 1). An integrative psychotherapy draws together overlapping concepts and strategies to create effective systems of psychotherapy. "Psychotherapy integration grew out of increasing dissatisfaction with the continuous creation of new schools of psychotherapy…" (Beitman and Manring 2009, p. 705). It may be of interest for readers to know that the following "schools" of psychotherapy (among others) are also considered integrative by the above authors:

- Acceptance and commitment therapy (ACT)
- Cognitive-affective behavior therapy
- Cognitive-analytic therapy (CAT)
- Cognitive-behavioral analysis system of psychotherapy (CBASP)
- Dialectical behavior therapy (DBT)
- Eye-movement desensitization and reprocessing (EMDR)

This list does *not* include the well-known therapy simply called cognitive therapy or CBT, but several variations thereof.

Doing psychotherapy with prisoners may have the same goals that it has with anyone else. It may also have goals that are specific to a person in prison. For example, you might be thinking, "Should I be helping this person to stop committing crimes, so he doesn't come back?" Table 1–5 shows what we think is a representative list of possible goals of individual psychotherapy with prisoners.

It should be noted that in their use of supportive psychotherapy, the Ancient Greeks were interested in achieving a calm, happy, and fulfilled state of mind called *eudaemonia* and not merely in eliminating diseases and errors of the mind. It took a while, but just about when supportive psychotherapy was celebrating its 2400th birthday, something else happened within the world of psychology: the birth of positive psychology, a school of thought developed by Seligman and his colleagues (Seligman 2002; Seligman and Csikszentmihalyi 2000), the aim of which is to help people to improve their lives whether or not they seek counseling for psychological problems or pathology. Jeste et al. (2015) discuss how these principles are used in psychiatry as well.

TABLE 1–5. **Goals of supportive psychotherapy**

General goals (without specific reference to criminal history)

Emphasize adherence to treatment plans

Decrease inappropriate behavior

Decrease dysphoric thought processes and content

Improve coping skills

Improve social skills

Resolve external conflicts

Prevent relapse, deterioration, or hospitalization

Enhance self-esteem

Improve regulation of emotions

Lessen impulsivity

Improve reality testing (of patient, others, and the world)

Strengthen healthy defenses

Weaken maladaptive defenses

Maximize family and social support

Lessen hallucinations, lessen depression, stabilize mood disorder, lessen anxiety, improve sleep, and so forth

Improve self-esteem (may coexist with goal of developing remorse at crime)

Lessen self-hatred or hatred at others

Lessen danger to self (self-harm or suicidality, attempts to escape, hoarding pills)

Improve job performance

Lessen "acting out" behaviors (e.g., needless use of services, unnecessary demands on providers)

Lessen unnecessary use of medical services (another kind of acting out or displaced behavior)

Lessen danger to others (risk of fighting or assault)

Learn not to see self as victim (part of trauma therapy)

Lessen behaviors leading to becoming a victim of sexual or emotional or physical or domestic abuse

Lessen rage at past parental figures

Improve interpersonal relationships with others in prison or outside

Learn altruistic behaviors or lifestyle

Improve existing family relationships (including with children)

Find productivity or meaning in daily life or in plans for future

Possible goals of individual psychotherapy with prisoners

Deal with crisis in getting arrested, sentenced, or entering prison

Deal with separation from family and friends and grieve losses of job and support system (includes dealing with disenfranchised grief; see Chapter 5)

Do more than just "kill time"

Develop healthy (nonviolent and as healthy as possible) compensations for isolation and rage at injustice and imbalance of power and institutional and personal oppression and dominance (from staff and/or other prisoners)

Develop a healthy lifestyle, including healthy nonvictim relationships and physical health

Prevent relapses and recidivism

Avoid fighting, discipline and rule violations, and conflict with correctional officers

Improve socialization and lessen isolation in prison

TABLE 1–5.	**Goals of supportive psychotherapy** *(continued)*

Offense-related types of proposed insight or awareness

Take responsibility for past crimes

Learn sources of "criminogenic" behavior and how to change

Benign "blame" of codefendant so as to be able to live with oneself for the terrible thing done

Symbolic payback to abusers (e.g., unwritten letters or activism for rights)

Forgive past abusers

Learn empathy/respect for other human beings

Increase victim awareness (often the object of a packaged program)

Forgive oneself for one's transgressions

Atone for crime and pay back specific victim or society

Faith-based coping (using existing faith but not being inculcated or forced to learn a new one)

Develop awareness of offense and remorse so as not to reoffend

Advance to a higher state of moral development

Effect rehabilitation of behavior and learn not to offend

Play a role in alcohol and drug relapse prevention

Prevent reoffending or reduce recidivism (offense central to therapy)

Improve coping skills, social skills, or job skills

Develop more self-control and anger or impulse management leading to lessening of violence

Serve as an adjunct to self-control groups (adjunct to anger management or domestic violence or sex offender groups)

Serve as an adjunct to victim groups (PTSD, nightmares)

Goals that are especially relevant to persons with severe mental illness (SMI)

Learn about their skills and so-called illness

Learn to trust and collaborate with providers

Make a rational decision whether to take medication or psychotherapy or obtain other services

Prevent self-harm and suicidal behavior

Learn social skills (a major lack in many individuals with SMI)

Learn prison skills: what to tell others when they hear their voices; how much to share with others; when to ask for help; follow safety plan

Goals that are especially relevant to persons with severe personality disorders

Learn not to use lying as a lifestyle

Learn feelings/empathy for others

Learn not to disrupt the treatment of others ("treatment-interfering behaviors")

Compensate for narcissistic injury leading to suicidality (while therapist attempts to treat the narcissism)

Learn noncriminal lifestyles

Learn that antisocial behavior has negative consequences to their narcissism (e.g., that one of their malignant personality characteristics conflicts with one of their other malignant personality characteristics)

Understand how one's genetics and childhood experiences shaped the person one is today

Explore interpersonal experiences

Explore inner experiences that lead to anger and rage and other behaviors

TABLE 1–5.   **Goals of supportive psychotherapy** *(continued)*

Goals that require some depth in the methods and are not usually possible with correctional patients

Achieve deep insight and self-understanding

Resolve intrapsychic conflicts

Restructure personality (although supportive psychotherapy is known to do this)

Like supportive psychotherapy, positive psychology can trace its roots back to the Ancient Greeks, although it is also an outgrowth of earlier medical and spiritual thinking. Seligman and colleagues explored what makes life worth living and how to use that as a motivation to solve problems their patients might have. They extrapolated from this to identifying those attributes and climates that amplify a person's strengths: positive experiences, subjective well-being, and self-determination, building on human needs for competence, and belongingness and autonomy (Seligman and Csikszentmihalyi 2000). Positive psychology identifies 11 primary goals: satisfaction in life, knowledge, excellence in play, excellence in work, excellence in agency, inner peace, relatedness (friendship and intimacy), community, spirituality (meaning and purpose), pleasure, and creativity (Wormith 2015). Interventions are intended to improve effective coping, help flow and creativity, increase curiosity and hope, and improve lives beyond alleviating mental illness, and to improve psychological wellness as do wellness programs in physical health (Peterson 2006). It many cases, positive psychology is based on moral values: doing good for oneself and others, and creating good out of bad experiences, such as using traumatic events to grow in understanding of oneself (Linley et al. 2009), building strength of character to lead to fulfillment and meaningful life, assessing prior success and positive relationships, and using positive emotions such as gratitude to broaden perceptions, thoughts, and actions. Many techniques are shared with other forms of psychotherapy, such as reminiscing and working through. Some special techniques include counting blessings, visualizing one's best self, expressing gratitude, and practicing using one's strengths (Cohn and Fredrickson 2009).

Both supportive psychotherapy and positive psychology aim to help patients deal with or overcome mental illness through training, education, and skills-building, focusing on overcoming the medical diagnosis, giving patients skills and tools to avoid past problems, and helping them to develop strategies for living a productive life under their own control. Therefore, there is much overlap in approaches, although this has not generally been written about except for one account that recognizes that supportive psychotherapy applies the same principles and attitudes toward emotions and experiences as does positive psychology (Summers and Lord 2015).

For example, achieving autonomy in one's decisions in life is a goal that is common to both supportive psychotherapy and positive psychology. Other goals found in positive psychology—such as achieving happiness—are a natural extension of the goals already found in supportive psychotherapy. This does not mean that you must or should try to instill happiness in your patients. The specific goals that you develop with your patients will depend on their treatment plans.

However, and especially when working with incarcerated populations, we do not feel we can accomplish our goals by solely developing strengths and positive emotions. A full discussion of the relationship between supportive psychotherapy and positive psychology is beyond the scope of this manual. For example, positive psychology eschews medical explanations, but we don't. We continue to use what Summers and Lord (2015) call the traditionally defining elements of supportive psychotherapy—for example, strengthening psychological defenses and avoiding psychodynamic interpretation.

A parallel development, well-being therapy, is an integrative psychotherapy that seeks to increase personal well-being and is especially suited for treatment of depression (Fava 2016). There is also an outgrowth of positive psychology called the Good Lives Model that was developed to lessen recidivism in sex offenders, a group of people who have typically been thought to be particularly resistant to treatment. The Good Lives Model has been used in working with people who have had traumatic experiences and with prisoners in programs that help them acquire skills and tools for coping with incarceration and, ultimately, reentry (Linley et al. 2009). We will say more about it later in this book.

Of the many possible goals of supportive psychotherapy with incarcerated persons, it is more than a theoretical interest to ask which of them might actually result in a reduction of future criminal behavior—for example, that all-important figure of recidivism and probably another important statistic, relapse to drug use, since drug use accounts for much criminal behavior. The answer depends on empirical evidence of what interventions really do work, and whether the interventions will be designed based on a theory of criminal behavior. Of several approaches, the risk-need-responsivity (RNR) theory of Bonta and Andrews (2017) has been the dominant one in the field.

- *Risk.* Bonta and Andrews present a group of "Central Eight" risk/need factors that account for crime and recidivism to further crimes and are (with one exception) the most important targets for intervention to prevent recidivism. The specific factors have changed somewhat as the data have developed, but the basic components have stayed the same (list below adapted from Bonta and Andrews 2017, p. 338; Latessa et al. 2015, p. 22):

  1. Antisocial/procriminal attitudes
  2. Procriminal associates and isolation from anticriminal others
  3. Temperament and personality factors (including impulsivity, poor socialization, risk-taking, and poor problem-solving skills)
  4. Criminal or antisocial behavior history (the one area that cannot be changed)
  5. Family/marital status such as poor parenting and abuse and neglect (the goals of intervention are to reduce dysfunction or conflict and build positive relationships with monitoring and supervision)
  6. Low levels of achievement in school and work, with unemployability and being unemployable seen to be criminogenic
  7. Leisure and recreation, with not being involved in prosocial leisure activities being seen as criminogenic
  8. Substance abuse

  In previous editions of Bonta and Andrews, the first four criminogenic factors were considered more important than the others, but subsequent research changed the assessment. These eight factors as a group and individually have received widespread acceptance as the main risk factors for criminal behavior. Interventions in these areas have been shown to reduce recidivism, provided that the interventions follow a set of principles that we will describe later in the book.

- *Need.* The need component of RNR programs focuses on the criminogenic aspects of risk factors to be addressed in programming for clients. RNR programs are oriented toward working primarily with criminogenic factors such as attitudes, lack of education, and lack of employment rather than with aspects of mental health and physical health.
- *Responsivity.* Responsivity refers to addressing the way in which a program interacts with the individuals involved. The major concept behind RNR programs is that intense structured programs of social learning and behavior change tailored to the individual work best (Latessa et al. 2015). RNR programs are primarily focused on cognitive-behavioral models with the goal of changing behavior by addressing criminogenic needs and thinking and helping participants to learn prosocial alternatives to behavior and attitudes.

What about possible factors that are not on the list? As Bonta and Andrews tell us, "The minor risk/need factors include the following: personal/emotional distress, major mental disorder, physical health issues, fear of official punishment, physical condition, low IQ, social class of origin, and seriousness of current offense" (p. 338). Now, it may concern you to find that the things you do best—ameliorate personal or emotional distress and major mental disorder—are not on the Central Eight list. That's what the research shows. The major part of the work we do is *not primarily for the purpose of preventing recidivism.* It may have some effect on recidivism, but that is not the primary purpose. Rather, we work to alleviate distress, dysfunction, or mental illness in our patients. To the extent that you want to address a patient's problems of criminal behavior, however, you can certainly make that part of your treatment plan. Just recognize that there will always be interventions that don't make much of a difference on the recidivism statistics but that may have a humanitarian purpose. These may include interventions that improve self-esteem, feelings of personal distress, major mental disorder, and physical health.

As mental health professionals, we find that the inclusion of mental health in the latter list does raise some interesting questions. Are they saying that the treatment of a prisoner with mental illness (e.g., of a person with schizophrenia) is a humanitarian activity that has no effect on that person's criminal behavior? Most RNR researchers do think that treating mental illness per se is not known to be a goal that lessens criminogenic behavior. The research on this issue is changing, but many researchers still believe that treating mental illness does not have a major effect on recidivism. In our opinion, the reason for this is a "pearl" of correctional knowledge that you probably know already but that we will tell you about when we discuss serious mental illness in Chapter 8.

To be sure, it seems hard to believe that treating mental illness would *not* reduce criminal recidivism, such as when delusions from mental illness led to commission of a crime. In fact, there are some data (see Chapter 8) that at times some persons with schizophrenia do commit crimes because of their mental symptoms. Most of the time, however, the connection between mental illness and crime needs to be understood as a secondary one. Insofar as treatment of some persons' mental health leads to prosocial attitudes and a prosocial environment, then it addresses criminogenic factors. And in a limited number of cases, if a person's delusions lead to antisocial behaviors, then treatment of the delusions may be anticriminogenic. In addition, it is a humanitarian belief that treatment of mental illness and physical illnesses is *prima facie* the right thing to do and even a constitutional right. We would be doing it anyway with or without the recidivism statistics.

Regardless of psychotherapy methods, caution is suggested in the treatment of persons with antisocial personality disorder or psychopathy: If these persons receive interventions to increase their self-esteem, they might become better able to rationalize their crimes and recidivism is increased. Therefore, if we are to apply this consideration to the treatment of other prisoners with mental illness, should you think twice before routinely "increasing the self-esteem" of your patients? Probably so. If you are routinely reassuring your patients with statements that help them to excuse or rationalize their criminal activity, you have misused that intervention. You will understand this better when we discuss such things as the use of confrontations. For example, increasing self-esteem may be a useful technique when the patient is suicidal. Later, as the patient approaches release, he may need confrontation about his thrill-seeking and desire to use drugs. It is a matter of timing. There are also some persons with psychopathy who do actually have low self-esteem that can be therapeutically addressed.

It should be obvious by now that the world of corrections incorporates a variety of programs and treatments. Many, such as the practice of incarceration itself, have been around for hundreds, if not thousands, of years, while others, including many psychotherapeutic methods, have been developed more recently. We thought it would be helpful to visualize these treatments in Figure 1–1, which characterizes them as more traditional and deficits-based versus innovative and strengths-based. We are not implying that a therapist should be avoiding the so-called traditional treatments. After all, one of the traditional treatments is incarceration, and presumably our readers work in those settings. Rather, we hope that this division illustrates some of the contrasting approaches now being used in corrections and the importance of knowing about them. Included are several of the programs we discuss in this book, such as RNR theory and positive psychology/Good Lives Model. For example, critics of RNR theory say that it is a deficit-based theory and does not address the positive human capacities of prisoners. Positive psychology does that and offers the Good Lives Model as a strengths-based model. Supportive psychotherapy, however, cuts across the deficits and strengths of patients. It can be used to remedy deficits, but it does not have to stop there. It can also be used to develop patients' strengths and capacities to be lawful, empathic, and moral human beings as proposed in the Good Lives Model. So it is that we find supportive psychotherapy to be in an excellent position to work with a variety of treatments, and we have placed it at the center of the presentation.

What Works?

People will talk about the purpose of laws and society. For example, a classical Greek view of law was called *virtue jurisprudence*, or the position that laws exist to guide people toward being virtuous or moral. But what does a society do when its citizens disobey the law? There are various forms of discipline, of which incarceration is only one, and the availability of alternatives to incarceration was reconsidered when the COVID-19 pandemic began. But given that we do have a criminal justice system that puts people in prison, and even sifting out the issues of when it does so unjustly and unfairly, we get to the question: Does prison work? That is, is prison effective in what prison is supposed to do? Some purposes of incarceration are said to be:

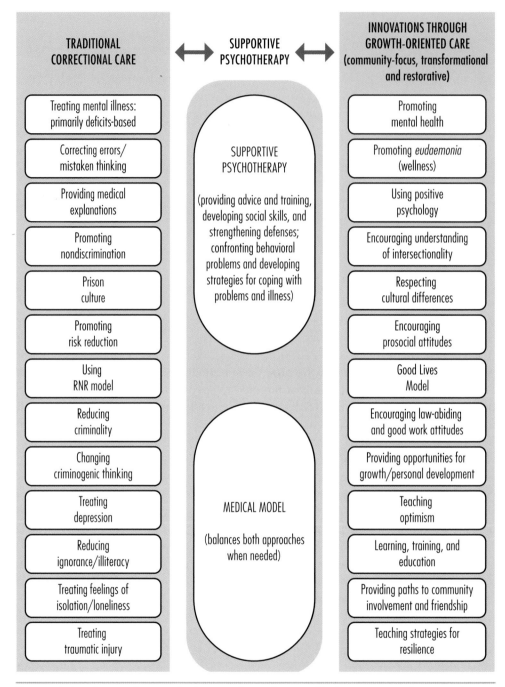

FIGURE 1–1. Supportive psychotherapy draws from and balances several approaches.
RNR=risk-need-responsivity.

- Punishment of persons who commit crimes, including development of remorse for their criminal acts.
- Retribution and/or restoration: society or government's moral or legal obligation to respond to the criminal act, perhaps on behalf of the victims (if there are known victims) or society as a whole for the offense to society and "restore" the balance.
- Containment or incapacitation (preventing the prisoner from committing a crime during the time he or she is imprisoned).
- Prevention, or what is called *individual deterrence* (e.g., of future crimes), by the same person or groups of persons released at a given time as measured by recidivism rates or likelihood that an individual will return to prison.
- Rehabilitation of the prisoner so that his or her character is prosocial, noncriminal, and so forth.
- Deterrence of future crimes by persons other than the criminal (often called *general deterrence*).

Recidivism rates do provide a measure of what many consider an important aspect of success of a prison system. However, many researchers think that general deterrence does *not* work, so prisons should not be relied upon to prevent nonprisoners from committing crimes. Depending on what statistics you gather, incarceration is probably partly effective in lessening recidivism, although longer stays may actually worsen it (Kuziemko 2013). This is discussed further in Chapter 14. However, the effectiveness of incarceration may be due to the programming that prisoners receive while there. Prison programs work, especially if targeted to specific offenses they are meant to prevent, and this even applies to the most serious offenses, including sexual assault of minors. To be sure, the popularity of specific programs has risen and fallen with policy, research, and political tides. For example, confrontational Synanon–type substance abuse groups went away a long time ago, and boot camps are on the way out.

Most such programs involve group work, although some have individual therapy components. However, when the RNR model is used as a basis for these programs, there is a stringent limitation on the effectiveness of such programs: in general, programs must target prisoners who have the highest level of risk with intense amounts of effort. Programs that target low-risk inmates with small amounts of services are generally ineffective. And (until some recent research found otherwise) it was said that programs that treat only mental illness do not reduce recidivism at all.

Rather than be dissuaded by this, take it that your function is to do what psychotherapists do everywhere—to treat the mental and emotional ills of your patients and ameliorate their distress, as already listed in the goals of supportive psychotherapy earlier. However, we do believe that you should direct some of your efforts to recognize the causes of criminal activity (e.g., what is called "criminogenic thinking") and utilize interventions to lessen criminogenic thinking in your patients. This raises some ethical questions, but most of them can be dealt with by including the patient in your plan—which is called *their* treatment plan for a good reason.

Although supportive psychotherapy is by no means limited in application just to patients with poor education, in crisis, with poor coping skills, or with difficulty learning new things, it is certainly an excellent choice for such patients. Those patients may benefit more than others from psychoeducational methods, suggestions, guidance, and repetition to ensure learning. Prisoners (not all but many) frequently have dis-

rupted lifestyles with characteristics such as poor or abusive relationships, poor education, difficulty in abstraction, and frequent life crises. Therefore, supportive therapy
is ideally suited to most prisoners, because it is more likely to work. If you do have
issues about reducing recidivism with your patients, we suggest you talk it out with
them. Some years ago, it was debated whether and how a therapist could adopt treatment goals not accepted by the patient. Yet consider that for many years there were
therapists who embraced the paternalistic principle that therapy was justified if it was
in the best interest of the patient!

As just mentioned, many prison programs do incorporate components of psychotherapy. But does prison psychotherapy work? Does supportive psychotherapy work?
Does supportive psychotherapy work in prison? The conclusion of many researchers
is that most types of psychotherapy work, despite their supposed theoretical differences. Their effectiveness is thought to be due to the generally supportive elements in
all therapies—those elements that we have already called the "stem" of the Y. Laugh
if you wish, but in all seriousness, the claim that most psychotherapies are equally effective has been called the "Dodo Bird conjecture" from a statement in Chapter 3 of
Lewis Carroll's *Alice's Adventures in Wonderland* that "Everyone has won, and all must
have prizes." A serious name for it is the "common factors theory of psychotherapy."
There are many discussions of this in the research literature (see, e.g., Wampold et al.
1997), and you can find a summary in Wikipedia. Supportive psychotherapy and other
types of psychotherapy work because they contain what are called *common factors*, including a trusting therapist-patient relationship, an expectancy of getting better, and
the skill of the therapist in establishing a relationship early in the course of treatment.
In fact, the American Psychological Association tried to identify psychotherapies that
were evidence-based in the late 1990s and came up with a list of more than 25 (out of
several hundred) psychotherapies that seemed to meet the criteria. However, they encountered so much criticism of this project that they never repeated it (also discussed
in Wampold 2019). Proponents of the common factors theory hold that there are many
valid and effective psychotherapies that contain common factors leading to success.
Many of the integrative psychotherapies we previously mentioned utilize common factors in their success. However, supportive psychotherapy can actually be seen as a
widely practiced day-to-day application of the common factors in psychotherapy, and
it is paradoxical that "it is the least theorized, recognized, regulated, or researched"
(Trijsburg et al. 2007, pp. 99–100).

To be more specific and emphatic, however, supportive psychotherapy does work
about as well as other therapies, and sometimes better, for the wide variety of conditions
you are likely to encounter in corrections. Despite the seeming dominance of cognitive-
behavioral therapies in the general field of psychotherapy practitioners, supportive
psychotherapy has proved equal and even superior in a number of studies. In our
previous book (Novalis et al. 2020), we discuss some of the superiority in head-to-head
studies. To cite several examples: A review of 26 papers concluded that supportive
psychotherapy was as effective as several other well-known therapies in the treatment of adult depression (Jacobs and Reupart 2014). Both supportive therapy and
mentalization-based therapy were found to be effective in treatment of bipolar disorder
(Meyer and Hautzinger 2012). Brief supportive psychotherapy was found to be as effective as short-term dynamic psychotherapy in high-functioning outpatients with
personality disorder (Hellerstein et al. 1998) and leads to improvement in interper-

sonal functioning (Rosenthal et al. 1999). General equivalences were found between transference-focused therapy, supportive psychotherapy, and dialectical behavior therapy in the treatment of outpatients with borderline personality disorder (Clarkin et al. 2007). Supportive-expressive psychotherapy (the kind associated with Luborsky [1984]) was found to be as effective as psychodynamic therapy in outpatients with Cluster C personality disorders (avoidant, dependent, obsessive-compulsive) (Vinnars et al. 2005). Both mentalization-based treatment and supportive psychotherapy were found to be highly effective in treating patients with borderline personality disorder (Jørgensen et al. 2013). Finally, mentalization-based treatment and a minimal therapeutic method called "structured clinical management" were both found to be effective in treating borderline personality disorder (Bateman and Fonagy 2009).

Does supportive psychotherapy work in prison? On common measures of psychotherapy, such as the improvement of mental illness, prison psychotherapy does work. A meta-analysis of 37 studies (Yoon et al. 2017) showed a modest advantage to CBT and mindfulness, but supportive psychotherapy was not specifically studied as a variable. In our own opinion of that article, the advantage was not very convincing, even for the two supposed leaders. But just as you may be tempted to brush up your skills using the supposed "therapy leaders" (i.e., CBT and mindfulness), there comes another study showing the benefit of interpersonal psychotherapy in prison (Johnson et al. 2019). Fortunately, the techniques used in supportive psychotherapy are fundamental to nearly all successful psychotherapies because they embody the common factors in successful psychotherapies everywhere.

As experienced therapists practice and learn, they acquire a repertory of methods. A typical supportive therapist would use supportive techniques (also those of positive psychology) as the basis of his or her techniques, buttressed by additional psychotherapy methods from mainstream schools of psychotherapy such as cognitive-behavioral therapy and so forth. See Figure 1–2 for a conception of how a supportive therapist might view his or her repertory of techniques. As our conception of supportive psychotherapy shows, it is an eclectic therapy that can draw from a variety of techniques and programs.

In addition to the usual goals of psychotherapy, there is the question of whether prison programs reduce recidivism. The answer is a chorus of "yesses" for multiple programs with multiple theoretical bases. Most such programs are intensive and group-based, but some have individual components. We listed many in Tables 1–1 and 1–2. Your institution has probably adopted one or more of these programs for specified groups of prisoners. As indicated in Figure 1–1, we think you can incorporate elements of these programs in your individual therapy sessions. You can also use many accessory materials, such as handouts addressing cognitive distortions, to reduce criminal recidivism for those patients who embrace that goal as part of their treatment. But except for the times when you're using specific antirecidivism methods, the majority of your time you might find yourself just doing "plain and simple" psychotherapy as adapted to prison conditions.

Can supportive psychotherapy be harmful? Any *therapist* can harm a patient by doing therapy in the wrong way. Schermuly-Haupt et al. (2018) discussed the negative outcomes in cognitive therapy, although we have not seen any study addressing risks in supportive psychotherapy. However, not everyone gets better in any type of therapy. Also, in prison situations, where prisoners can blame therapists and providers of

ACTIVE SUPPORTIVE PSYCHOTHERAPY

Positive psychology methods

Supportive counseling and nondirective counseling

General conversational skills

Additional methods chosen by the therapist as part of favored repertory

Mainstream therapies that should be well known (e.g., cognitive-behavioral therapy, interpersonal psychotherapy)

Isolated techniques that can be incorporated into anyone's therapy, including homework, letter writing, journaling, guided imagery, progressive muscle relaxation, behavioral treatment of nightmares, etc.

Sparing use of psychodynamic methods, interpretation of unconscious material

Items selected from group training programs specific to inmates

Educational and training methods (e.g., skills training for schizophrenia)

FIGURE 1–2.   Building blocks of a typical supportive psychotherapist.

all disciplines for any negative outcome, we have taken pains to qualify and limit any directive interventions that by any stretch of the imagination could be blamed for a negative outcome. In cases where you have a concern, you should qualify the giving of direct advice so that the patient must take the final step in decision-making and cannot "blame" it on the therapist. Finally, as we have mentioned, interventions to raise self-esteem do need to be chosen carefully when used with antisocial persons and with respect to criminal actions. This will be discussed further in Chapter 10.

What Ethical Issues Are Raised by Providing Supportive Psychotherapy in Correctional Settings?

The formulation of goals of supportive psychotherapy in corrections inevitably brings up ethical issues. Many therapists who trained in the past, and even some training now, are told that therapy is "value free." Not counting psychoanalysts, there are also, less common these days, nondirective therapists who mostly listen but, as the name implies, do minimal forms of interpretation or direction. The attitude conveyed may be something like "You can do what you want in your life, and I'm just here to help you do it better (e.g., resolve your conflicts but not create any goals you don't have already)." Researchers on recidivism, we assure you, have nothing positive to say about nondirective therapies. Maybe people outside of prison can change for the better without much direction, but not prisoners. Most people involved in correctional work conclude that it cannot be value-free. Goals such as being or becoming prosocial (rather than antisocial) and avoiding criminal activity would seem to be desirable when doing psychotherapy in prison. Historically, the American Psychological Association raised the question of "Who is the client?" when working in the criminal justice system, urging therapists to make the goals of treatment transparent to the criminal justice client (Brodsky 1980; Monahan 1980). Thus, correctional treatment has been described as a "unique hybrid" that balances traditional elements of public health treatment and correctional activities such as rehabilitation. "At times the partnership is uneasy and conflictual, but in the best of all possible worlds it is *synergistic*" (Scott and Crime and Justice Institute 2008, p. 7). Furthermore, "The hallmark of correctional treatment is that it addresses both the behavioral healthcare condition as well as the criminality" (Scott and Crime and Justice Institute 2008, p. 16).

The supportive psychotherapist should not view herself as an agent of punishment or retribution and is not the agent of containment (which falls to custody staff or "the ones with the keys"). But we do think a therapist must consider the values of the society in which she lives. Prevention of recidivism is an implied goal of the correctional institution in which the therapist is working. Does it become the therapist's job to increase rather than lessen the distress created by someone's past criminal acts? Therapists may have strong criticisms of their jurisdiction's current correctional system or the correctional institution in which they work. They may even share those concerns with their patients. For example, "I wish we did have a literacy program for you…I wish we did have some college courses you would like." Or perhaps, "It seems to me that you shouldn't have been put in prison for what you did."

Many correctional systems are underfunded, and the people who run them are less than perfect and sometimes downright sadistic. There are problems in systems of justice running the gamut from community police, to the courts, to correctional officers. But the reality is, our patients are where they are, and we are where we are. And as long as you work in corrections, you can choose to be, as you see fit, an iconoclast and a reformer, but not a subverter and destroyer. You are there to get patients through it and to keep them from coming back—with the proviso that you don't want to make them better criminals.

We believe that supportive psychotherapists should support the rule of law and the system of justice and abide by the general rules of their correctional institution, although not necessarily every one of its policies. This is consistent with but goes well beyond the tenet of the American Correctional Association Code of Ethics which states that "[m]embers shall respect and protect the right of the public to be safeguarded from criminal activity" (American Correctional Association 1994). Exceptions to these guidelines ought to be thought out carefully, especially if they bring you into conflict with the rules of your institution. Since we do think that therapists are often models of behavior for their patients, it would be a strange situation in which you expect your patients to "do as I say but not as I do." You can certainly give them the message that you expect them to be self-assertive toward institutional change, but not to undermine the institution in a way that would incur discipline.

That said, most therapists would agree that the American system is not always fair and is often racially and ethnically and culturally biased (including being against women) and underfunded and understaffed. Punishments may still be cruel and unusual. Some people think that most nonviolent persons should not be imprisoned. Some people think that even violent criminals can be treated in the community, and there is a prison abolition movement. And while much violence in prison is prisoner-to-prisoner, there are those who see it as the expected result of turning people into prisoners. Some also think that the "labeling" of people as criminal at the time of their first offense creates a self-fulfilling prophecy that leads to their recidivism.

We suggest three principles that should apply to *all* therapists:

- *Strive to practice in a culturally sensitive manner.* This includes sensitivity to race, language, national origin, ethnicity, gender identity, and/or sexual preference. That is, in general, we do think therapists should embrace diversity, but not moral deviance.
- *Strive to practice in accordance with ethical principles of their professional organization(s).*
- *Practice in accordance with principles of enlightened multiculturalism and common morality so as to foster justice in the society, the correctional institution, and the patient.* "Common morality" is a concept that has been described by ethicists to provide a cross-cultural understanding of what is right and wrong (e.g., that in general murder is wrong; that suppression of some particular group in a population such as women is wrong). We believe that therapists can celebrate multicultural diversity but with a common morality in mind. We will say more about common morality in Chapter 13.

Examples of behavior governed by ethical rules would be: A therapist should not have a sexual relationship with his or her patient. The therapist should not condone murder.

The therapist should not help the patient to excuse his past crimes and disregard the impact they had on the victims. The therapist should not aid the patient in escaping.

However, some correctional goals as rehabilitation may not or may not yet be accepted by the patient himself. Many patients hold that they are innocent and hence not in need of any form of correction. Does your patient admit to having committed a crime? Does he even want to talk about his crimes or his feelings of remorse (or lack of such feelings)? These questions will be asked and answered in the early stages of psychotherapy and will help formulate the treatment plan. If your patient is never willing to talk about his crime or claims to have "blacked out" during commission of it, you will never talk about the specifics of it. However, you will still have the opportunity to talk about many other aspects of his life, including what we describe as "criminal thinking patterns." But if you do not believe that your actions as therapist are moral or just, should you be working in a correctional institution? We understand that therapists do not want to view themselves as agents of an oppressive carceral state. Therapists may not believe in the drug laws that led to their patients being imprisoned, and so forth. Therapists can differ from the "official" policies of society. But there are limits.

As with most ethical issues, there are disagreements and no easy answers to many of the concerns that are raised when working in corrections. However, there is guidance: "Simply put, for oppressed people, advocacy is required for true recovery. Although it is true that in most cases, the complete restoration of justice is far beyond our ability, it is also true that in most cases, furthering justice—in some way—is well within our reach" (Cyrus and Vinson 2021, p. 226). Learning more about one's power orientation in therapy (vitally important in a prison) and how to advocate for social justice is part of the process. The American Counseling Association, for example, has as one of its principles: "When appropriate, counselors advocate at individual, group, institutional, and societal levels to address potential barriers and obstacles that inhibit access and/or growth and development of clients" (Standard A7.a.; Herlihy and Corey 2015, p.159).

Key Points

- In the United States, more so than in the rest of the world, millions of persons are housed in jails, prisons, and detention centers, or under correctional supervision. The U.S. system also suffers from racial and ethnic inequalities and a high recidivism rate.

- The dominant theory of correctional treatment believed to prevent recidivism is known as the risk-need-responsivity (RNR) theory. It identifies eight criminogenic factors, most of which can be modified to reduce recidivism.

- Supportive psychotherapy has been around in practice since the Ancient Greeks and has been elaborated for more than a hundred years by modern practitioners, including Sigmund Freud himself.

- Supportive psychotherapy is an evidence-based set of psychotherapy techniques that are especially suited to persons with limited cognitive and coping skills and poor control of their emotions, and the need for repetition and practice to learn new things, and applicable to persons in criminal justice settings.

- The techniques of supportive psychotherapy can be compared to the stem of a "Y," or better yet a flower, which serves as a common core of techniques used in therapies of most schools of psychotherapy.

- The goals of supportive psychotherapy are similar to the goals of positive psychology, which in turn serves as the basis for a well-known program for primarily treating sex offenders called the Good Lives Model.

- Correctional psychotherapists face many challenges in addressing both the needs of patients and the stated purposes of the correctional systems for which the psychotherapists work.

- Supportive psychotherapy may serve the purpose of reducing recidivism, but it also serves a humanitarian need.

- Theories of criminology have been around for hundreds of years and continue to evolve in order to explain the complexities of human criminal behavior and its amenability to deterrence and rehabilitation.

- Psychotherapy in corrections raises ethical issues that can be addressed in part by reference to the ethical standards of professional organizations and a belief in principles of common morality.

References

Alper M, Durose MR, Markman J: Update on Prisoner Recidivism: A 9-Year Follow-up Period (2005–2014). Special Report. NCJ 250975. Washington, DC, Bureau of Justice Statistics, May 2018. Available at: www.bjs.gov/content/pub/pdf/18upr9yfup0514.pdf. Accessed November 12, 2020.

American Correctional Association: Code of Ethics. Adopted by the Board of Governors and Delegate Assembly, August 1994. Available at: https://www.aca.org/ACA_Member/About_Us/Code_of_Ethics/ACA/ACA_Member/AboutUs/Code_of_Ethics.aspx?hkey=61577ed2-c0c3-4529-bc01-36a248f79eba. Accessed November 28, 2020.

Andrews DA, Bonta J: The Psychology of Criminal Conduct. Cincinnati, OH, Anderson, 1994

Bateman A, Fonagy P: Randomized controlled trial of outpatient mentalization-based treatment versus structured clinical management for borderline personality disorder. Am J Psychiatry 166(12):1355–1364, 2009 19833787

Battaglia J: Doing Supportive Psychotherapy. Washington, DC, American Psychiatric Association Publishing, 2019

Beitman BD, Manring J: Theory and practice of psychotherapy integration, in Textbook of Psychotherapeutic Treatments. Edited by Gabbard GO. Washington, DC, American Psychiatric Publishing, 2009, pp 705–726

Bonta J, Andrews DA: The Psychology of Criminal Conduct, 6th Edition. New York, Routledge, 2017

Brodsky SL: Ethical issues for psychologists in corrections, in Who Is the Client? The Ethics of Psychological Intervention in the Criminal Justice System. Edited by Monahan J. Washington, DC, American Psychological Association, 1980, pp 63–92

Bronson J, Berzofsky M: Indicators of Mental Health Problems Reported by Prisoners and Jail Inmates, 2011–2012. Special Report. NCJ 250612. Washington, DC, Bureau of Justice Statistics, June 2017. Available at: www.bjs.gov/index.cfm?ty=pbdetail&iid=5946. Accessed November 12, 2020.

Bronson J, Carson A: Prisoners in 2017. NCJ 252156. Washington, DC, Bureau of Justice Statistics, April 2019. Available at: www.bjs.gov/index.cfm?ty=pbdetail&iid=6546. Accessed June 12, 2019.

Clarkin JF, Levy KN, Lenzenweger MF, Kernberg OF: Evaluating three treatments for borderline personality disorder: a multiwave study. Am J Psychiatry 164(6):922–928, 2007 17541052

Cohn MA, Fredrickson BL: Positive emotions, in The Oxford Handbook of Positive Psychology, 2nd Edition. Edited by Lopez SJ, Snyder CR. Oxford, UK, Oxford University Press. 2009, pp 13–24

Cyrus KD, Vinson SY: Social justice and advocacy, in Social (In)justice and Mental Health. Edited by Shim RS, Vinson SY. Washington, DC, American Psychiatric Association Publishing, 2021, pp 225–238

Dean ME: Pros and cons of the eclectic approach to therapy. BetterHelp.com. Updated May 19, 2021. Available at: www.betterhelp.com/advice/therapy/pros-and-cons-of-the-eclectic-approach-to-therapy. Accessed April 1, 2022.

Fava G: Well-Being Therapy: Treatment Manual and Clinical Applications. New York, S Karger, 2016

Freud S: Lines of advance in psycho-analytic therapy (1919[1918]), in The Standard Edition of the Complete Psychological Works of Sigmund Freud, Vol 17. Translated and edited by Strachey J. London, Hogarth Press, 1955, pp 157–168

Hellerstein DJ, Rosenthal RN, Pinsker H, et al: A randomized prospective study comparing supportive and dynamic therapies. Outcome and alliance. J Psychother Pract Res 7(4):261–271, 1998 9752637

Herlihy B, Corey G: ACA Ethical Standards Casebook, 7th Edition. Alexandria, VA, American Counseling Association, 2015

Hernández KL, Muhammad KG: Introduction: constructing the carceral state. J Am Hist 102(1):18–24, 2015

Jacobs N, Reupart A: The Effectiveness of Supportive Counselling, based on Rogerian Principles: A Systematic Review of Recent International and Australian Research. Melbourne, PACFA (Psychotherapy & Counselling Federation of Australia), May 2014. Available at: www.pacfa.org.au-wp-content-uploads-2012-10-PACFA-SupportiveCounselling-literature-review-2014-Final.pdf. Accessed November 14, 2020.

Jeste DV, Palmer BW, Rettew DC, Boardman S: Positive psychiatry: its time has come. J Clin Psychiatry 76(6):675–683, 2015 26132670

Johnson JE, Stout RL, Miller TR, et al: Randomized cost-effectiveness trial of group interpersonal psychotherapy (IPT) for prisoners with major depression. J Consult Clin Psychol 87(4):392–406, 2019 30714749

Jørgensen CR, Freund C, Bøye R, et al: Outcome of mentalization-based and supportive psychotherapy in patients with borderline personality disorder: a randomized trial. Acta Psychiatr Scand 127(4):305–317, 2013 22897123

Kaeble D, Cowhig M: Correctional Populations in the United States, 2016. NCJ 251211. Washington, DC, Bureau of Justice Statistics, April 2018. Available at: www.bjs.gov/content/pub/pdf/cpus16.pdf. Accessed August 17, 2019.

Kourkouta L: Ancient Greek psychotherapy for contemporary nurses. J Psychosoc Nurs Ment Health Serv 40(8):36–39, 2002

Kuziemko I: How should inmates be released from prison? An assessment of parole versus fixed-sentence regimes. Q J Econ 128(1):371–424, 2013

Latessa EJ, Listwan SJ, Koetzle D: What Works (and Doesn't) in Reducing Recidivism. New York, Routledge, 2015

Leichsenring F, Leibing E: Supportive-expressive (SE) psychotherapy: an update. Current Psychiatry Reviews 3:57–64, 2007

Linley PA, Joseph S, Maltby J, et al: Positive psychology applications, in The Oxford Handbook of Positive Psychology, 2nd Edition. Edited by Lopez SJ, Snyder CR. Oxford, UK, Oxford University Press, 2009, pp 35–48

Luborsky L: Principles of Psychoanalytic Psychotherapy: A Manual for Supportive-Expressive (SE) Treatment. New York, Basic Books, 1984

Math SB, Murthy P, Parthasarathy R, et al: Minds Imprisoned: Mental Health Care in Prisons. Bangalore, India, National Institute of Mental Health and Neuro Sciences, 2011

Meyer TD, Hautzinger M: Cognitive behaviour therapy and supportive therapy for bipolar disorders: relapse rates for treatment period and 2-year follow-up. Psychol Med 42(7):1429–1439, 2012 22099722

Miller J: Getting Played: African American Girls, Urban Equality, and Gendered Violence. New York, NYU Press, 2008

Monahan J (ed): Who Is the Client? The Ethics of Psychological Intervention in the Criminal Justice System. Washington, DC, American Psychological Association, 1980

Novalis PN, Rojcewicz SJ, Peele R: Clinical Manual of Supportive Psychotherapy. Washington, DC, American Psychiatric Press, 1993

Novalis PN, Singer V, Peele R: Clinical Manual of Supportive Psychotherapy. 2nd Edition. Washington, DC, American Psychiatric Association Publishing, 2020

Peterson C: A Primer in Positive Psychology. Oxford, UK, Oxford University Press, 2006

Pittaro M: Criminology (Quick Study Academic). BarCharts Inc, 2010

Plakun EM, Sudak DM, Goldberg D: The Y model: an integrated, evidence-based approach to teaching psychotherapy competencies. J Psychiatr Pract 15(1):5–11, 2009 19182560

Pohl J, Gabrielson R: There has been an explosion of homicides in California's county jails. Here's why. ProPublica. June 13, 2019. Available at: www.propublica.org/article/explosion-of-homicides-in-californias-county-jails-heres-why. Accessed June 14, 2019.

Renner B: Nearly half of Americans have had immediate family member incarcerated. StudyFinds.org March 9, 2019. Available at: www.studyfinds.org/half-americans-immediate-family-member-imprisoned. Accessed August 10, 2019.

Rosenthal RN, Muran JC, Pinsker H, et al: Interpersonal change in brief supportive psychotherapy. J Psychother Pract Res 8(1):55–63, 1999 9888107

Sawyer W, Wagner P: Mass incarceration: the whole pie 2020 (press release). Northampton, MA, Prison Policy Initiative, March 24, 2020. Available at: www.prisonpolicy.org/reports/pie2020.html. Accessed May 10, 2020.

Schermuly-Haupt M-L, Linden M, Rush AJ: Unwanted events and side effects in cognitive behavior therapy. Cogn Ther Res 42(7):219–229, 2018

Schram PJ, Tibbetts SG: Introduction to Criminology: Why Do They Do It? Thousand Oaks, CA, Sage, 2013

Scott W, Crime and Justice Institute: Effective Clinical Practices in Treating Clients in the Criminal Justice System. Washington, DC, U.S. Department of Justice, National Institute of Corrections, 2008

See E, Kieser E: Student Study Guide for Criminological Theories: Introduction, Evaluation, Application by Akers RL and Sellars CS. New York, Oxford University Press, 2013. Available at: https://global.oup.com/us/companion.websites/9780199844487/guide1/study_guide.pdf. Accessed June 6, 2020.

Seligman MEP: Authentic Happiness: Using the New Positive Psychology to Realize Your Potential for Lasting Fulfillment. New York, Free Press, 2002

Seligman MEP, Csikszentmihalyi M: Positive psychology. An introduction. Am Psychol 55(1):5–14, 2000 11392865

Sharpless BA: Psychodynamic Therapy Techniques: A Guide to Supportive and Expressive Interventions. New York, Oxford University Press, 2019

Solis D: Immigration detention centers are emptying out as the U.S. cites coronavirus for removals: the plunge raises questions over how necessary prison-like detention is for immigrants. The Dallas Morning News, October 2, 2020. Available at: www.dallasnews.com/news/immigration/2020/10/02/immigration-detention-centers-are-emptying-out-as-the-us-cites-coronavirus-for-deportations. Accessed November 28, 2020.

Summers RF, Lord LA: Positivity in supportive and psychodynamic therapy, in Positive Psychiatry: A Clinical Handbook. Edited by Jeste DV, Palmer BW. Arlington, VA, American Psychiatric Publishing, 2015, pp 167–192

Trestman RL: Is justice really blind? Non-dominant groups in the American justice system. J Am Acad Psychiatry Law 46(4):416–418, 2018 30593470

Trijsburg RW, Colijn S, Holmes J: Psychotherapy integration, in Oxford Textbook of Psychotherapy. Edited by Gabbard GO, Beck JS, Holmes J. New York, Oxford University Press, 2007, pp 95–107

Vinnars B, Barber JP, Norén K, et al: Manualized supportive-expressive psychotherapy versus nonmanualized community-delivered psychodynamic therapy for patients with personality disorders: bridging efficacy and effectiveness. Am J Psychiatry 162(10):1933–1940, 2005 16199841

Walsh A, Jorgensen C: Criminology: The Essentials, 4th Edition. Thousand Oaks, CA, Sage Publications, 2020

Wampold BA: Principles of Psychotherapy. Washington, DC, American Psychological Association, 2019

Wampold BA, Mondin GW, Moody M: A meta-analysis of outcome studies comparing bona fide psychotherapies: "All must have prizes. Psychol Bull 122(3):203–215, 1997

White J: The Galactic Gourmet: A Sector General Novel. New York, A Tor Book, 1996

Wikipedia: Dodo bird verdict. Available at: https://en.wikipedia.org/wiki/Dodo_bird_verdict. Accessed August 23, 2017.

Winston A, Rosenthal RN, Roberts LW: Learning Supportive Psychotherapy: An Illustrated Guide, 2nd Edition. Washington, DC, American Psychiatric Association Publishing, 2020

Wormith JS: RNR and GLM: Shall (or should) ever the twain meet (Slide 23)? 2nd Annual IACFP Edwin I. Megargee Lecture at the International Community Corrections Association (ICCA) Conference, Boston, MA, November 8, 2015 Available at: https://cfbsjs.usask.ca/documents/SW_RNR_GLM.pdf. Accessed October 27, 2019.

Yoon IA, Slade K, Fazel S: Outcomes of psychological therapies for prisoners with mental health problems: a systematic review and meta-analysis. J Consult Clin Psychol 85(8):783–802, 2017 28569518

2

The Techniques of Supportive Psychotherapy

In this chapter we present techniques of supportive psychotherapy, especially as applied in the correctional environment. We divide our techniques into two types, *communication* (Table 2–1) and *direction* (Table 2–2). Techniques we rarely use are mentioned in Table 2–3 but will not be discussed in any detail. Supportive psychotherapy is an active therapy and does not hold the assumptions of so-called nondirective therapies, although we do use several techniques of the historically nondirective therapies such as *generating empathy* and *active listening*.

The supportive patient-therapist relationship is generally a warm one but not a friendship, especially in prison. We will say more about the nature of this relationship, along with the issues of transference and countertransference, in Chapter 4. For example, although some therapists share some personal information, we recommend that you rarely give out any personal information such as a religious affiliation. But it is okay to express a personal interest. For example, "I'm glad to see you because we missed our last session due to the lockdown." Or "Thanks for coming back so soon; I realize that when you left our last session you were angry at me." Reactions should be warm but not effusive. Many prisoners have severe deficits in personal relationships, either moral or simply related to practical skills, and may have inappropriate reactions to the prison environment and other prisoners. Strong positive emotions, or even false sympathy or empathy, can be as problematic as strong negative reactions.

TABLE 2–1.   Techniques of supportive psychotherapy: communication

First level: Listening

Listening

  Personal

  Professional

  Active

Questioning

  Closed ended

  Open ended

  Exploratory

  Provocative

Generating and conveying empathy

Conducting trauma-informed therapy

Helping the patient to test reality

Reassuring (its cognitive aspects)

Observing

Expressing interest and concern

Echoing

Tracking

Commenting

Restating or "replaying"

Eliciting current life reports (here-and-now emphasis)

Obtaining the interval history (what has happened since you last met)

Encouraging ventilation and expression of affect (balance with control of affect, a directive technique)

Generating a feeling of safety

Creating an expectation of success

Creating a healing environment

Managing the transference (see Chapter 4)

Second level: Confrontation

Looking at issues together

Directing attention to inconsistencies between and among different behaviors, beliefs, and purported values

Directing attention to conflicting goals and motivations

Third level: Explanations (at times may be called interventions, clarifications, or interpretations)

Providing information available to the patient but of which he or she is not aware

Offering mechanisms responsible for patients' behavior

Fostering benign projections and introjections

TABLE 2–1.	Techniques of supportive psychotherapy: communication *(continued)*

Third level: Explanations (at times may be called interventions, clarifications, or interpretations) *(continued)*

Providing certain kinds of explanations

    Of defenses

    Limited or inexact

    Avoided, delayed, softened, and controlled

    Displaced, universalized, generalized, normalized, and metaphorical

    Of transference (limited)

    Of dreams (limited)

Working through

Discussing the "criminal" and "noncriminal" parts of a person

Communicating: From Listening to Explaining

Communications work at different depths, from the surface down. We divide them into three levels: listening, confrontation, and explanation. Perhaps you already use them but have given them different names or have not thought of them in a hierarchy.

Let us start, as you do in therapy, with listening. At this level, listen, but also ask questions, get answers, develop your database, and begin to move the therapy in the direction you want it to go. (One technique, managing the transference, is discussed in Chapter 4. It is a communication technique because it involves conveying attitudes and information to the patient to maintain a positive relationship.)

Listening and Asking Questions

Listening and asking questions are fundamental. Questions can be closed ended (yes, no, or a numerical answer) or open ended ("What did you think about your father?"). They have the purpose of acquiring information or of provoking, confronting, exploring, or instilling awareness and insight. As you ask questions, you will be listening. *Personal listening* begins by learning about a patient's life from his point of view and by beginning to develop feelings and reactions to the patient. You might compare this process to listening to the overture of the symphony without reference to any knowledge of music theory. A component of personal listening is what Harari (2014) calls "emotionally attuned listening." *Professional listening* consists in applying structures and categories to the patient's statements, just as a professional musician would discern the underlying themes and orchestration of a musical composition. Because a major task of supportive therapy is to understand defenses and coping behaviors, whether ordinary or criminal, you must begin to categorize (and formulate future questions about) those behaviors. Professional listening is the basis for future targeted interventions, and it is what makes supportive therapy more than a succession of friendly chats.

Communicative techniques were discussed and developed in depth by Carl Rogers, whose approach was based on understanding his patients and their circumstances and establishing a relationship with them. His theory of communication was

TABLE 2–2.   **Techniques of supportive psychotherapy: direction**

Suggestion

Advice and guidance

  Permission giving

  Reassurance (its guiding and encouraging aspects)

Strong advice and (sometimes for appropriate patients) explicit direction

Limit setting

  Inside the therapy (e.g., when a session will be terminated)

  Outside the therapy (e.g., in cell block or interactions with staff)

Reframing

Instilling of hope (see text)

Teaching self-soothing

Helping patients to manage their affects and impulses

Dealing with other prisoners

Dealing with correctional staff and administration

Communicating with outside professionals (caseworkers, attorneys, etc.—not meant to
  include legal advice)

Education within and outside the institution

Parenting skills (remote parenting or later in person)

Dealing with family issues

Social skills training (discussed more in Chapter 8 for patients with serious mental illness)

Work and work skills

Scheduling activities

Cognitive restructuring/behavioral and experiential learning

Modeling and identification with the therapist

Homework

Journaling

Writing a letter that is not sent

Prescriptions for exercise

"Work" prescriptions

Diversions and substitutes

Reinforcement of desirable behaviors

Referral to other providers (e.g., for psychological testing, medication)

Problem-solving

Environmental interventions (e.g., encourage use of outside supports)

called *active listening*, which has been applied to therapy as well as managerial and other interpersonal communications. With active listening, the therapist is listening to the words, the intonation, and the meaning behind the patient's statements, and, built on previous understanding of the patient, modifying and reassessing along the way as needed (Kirschenbaum and Henderson 1989). One of the goals of active listening is to show the patient that you are invested in the relationship and understand the patient's point of view. As enumerated by Rogers (Rogers and Farson, 2015, pp. 9–13), it includes:

TABLE 2–3.   **Techniques used rarely or never in supportive psychotherapy**

Never	Rarely
Anonymous therapist	Deep interpretations (of unconscious content)
Abstinence, neutral attitude	High anxiety-provoking interpretations (but may use mild and moderate anxiety in therapy)
Total therapeutic or technical neutrality	
Total professional detachment	
Freud's "blank screen"	Dream associations or analysis (rarely, but will actively treat nightmares and repetitive anxiety dreams that can be rescripted)
Uninvolved, inactive attitude	
Nondirective attitude	Encouraging fantasy
Getting the patient to "break down"	Interpreting daydreams
Demeaning, screaming therapist	Fostering free association
Instilling supposedly lost memories of abuse (in the manner of previously debunked therapies, not in a current trauma-informed manner)	Encouraging regression

- Listening for total meaning: the content and feeling in what is being said.
- Responding to feeling as well as content.
- Noting all cues, verbal and nonverbal.
- Testing for understanding by getting feedback from the patient and testing your own responses by rephrasing the meaning and discussing it with the patient.

You build upon the basic techniques of empathic and active listening and talking by *observing* your patient. Other than the standard uniform, what draws attention to her appearance (e.g., tattoos, makeup, accents)? How are her feelings and moods related to the conversation? To encourage communication, *expressing interest and concern honestly* is fundamental. *Echoing* the patient's statements, in the same or slightly altered words, is the simplest form of acknowledgment. Emotions, too, can be echoed empathetically. *Tracking* is the indication, by words or gestures, that you are following the patient's account. *Commenting* on the patient's behavior (as in, "You seem really anxious today") may simply convey understanding, or it may be part of a more thoughtful plan to relate different aspects of the patient's behavior in a later interpretation. *Restatement*, which involves reformulation of the patient's remarks, is the beginning of the process in which you uncover hidden aspects of the patient's situation or infer thoughts that the patient is unable or unwilling to express. Simple restatements may be equally powerful in helping patients to understand themselves both as individuals and as social beings. Many chronically mentally ill patients lack basic communication abilities; others are quite verbal but *mis*communicate their intentions and, as we said above, *mis*interpret the intentions of others. Both have trouble communicating realistically so that their needs can be met by social negotiation. The therapist's ability to restate the patient's needs, even without embellishment, reflects the therapist's understanding back to the patient.

Such techniques provide feedback that you are listening attentively and trying to understand and are consistent with the common factors theory of psychotherapy, which holds that communication per se is of therapeutic value. Restatement and echoing also serve to convert affects into words, a helpful technique for a patient who is expressing extremes of affect such as hatred, rage, anxiety, or depression and helplessness.

When either affect or cognitive information needs to be expressed but is not forthcoming, you may need to *encourage ventilation of feelings and expression of affect*. Indeed, the rediscovery and expression of isolated or repressed affects are central to psychoanalytic abreaction. However, this process must be used judiciously, particularly in prisoners with poor reality testing or poor self-control. Know what your patient can handle, and don't ask them to unload "all your feelings."

As we listen, even at this stage with minimal value judgments but openness, we (i.e., we *therapists*) can be subject to manipulation by criminals, and especially antisocial and psychopathic persons. Many criminals lack empathy for others and see them as means to an end. They may not care about the consequences of their impulsive actions, and thrill-seeking and excitement go hand-in-hand with their impulsivity. Also, as you listen to criminals (not everybody, but criminals), you will find that their patterns of thinking can be categorized into what are called *criminogenic* thinking styles.

Confrontation

Even in the future world of Sector General Hospital, psychologists feel the conflict between doing what helps a patient versus being friendly to them. As healers, they were taught to give comfort, but as the saying goes (since they still read Shakespeare), they sometimes have to be cruel to be kind. But how much of this supposedly cruelty is actually justified (White 2002, p. 586)?

As you begin to deal with inconsistencies between your patients' stated beliefs and behaviors, contradictions between different beliefs, or conflict between the stated goals of their actions and the actual results, you employ the second level of communication, or *confrontation*. Confrontation is helpful when you are talking about discrepancies between a patient's behavior or statements. In corrections, it's easy to find such discrepancies, so the challenge is usually not in finding them but in deciding which ones to discuss and when to discuss them. For example, it would be easy to say, "You wanted some money and you robbed a convenience store...but what were the consequences of that?" In the world outside of corrections, we used confrontations carefully and even hesitantly and tentatively so as not to alienate our patients. When we moved into the correctional setting, we found that prisoners handle confrontations quite well. Why? Because correctional environments are confrontational in their very nature. Prisoners are confronted practically every minute by officers and other prisoners. "Stand up for count." "Show me what's in your hand." "What is this thing we found in your cell?" "Don't you know you can't have more than two oranges?" "Visiting time is over!" "I will pat you down for contraband." Therapeutic confrontations, however, are not meant to instill resentment or hostility or obedience or compliance, but it is true that they probably have a greater applicability in prison settings than in other settings. In the prison setting, we agree with another of the sci-fi characters from Sector General Hospital Chief Psychologist Dr. O'Mara, who reflects, somewhat crudely, that his job is to shrink heads, not swell them (White 2001, p. 160)!

Confrontation implies the existence of conflict. Some therapists limit the term to a forceful or insistent presentation of painful truths to the patient. Others believe that the patient must be confronted with behaviors and self-concepts that he or she finds unacceptable or has long ago disowned. Such direct confrontations may also oppose the patient's current plans, beliefs, or ideas. For example: "You can't continue assaulting people." This type of confrontation is often necessary for a patient who commits destructive acts, and you should not shy away from such directness when he needs to be told the truth. As Hamlet says to his mother, "I must be cruel only to be kind," repacking an old piece of wisdom that good medicine sometimes has a bad taste (*Hamlet*, Act 3, Scene 4). Hold back on the cruelty a bit, however. Prisons have enough of that already.

Being blunt as in the style of "You're totally wrong about that" might even work with certain patients if that is the style you have developed with them. However, in severely mentally ill patients, such total rejection of their viewpoint (i.e., challenging a delusion) can create opposition, anger, and even violence.

Sometimes it is helpful to think of "confrontation" in its other meaning of "comparison." In fact, an older meaning of the word *confront* itself is to look at something *together*, and this is an attitude you can convey with your confrontations (i.e., the patient should feel that she and the therapist are facing the problem together). For example, you might confront a patient's desire to stop using drugs while she continues to hang out with her drug-using friends, explaining you feel that there is a problem there that needs to be worked out.

The mention of substance use brings to mind that many therapies are available for it. Motivational interviewing was developed during the 1980s from the work of William Miller and Stephen Rollnick with problem drinkers (Miller and Rollnick 1991). Supportive psychotherapy was also being developed during this time, such as in the monograph by Werman (1984) and our own article (Novalis 1989). Both motivational interviewing and supportive psychotherapy evolved in part from the person-centered approach of Rogers. Motivational interviewing includes many of the techniques we have described above, sometimes with different names. Motivational interviewing uses four core interviewing techniques, called OARS:

- **O**pen-ended questioning
- **A**ffirmations
- **R**eflecting (reflective listening)
- **S**ummarizing

Motivational interviewers express empathy, avoid arguments, and support self-efficacy (a psychological concept developed by other researchers); they initially used a technique calling "rolling with resistance" but later recommended avoiding the concept of resistance entirely (Miller and Rollnick 2012). Although motivational interviewing was not initially adapted for use with mentally ill persons and prisoners, it has since been used with such groups.

However, there are important differences between motivational interviewing and supportive psychotherapy:

- Motivational interviewing avoids confrontations that we, as supportive therapists, feel are necessary to work with an incarcerated population. To use another of our sci-fi references, you shouldn't have to be tactful when you tell someone not to kill himself (White 2001, p. 437)!

- Motivational interviewing takes a nondirective approach to institutional change in patients, developing discrepancies between their stated goals and their actual behavior or fostering ambivalence between conflicting goals.
- Motivational interviewing certainly proved itself in the population of problem drinkers who come to realize that drinking is a seriously damaging habit or behavior that is interfering with their life goals. But that population is quite different from criminal offenders and mentally ill persons.
- Criminals need direction, prosocial modeling, and a host of other techniques that are avoided in motivational interviewing. Also, mentally ill persons often need explicit advice and direction to deal with their illness and accept treatment.

Despite the limitations noted, there is certainly merit in the methods of listening and expressing empathy used by motivational interviewing. Recall, though, the discussion (in Chapter 1) that many kinds of psychotherapy (even those that are quite different in their premises and "philosophies") work because of their common elements. We emphasize that supportive psychotherapy is the approach we think is best in the correctional setting for the reasons we just mentioned.

Explanation

Moving on: At the third level of communication techniques, you will offer *explanations* of your patient's experiences, life history, and behaviors. Simple explanations can be called *clarifications*, and complex communications involving what is thought to be unconscious material in the patient may be called *interpretations* in psychodynamic psychotherapy. In the past, we have referred to complicated explanations as interpretations, but we have found that doing so creates some confusion with the psychodynamic therapists' use of the term, so we usually speak instead of explanations in this book. We use explanations to help patients understand things they are not aware of. To apply these to a hypothetical patient: these things may be consciously available but unappreciated (e.g., that the patient hasn't talked to his cellmate for a week), preconscious (something that he can become aware of by focusing his attention on it, like the fact that he is angry at his therapist), or things that he is not aware of (e.g., that he is sadistic and unfeeling). But if it is just some fact that he doesn't know (like who won the 1953 World Series), we would not call it an explanation but just "learning a fact."

We turn now to some important concepts that affect the way you will work with prisoners, and we'll say more about communication after that.

Defenses and Coping Behaviors

When Freud theorized that some mental contents are unconscious, it was a revolutionary idea, but one that was soon widely accepted. Freud also believed that people employ psychological defenses, which are ways of thinking that allow them to avoid or "repress" conscious knowledge of their behavior. Freudian theory has undergone much development in the past 100 years, and it is by no means necessary for you to accept classic Freudian theory. *We* certainly don't. However, the notion of psychological defenses is still a particularly useful one that helps us to understand why ordinary people (like you, like us) are unaware of unconscious information which affects our lives.

Example 1 (well-worn)

A man has a fight with his wife and is angry at her. The next day he "forgets" it is their anniversary and even finds it "necessary" to work late and arrive home long after she has gone to bed. His mind has used the defense of forgetting, but at no time does he consciously decide to forget. Of course, it is possible that a man in his situation could deliberately stay late at the office to avoid dealing with the anniversary, but this is not the case with him. When his wife "mentions" to him the next morning that he missed their anniversary, he is surprised and apologetic. Perhaps he realizes that the argument the previous day left him with some anger, and he admits that to his wife and tries to make it up to her.

Example 2

Although there is no rational reason for it, a paranoid prisoner thinks that his cellmate is planning to kill him. He decides to make a "preemptive strike" against his cellmate to protect himself. This patient is unconsciously using the defense of *projection*. He has projected his own hostility onto his cellmate and in this case may actually kill his cellmate in his protective reaction.

As a therapist, it helps to appreciate how psychological defenses operate in people's thinking and actions. It also turns out that the traditional "collection" of psychological defenses evokes many similarities to the thinking styles that habitual criminals use to justify their behavior. For the use of supportive psychotherapy in corrections, we have organized a list of defenses and coping behaviors in Table 2–4, ranging from what most researchers would consider mature to what are considered immature or even "primitive." Defenses utilized or favored by criminals are illustrated.

To use a sports analogy, defenses are a person's "playbook" for actions: planning them, doing them, justifying them to oneself, and explaining them to others. Defenses enable people to ward off unpleasant feelings such as anxiety, guilt, or fear. They help us to preserve some dysfunctional aspects of ourselves that we can't or don't want to change.

Depending on how they are used, psychological defenses can preserve function in low-functioning people or cause great dysfunction in high-functioning people. Highly functional and successful people are not without their moments of denial, projection, splitting, and regression—defenses in the low-functioning constellation. Similarly, humor can be cruel and sadistic or gentle and provocative. Rationalization, a defense in the middle group, can flout the laws of logic in a psychotic individual or simply deny basic facts in a sentenced prisoner. So the dysfunction expressed and created by a defense can vary considerably. After all, there are little lies and big lies, and so forth. Because many defenses involve forgetting or avoiding the thought of something, the thing that is avoided or forgotten (or repressed in psychoanalytic terminology) usually affects the seriousness of the defense. Thus, a patient who "forgets" that he didn't pay for something in the store is doing something more serious than the man mentioned above who forgets his anniversary.

The term *coping behaviors* refers to the most observable type of defenses. Often, coping behaviors are appropriate to the situation or threat that evokes them. For example, during the coronavirus pandemic, many people coped by wearing face masks, following rules for social distancing, and washing their hands frequently. If they were asked to explain why they did those things, they would explain them on the basis of

TABLE 2–4.   **Classification of defenses and coping styles useful in corrections**

Defense	How normally used	How offenders use
Mature		
Dealing with the world as it really is; facing and accepting truths about the world and yourself, however upsetting or unpleasant; genuine altruism; humor	Rational and mature people face and accept life as it is and give back to others. They can take themselves "with a grain of salt" and laugh at their own foibles.	As a "sop" to altruism, criminals do small deeds or give a little to good causes as "sentimentality." They laugh at others and their crimes, but not in the self-reflective way that mature people use humor.
Usually mature		
Suppression and sublimation	People work hard, go to school, and so forth, and put off the pleasures of the future.	Criminals do the opposite and put off thinking about the bad things they do.
Intermediate		
Obsessional Isolation Isolation of affects Doing and undoing	At times we all avoid thinking about unpleasant things. We can do things repetitively to avoid anxiety about other things.	Criminals become all-absorbed and obsessional about doing their crimes but isolate and avoid genuine feelings of remorse.
Neurotic		
Reaction formation Projection Dissociation Displacement Minor forgetting Minimization	We sometimes blame others for own fault and can project own impulses onto others; we may "kick the dog" when we get home instead of kicking the boss at work. We may minimize the importance of something stupid that we did.	Using "externalization of blame," criminals routinely accuse others of forcing them to do it (or of victims asking to be victims by their own behavior), having bad motives, or being more criminal than they are; they forget things when it is convenient to do so. They frequently minimize serious consequences, as in "It was no big deal, nobody died, they won't miss the money."
Narcissistic		
Grandiosity Selfishness Omnipotence Devaluation of others	At times people like to think of themselves as more important or consequential than they really are, but this is usually corrected by reality.	Part and parcel of the power orientation seen in many criminals, they put themselves first and devalue other human beings. Many fulfill the diagnostic criteria for narcissistic personality disorder, antisocial personality disorder, or a mixed personality disorder.

TABLE 2–4. **Classification of defenses and coping styles useful in corrections** *(continued)*

Defense	How normally used	How offenders use
Low-level		
Splitting Dissociation Passive aggression Projective identification Somatization Rationalization Autistic fantasy	Persons with borderline personality disorder (often seen in corrections) see others as all-good or all-bad, which results in staff infighting (splitting). Many of us have a tendency to drag our feet or avoid unpleasant work (passive aggression). We all seek to give the best possible explanation for what we do, sometimes avoiding the real facts (rationalization).	Criminals can be work-avoidant and do things poorly or slowly while trying to give the impression that they are working hard. They can deliberately try to get staff working at cross-purposes by telling them different things at different times. Rationalization is the mainstay of criminals who blame others individually or society. They may use situational necessity ("I had to do it—I needed the money"), social necessity ("Nobody would give me a job"), or psychological necessity ("I'm impulsive and I couldn't stop myself").
Negating and delusional		
Psychotic denial Repression of major memories Major distortion Delusion Fabrication Pathological lying "Blacking out"	Sometimes we just don't want to remember painful things, and we may forget without knowing we have forgotten. Psychotic persons may genuinely be unable to remember what they did, including a criminal act.	Criminals routinely deny committing crimes (this may be true sometimes), claim to have "blacked out," or just lie repeatedly about most matters in their lives; they may run away from confrontations in real life or abruptly leave a therapy session. Denial (of facts or external reality) can be used to avoid confrontation about criminal behaviors or to avoid remorse. They will distort the details and rewrite their personal histories or fabricate incidents "out of whole cloth."

Source. Based on Di Riso et al. 2011, p. 62, and the 7-level Defense Mechanisms Rating Scale (Perry 2002; Di Giuseppe et al. 2020); and in part on Vaillant 1988, p. 203.

what their leaders or the experts had advised them to do, or of what they had personally decided to do after considering the evidence.

Defenses and coping behaviors are utilized extensively by persons who are criminals to defend their past behaviors and plans for future behavior. You will be faced daily with explanations of why your patients did what they did, said what they said, believe what they believe, and plan to do what they are going to do when they go back to their cell in 15 minutes. It is simply amazing to contemplate the "reasons" people give for their antisocial attitudes and dangerous and unlawful behaviors.

Psychological defenses are addressed in long-term psychotherapy and improvement of defenses correlates with improvement in personal function (Perry and Bond 2012). Your work with defenses will be limited, but we do feel that that is one area of psychological function that can be improved in prisoners, not just those with criminal thinking patterns. Hopefully you can reduce the use of patients' defenses that support their criminality, improve the maturity of defenses, and make it less likely for them to utilize immature defenses. Some insight and understanding will be required on their part, but a little bit at a time.

As you notice dysfunctional or immature defenses. you should try to learn more about the patient's general pattern of defenses rather than immediately criticize a specific defense. Because attacking (or even appearing to attack) defenses creates anxiety that is disturbing to patients whose defensive structures and personalities are already deficient, criticisms as well as explanations of defenses must be offered carefully to blunt their full force.

When we began correctional work, we noticed that the psychological concept of defenses was closely related to another empirically validated collection of beliefs known as "criminogenic beliefs" or "criminal thinking." The relationship, of course, is not coincidental, since criminal thinking is a defensive style of thinking that arises from psychological defenses. Therefore, patients who are criminals or who have some characteristic of criminals should receive a more detailed assessment of their criminal thinking patterns. However, keep in mind that many of your patients may not be criminals at all. They may be innocent but accused people with no other criminal record, or a person with a record who is innocent of the current charge. This may be the first time they've been accused of a crime, or they may be in for the 10th time. Know your patients individually. Criminals will say many things that you will individually recognize as distortions, negations, or outright denials of "correct" beliefs. Criminals are people with an established criminal lifestyle. *Criminal* is the term that is consistently used by developers of programs to treat criminality in prisoners. We use this term with qualification, since some researchers are concerned that labeling people as criminals has a self-fulfilling component that is undesirable.

Should a person who has committed many crimes be *called* a criminal? Should a person with schizophrenia be called a "schizophrenic" and a person with bipolar illness a "bipolar"? In the latter two cases we try to avoid the nouns "schizophrenic" and "bipolar." A person may have a disease, but a person is not the disease. Some schools of therapy, including feminism and motivational interviewing, also try to avoid labels. We recognize that a person who commits only a few crimes will fare better if not labeled a "criminal"; in such cases, the person could be called an "offender" but not a "criminal," which implies a habitual criminal with a criminal lifestyle. Therefore, if someone has committed a crime or two, or maybe three or four, we might call them an offender, and when we see someone like that, he or she will be a prisoner and a patient, but not necessarily a criminal. For example, Boyd Sharp, a psychologist and program administrator who wrote for the American Correctional Association, tells us that he uses the word "criminal" in the nonderogatory way that others use the word "alcoholic"—that is, to refer to a past behavior that allows one to be in a state of recovery. He believes this is important so that criminals are discouraged from reverting to their previous criminal behaviors. However, he does acknowledge that the term "criminal" is still offensive to some people (Sharp 2006, p. 104).

That being said, persons with significant criminality are usually different from those people who usually do not commit crimes. To be sure, in much of their lives they do have unconscious defenses and are unaware of using them. However, in regard to their criminal activities, they frequently use psychological defenses verbally and knowingly, whether in thinking about the matter to themselves or in explaining their behavior to others (including their peers and their therapists). For example, they frequently *rationalize* their criminal behaviors using a variety of excuses. When they do that (e.g., rationalize their behaviors), their behavior is usually conscious. They know when they are breaking the law, they know when they are breaking someone's arm, and so forth. When we examine the causes of their behavior, of course, there may be other factors, such as social inequities, and not just individual criminal thinking.

Case Vignette

A 25-year-old man drives a delivery truck in his regular job. The driver's side of the truck is fairly open for making the deliveries easier. One day his truck is on the side of the road in a residential neighborhood. He is parked near some young girls who are playing in a wading pool. One of the neighbors walks by the truck and notices that he has exposed himself. The neighbor is offended by this and calls the police, and the driver is arrested. From the presentence investigation, the psychologist obtains a lot of information about him. He hears that the patient considers himself a fairly normal person. He has had a girlfriend for a year. However, he has been arrested twice before for some type of exposure, which he "explains away" as a misunderstanding. As they go through the details of what happened on the day of the crime, the patient says that he cannot remember the incident he is accused of. He does not even remember parking the truck in that neighborhood or exposing himself. When confronted with the eyewitness testimony that convicted him, he just shrugs and says, "That's what they said, but I don't remember it." He is convicted of the crime. Much later, when he is in prison and treatment is offered as a way of hastening his release, he begins to remember what happened.

It might be possible that this man has "repressed" his memory of the incident because it was so painful. If he were suffering from a psychotic disorder, he might have what is called "psychotic denial" of the incident. However, since he has no mental illness, it is much more likely that he just did not want to talk about the incident until such time as it began to benefit him to talk about it. And how soon he talks about it, and how soon he begins to deal with what has happened in his life, may depend on his psychotherapist.

Criminals use psychological defenses frequently and consciously and run the gamut of defenses. They defend their criminal attitudes and slant the historical interpretation of their criminal record. They may deny their behaviors outright or rationalize them if they acknowledge them. They may laugh off their offenses. They may suppress their inclinations to follow the law. Often these are not unconscious defenses that need explanations but criminal excuses that need calling out. For example, they frequently perceive themselves as "good" people despite the injuries they have caused to others.

The expert criminologist Walters (1995a, 1995b, 2010) identified eight criminal thinking styles. Like the eight risk-need-responsivity (RNR) factors described by Andrews and Bonta, this is another important "gang of eight." Basically, these styles involve combinations of psychological defenses, mostly rationalizations and denials. This list of eight is widely known, and there are many presentations of it, but we present our own in Table 2–5.

TABLE 2–5.   **Eight criminal thinking styles**

Criminal thinking style	Definition	Examples of things criminals say or do
Mollification	Similar to the psychological defense of rationalization: they blame others and minimize the importance or damage.	"She asked for it." "Nobody got hurt." "What's the big deal; they're not going to miss a few dollars." "Everybody does it." "Everyone else I know is worse." "If you were in my position, you'd do the same thing."
Entitlement	They believe they are entitled to the fruits of crime without effort and that they are entitled beings with special privileges. They confuse wants with needs and necessities that must be acquired regardless of the cost to others.	"I deserved that money, and I took it." "I deserve to be rich." "Nobody has the right to deprive me of this."
Power orientation	Power is all-important to them. They must have power over others. They think the world is divided into the weak and the strong. Without power they feel they are in a "zero" state that is utterly intolerable for them.	"You'd better do this or else…." "I can make you do this." "Submit, you f---head!"
Cutoff	They cut off consideration of the seriousness or morality of behavior by just impulsively doing it. They lack reflection or self-control. Or they use drugs to dull their reasoning abilities prior to the act.	"What the hell…" "Ya know, just f--- it. I am going to hit the guy."
Sentimentality	They have a soft spot for charities or wounded animals or doing little things that make them feel they are good people and compensate (perhaps unconsciously) for the bad things they do.	"I'm a good person…I take in lost dogs…I donated to the Save the Whales people. I give money to homeless guys on the street. I may be a gang leader, but I contribute to my community center."
Superoptimism	They will ask for things or assume they can get things for which they are clearly unqualified (e.g., apply for jobs without caring to meet the prerequisites).	"They'll never catch me for these burglaries…I'm too smart for them." "I know a lot about drugs…I can teach your relapse prevention course."
Cognitive indolence	Their decisions do not show the normal attention to facts and logic. They do not think things through. They discount or do not appreciate the amount of work that is needed to accomplish a task.	"I know everything I need to know to pass this course…I don't have to attend the classes…and I don't have to bother with doing the homework."

TABLE 2–5.	Eight criminal thinking styles *(continued)*	
Criminal thinking style	Definition	Examples of things criminals say or do
Discontinuity	They fail to see the conflicts between their criminality and the need to obey the law. They don't have the unified, consistent personality that non-criminals strive for.	"I'm a good person, I don't know why you always call me a criminal…My rap sheet is only 5 pages." They may glory in their impulsiveness as "I'm the kind of guy who if I just think of something I do it."

Source. Based on Walters 2001, 2005, 2010.

Criminals' rationalizations are, of course, anything but rational. For example, the sentimental criminal may reason that "since I gave a few dollars to charity, I am really a good person even though I steal and assault people." No one except the criminal (or some of his friends) actually believes that. Because of the research behind criminal thinking styles, when we are working with a habitual criminal, we remind ourselves of Walters' list or the similar lists developed by others.

As it affects therapy, therefore, the advice is:

1. When dealing with noncriminal issues, think about the psychological defenses a patient is using.
2. When dealing with issues of criminality, think in terms of Walters' list.
3. Try to identify other excuses, defenses, or rationalizations to determine if they are conscious and deliberate or unknown to your patient.

In supportive psychotherapy, you can do much to change criminogenic thinking and some work to reduce recidivism. You can at least try to affect some of the eight RNR risk factors discussed in the previous chapter except the first one (the criminal history). You probably won't change an "unmarried" risk factor, but you can address the family instability. You can help patients improve their employment, education, and prosocial leisure activities through the advisory and directive interventions that we shall describe later. The "proof" that such interventions work is in the research studies on programs that use structured protocols and high "doses" of intervention. However, you can use many similar interventions in your regular therapy. Andrews and Bonta (2010) specify interventions that do and don't work in targeting recidivism. On the basis of their presentations (which most but not all practitioners accept), the interventions that don't work are said to be:

- Using interventions that increase self-esteem without reductions in procriminal attitudes and associates.
- Addressing vague personal or emotional complaints that don't affect criminal conduct.
- Increasing conventional ambition without providing the means to achieve it (in work or schooling).
- Trying to make people "better."

But there are some typical therapeutic interventions that do work, as noted by Andrews and Bonta (2010), and these include:

- Changing procriminal attitudes.
- Reducing angry, hostile feelings.
- Increasing self-control, self-management, and problem-solving skills.
- Providing mentally disordered offenders with housing appropriate for them.

Most correctional systems can provide you an assessment of your individual patient's eight factors using risk/need assessment instruments. There are many such instruments, such as the Ohio Risk Assessment System (ORAS; Latessa et al. 2009). To give one example, the ORAS–Reentry Tool measures several factors in criminal thinking:

- Criminal pride
- Belief that it is possible to overcome the past (rated as criminal if "no")
- Use of anger to intimidate others
- Ability to walk away from a fight (rated criminal if unable)
- Belief that it is possible to overcome the past (criminal if no)
- Problem-solving ability (poor in criminals)
- Ability to express concern about others' misfortunes (criminals don't)
- Belief in "Do unto others before they do unto you"

In other scales, the ORAS also recognizes criminal lifestyle factors, which include

- Being able to control anger (scored high if poor).
- Acting impulsively.
- Feeling lack of control over events.

Since criminal thinking affects future actions, criminal lifestyles are measured by several validated assessment instruments that your institution may use already. Two of them are the Psychological Inventory of Criminal Thinking Styles (PICTS) and the Measure of Criminogenic Thinking Styles (MOCTS). The PICTS is an 80-item scale, appearing in multiple versions (Walters 1995a, 1995b,1998, 2001, 2010), that provides a variety of information, including an overall scale of general criminal thinking and it sorts into Walters' eight individual criminal thinking styles (Walters 2001, 2005, 2010; see also Gavel 2017). The MOCTS (Mandracchia and Morgan 2011, 2012) is a 70-item self-report measure of maladaptive thinking styles that are influential in the development and maintenance of criminal behavior. It contains subscales for three types of maladaptive thinking:

- *Cognitive immaturity* assesses the tendency to engage in judging, blaming, and self-pitying thoughts.
- *Control* addresses the need for expression of power over oneself, others, and the environment.
- *Egocentrism* assesses the tendency to view oneself as important or the center of attention in situations (Gavel 2017, p. 31). (The dissertation by Gavel discusses the relationships between measures of criminal thinking and attitudes.)

An instrument developed by Andrews and others for assessment of services needed is the Level of Service Inventory—Revised (Andrews et al. 2020). There is also much didactic or educational material for use with prisoners. For example, Hazelden Publishing and the Minnesota Department of Corrections developed a program addressing criminal thinking (Hazelden Foundation 2019).

We recommend that you become familiar with assessment instruments, and especially the ones in your institution. Read the assessments and get a general picture of thinking patterns of your patients. As is frequently claimed, criminal thinking can involve cognitive errors, but we emphasize that this is also a matter of perspective. It could be sardonically claimed that a serial killer has committed the cognitive error that "It is a good thing to kill people repeatedly" and simply needs to be "educated" that his thinking is erroneous. Experts would point out that this is a gross oversimplification; no one would claim that serial killers merely need to correct their thinking errors. However, to a lesser extent, that is what the cognitive therapy programs claim to do for offenders with multiple convictions and a criminal lifestyle. In other words, we think it is a little too easy to blame everything "wrong" that a person does on cognitive errors.

Whether or when to talk about criminal thinking patterns with your patients is a judgment call. You may ask them when they feel ready. They may never be ready, or it may not matter much if they have a long sentence. When they are beginning to think about the end of their sentence, they may be more amenable. Or it may not be relevant to the reasons they committed a crime. Decisions to commit crimes also involve differences in moral values. They may involve adherence to criminal peer group values rather than social values. We must help an offender to consider that their peer group ought not have the right to assert its superiority over society as a whole. An exception to this may occur in the case of civil disobedience, which probably few of your patients are asserting. They may assert that ours is an oppressive society and that they have been prevented from having the opportunities that others have gotten. As we develop our adult sets of beliefs, we put together a variety of facts and beliefs to support our positions in life. This includes what many would call mainstream political positions and also deviant positions (e.g., that sexual relationships with children are a good thing despite society's repression of it). If you are interested in learning more about this, the way that world views can be justified and held against all opposing arguments was described some years ago by the American philosopher Willard Van Orman Quine (Quine 1978). In a similar vein, the American philosopher George Lakoff argued that there are defining metaphors to persons of different political affiliations, with conservatives adhering to a strict father model and liberals to a nurturant parent model (Lakoff 2016). We mention these issues because we urge you to think about the assumptions you hold about people, behavior, and criminality.

To simplify matters, however, we would suggest that you organize the beliefs of your patients around Walters' eight criminal thinking styles. Examples of such an approach are given in Table 2–6. Relating this to the things we have said about defenses and coping skills, many criminal thinking patterns involve low self-esteem and negative self-images combined with compensatory grandiosity and other pathological defenses. In persons with these patterns, their low or nihilistic self-esteem is related to their power orientation. Their grandiose beliefs are related to their criminal style of entitlement, and so forth. You can certainly use your own mental or written checklists as you do psychotherapy and encounter criminogenic thinking.

Lack of prosocial attitudes is a criminogenic factor. Even though the opportunities are limited in a prison society of criminals, it is of benefit to encourage your patients to engage in these activities. If you have a therapeutic community, you have a mini-society governed by rules and laws that must be obeyed and respected.

Bonta and Andrews (2017) address a question that frequently arises: Do special subgroups of criminals such as domestic abusers or sex offenders differ in some fundamental ways in their risk factors? For example, are they "specialists" who are only likely to reoffend in their particular areas of crime? The answer is "mostly no." They often have other criminal records and reoffenses. That means that if you do treat them and don't provide a specialized program for them, you can treat them as you would treat other criminal inmates. In general, Bonta and Andrews also state that recidivism in women can be treated just like in any other defined group of offenders, but we do find that there is controversy about this point.

Reality Testing

In our account of defenses, we consider it a sign of maturity to deal with the world or "reality" as it really is. But patients, such as depressed and anxious ones, often by utilizing psychological defenses, usually have some disturbance in reality testing. Seriously mentally ill persons often have alterations in perception (hallucinations) and belief (delusions) that cannot be validated by independent observers of the same culture. And we do admit that there are some errors in criminogenic thought processes that might be corrected by learning. Since the development of beliefs involves cognitive processes, there are many aspects of what is now called cognitive-behavioral therapy (CBT), which is being used to change criminal attitudes and behavior. Structured programs involving CBT do have an evidence basis for success in preventing recidivism and of course we encourage them. Most of the procedures in CBT are transparent to the patients (e.g., there is not some "secret game" going on by which the therapist manipulates them). The supportive psychotherapy techniques we describe are certainly compatible with CBT programs and are presented here not as a structured or packaged program, but as the techniques you need to use for all your patient's issues, not just when attempting to prevent recidivism.

Current research in preventing recidivism, however, leads to a mixed and somewhat unsettling picture. To recap: According to the RNR model, there are three important components to any program that attempts to lower recidivism (Andrews and Bonta 2010):

- *Risk:* The level of service is matched to the offender's risk to reoffend.
- *Need:* The program determines and treats the offender's specific criminogenic needs.
- *Responsivity:* The interventions are matched to the offender's capabilities (i.e., his learning style, motivation, abilities, and strengths).

As we have mentioned, however, a limitation of the RNR approach is that *prisoners respond only to high levels of therapeutic programming.* For example, persons with a high risk of reoffending might require 200–300 hours of programming over 6–12 months, and those

TABLE 2–6.	Examples of beliefs related to criminal thinking styles

Criminal beliefs related to mollification

If I was white, I wouldn't have been stopped. (Worth discussing. Were they breaking the law?)

If racism was involved in their apprehension, what is the proper response now? How can they deal with the racism that has created disadvantage in their life?

Rules don't count.

Methamphetamine should be legal. (This may be true of marijuana, and states may be legalizing possession of small quantities, but it is unlikely that selling large quantities of methamphetamine will be made legal.)

Criminal beliefs related to the factor of entitlement

I am unique.

I am superior.

Rules don't apply.

I am an exceptional person.

No one recognizes my talents.

Because I was so poorly treated, I am entitled to break the law.

The world owes me a living.

Money is all that matters.

And…how you get the money doesn't matter.

Criminal beliefs related to power orientation

I am nothing.

I am a zero.

I am worthless.

My parents taught me that I am a piece of sh--.

I have only criminal friends.

My criminal friends are the only ones that appreciate me.

Being strong is all that matters.

I hate weak people. They are disgusting.

with a moderate risk may require 100 hours over 3–6 months (National Parole Resource Center 2022); the intensive RNR program should not be used for low-risk offenders because it is costly and ineffective and may increase recidivism (Andrews and Bonta 2010). Use of the RNR program can reduce recidivism, but by how much? The National Parole Resource Center (2022) says that the effect can be as much as 30%, but keep in mind that low-risk prisoners need different programming, because their criminal behavior may actually worsen from RNR interventions. Also: Mental illness per se is not a criminogenic factor. Therefore, it may be of humanitarian value to treat low-risk and mentally ill prisoners, but such treatment in and of itself may not reduce recidivism.

If the patient's world view is pathologically distorted, you should help to correct his view and possibly help him understand how the distortion came about. Doing this work is described as "correcting cognitive distortions" (Sun 2012). Sometimes, this reality-enhancing work is simply a matter of supplying missing information. A patient who is fearful of going to her first day of vocational training may simply need some help in learning what the classes are like and that they may actually be fun. Another patient, burdened by depression after a month in prison, may be helped by knowing that there is a likelihood that medication will relieve it.

A further step is to involve the patient in activities that lead to greater opportunities and satisfactions in life. She may need guidance or encouragement in

- Learning new skills that will be helpful in the community.
- Trying out new behaviors and experiences.
- Overcoming avoidant or phobic behaviors toward feared situations.
- Giving up dysfunctional behaviors.
- Thinking about herself in more positive terms.

We find that prisoners frequently have what we refer to as serious paranoid distortions of reality that are caused by the defense mechanism called *projection* (i.e., they attribute evil motives to others arising from their own hatred of others). But paranoia can also be interpreted as partly the result of illogical generalization from a history of abuse and mistreatment. It is hard for the patient to trust, and often this is for good reasons. When the patient attributes motives or reasons for action to others, at first it is usually advisable not to weaken the defensive operation (i.e., projection) but to approach it as a cognitive error, suggesting that other motives might be operational.

Case Vignette

A prisoner complains vociferously of his mistreatment by one particular officer. This officer, he says, must be a racist. He complains that the officer tosses his cell for contraband but leaves the others alone. He does pat downs every time this person leaves culinary.

A therapeutic reaction to this scenario might draw on your knowledge of criminogenic thinking, the pathology of paranoia, and what you know of the patient's personal history. At first you might just listen and see the purpose of the session as ventilation. Perhaps the patient really doesn't think you are going to do something about the officer, as he has already filed a grievance about the officer and talked to the associate warden. Maybe he just wants you to hear him out and sympathize (or as you would say, empathize). Maybe he wants to confirm that the officer and officers in general are racist, and so are you, because you are not of his race, so you could not personally understand what he had gone through in his life.

A psychodynamic therapist might interpret this behavior as the projection of the patient's own hatred onto the correctional officer, but in supportive therapy it is approached as an appreciation of the consequences of his actions. You can stress the patient's power to antagonize the officer further and make the situation worse by incurring unfair discipline. He is welcome to file his grievances, but if he mouths off to the officer every time he sees him, he will get written up for it. After you get the facts, you may be able to conclude: "Don't take it personally." Maybe this officer pats down a lot of people every day, more so than the other officers. If the prisoner implies that you are racist, you may or may not want to bring this up for discussion. This is an interpretation of transference and is discussed in Chapter 3. Since it is a negative transference that might threaten the trust in your relationship with the patient, it probably needs discussion but how and when is a therapeutic decision.

Externalization of blame ("It was someone else's fault") is a common defense in criminals. In the traditional meme of criminal behavior, the car thief explains his behavior by saying, "They deserved it because they left their keys in the car." Some will just say they were "impulsive," as if that was an excuse for the behavior. Other issues, for example, may involve the thrill-seeking component of criminal thinking. It can be pointed out that nearly anything can be "enjoyable" if you develop an interest in it, but when it is antisocial or criminal it could get you into trouble. Sometimes the blaming can be a generalization, such as "I can't work, because nobody likes me." You can work with this in the usual way of diffusing generalizations as cognitive errors, or in finding that the patient's boss in particular is a difficult person, but everybody doesn't hate the patient!

Reassurance and Enhancement of Self-Esteem

We have seen that interventions that improve self-esteem are not necessarily going to reduce recidivism in our patients. Bolstering self-esteem in antisocial prisoners is neither necessary nor desirable. *Enhancing self-esteem* in general is not necessarily a desirable goal for all prisoners since it depends on their criminal attitudes and thinking. A criminal who thinks he is the smartest and strongest fellow in the place does not need his self-esteem enhanced; rather, he may need to understand that his self-esteem is falsely inflated and a defense again past victimization or treatment by his family. However, many prisoners, including many criminals, actually have very negative self-images and self-appraisals for which their grandiosity is a compensation. Improving self-esteem is often desirable in doing supportive psychotherapy with low-functioning patients who have faced problems due to deficiencies in self-esteem from their upbringing or past life experiences.

1. Improved self-esteem and its consequence, self-confidence, are recognized as factors that promote adequate performance (see, e.g., Beck and Emery 1985, p. 76). A patient who gains in *realistic* self-esteem can therefore overcome previously disabling unrealistic fears.
2. "Disbelief in oneself" is a self-fulfilling prophecy of failure that in turn leads to even lower self-esteem.
3. The cognitive *anticipation of failure* can generate excess anxiety that impairs performance.

Reassurance involves more specific statements about the patient's beliefs and behaviors. Reassurance may involve simply pointing out that the person has been an effective parent, despite now being separated from her child. This should involve an emphasis on positive or hopeful elements in her life that she may have neglected. Or just saying, "I know a year sounds like a long time, but you'll be back there for them before you realize it!" Here you can provide what your patient lacks: the longer time perspective that makes suffering more endurable and happiness more tenable. And while we don't recommend false reassurances that will fall flat in a week or two, it depends. If you are trying to prevent a suicide, you may need to varnish the truth by saying, "Hey, it's going to be okay! We'll get you through this!" There are also reassurances where the facts don't matter because they can be self-fulfilling prophecies such as "I know everything will be all right because you will make the right decisions." Sometimes you need to give reassurances that have a basis in fact and sometimes just hope, possibly when your patient laments:

- I will never get parole.
- No lawyer will ever help me.
- My husband is going to divorce me.
- I will never get a job when I get out of here.
- I am going to get 60 days in the hole for nothing.

You should assess 1) the factual validity of the fear, which may range from imaginary to entirely justified; 2) its consequences, which may be exaggerated in the patient's opinion; and 3) its emotional validity, which should be acknowledged but not necessarily accepted at face value, either, because it may represent a displacement from another fear. For example, a fear of loss of job might really be a fear of losing the ability to support her child. Proper reassurance can reduce guilt for encountered loss. This is important in working with mentally ill people who blame themselves for their own illness, physically ill people who do the same, or parents who have lost custody of their children. Alleviation of guilt raises self-esteem. It is proper to do so when dwelling on the past makes the patient worse. But it is not necessarily proper to alleviate guilt or raise self-esteem when looking back on criminal acts. Therefore, you will frequently be making a choice about what to reassure and when. The utility of an informed reassurance cannot be overemphasized. However, bland reassurances, not based on an understanding relationship with the patient, are bound to be taken as insincere.

Self-esteem is ultimately enhanced through feedback to patients about their behavior as they are guided into increasingly productive and rewarding activities. We wish there were more such activities in prison, since we know that competence, mastery, and success raise self-esteem more effectively than talk. Sometimes, the best we can do is help them to remember past successes and to build on them.

Explanations and Clarifications

As mentioned earlier, we use the general term *explanation* to describe communications that are specific to the patient. Explanations may be "genetic" (which in psychotherapy includes early life and family influences, not just influences involving genes) or contemporary (i.e., explaining one current process by another one). They are useful agents of therapeutic change, not necessarily via insight, but because they result in changes in the patient's self-esteem, feelings, and repertory of behaviors. Explanations may refer to the offering of causes, contributing factors, motives, reasons, mechanisms of action, and processes behind or antecedents to the patient's feelings, thoughts, and behaviors. A somewhat simpler type of interpretation, often called a *clarification*, is a relatively superficial explanation that reveals unknown or unacknowledged aspects of the patient's life without delving deeply into the patient's hidden motives, fears, wishes, or defenses.

We recommend that the *level* of an explanation be kept superficial, and, in general, the *force* (or critical import) needs to be blunted in a number of ways. The *pacing* and *timing* of explanations are also crucial. Premature explanations may be erroneous and therefore unhelpful and misleading. Even when correct, a premature interpretation may be ineffective or disregarded. Worse yet, it may anger the patient, create anxiety, and disrupt the therapy. You will work with fragile patients who can be frightened by premature or deep explanations. Knowing this, you may be tempted to "tread lightly" to the point that your therapy is ineffective; you need to counteract this by drawing from the available techniques that offer explanations effectively. You can use *limited or inexact explanations*, which are partly true but not entirely so. For example, consider a prisoner who was previously heterosexual who now has to deal with fears of rape or with homosexual feelings toward another prisoner. Beginning with "surface" explanations, you might discuss feelings toward another person as a normal type of friendly feeling. Later, you may need to think it is appropriate to explain that persons have a potential for heterosexual and homosexual behaviors and that the confinement in prison leads many individuals to find new ways to express their sexuality.

When to Give an Explanation

When you want to say something that might create anxiety, it helps to "soften the blow." For example, you can preface a confrontation with a small item of praise. "You are really doing well at work. But I did get this note from your supervisor that we should discuss." It also helps prepare for the future by announcing plans to talk about a difficult subject. "I know it's painful to talk about your drug use, and I see that you don't want to talk about it now. So, let's put this off for a while until you feel ready." A statement like this is preferable to an unstated collusive bargain in which you simply avoid the topic.

Patients may also introduce topics at an inappropriate time. The patient may say: "I want to tell you about Mary, my first wife." You may have to say: "I would like to hear about her, but we only have 5 minutes left. Why don't we plan to do that the first thing next time?" Patients frequently introduce problems at the very end of the session or make "staircase" pronouncements—so-called because Freud saw patients upstairs in his house and found that they frequently said such things on the way down. Patients may declare they are suicidal or that they have just been rolled up for discharge. And be prepared for Parthian shots, named after a tactic of ancient archers of shooting back while retreating. Develop your preferred procedure for dealing with these at the time, and for talking about them later.

Another rule is to "strike while the iron is cold" (Pine 1986). While psychodynamic therapists may strive to offer explanations when feelings are fresh, the supportive therapist may prefer to wait until the patient has emotionally cooled off. This tempers the potentially critical or humiliating impact of the explanation. For similar reasons, you can limit or close off the patient's associations to the explanation, introduce explanations tentatively, give the patient the opportunity to stop the discussion, and prepare the patient for the explanation by letting him or her know earlier in the session that the subject will be discussed later (Pine 1985).

Displaced Explanations

When a group and its therapist address one patient's problems, the entire group benefits. Explanations can be delivered effectively when you are in a group situation or talking to several people together by directing them (*displacing* them) to someone other than the person who is merely "listening in." You should always be aware that you are "in role" when conducting a conversation in a group. This technique can be used in individual psychotherapy, for example, by discussing stories in the public press regarding the mental illness, or substance abuse problems of celebrities. You can use anonymous examples, such as: "I had a patient last year who was embarrassed about not knowing how to read, but he went to the literacy program and did really well." When we do so, we do explain that we have "anonymized" the story and we never talk about a current prisoner.

Just as it is safer, proverbially speaking, to kick the dog instead of one's boss, it is safer to talk about one's problems in displacement. You can take advantage of such displacements in many ways. *Vicarious discussion* is familiar as the use of topics that have personal relevance to the patient's pathology. Prisoners can talk about violence and aggression in current events, which may include gun violence, war, and physically combative sports. The displaced discussion may by itself serve a ventilatory purpose, or an introduction to the violence in their own lives—the violence that they have experienced or the violence they have perpetrated. You may go on: "You have seen a lot of violence yourself, haven't you?" "Oh yeah (*angry*). My father practically killed my mother one time, and he would have, if I hadn't stopped him, the bastard!" You may follow up on the facts or the feeling. Or the patient may observe: "You know, I can imagine being angry enough to get a gun and go kill a bunch of strangers!" You may explore that or not depending on your sense of readiness to go farther. In later sessions, as your patient has learned to feel comfortable (or enjoy?) talking about the violence in his past, you may say, "You know, you've mentioned that some of your crimes are violent." The answer may be, "You bet, but that so-called assault was self-defense. Don't you be accusing me of just hitting people for no reason. I don't do that, and I've never done that!" You will now need to manage the emotions in your subsequent therapy. You may not be able to do *anything* about it, ever. Perhaps these topics will never be safe to explore, and you may even feel physically threatened to explore them if you are working with a bullying and threatening antisocial prisoner. If so, do what is safe and move on to other topics. You need to decide if you are personally going to try to prevent him from reoffending. Of course, we are implying that the answer in the current case is "No." Unless you facilitate one of the structured and packaged programs to prevent reoffending, it is not your personal project to address reoffending at every turn.

You can also ask patients to tell you about other people, although in general you can't expect them to reveal confidences. Or ask them to tell you what they think "in general." For example, "Do you think most people succeed in the community? Do you think they all fail, or do some of them succeed?"

Keep in mind that explanations may require repetition to be effective.

We sometimes draw an analogy between making explanations and opening doors. The physical plant of a prison provides some new metaphors by which to discuss the way to make interpretations. Imagine that your patient's mind is itself like a prison with many cells and behind each are several related beliefs, issues, concepts, or memories. The prison unit has a "day room" that represents the patient's current attention to the issue. Since cells have doors or windows to see what is inside, when you offer an explanation, you may be looking into a cell to get a glimpse of what is behind the door or opening the door. Guidelines for the delivery of interpretations are summarized in Table 2–7 using the metaphor of cell doors on a prison unit.

TABLE 2–7.   **Giving an explanation is like opening a cell door on a unit**

Rule	Rationale
Don't open a hot door.	If you already know that a topic is a hot one and the patient will be very confrontational or resisting, consider waiting until the issue cools off so you can "strike while the iron is cold."
Take a look inside first.	Try to get a general idea of what your explanation is going to sound like before you say it!
See who is out on the unit already.	Before you start a new topic, make sure you have taken care of old or pending business.
Open a cell door slowly.	The patient may have multiple reactions to your explanation, so consider slowing down his responses. Observe what happens and change your plans based on what you see behind the door.
Open it cautiously and be prepared to close it.	Change your tactics or direction if it turns out your explanation is premature or too threatening. Put your explanation back in that cell and save it for a subsequent session!
Let the patient know you are going to open it.	Consider warning the patient. This allows her to anticipate things.
Allow the patient to open and close it himself or herself.	Let the patient "come out of his cell" and "go back into his cell" under his own control, not yours. Giving the patient control over the discussion of sensitive material allows him or her to maintain defenses.
Sometimes you must close the cell door when the patient wants to open it.	Be prepared to limit the discussion if the patient decompensates or regresses or it makes her violent.
Make the room comfortable.	Present explanations in a supportive environment or soften them when you present them.
Open the door repeatedly.	Repeat interpretations and present in small doses to overcome resistance.
Try to open only one door at a time.	Don't try to get by with too many explanations in a single session.
Talk about what you will let out tomorrow.	Prepare the patient—if that makes it easier for him.

Genetic and Historical Explanations

We mentioned above that genetic interpretations relate current conflicts to early life and family influences and not just heredity. While we do not talk about repression and the unconscious in prison conversations, we do frequently talk about the origins of our patient's criminal behavior in family treatment and dysfunction, which are both historical causes of criminal behavior and correctible causes of future criminal behavior under the RNR model. However, while historical explanations may lessen the patient's guilt or blame for his condition, their use needs to be judicious, since this is typically how patients with character disorders (such as antisocial personality disorder) defensively invoke such explanations to protect themselves from responsibility (Arlow 1981).

"Upgrading" a Patient's Defenses

We have discussed how prisoners, and especially criminals, use a variety of dysfunctional psychological defenses to justify their self-images and criminal behaviors. In supportive psychotherapy we hope to teach prisoners that their defenses have outlived their usefulness and are generating negative consequences such as imprisonment and loss of intimate human relationships. "Upgrading" defenses refers to the offering of explanations that strengthen a mature defense or weaken an immature defense. Since prisoners typically use rationalization for their past acts, we may agree in part with their rationalization of past acts as a necessary action given their beliefs at the time but go on to say, "Behaving like that seemed to be the right thing at the time, but you know better now." Some of the researchers who work with the recidivism prevention programs do also think that many prisoners need to develop a sense of *disgust* at their past behaviors in order to change.

Stories and Dreams

Myths, biblical stories, fables, the classics of literature, historical precedents, examples from popular entertainment, Broadway musicals, and comic strips can be used to illustrate a patient's predicament. Fairy tales, for example, deal with universal human problems and situations, primitive feelings, and existential dilemmas; they often foster strong identification with the main characters (Bettelheim 1976).

Listening is a fundamental skill for therapists and so is storytelling. Stories by others in similar circumstances, such as prison and jail, can show your patient the ways in which others have coped, learned from experience, and improved their understanding of problems and perhaps, even benefited from insights. Several such books, such as *Chicken Soup for the Prisoner's Soul* (Canfield et al. 2012) and *Serving Productive Time* (Lagana and Lagana 2009), collected stories about experiences in prison that inspired and improved the attitudes and even the physical circumstances of the individuals who contributed to each book. Stories serve several purposes for helping your patient process and understand the current circumstances, feelings, and events in his life. Whether autobiographical or fictional, reading, writing, or telling a story provides the author with an outlet, provides the listener with some insight, and gives each validation that his story is important. In therapy we usually ask the patient to tell us something about his past and current problems. Having someone to listen empathetically is a first step in developing a good therapeutic alliance; telling the story is a way of organizing thoughts. Reading or listening to someone else's story is a way of connecting to another person and perhaps gaining some inspiration for one's own thinking and problem solving. An example of a simple story that can illuminate and provide inspiration for exploring relationship problems is found in *Serving Productive Time*. An incarcerated man called his father simply to say he needed him. This reestablished their relationship and enabled them to rebuild their trust (Lagana and Lagana 2009, p. 37). Literary devices such as aphorisms, similes, and metaphors can be effective when working with prisoners. Metaphors such as describing the patient's journey as a trip into a dark unknown wilderness or an aphorism that "addiction is spirituality that went to the wrong address" can be used in treating substance abusers (James and Hazler 1998, p. 128). Or the therapist can wryly observe that the patient is still being controlled by his or her addiction as if wearing a dog collar (Romig and Gruenke 1991). Metaphors, myths, and stories do have a special place in therapy with men, and we will say more about masculinity issues in Chapter 12, but we regret that there is only so much space. So, if you are doing therapy in prison with men, learn about therapy with men and keep a repertory (e.g., of sports quotes):

> I've missed more than 9,000 shots in my career. I've lost almost 300 games. 26 times, I've been trusted to take the game winning shot and missed. I've failed over and over and over again in my life. And that is why I succeed. (Michael Jordan, quoted in Scott 2019)

Or a patient might complain how slow his progress is in school, and you might compare that to the race of the tortoise and the hare. "Slow and steady wins the race," you point out. "Other people get careless and don't apply themselves like you do, and they start fast but drop out because they don't have your determination."

Here is another Aesop's fable we find useful:

The Scorpion and the Frog

A scorpion can't swim across the river, so he asks a frog to carry him. "Are you crazy?" the frog exclaims. "If I carry you across the river, you'll sting me!"

"Oh no," says the scorpion. "If I sting you, we'll both drown, so I wouldn't do that!" So the frog carries the scorpion into the river, and guess what? Halfway across the river, the scorpion stings him! As the frog is dying, and they both sink into the river, the frog gasps, "Why did you do that?" And the scorpion answers, "It's my nature!"

We tell this story when a patient reports being disappointed or double-crossed by someone else with whom he committed crimes. "That's what criminals are. Haven't you ever done that to someone else who trusted you?" Or more briefly, "There's no honor among thieves!" These are interventions to address a person's choice of criminal associates and the consequences of doing so.

Patients will report dreams, but it is usually best to divert attention elsewhere. Showing interest in a dream and spending time on its explanation will, by simple reinforcement, result in more dream reports. It is usually best to point out that dreams are difficult to interpret and of uncertain relevance to the patient's life.

There is one type of dream, however—the anxiety dream or nightmare—that lends itself to treatment with behavioral methods rather than dream interpretation. Freud himself found anxiety and trauma-inspired dreams problematic because they did not appear to fit his theory of representing wishes. Some of the behaviorists who treat nightmares explain them as *failed* attempts through repetition, or kind of a sound loop, of an initially positive but now distressing attempt to master a problem. We have found that repetitive nightmares can be treated individually or as a symptom of PTSD with behavioral methods (Krakow 2020). This is accomplished with a structured program of 12 sessions that can be either professionally led or self-guided. When we encounter repetitive dreams or nightmares, we do guide our patients to rewrite their dream scripts before they go to bed. This is done only if they are comfortable with the material in the dreams. For example, a person whose dreams involve rape may not want to think about the experience even briefly, whereas a person who is being chased may feel comfortable rescripting the dream by chasing away the pursuer. This usually works best with patients whose dreams are repetitive and have the same "plot." The patients are also fully informed about the theory behind rescripting ("Your mind has been trying to solve this problem but has not worked out a solution").

Induced Dichotomy

Induced dichotomy of personality (Ermutlu 1977) is the attribution of the patient's conflicts to "sick" and "healthy" parts. We used this for many years in community mental health patients but then found it helpful in dealing with prisoners who do have conflicts of values. We discuss the "criminal" and "lawful" parts of their personalities (as metaphorical) and ask them how they would propose strengthening the lawful part. Dichotomized interpretations can be used in the way that Ermutlu (1977) proposes, but can also be introduced without value judgments—for example, "It seems that a part of you would like to get your G.E.D. now, but another part just wants to get some work experience first." Of course, this talk about dichotomies parallels the emphasis in programs designed to increase prosocial versus criminal behaviors.

Directing: Advising and Telling

We complete our discussion of techniques with *directive interventions* (see Table 2–1). One of these, a major one in corrections, is education. Throughout this book we've discussed the ethical issues that can be raised by attempting to change the lives of criminal offenders. The therapist may be uneasy in giving some types of advice. For example, if the therapist believes that the patient made a genuine mistake in committing a crime and no further learning is necessary, what more information needs to be taught? "Don't get caught next time?" We hope not. Most directive interventions should be accepted by patients as part of their agreed-upon treatment plans, but some may not, and the differences can be noted in your progress note or in the treatment plan by their signatures.

Determining Your Patient's Interests

At times you may believe that there is a conflict between the patient's interests and society's interests. Is it in society's interest for the patient to provide restitution or meet with the victim according to a program of restorative justice? Is it in the patient's interest to find some subtle way to avoid the payments (e.g., by changing his identity)? Are there things like this that a therapist could by some stretch of the imagination come to support? We also know that therapists are not necessarily in agreement with all the goals of their institution. For example, many therapists believe that prisoners who work should be paid a higher wage or a statutory minimum wage.

When you tell a distraught patient in no uncertain terms to tell their dormitory officer to call you or the clinic before acting on a suicide plan, you are acting in the patient's interests. Many systems employ a written "crisis response safety plan" that the patient keeps with himself. In succeeding chapters, we will describe how to make these plans in circumstances involving suicidal behavior, trauma, and community reentry. Similarly, directive interventions when the patient is not in crisis should be guided by your rules of meeting the treatment objectives. Many prisoners have impaired impulse control and judgment and will not make safe or legal or moral decisions when left to their own devices. As you get to know your patient, you will know to offer *what* the patient needs *when* the patient cannot provide it himself.

Offering Advice

Advice can gently guide a patient toward a goal or be blatantly obvious and directive. Patients who cannot make rational decisions may need more directive advice. If a patient does not really need advice, you can encourage him to make a decision by himself without your opinion. But let's say that your patient reports a conflict with her supervisor in the kitchen and wants to quit. You may want to explore the situation: the details of the incident, the patient's vulnerability to criticism, her personal feelings about the supervisor, and so forth. But your time is limited. You can, of course, delay the issue or schedule an extra session to consider the issue. But if it is clear that quitting the job would be a major setback in the patient's treatment progress, you should be prepared to give your advice, qualified as usual based on your knowledge of your patient.

Giving advice is problematic in some circumstances, but especially in correctional environments, even though you might think the choices in those environments are limited. Examples of advice we think are correct in all environments include recommending to a patient with alcohol use disorder and/or a substance use disorder that he cut down and, in most instances, stop using alcohol or illegal substances. You should point out that returning to drug-using environments is much more conducive to relapse than returning to drug-free settings. You may point out to the person with an alcohol use disorder that living in an alcohol-free home is much better than living in one where alcohol is readily available. You can recommend education courses based on the patient's capacity, keeping in mind the patient's traits of superoptimism and cognitive indolence.

While much has been said about cultural competence in psychotherapy, less has been said about religious competence. In a helpful source, two clinicians point out the low levels of religiosity (compared with the general American population) of psychiatrists and hence their reluctance in dealing with religious issues. They describe components of religious competence as including taking a spiritual history and respecting and supporting a patient's spiritual beliefs (Whitley and Jarvis 2015). We do think that advising a detainee to utilize faith-based coping using her established faith is reasonable. The previous authors do go further and with the patient's permission suggest challenging beliefs or praying with a patient. However, their advice is not presented in a correctional context. In correctional environments, we think it is best to refer complex or controversial issues to the chaplain.

Be familiar with the legal and documentation requirements of your setting. Work with your department team and be aware of what types of complaints are made (e.g., to licensing boards) and what types of litigation take place. Although many complaints are directed toward prescribing providers, therapists can be sued or referred to licensing psychology boards because of complaints even about the giving of "wrong advice." The majority of complaints are eventually dismissed as frivolous, but it can be stressful and time-consuming while they are being reviewed or adjudicated. Therefore, given your understanding or your patient's character and history, any advice-giving may have to be carefully documented with qualifications such as "Based on your history, you would be a good candidate for the anger management group, but only if you're sure you can handle the stress. Don't sign up for it unless you've really thought about it and you're always going to be responsible for your own behavior." This would forestall an antisocial prisoner from complaining that he was given advice to join an anger management group "when I wasn't ready for it" and then assaulted another prisoner. In fact, it should be part of your disclaimers for antisocial patients that "you should only do what you think you are ready for," and your documentation should have a similar disclaimer explaining the limitation on your advice (e.g., that it is professional advice based on your available knowledge but that an outcome can never be guaranteed).

Never give advice that could be construed as being outside your field of expertise (e.g., advice that is legal or quasi-legal in nature). Phrase advice in terms of probabilities and document it as such (e.g., "You would probably be better off getting a day job because you have had problems staying awake when you are on the night shift, don't you think?"). If your relationship with the patient is too hostile for advice giving yet you still want to do some sort of therapy with them, then stop giving advice and qualify all your "advisory" statements as such: "I can't give advice on this, so you'll have to make your own choice. All I can tell you is what I know about XYZ."

Supportive therapists in corrections often contend with ethical issues when they try to help patients strengthen coping skills and defenses. How does one, or should one, shore up a patient who experiences remorse over her crime? On the other hand, how does one address the patient who has no remorse? It should help to explore the patient's value system and see if this is reasonable and conventional or too extreme to work with. You should find areas where you can work productively using conventional values, or areas that are value-free. The patient may have interests to pursue, relationships to discuss, and plans to make. If she is not amenable to therapeutic assistance, then she will not be a candidate for therapy. This problem often solves itself, as many patients who find therapy unhelpful reject the service anyway.

Strong Advice and Explicit Direction

It is possible to phrase directions in various forms depending on the patient's best interests (see Table 2–8). Knowing which form to use is a skill and an art, yet it is based on our earlier proviso: use the strongest form that the patient needs. Some patients may benefit from strong or barely cloaked advice such as "I really think you should go to the GED class" or "I don't want you missing your therapy appointments." Often explicit direction can be limited to situations when the patient's behavior threatens the integrity of the therapeutic process (as in the section on limit setting). However, there is a wider role for strong advice or explicit direction with many patients who have impaired judgment or skills.

Making Suggestions

In Jonathan Kellerman's detective novel *Museum of Desire*, psychologist Alex Delaware is chided about his interview skills, and it is suggested that it is better to hint at answers than to tell people outright (Kellerman 2020, p.185). We agree: Hinting or suggesting can be more effective than saying something outright. In the ordinary sense of *suggestion*, you can suggest new strategies, behaviors, or activities to the patient to meet his needs: "Have you thought about taking a college course while you are here?" "Do you think you should talk to your brother whom you have been avoiding since you got here?" Such suggestions are nothing more than qualified advice. But other suggestions also work unconsciously, as evidenced by their historical use in hypnosis.

TABLE 2–8.	The many faces of direction in dealing with a patient considering leaving his or her job
Direct advice	"Don't quit your job."
"Objective"	"You have got to keep working."
Invoking of facts or motivators	"Think about what it would mean to lose your commissary money. Think of what your mother is going to say. What are you going to do all day in your cell?"
Generalization	"We find that it often helps for prisoners to stay on the job to pass the time."
Suggestion/temporization	"I know you feel like quitting right now, but I would suggest that you stick with it and you will feel better in a few days."
Probabilistic but specific to the patient	"You'll probably feel better if you go back and work out the problem."
Use of therapist's influence	"Keep working. Trust me, you'll thank me later for this."
Hands off	"I can't make your decisions for you."
Exploration and clarification	"It seems that you want me to make the decision for you."
Rhetorical question	"Don't you think it's better to hang on to the job and your income? You really need it now."
Open question	"Do you think you should be quitting work? What will you do?"
Indecisive	"I wonder if it would help to quit now."
Oppositional	"You can keep working if you want, but I don't think you can handle it!"
Permissive	"It's okay to quit if you feel that's best. I know you've been under terrible stress lately." (Used for those patients who would seem to need permission to stop and should.)
Delay	"Keep working a little longer, and we'll talk about your decision next week."

Giving Permission

Giving permission is a useful variation of advice. For example, you might want to give the previously mentioned patient permission to quit his job if you believe that a psychotic illness is interfering with his performance. "You can get your job back later, and in fact I will recommend it, but first we need to take care of your hallucinations." You may have to give patients permission to grieve the loss of a family member, the loss of custody of a child, or similar losses.

Setting Limits

Limit setting, or the outright, nonnegotiable prohibition of certain types of behavior, is often necessary in corrections. It is often essential to the safety of the institution, the safety of other prisoners and staff, and, not least, your own safety. Violence, sexual assault, and disruption of the treatment site may occur if you fail to heed the warning signs of escalating behavior or respond to such behavior inappropriately. And while setting limits asserts your own rights (and those of the institution) and the patient's need to respect them, it can also be used to convey your concern for your patient's well-being, such as not getting into a violent confrontation.

Some therapists fail to set limits because of a desire to be liked or loved. That can be dangerous in a correctional setting. In fact, limit setting often improves the therapeutic relationship, making it safer and more predictable. Limit setting shows prisoners that you are not frightened but instead capable of containing their behavior. For example, you need to write up and report a person who makes a sexually inappropriate remark or touches you "accidentally." These are well-known manipulations that are designed to test the tolerance of staff for their rule violations and to progressively compromise staff. If you are *really* not sure, give a warning. But at the minimum we would suggest you say, "We have a zero-tolerance policy for touching or for suggestive remarks. As far as I am concerned, there are no such things as an accidental touch or an innocent suggestive remark. Is that clear?"

While we emphasize that limit setting should not be delayed by a fear of "loss of love," it is true that your ability to set limits should actually be enhanced by a preexisting positive (professional) relationship with your patient. Of course, if you think your patient is simply ill-informed about the rules, you should give him an opportunity to exercise self-control before issuing some type of punishment such as rescheduling them if they are late for an appointment.

Limits Within the Therapy and Clinic Must Be Firmly Set

Limits must be absolute for physical abuse and threats of it. If the patient begins to lose control, the session may be terminated; you probably got specific training for that in your institution. We do not believe that therapists in corrections should tolerate a great deal of verbal abuse; they can be reasonably tolerant of ventilation or a certain level of criticism but not direct abuse. If you find yourself tolerating a lot of abuse, you should ask yourself what purpose it serves. Also think about whether you have learned to tolerate excessive abuse from a particular patient. That is, do you have special (higher) limits just for them. If so, why? Do you like him more than you should or are you more afraid of him than you should be? Also distinguish ventilation that is a *substitute* for action from ventilation that is a *prelude* to violence.

Limits Outside the Therapy Session (Behavior in the Prison)

In the world outside the institution, a patient may violate behavioral codes and the law and talk honestly about the violations. However, within an institution, you cannot generally condone misbehavior and rule breaking. Here are some do's and don'ts of limit setting (based on Green et al. 1988):

- DO distinguish between absolute (i.e., nonnegotiable) and relative (i.e., negotiable) limits. For example, maybe you will let patients get loud once in a while.
- DO convey the limits to patients both verbally and nonverbally. Use the appropriate expressions and emotions when you convey limits, but never in a way that suggests you have lost control or are fearful or afraid, just firm and stern.
- DON'T give mixed signals (e.g., verbally prohibit, nonverbally encourage).
- DO examine the countertransference implications of limit setting (e.g., manipulative, punitive) or failure to set limits (e.g., reaction formation, being overly nice, desire to appear permissive, need to be loved).

- DON'T assume that it is sufficient to tell the patient once. But most "normal" (not seriously impaired) prisoners should learn the absolute rules (e.g., "no touching me even by accident") the first and only time you have to tell them.
- DO (within reasonable limits) examine the patient's responses to limit setting and be willing to change your limits. For example, if the patient tends to get out late from her culinary job and that makes her late for your session, you might have a reason to be more flexible.
- DON'T take on the job of limit setting when it belongs to someone else, such as another therapist, the prescribing provider, or custody staff. For example, the corrections officer is certainly capable of setting the limits of behavior on the unit, so your patient should not be asking you what the rules are.

Limit Setting Implies That There Will Be Limit Testing

For many reasons, such as personality disorder or severe mental illness, prisoners will test the limits that are set for them. Especially for personality-disordered patients who do not have a severe mental illness, be prepared to defend the limits that need defending and do not cave in the first time you are tested. We realize that this is difficult to do in circumstances such as chronic self-cutting or suicidal thoughts or behavior. Behavioral management programs and team management meetings may be required.

Helping Patients to Manage Their Emotions

Prisons, like bars late at night, are full of people who cannot control their emotions. In a bar, patrons may suffer the disinhibiting effect of alcohol, but many prisoners suffer disinhibition from mental illness or personality disorder. In your individual sessions, you will still have opportunity to discuss how they control their emotions, such as to avoid fights and disciplinary sanctions. As happens in bars, some patrons get drunk in order to become disinhibited. Prisoners learn to provoke one another to find excuses for assaultive behaviors and they need to be called out when you see that happening.

Strategies for dealing with impulsive behavior are:

- Elaborate the unwanted and self-destructive consequences of impulsive behavior.
- Pit self-destructive consequences against equally powerful motivators.
- Note that condemnation only reduces a patient's self-esteem further.
- Address and empathize with the affect that generates the impulses.
- Find more appropriate ways to satisfy the need that generates the impulse.

Work Skills

There is not a lot to do on many days in prison, but working is one of those things. Patients in corrections have frequently had problems with work in the past and will experience similar problems in prison. To make matters worse, the other workers on the detail are also prisoners with their own problems, and the wages are usually below standard. Nevertheless, work is something that most people have done or aspire to, and something they think about doing and are willing to talk about. It is true that prison jobs are not fully representative of the outside world. Maybe your patient cannot be a janitor but would be a good computer repair technician (i.e., a job that actually requires a higher level of education and skill and pays better). So you cannot view prison work as the crucible in which all work skills are judged, but failure there should be examined. If it is due to abject mental illness, then the patient should be involved in a discussion of receiving treatment. If failure at work is due to inability to handle authority (a frequent issue), then solutions need to be addressed, including working with both the patient and relevant staff to make mutual adjustments in behavior. Looking ahead, when the patient is released, he may need to get into community college, vocational training, or a supported employment program.

To most people, work has positive connotations, and most prisoners want to succeed in work, but some may want to fail in order to prove they are worthless or hopeless, or simply because they don't want to work (e.g., for the wages offered) or because of the criminal trait of "cognitive indolence." You can offer validation to prisoners who think the current assignment is "beneath them" by explaining the importance in their overall program and the value of positive evaluations even if it is just a maintenance job. Therapists are often asked to approve lay-ins (work excuses) in institutions where work is an ongoing requirement. When required to work, some prisoners hope to create enough disruptions and discord to permanently exempt them. When in doubt, seek the assistance of a vocational counselor. The counselor may be better able to determine whether your patient has the ability to sustain attention to work part time or full time or follow complex instructions, or would be better off working alone, such as stocking shelves late at night. Many of our patients have very good telephone skills and can work in call centers.

A patient's ambivalence about work does not usually reflect a fundamental conflict of values; instead, it represents the operation of understandable fears and anxieties about performance. Because of grandiosity and entitlement, some prisoners will aspire to jobs for which they are clearly unsuited by training or temperament. Some will actually show an interest in occupations for which they have no intrinsic interest just because it reflects their grandiosity. Prepare yourself to deal with all the variations of these problems.

Modeling and Identification With the Therapist

The therapist's role as a model for the patient has always been emphasized in psychotherapy. In correctional settings, this is called *prosocial modeling* and is a source of social learning as well as a component of programs designed to correct criminal thinking.

Incorporating Homework

Some proponents of supportive psychotherapy avoid assigning homework because such assignments can overwhelm patients with limited skills (Markowitz 2014). However, homework has proved its purposes in correctional populations with poor education and motivation, and it is standard fare in CBT. Homework also ties their memories back to the therapy sessions and reinforces learning. You should inquire if your patient does his homework. If he routinely cannot do it, then change your strategy. Note that cognitive indolence, one of the eight criminal thinking styles, is a major problem in getting people to do homework. Resources for homework are numerous, including the well-known series by Jongsma (2016).

Providing defenses (such as rationalizations) *for social use* is also important, because peer group influence and the fear of losing peer group approval are responsible for (or at least partly responsible for) many criminal behaviors. Fears or projections of peer group opinions may also be exaggerations of realistic concerns about acceptance, or defensive covering of deeper fears such as loss of control. For example, one of our patients explained to us that he wanted to drop out of the gang but it was too dangerous for him to do so. He requested we discipline him so it would appear that he was in protective custody for the rest of his stay. We referred this to our security threat group director, and he worked out a plan.

Paradoxical interventions, in which the therapist advises the opposite of the intended behavior, are sometimes used with patients in the community but are generally to be avoided.

Giving Praise When Appropriate

Praise can put you in a parental role and can create dependency and control issues. However, it may also be necessary for patients with self-esteem problems. Praise can be misused by criminals who remember forever that you praised them on one particular issue and one particular day and take the praise as a message that "inoculates" them from future criticism. That is, you criticize them and they respond with, "Didn't you say yesterday that I was a really generous person?" Make your praise concrete and tied to specific behaviors (Sharp 2006, p.121).

Key Points

- Supportive psychotherapy uses communication and direction.

- Therapy starts with communication that uses several types of listening, which we describe as *personal*, *professional*, and *active*.

- Prisoners are used to confrontations, which may be used to expose inconsistencies in thinking.

- Supportive psychotherapy and motivational interviewing do have some techniques in common, such as generating empathy, but there are also some differences that we think make supportive psychotherapy better suited to work with prisoners.

- Using your knowledge of your patients' personal defense styles, you should strive to correct your patients' distortions of reality and psychological defenses.

- In general, giving advice in correctional institutions needs to be qualified, especially when you are working with antisocial or litigious patients.

- Everybody has a repertoire of psychological defenses and coping styles, but persons with criminal lifestyles, whom we call "criminals," can be characterized as using eight types of thinking styles: mollification, power orientation, entitlement, cutoff, sentimentality, superoptimism, cognitive indolence, and discontinuity.

- Some of the explanatory techniques that make therapy supportive include giving reassurances and enhancing self-esteem.

- There are numerous ways in which confrontations and explanations can be weakened, softened, delayed, or displaced so as to make them more effective.

- Risk-need-responsivity–inspired programs typically require hundreds of hours, and their goal (of reducing recidivism) is not necessarily met by individual psychotherapy.

- Some psychotherapy goals, such as enhancing self-esteem, do need modification when working with criminals, and most psychotherapy goals may meet humanitarian needs but may not necessarily reduce recidivism.

- All therapy requires limit setting both inside and outside therapy sessions, and this is especially important in corrections.

- Using your institution's assessment instruments can give you a more detailed picture of your patient's thinking styles and therapy needs.

- Since most prisoners work, and most worked before prison and will work after prison, it is usually helpful to explore and improve work skills in patients.

- Aphorisms, metaphors, and fables such as "The Tortoise and the Hare" can help you to impart ideas in therapy. Stories and quotes from famous sports personalities can also help.

- Other interventions that should be in your repertoire include modeling and identification with the therapist, homework, and reinforcement of desirable behaviors.

References

Andrews DA, Bonta J: The Psychology of Criminal Conduct, 5th Edition. New Providence, NJ, LexisNexis, 2010

Andrews DA, Bonta J, Wormith S: LS/CMI Level of Service Case Management Inventory. North Tonawanda, NY, MHS, 2020

Arlow JA: Theories of pathogenesis. Psychoanal Q 50(4):488–514, 1981 7302039

Beck AT, Emery G (with Greenberg R): Anxiety Disorders and Phobias: A Cognitive Perspective. New York, Basic Books, 1985

Bettelheim B: The Uses of Enchantment: The Meaning and Importance of Fairy Tales. New York, Knopf, 1976

Bonta J, Andrews DA: The Psychology of Criminal Conduct, 6th Edition. New York, Routledge, 2017

Canfield J, Hansen MV, Lagana T: Chicken Soup for the Prisoner's Soul: 101 Stories to Open the Heart and Rekindle the Spirit of Hope, Healing and Forgiveness. Cos Cob, CT, Backlist LLC, 2012

Di Giuseppe M, Perry JC, Lucchesi M, et al: Preliminary reliability and validity of the DMRS-SR-30, a novel self-report measure based on the Defense Mechanisms Rating Scales. Front Psychiatry 11:870, 2020

Di Riso D, Colli A, Chessa D, et al: A supportive approach in psychodynamic-oriented psychotherapy: an empirically supported single case study. Res Psychother 14(1):49–89, 2011

Ermutlu I: Induced dichotomy of personality as a technique in supportive psychotherapy. Psychiatr Forum 7:19–22, 1977

Gavel DW: More Than Mere Synonyms: Examining the Differences between Criminogenic Thinking and Criminogenic Attitudes. Dissertations 954. University of Southern Mississippi, 2017. Available at: https://aquila.usm.edu/dissertations/954. Accessed July 4, 2020.

Green SA, Goldberg RL, Goldstein DM, et al: Limit Setting in Clinical Practice. Washington, DC, American Psychiatric Press, 1988

Harari E: Supportive psychotherapy. Australas Psychiatry 22(5):440–442, 2014 25183321

Hazelden Foundation: Criminal and Addictive Thinking, 2nd Edition. Center City, MN, Hazelden Foundation, 2019

James MD, Hazler RJ: Using metaphors to soften resistance in chemically dependent clients. J Humanist Educ Dev 36:122–133, 1998

Jongsma A: Adult Psychotherapy Homework Planner, 5th Edition. New York, Wiley, 2016

Kellerman J: The Museum of Desire: An Alex Delaware Novel. New York, Ballantine Books, 2020

Kirschenbaum H, Henderson VL (eds): The Carl Rogers Reader. Boston, MA, Houghton Mifflin, 1989

Krakow B: Turning nightmares into dreams. 2020. Available at: https://barrykrakowmd.com/product/turning-nightmares-into-dreams. Accessed November 13, 2020.

Lagana T, Lagana L: Serving Productive Time: Stories, Poems, and Tips to Inspire Positive Change From Inmates, Prison Staff, and Volunteers. Deerfield Beach, FL, Health Communications, 2009

Lakoff G: Moral Politics: How Liberals and Conservatives Think, 3rd Edition. Chicago, IL, University of Chicago Press, 2016

Latessa E, Smith P, Lemke R, et al: Creation and Validation of the Ohio Risk Assessment System: Final Report. Cincinnati, OH, Center for Criminal Justice Research, School of Criminal Justice, University of Cincinnati, July 2009. Available at: www.ocjs.ohio.gov/ORAS_FinalReport.pdf. Accessed July 4, 2020.

Mandracchia JT, Morgan RD: Understanding criminals' thinking: further examination of the Measure of Offender Thinking Styles—Revised. Assessment 18(4):442–452, 2011 20660469

Mandracchia JT, Morgan RD: Predicting offenders' criminogenic cognitions with status variables. Crim Justice Behav 39(1):5–25, 2012

Markowitz JC: What is supportive psychotherapy? Focus 12(3):285–289, 2014

Miller WR, Rollnick S: Motivational Interviewing: Preparing People to Change Addictive Behavior. New York, Guilford, 1991

Miller WR, Rollnick S: Motivational Interviewing: Helping People Change, 3rd Edition. New York, Guilford, 2012

National Parole Resource Center: Setting Parole Conditions to Achieve Public Safety. Action Guide Series. 2022. Available at: https://nationalparoleresourcecenter.org/action-guide-series-parole. Accessed March 7, 2022.

Novalis PN: What supports supportive therapy? Jefferson J Psychiatry 7(2):17–29, 1989

Perry JC: Defense Mechanism Rating Scale (1990), in I Mechanismi de difesa. Edited by Lingiardi V, Madeddu F. Milano, Rafaello Cortina, 2002

Perry JC, Bond M: Change in defense mechanisms during long-term dynamic psychotherapy and five-year outcome. Am J Psychiatry 169(9):916–925, 2012 22885667

Pine F: Developmental Theory and Clinical Process. New Haven, CT, Yale University Press, 1985

Pine F: Supportive psychotherapy: a psychoanalytic perspective. Psychiatr Ann 16:526–529, 1986

Quine WVO: The Web of Belief. New York, McGraw-Hill, 1978

Rogers CR, Farson RE: Active Listening. Mansfield Centre, CT, Marino Publishing, 2015

Romig C, Gruenke C: The use of metaphor to overcome inmate resistance to mental health counseling. J Couns Dev 69:414–418, 1991

Scott N: The 40 best sports quotes of all time. USA Today, December 3, 2019. Available at: https://ftw.usatoday.com/2019/12/best-sports-quotes. Accessed January 15, 2021.

Sharp BD: Changing Criminal Thinking: A Treatment Program, 2nd Edition. Washington, DC, American Correctional Association, 2006

Sun K: Correctional Counseling: A Cognitive Growth Perspective, 2nd Edition. Bolingbrook, IL, Jones & Bartlett, 2012

Vaillant GE: Defense mechanisms, in The New Harvard Guide to Psychiatry. Edited by Nicholi AM Jr. Cambridge, MA, Harvard University Press, 1988, pp 200–207

Walters GD: The Psychological Inventory of Criminal Thinking Styles, I: reliability and preliminary validity. Crim Justice Behav 22(3):307–325, 1995a

Walters GD: The Psychological Inventory of Criminal Thinking Styles, II: identifying simulated response sets. Crim Justice Behav 22(4):437–445, 1995b

Walters GD: Changing Lives of Crime and Drugs: Intervening with Substance-Abusing Offenders. New York, Wiley, 1998

Walters GD: The Psychological Inventory of Criminal Thinking Styles, Version 4.0. Unpublished measure, 2001

Walters GD: How many factors are there on the PICTS? Crim Behav Ment Health 15(4):273–283, 2005 16575848

Walters GD: The Psychological Inventory of Criminal Thinking Styles (PICTS) Professional Manual. Allentown, PA, Center for Lifestyle Studies, 2010

Werman DS: The Practice of Supportive Psychotherapy. New York, Brunner/Mazel, 1984

White J: Beginning Operations: A Sector General Omnibus. New York, Tor Books, 2001

White J: Alien Emergencies: A Sector General Omnibus. New York, Tor Books, 2002

Whitley R, Jarvis GE: Religious understanding as cultural competence: issues for clinicians. Psychiatr Times 32(6):13–18, 2015

3

Entering the Institution

Abandon hope, all ye who enter here.

Dante Alighieri[1]

According to Dante, the nine sins that get a person into Hell are Limbo, Lust, Gluttony, Greed, Wrath, Heresy, Violence, Fraud, and Treachery. Some of these might even get a person into prison these days. And although many historical places have been likened to the gates of Hell, prisons could also make similar claims.

Let's Start the Show!

To start therapy, you could just get going. After a while, things would either stay the same, get better, or get worse. Some patients will not want to see you again, and you will have to work hard to keep them in therapy if you are convinced that they would benefit from it. Other patients will be happy to see you so they can abuse you, or flirt or sexualize the therapy, or maybe just get out of their work assignment. However, we recommend that you read the next chapter before you actually get going! There are many things you can do to establish a working relationship with your patients and to keep your relationship viable.

Entering or reentering jail or prison can have different meanings for different people. Table 3–1 mentions typical reactions to entering the institution (from the standpoint of someone who has physically entered the building). Because of recidivism, many are returning; some are relieved, and some see it as confirmation of their failures in life. Since returning can have different meanings, you should ask your patients about the personal meaning to them. Give them a blank piece of paper and ask them

---

[1]According to the medieval Italian poet Dante Alighieri (1265–1321), in his *Inferno*, that inscription (translated from Italian) is above the gates of Hell. The gates are also inscribed: "Through me you pass into the city of woe:/Through me you pass into eternal pain:/Through me among the people lost for aye" (Phrases.org 2020).

to list five negative meanings of entering and then five positive ones. Take the negative ones and argue against them. Take the positives and capitalize on them.

We should pause here and consider the role of trauma in initial interactions and continuing interactions with prisoners. We give you a multiple-choice question to consider in Table 3–2. We hope you get the idea that all interactions with offenders should be trauma-informed and that the effects of trauma also apply to you as a therapist—*all the time*. And whatever you think of latte-drinking, pluggable car–driving therapists, it may help you to drink a latte once in a while (if you can afford one on your public servant salary) to calm down and prevent personal burnout. It will also help you, if not to drive an electric car, to be ecologically sensitive to what we called the immersive or alien environment of the prison and the trauma it can wreak on your patients and as secondary trauma on you.

It can be hoped that trauma-informed care started with your patient's first interactions with criminal justice—that is, with the arrest and any incarcerations and trial prior to meeting you. In learning about trauma-informed care, there are available a set of TIPS (Treatment Improvement Protocols) from the Substance Abuse and Mental Health Services Administration (SAMHSA). Now, when we think of a "tip," we might be inclined to think of somebody at the 2020 Kentucky Derby whispering the words, "Tiz the Law" to us (the name of the favorite, who ends up coming in second), which would also be a really poor and flippant response to someone in a therapy session asking why she was put in jail. However, when SAMHSA gives you a TIP, it is usually about 343 pages. There are even summaries of TIPS and TIPS about other TIPS. Mythology holds that the world is supported by an elephant standing on a turtle, but the world of therapy is supported by the famous elephant in the room standing on a pile of SAMHSA TIPS. To answer the question of what supports the TIPS, it is not "turtles all the way down" but TIPS all the way down to the bedrock of government statistics. We will discuss SAMHSA TIPS about trauma in Chapter 6.

Trauma in the histories of prisoners is substantial. Trauma-informed care should begin on admission and continue even if the individual does not report a personal history of trauma. Incarceration is a disempowering experience and recreates and rekindles the trauma of the person's past. Miller and Najavits (2012) call it "institutional trauma" (the trauma of being institutionalized). But many prisoners will not talk about their traumatic history to anyone, much less their new psychotherapist. Statistically, more women than men report trauma, typically childhood sexual abuse or intimate partner violence. Many men, however, have had significant trauma in the form of witnessing violence, and physical assault, and have also suffered childhood sexual abuse. Many experts include the cumulative effects of smaller traumatic incidents, such as the effects on persons of the historical treatment of their race or social group as shown throughout their individual development and interactions with others outside the family, including but not limited to their interactions with police. And not just their own personal interactions. In the United States, in the spring of 2020, a young Black woman named Breonna Taylor was killed by police during a botched no-knock raid. As the details of the raid surfaced, and there were delays and outrages from the resulting inaction and lack of prosecution for the police in the raid, there was national outrage. A trauma specialist reported that Black women in therapy experienced vicarious or secondary trauma from hearing about the Breonna Taylor case and worried that these things could happen to them (Burnett-Ziegler 2020). For a newly admitted

TABLE 3–1.	Entering the institution

Immediate reactions

Oh f---!

Here I go again *or* Here I am again.[a]

I'm safe again. (I was unsafe outside.)

I'm not safe again. (I was safer outside.)

I'll be fed.

It's nice to go to a place "where everybody knows your name."[b]

I'll be retraumatized. (See text.)

I'll be off drugs and alcohol. (This can be positive or negative.)

I'm withdrawing and craving drugs and alcohol.

I miss my family/friends.

I have lost/will lose my job/income/spouse.

What is my spouse/dependent mother/other family going to do?

Who will take care of my children?

People are disappointed in me/I am disappointed in myself.

At least I can get back on my medicine now.

I don't want to be forced to take medicine.

I can get treatment for my mental illness now.

I can get back into therapy.

I can get medical (nonpsychological) care at last.

I can give birth to my baby in a safe place, but will I be able to keep her?

I won't be able to get pain relief anymore in a prison clinic.

I won't be able to see the specialists I usually see.

Blaming

It is all my fault.

It was partly my fault, but I shouldn't be in prison for this.

I am totally innocent, and I don't even know why I was picked up for this crime.

It's my parents' fault for raising me the way they did, abusing me the way they did, etc.

It is all someone else's fault.

My co-offender tricked/used/manipulated me.

My co-offender didn't really love/care for me anyway.

The public defender was incompetent.

The judge was evil/prejudiced/sexist/ignorant.

The system/judge/jury was rigged against me (personally or others like me in race, national origin, LGBTQ status, or others).

Society as a whole is to blame for systemic racism and for putting a third of my community into the criminal justice system.

I have remorse for the person I hurt.

I want to make amends to the victim, but I don't know how I would even speak to him.

[a]A 1982 song by the British band Whitesnake that was recycled a few years ago in a GEICO motorcycle commercial, but the phrases "Here I go again" or "Here I am again" are a common theme in song titles, first lines, and even for entire albums. The humorist Shel Silverstein wrote, "Here I Am Again," which was sung by Loretta Lynn in 1972. Scores of others have used these phrases. Sweet, bitter, or bittersweet as the thought or feeling may be, it expresses a theme in people's lives as they deal with resurgences of "the Good, the Bad, and the Ugly" (which was a 1962 film starring Clint Eastwood).
[b]Aka "Theme from Cheers." For many, there are comforts in being institutionalized, including the fact that everybody does know you (but no alcohol!).

TABLE 3–2.   **Trauma: a multiple-choice question**

More than one answer may apply (for discussion, see text)

Trauma-Informed Care

   a.   Is something invented by latte-drinking, pluggable car–driving therapists.
   b.   Is not particularly relevant to my practice because I do not directly experience trauma in doing psychotherapy, even if I might hear about it.
   c.   Is something I have heard about but could always afford to learn more about if I can make the time.
   d.   Is probably going to apply to people, especially women, who have had previous trauma in their lives.
   e.   Should probably start or be put in the treatment plan when a patient relates a history of previous trauma.
   f.   Should start the moment I meet a patient, regardless of whether he or she relates a history of trauma.
   g.   Should start the moment I open any chart before I meet a patient (if I actually get to see their chart before I meet them).
   h.   Should start the minute I get up every morning because it applies to both myself and all my patients.
   i.   Needs to be with me 24 hours a day because it applies to both me and my patients 24 hours a day.

Black woman, now in therapy, it might be expected that she would relate her experience to injustices in general that Black women have experienced as well as to any recent ones. Important things that have been learned from studying trauma are that:

- Trauma plays a role in criminal behavior via violence and substance abuse.
- It impairs institutional adjustment—for example, via numbing and dissociative features of traumatic reactions—and creates additional risks for institutional discipline and violence via anger, hostility, and hyper-response to threats.
- It impairs the ability of a patient to benefit from the various therapies. For example, "Women who have limited coping skills do not fully engage in or benefit from the cognitive-behavioral therapy interventions often implemented in prison" (Whitten 2014, p. 2, based on Miller and Najavits 2012).
- A single therapeutic alliance (e.g., with you) can make a profound difference to a traumatized person (e.g., a man with a history of abandonment). In the famous quote of Chesterton: "[T]here are no words to express the abyss between isolation and having one ally. It may be conceded to the mathematician that four is twice two. But two is not twice one; two is two thousand times one" (Albany Chesterton Society 2020).

As individuals enter institutions, they are often referred to individual psychological therapy. This may be done routinely (e.g., for a person with known mental illness) or because of a crisis. Be sure you know the reason for the referral—that is, if there is a specific issue you were asked to discuss (e.g., a traumatic event they want to talk about). Also, as you begin therapy, you should be aware of the person's classification level, housing assignment, and other programs to which she has been referred, or be prepared to make other referrals yourself.

In some cases, you will have a new patient and have to start, as they say, *de novo*. In other cases, you will find a presentence investigation or intake done by someone else. We do think it helps to read those things. Sure, they might bias the initial impression you get from the patient. But as we said, your time is limited. Maybe you need to learn that your patient has a rap sheet 20 pages long, no part of which he relates to you in the session, because he is figuring out what you know and how much effort you are willing to make to know him.

Or you may inherit a caseload from a departing therapist.

Dialogue

> THERAPIST: Soooo, it looks like you have been seeing Dr. Smith for 2 years.
> PATIENT: Oh yes, Dr. Smith was a moron and an a-hole.
> THERAPIST. Oh, I see. Well, that's two different things, isn't it? He was both stupid and a jerk. How so?
> PATIENT: He never remembered what I told him about my father, and I told him five times.
> THERAPIST: Okay, so he was stupid, or lazy, or whatever. How was he a jerk?
> PATIENT: He made fun of my job. He said it was beneath me to clean stores at night.
> THERAPIST: Well, okay, he was stupid and a jerk. I will try not to be both. So, did you want to get started?

Now, Dr. Smith might be your best friend in the department. And you recognize that the patient may have a borderline or narcissistic personality and may be splitting the treatment team. But it probably does not help you to defend Dr. Smith at this minute. The patient is directing his negativity toward the previous therapist. You are lucky that you are not the target, and you can try to build a positive relationship. We will show you how to do that in the next chapter.

Of course, the opposite scenario could occur, and Dr. Smith might be described as "the most wonderful person in the world." Now you have a lot to live up to, and you are probably going to fail. But you have an opportunity to find out what your patient liked about Dr. Smith so you can make use of that knowledge to continue the therapy.

Some patients have had years of therapy from multiple providers. Some have had none; it is certainly fair game to talk about the who and the what, and the good and the bad (and the ugly), of their previous therapy sessions. We usually ask our intakes with such history what they learned from their previous therapist. Name one thing. Name five!

"What's Past Is Prologue"

The stereotypical psychotherapist seems obsessively interested in your past and especially your early childhood. She wants to talk about your toilet training and other embarrassing episodes in your early life. Then, there is another group of therapists who want to confine their talk to the "here and now." This can make sense when patients who have committed crimes misuse their (usually disadvantaged) past to muddle the therapy and blame their upbringing. Although some people have come to think that the above quote means that the past controls the future, the actual meaning of Shakespeare's "What's past is prologue" is that the past is gone and over with. (In *The Tempest*, Act 2, Scene 1, Antonio is trying convince Sebastian to kill his sleeping father so he can become king.) That is what you need to tell most of your patients who

TABLE 3–3.   **Therapist checklist (opening agenda) when meeting patients**

Clarify the mechanics.

Discuss time, flexibility, and availability.

Discuss confidentiality rules; what is normally and what is not normally confidential.

Discuss that the "circle of care" can and does include custody staff when certain issues such as suicidality and violence are at stake.

Discuss what you will do when the patient says, "Don't write this down, but…" (See the next item for a partial answer.)

Decide (as you go along or at the end of the session) what to document. Keep in mind that "anything can be subpoenaed, even your memories!"

Learn your patient's social and criminal history (at least some of it prior to meeting him or her).

(Probably later): Determine your patient's attitude toward their criminal history; do they admit to the crime at all, or any crimes at all?

(Probably later): Construct their life narrative. How is it that they now find themselves here at this age and this point in their life?

Determine (triage) immediate needs—crisis, suicidality, and so forth. What about their family, including children?

Build your own history (piece by piece).

Divide session time between history gathering and immediate needs.

Using active listening, form an emotional impression.

Learn your patient's psychological defenses and criminogenic beliefs (either from assessment instruments or your personal assessment). Which defenses predominate?

Learn your patient's strengths and weaknesses. Utilize strengths in a strengths-based treatment approach.

Learn your patient's longer-term goals in life (especially if you are interested in positive psychology).

Now do your homework: what do you need to learn about the patient's culture, history, and diagnoses before the next session?

are constrained by abusive, traumatic, or criminal pasts. "The past is over and done. It does not determine your whole future. You can make new decisions and act differently now." They need to understand how they got here, develop self-control, and learn that they cannot use their past to justify future criminal behavior.

In the previous chapter, we compared listening to hearing the overture to a symphony for first time. Like symphonic overtures, initial meetings in supportive therapy may set the mood and tone and introduce the themes for the succeeding exposition. Your opening agenda (see Table 3–3) must eventually cover the mechanics and business arrangements, but these should be worked into the session piece by piece.

Referrals to Group Therapy

Even as an individual therapist, you will be involved in a number of activities related to group therapy with your patients. You will be:

- Deciding when to refer to groups and which groups to refer to.
- Deciding whether to defer certain issues to the group rather than deal with them in individual therapy.

TABLE 3–4.	**Advantages of group psychotherapy**

The group is a kind of family (and psychodynamically serves many purposes as such).

The group reinforces positive values and prosocial culture.

The group can counter attitudes of prison culture.

The group utilizes peer pressure, which is a different mechanism than used in individual therapy.

Members hear from others who are farther along in learning.

Members get advice from multiple sources not limited to the group leader.

Members realize they are not alone in their problems or suffering.

Members can experience an emotional catharsis in expressing feelings to the group.

Members can (with professional guidance) ventilate complaints about the prison and formulate solutions, if possible, for management.

Some groups can even be a forum for guest speakers from management if there are certain issues that need to be discussed.

Members serve as role models to one another and can learn from one another by social learning.

Some members (especially those with antisocial personalities) learn best from their peers.

Some members (especially those with antisocial personalities) can be more effective than the group leader in pointing out the avoidance and game playing and self-delusion of the member when confronted by the group about something they did.

Source.   Pollock 1998, pp. 124–135, referencing several others.

- Discussing what happened in the group.
- Preventing the patient from defeating the group process.
- Probably running some of the groups yourself.

If nothing else, group therapy is efficient. It is a way to "dose" psychotherapy to 5– 10 or more people with one or two staff members. Groups can also be structured around specific topics and manualized learning programs. Self-directed support groups like AA also have a special effect. And *group processes can do some things that individual therapy simply cannot do.* Moreover, you should not as a matter of efficiency take on personally any of the tasks that really ought to be done in a group setting. For example, if your patient is going to learn job skills in her group, it should not fall to you to provide that training. (However, you should work with his fears or resistances to working.) As a reminder to you in making your referrals, Table 3–4 shows some of the advantages of the group process.

One supposed advantage to groups is that it takes less skill to be a group leader than to be an individual psychotherapist. It is true that it does not take a lot of skill to just sit there and keep people from yelling too loudly or hitting each other. But it takes considerable skill, which can be learned from other teachers and practice, to do group therapy in prison, so it is not something we have space to cover in this book. Leaders must be skilled in keeping obnoxious or manic members from dominating the group or keeping the group from endorsing the prison culture and opposition to custody. Some members will just play mind games and otherwise waste the time deliberately. Others will be quiet and avoidant and make no contribution whatsoever. In the group progress notes, the leader may attribute some progress to them ("listened attentively and followed the group process"), but this might be a matter of conjecture. It can be a subject of your discussion with them in individual psychotherapy. Finally, there are many things that people do not want to speak about in groups, such as their criminal acts. They may feel that they are subject to uncomfortable peer pressure to discuss such things. Even though groups are supposed to share a sphere of confidentiality, this may be violated; even if such violations do not occur, there will be some events that group members do not want to share "in public" (Pollock 1998).

Consent and Confidentiality

In the world of Sector General Hospital, confidentiality is taken for granted. This is because the healing art is unique in its need to explore personal and delicate states of mind, including forbidden and dangerous behaviors that the patient would otherwise not be inclined to reveal. The healer may not normally be allowed to share this information except in the best interests of the patient (White 2002, p. 442). As this suggests, issues of confidentiality are important and apply to all types of therapy. James White does not elaborate his fictional account of the importance of confidentiality in order to encourage psychotherapy, but you know that if you are encouraging discussion of sensitive material, such as a patient's recollection of his motives for committing a crime, you want the rules made clear about your duty to report or not to report what you hear. Follow the rules for your department or institution, and you must have a policy for patients who express their objections and do not wish to formally consent to psychotherapy. Such persons still need assessments for safety and security purposes, but you would not engage them any further in the therapy processes.

Consent involves a discussion of the limits of confidentiality. You can briefly explain who has access to the medical record, and a pithy line that we often hear is that "anything can be subpoenaed, even my memories." So it is not just what you write down, but what you have heard and observed about them that could come to the attention of a court. Obvious exceptions to confidentiality are PREA (Prison Rape Elimination Act) violations, future crimes, and abuse of children or other vulnerable persons for which you are a mandated reporter. You will receive extensive training about such things. Custody staff may not read medical charts, but they may be at times within the "circle of care," such as needing to know when patients are suicidal or whether they have threatened other prisoners or staff. Also, and something that many do not know, is that when a request for outside information about an individual is made, there is a correctional exception to the normal HIPAA requirements.

Initial Assessments

If the initial assessment was done by someone else, you should review it, and if there is not time beforehand you can scan it with the patient. For example, "Ms. Smith, the intake worker, said you are having a lot of anxiety. Is that your most important problem?" If your patient is in crisis, your first session may be a crisis evaluation and initial treatment, delaying the completion or elaboration of your initial assessment. We will talk about this below, but we also address it in Chapter 5 when we talk about treatments for crisis, self-harm, and suicidal behavior.

Because of PREA regulations, all correctional institutions assess for various types of previous abuse, especially sexual abuse and especially in previous correctional institutions. Assessment of young, old, small, shy, weak, or disabled persons is included. Prisons have predators. A classic study of assaultive street predators showed that they could identify vulnerable potential victims in 7 seconds from a videotape based on their rate and manner of walking, balance, posture, and other visible features (Dumond and Dumond 2010, citing Grayson and Stein 1981). Consider how much more time is available to a prison predator sizing up a new "Fish."

By the time newly admitted prisoners get to you, we hope they have gone through a safety-ensuring intake process, been offered protective custody if they have been abused or seem vulnerable now, and know what to do if they are threatened in the future. However, it is still important to ask: "Do you feel safe? Is anyone threatening or taking advantage of you?"

Documentation standards for assessments and psychotherapy notes vary widely and are addressed by your institution's, department's, and profession's policies. However, for use in supportive psychotherapy, we ask you to try to gather information about your patients' general level of education, intelligence, and coping skills in general. What is their family history? What is their social history in working and parenting? Do they obviously need working and parenting skills? And last but not least (as from the presentencing report), what do you know about their criminal history? Does it tell you if they have (or do you believe they have) an antisocial personality disorder or are a psychopath? Those two characteristics in our opinion do "set patients apart" in determining appropriate modes of treatment. If they do receive individual treatment, the goals of that treatment might be limited (e.g., to a suicidal crisis but not to prevention of recidivism in general). Two other groups that are well studied are sex offenders and (nonsexual) child abusers. If you treat anyone in these groups, you should acquire special expertise, and we will briefly mention one particular program for sex offenders. We have also mentioned trauma. Trauma affects the way that patients respond to authority figures and also the way they respond to confinement or restraint.

Keep in mind that patients can have multiple and conflicting diagnoses from different providers. Some systems require you to identify primary and secondary diagnoses as well as resolved diagnoses. The most common type of a resolved (nonsubstance) diagnosis would probably be an adjustment disorder.

The treatment plan is another standard feature of psychological therapies. There are well known resources, but we will discuss treatment plans in Chapter 4. In Chapter 1, we discussed several ethical issues of treatment goals such as reducing criminal behavior and recidivism. We pointed out that many prisoners will agree with such goals and so that should remove any controversy in your mind in proposing those goals. If not, however, you (i.e., the treatment team) have the opportunity to propose such goals in the plan and let them discuss them with you.

You will have some leeway in setting up your sessions, but we advise you to keep in mind the data about interventions and recidivism. The patients you find most "enjoyable" to treat may be the ones who will least benefit (in terms of the endpoint of recidivism, not necessarily personal growth) from therapy, at least according to the statistics. Frequency and length of sessions should vary depending on the principles of triage, but you may be bound by institutional rules that certain persons have to be seen weekly for 20–30 minutes and so forth, and there will be minimum requirements for patients at risk or in crisis.

The Relationship Between Supportive and Cognitive-Behavioral Therapy

As indicated in Table 3–1, prisoners may be overwhelmed with thoughts and feelings when entering prison, even if it is not for the first time. Putting their thoughts in a table (rather than, say, describing their nonverbal emotions) leads us to think that there must be some cognitive "answers" to their thoughts. This is, indeed, the spot to remind you of the premises and techniques of cognitive therapy, or what is now being called CBT or cognitive-behavioral therapy. The premise of CBT originally was that psychological dysfunctions come about from cognitive errors in the perception of and reasoning about our experiences. It took a while, but the cognitive paradigms for treatment eventually added a box for emotions, not just thoughts. Originally without the "behavioral" appellation, cognitive therapy amassed a wide range of therapeutic techniques, including behavioral types of learning. It also includes many interventions that are basically educational in nature and do not actually involve the correction of errors but the inculcation of knowledge.

Modern-day CBT encompasses a great number of techniques. It is a natural adjunct to supportive therapy as well as many other schools of psychotherapy, even if those other schools embrace a different premise as to the cause of psychological illnesses. For example, schizophrenia is a biological illness that is not *caused* by errors in cognition, but shows itself in such errors, many of which can be lessened by the techniques of cognitive therapy.

CBT is effective for many disorders. A specific program of cognitive therapy involves more structured elements than will be discussed here, but many cognitive and behavioral techniques are already being used successfully by therapists without conducting a complete or exclusively cognitive therapy program. In Beck's theory of depression, for example, the patient suffers a cognitive triad of negative self, world, and the future, created by underlying internalized, irrational core belief systems (also called *cognitive schemata*) that are expressed in numerous cognitive distortions of events in the patient's life. CBT therapists also ask patients to identify "automatic thoughts" that occur and can be argued against once recognized.

In Table 3–5 we have given instances of both immediate and long-standing beliefs typically held by prisoners and the names of the cognitive distortions that may apply to them. This is not to say that all such beliefs are entirely erroneous. Rather, there may be a truth in many of their beliefs. These prisoners have probably committed a crime. They may have been poor parents. The judge may not have been sympathetic. Their public defender may have been less than perfect. And so forth. You will probably recognize many of these distortions immediately, although you may not have had names for them. These errors are discussed in many texts, such as those by Freeman (1987), Beck and Emery (1985), Beck (2011), and Wright et al. (2017).

The patient's cognitive distortions are accompanied by typical response patterns. Patients with anxiety disorders, for example, are essentially "prisoners" to involuntary

TABLE 3–5. **Typical cognitive errors leading to psychological distress in jail or prison**

Cognitive error	Example
Selective abstraction	"My cellie is mad at me, so my day is ruined."
Catastrophizing	"Going to prison means the end of my life."
Arbitrary inferences (includes negative predictions and mind reading)	"The culinary supervisor didn't talk to me this morning; she must be mad at me."
Homogenization	"Everyone needs to like me, including my druggie friends."
Centering	"Everyone here always talks about me. They never leave me alone."
Absolutist (all-or-nothing) thinking	"A CO is either going to respect me or he isn't. It's that simple."
Overgeneralization	"Having committed a burglary makes me a failure as a human being."
Disqualifying the positive	"I've raised three children successfully, but I have abandoned my fourth child by going to jail."
Magnification or minimization	"My coworker is so much better than I am" (magnification applied to others). "I can never get any work done" (minimization applied to self).
Should/must/ought statements	"I should diet, exercise, work harder, be nice to people, etc."
Labeling and mislabeling	"I'm just a low-life criminal. I'm never going to do any better."
Personalization	"That officer just picks on me and leaves the other guys alone."

Note. CO=corrections officer.
Source. Categories are from Beck and Emery 1985 and Wright et al. 2017. The examples are ours.

negative associations to events. Their automatic thoughts and images, which dwell on the harmful meanings and consequences of events, can be recorded and scrutinized with the help of the therapist. Patients may also generalize potentially harmful stimuli to include a wide range of events. For example, a person hearing a car horn may think of an accident.

The cognitive therapist directs the patient's attention to the latter's automatic responses, both cognitive and behavioral, attempting to increase the patient's voluntary control. This requires repeated exercises in which the patient learns how his experiences are linked to cognitive distortions and develops alternative interpretations that are less threatening. Because the therapist explores these associations when the instigating situation has "cooled off" (or, as Pine [1986] would say, when the "iron is cold"), the connections can be seen more objectively.

At a deeper level, patients typically hold a constellation of cognitive schema or core beliefs that can cause them considerable suffering (Beck and Emery 1985; Branch and Willson 2012). For example, they may believe that "I have to please others." The cognitive therapist helps the patient to draw out these beliefs and develop counterarguments.

To be sure, some of us in mental health have core beliefs or "should statements" that can be dysfunctional at times, such as "I have to be the best at whatever I do" and "I've got to get everybody to like me," the latter being unrealistic when working in a prison.

Despite the widespread applicability of many techniques of cognitive therapy, some points should be recognized:

- Although used in schizophrenia, cognitive therapy is not always appropriate for such patients, whose illogicality is far reaching.
- Cognitive therapy requires a level of task orientation and motivation that many patients may not be able to meet.
- Cognitive therapists usually prescribe homework that may be beyond the capabilities of many prisoners.
- Cognitive therapy professes not to believe in any of the traditional psychological components, such as the psychological defenses that we feel are central to criminal thinking and behavior (e.g., blaming), as in Table 2–4.
- Cognitive therapy also likes to talk about the "here and now," but supportive therapy draws connections (both positive and negative) from past influences such as family life and traumatic experience and criminal associations leading to a criminal lifestyle.
- Cognitive therapists have appropriated many useful or educational therapeutic techniques and call them cognitive. They will teach guided imagery, progressive relaxation, and so forth. All these techniques work but are not unique to cognitive therapy.
- You can "prove" that a wide variety of therapies work because "everyone has won and all must have prizes" (i.e., the common factors theory of successful psychotherapy).
- Despite its apparent status of being a juggernaut (there's that wagon again) that is rolling over every other therapy in its path, cognitive therapy uses similar supportive techniques at its core to establish and run therapy.
- Cognitive therapy has negative studies of its own when compared with even supportive psychotherapy, interpersonal psychotherapy, and many others.
- Many cognitive and behavioral techniques can, however, be employed directly and can be buttressed by specific supportive interventions.

In patients with anxiety disorders, for example, these interventions include the fostering of positive but less restrictive basic assumptions that enhance the patient's self-esteem. For example, the patient needs to believe that "I can feel good about myself even though I committed a crime" rather than "I'm a failure because I committed a crime." Improved self-esteem, in turn, affects the generation of automatic thoughts in anxiety-provoking situations. The patient is less likely to succumb to a mild threat if she is able to generate self-reinforcing responses to the threatening stimuli. However, as we have mentioned, this is not necessarily a desirable process in antisocial and psychopathic prisoners.

To prioritize your tasks, you can now

- Complete your initial assessment.
- Use techniques to build a positive therapist-patient relationship.

- Look forward to what your treatment plan will be.
- Identify crisis situations and suicidal risks due to prison entry.
- Identify any immediate beliefs or feelings that might need reworking.

For example, a precipitous drop in self-esteem might need some immediate shoring up. You can use the techniques of cognitive therapy to identify and rebut cognitive distortions, especially the catastrophizing that occurs upon prison entry. (For example, "My life is over…it's hopeless…why go on…I might as well kill myself.") You can also use supportive techniques such as reassurance ("I know you will get through this") and diversions ("You don't have to think this every minute. Do some exercise, read some books, just watch the TV for a while.").

Extended Case Vignette Showing a Combination of Cognitive and Supportive Techniques

This is the therapist's first session with Roberto Lopez, a 35-year-old married Latino man. Mr. Lopez does not have a history of mental health treatment, but he was referred by the intake coordinator after making despondent statements and possibly suicidal ones. Mr. Lopez has been married for 13 years. Both he and his wife, Maria, are U.S. citizens. His parents came here from Mexico before he was born. Mr. Lopez's father had a roofing business, and Mr. Lopez worked with him until the father became disabled and now lives off disability. Maria is a naturalized U.S. citizen, having acquired her citizenship because of her marriage to Roberto. Maria's family is in Mexico. The Lopezes are safe and comfortable. They have three children: daughters ages 10 and 8 and a 6-year-old son. Mr. Lopez has an older brother, Raul, who was a powerful role model for him. "Never get involved with the gangs," Raul said, but he did not follow his own advice and is now in prison for a gang-related shooting.

Mr. Lopez avoided the gangs by working in his father's business After his father was disabled, he went to work for another roofer and has been busy and well paid, although he has lost some working time because of his involvement with drugs. He has had a few run-ins with the police over methamphetamine. What got him into prison was marijuana—100 kilos of it—wrapped in a tarp in the back of his truck, that was discovered at a police stop. There were arguments in the court about probable cause for them to search the truck. They said they smelled the marijuana, although it was clearly shown to be tightly wrapped. After 9 months in jail, Mr. Lopez was advised by his attorney to plea bargain for 3 years rather than take his chances in front of a jury given his rap sheet of misdemeanors.

Mr. Lopez says he loves his family and dotes on the kids. He believes that he loves and is faithful to his wife, but they have had some quarrels. In one of them, he pushed her and she fell down and she had to wear a back brace for 4 months. The police were called (although his wife said it was a neighbor who made the call), and he was ordered into domestic violence courses, which he almost finished but got angry at about having to attend and skipped the last one. Mr. Lopez's probation was violated and he was jailed briefly, but since it was the last session, the judge let him out and he finished the course. He says he did learn a lot from it. Mr. Lopez does hang out with his male friends, and that is probably why he picked up the misdemeanor drug convictions. He does not normally deal marijuana, but that last "gig" was a favor to a friend to transport a "little package" out of state where marijuana is still not legal.

Let's look at the therapy after the preliminaries and paperwork.

> THERAPIST: Please go over what you said to the intake coordinator. (Therapist kind of knows already but wants to hear first-hand.)
>
> MR. LOPEZ: I told him that my life is over…which it is…with this prison term.
>
> THERAPIST: Wait a sec, 3 years is not great, but it's not a lifetime. (Cognitive therapy to correct catastrophizing.)
>
> MR. LOPEZ: I already spent 9 months in figuring that this nightmare would end, and every day I was hoping it would. Now this…
>
> THERAPIST: I can see how disappointing that was after basically waiting every day to be released (empathic comment, supportive). But now it is important for me to know a little more about what you have been feeling and why you said that.

The therapist uses a version of the Columbia Suicide Severity Rating Scale to obtain additional details about Mr. Lopez's suicidal thinking for the past month (Columbia University 2020; National Suicide Prevention Lifeline 2020). The answers are all negative except for Mr. Lopez saying that he had thought about not waking up one morning. Protective factors are his love of his wife and children and family and his religion. And he can have a sense of humor and some distancing "observing ego." Risk factors appear to be anger, usually directed at others but sometimes at himself.

> THERAPIST: Thank you for answering those questions. That has really helped me to understand you! (Relationship building, reciprocity.) Now let's get back to your situation. Is your case on appeal? (Hope and positive outlook.)
>
> MR. LOPEZ: Of course it is! They stopped me for speeding, but they had no right to look in the back of the truck. We're appealing for an evidentiary hearing.
>
> THERAPIST: So maybe you'll get out sooner. (Not likely, but it can get Mr. Lopez to think about some alternatives the way he did while he waited in jail.)
>
> MR. LOPEZ: Well, you know how long appeals take.
>
> THERAPIST: Yes, you're right about that. (Simple empathic comment that supports patient's knowledge.) But what does the 3 years mean rather than the 9 months you already spent away from home?
>
> MR. LOPEZ: Well, my wife will never take me back, and I'll have to live with my parents forever.
>
> THERAPIST: I'm sorry, I'm confused. I thought you lived with your wife.
>
> MR. LOPEZ: Well, she kind of kicked me out after that DV [domestic violence] charge. I went to live with my parents a few months before I went to jail for the marijuana case.
>
> THERAPIST: I guess you "forgot" to tell me that. (Not really supportive, but the patient can't see the quote marks. In subsequent sessions, it can be pointed out that Mr. Lopez does want to appear to be a good person and loving husband but often glosses over the things he has done, such as the crimes and DV incidents. These are psychological defenses that support criminal thinking styles, but cognitive therapists would avoid the psychological causation and just question the erroneous belief "I have to make myself look good to other people.")
>
> MR. LOPEZ: Yes, well, I forgot to tell you that. But what good is all this talking anyway? You can't get me out of here by talking.
>
> THERAPIST: Of course not, but I am trying to deal with your feelings of being overwhelmed, and maybe we can come up with some ideas together. (Supportive and giving hope he can benefit from crisis therapy. Introduces a kind of "editorial we.") Don't you want to calm down and deal with the situation a little better?

MR. LOPEZ: Yes, okay, if it helps. So what do you think you can do for me?

THERAPIST: I see here you had finished your DV course, but what about a parenting course? You can tell your wife about it and get a certificate. That might show your commitment to your kids and get you back home.

MR. LOPEZ: That might help, yeah. But I think she'll never take me back.

THERAPIST: You know what they say: "Never say never." I know a guy who was kicked out five times, but he got back. (Gently opposing patient's cognitive error or selective conclusion that once being kicked out no one ever returns.)

MR. LOPEZ: Yes, that's how women are, aren't they? (Asking for a confirmation of something that the therapist will certainly not confirm.)

THERAPIST: Well, that's kind of a generalization. We can talk about that later. (Save this material for later.)

MR. LOPEZ: What about my wife, then? What can we do to impress her? (Has a sense of humor about this.)

THERAPIST: I don't know if we can do both, but maybe anger management, too.

MR. LOPEZ: I don't know. There was a lot of that about in the DV course.

THERAPIST: When we get time, I'd like you to tell me what you learned in that course. (Supportive and shows a commitment to future meetings; increases patient's belief that therapist is genuinely interested in his history.)

MR. LOPEZ: Yes, I'd like to tell you. But this thing about the 3 years gets to me…

THERAPIST: Okay, I hear you. It's 3 years you didn't intend to spend. (Echoing and tracking.)

MR. LOPEZ: Yes, 3 years just seems too long to handle.

THERAPIST: We'll deal with it one step at a time. (Repeating reassurances and hope to mirror patient's own repetition of complaint.)

MR. LOPEZ: Well, I just get so mad about it…I am so mad about it! (*laughs*)

THERAPIST: I do understand how mad you are about it. (Another empathic response.)

Discussion

This first session has to cover a lot of ground. Suicidal ideation needs to be cleared. Cognitive errors, catastrophizing thoughts, and automatic thoughts like "My life is over" are addressed. Supportive interventions are frequent, with echoing, tracking, reassurances, hope, and even a little humor that mirrors the patient's own sense of humor and not something that grates on it. A CBT therapist would probably look for cognitive errors underlying Mr. Lopez's worldview or core schemas. But does the CBT therapist think that criminal behavior is just one thing people will stop once they see the cognitive errors involved in choosing to offend? Is the information in a DV course solely the property of CBT, or do all therapies do education? A supportive therapist looks for opportunities, especially in this first session, to build rapport and keep the work going. Mr. Lopez might be putting the therapist into the role of "agony aunt" or a listener to his complaints who doles out upbeat advice. But the therapist is also beginning to look at Mr. Lopez's deficits (several criminal convictions, susceptibility to drug use—is he self-medicating some depression—DV) as well as strengths (hard worker and loyal to his boss, good father, loyal to parents and his brother).

Question 1

Do we need to talk about culture? Of course. It is obvious that the therapist is not Latino. There are cultural differences in marriages and relationships between men and women. Mr. Lopez makes a comment about women that the therapist lets pass for the time being. At some point, and in their discussions of how Mr. Lopez might have to "earn" his way back home, he may have to convince her that he will be a safe and loving husband and father. They should review what he learned in his DV course, relearn the lessons, or learn some new things.

Does the therapist believe that Mr. Lopez has a cultural "free pass" to treat his wife differently than other husbands? But he is an American husband, isn't he already? Does being from Latino culture give Mr. Lopez the right to push his wife onto the floor once in a while because she disrespects him?

Cultures change. We would probably not be having this discussion were it not for the man who invented the Oedipus complex, namely, Sigmund Freud. The story of Oedipus is a myth, but according to the myth, his father, Laertes, placed his son out to die to avoid fulfilling a prophecy that his son would kill him. Infanticide was widely practiced in the past (on both male and female infants, for example, when an infant was deformed), although it does appear that all contemporary societies officially condemn it. We spoke favorably of the Ancient Greeks for inventing rhetoric and supportive therapy, but they also had a practice of committing infanticide by exposure rather than murder, and so in the myth Laertes had his son hanged by the feet. Oedipus was rescued by a passing shepherd who gave him his name, which means "swollen feet."

Many cultural practices have changed over time, and as we mentioned in Chapter 1, we would like to believe there is a common multicultural morality toward which the world is slowly evolving. So we do not think that Mr. Lopez can claim that it is "okay" to push his wife. Possibly he can use his cultural background to explain why he pushed his wife in the past, but he cannot use that as a justification in the future.

Question 2

Does Mr. Lopez have to deal with his drug use problems? Of course. It looks like he has a major drug problem that (at least the criminal aspects of which) looms large in his life. A motivational interviewer might have started on this already in the interview, getting him to question his past decisions to use drugs with his friends and "give in" to a request for the marijuana run. Of course, Mr. Lopez is likely to say that he "doesn't have a drug problem anymore." He has been off the methamphetamine for at least 9 months, and he regrets the marijuana run. The therapist is still going to talk about relapse prevention classes in the prison (do we have enough classes lined up yet?) and linkage to AA and NA when he gets out. Mr. Lopez may resist that by claiming that he no longer needs them. He probably needs more insight about that. His working habits are probably somewhat overrated since he misses time because of his drug-using nights with his friends.

Question 3

Do we know enough to arrive at a diagnosis? The treatment plan will come out of this. Doesn't Mr. Lopez need some drug treatment? The therapist recommended parenting and anger management classes, but the drugs and the criminality are what got Mr. Lopez locked up, not his parenting skills or anger. Well, maybe the anger. It turns out that avoiding the police on a speed run was one of the charges he had plea bargained on.

Does Mr. Lopez have another diagnosis? Does he have an adjustment disorder? It would have to go on for 2 weeks to be major depressive disorder. The therapist needs to go through the features of depression. Is there a sleep disturbance, change of appetite, poor concentration, guilt, and suicidality (passive at least)? When did Mr. Lopez's symptoms start—earlier in jail, or the week before transfer when his case was lost?

Does he have a DSM-5-TR diagnosis, or something less? (See the section "Diagnostic Issues" below.) There are acute stress reactions that might be consistent with his catastrophizing presentation at entering these what he perceives as his personal "Gates of Hell" even though it is not an eternal sentence but merely 3 years. All sessions, even the first one, present with a host of unlooked-for opportunity and teachable moments. You need to determine which of these to tackle now and which are not yet ready for prime time. Should Mr. Lopez be referred for medication? It does not seem so, or at least it seems too early to consider it, but follow the policy of your institution.

Question 4

Where do we go from here? In subsequent sessions, the therapist may not necessarily control the whole process. He may use a psychodynamic technique that they call following or pulling "the red thread" or the theme that the patient naturally adheres to. But no therapist gets into his chair like getting into a car with a wild cab driver or ride-sharing driver (the patient) who takes him to some unknown destination. Supportive psychotherapy is directive, and the therapist does a lot of the direction. (In private practice and in psychodynamic psychotherapy, patients might assume otherwise, i.e., that they are there to talk to an audience and the therapist is supposed to listen for the most part.)

This introduction illustrates a combination of supportive and CBT techniques. See Table 3–6 for a comparison of how we look those approaches. At no point do we suggest that supportive psychotherapy is merely an introduction or segue into CBT techniques—we do suggest that they can be used together.

"I Can't Sleep"

Some things never change. In James White's *Tales of Sector General*, doctors tell us that chronic lack of sleep causes irritability that can turn into a permanent disorder (White 1999, p. 549).

We have an axe to grind about sleep, or actually several axes. True, it was the sound of a nearby sawmill, not the axes themselves (although they had some of those to chop the lumber), that kept the composer Ravel awake all night as he wrote his famous piece "Bolero." You can hear the sound of the saws in the music, but you probably know that story. Here's the 411 about being unable to sleep until 4:11 A.M.

From what we can tell, the most frequently reported problem of new arrivals in prison is difficulty sleeping. Many prisoners report at least temporary insomnia. Some of them had insomnia prior to incarceration, and many have taken medications ranging from over-the-counter remedies to high doses of controlled substances.

In the past, their diagnosis was just "insomnia." However, DSM-5 made major changes in classifying sleep disorders. Insomnia disorder is now one of many sleep-wake disorders, and it can be comorbid with depression, anxiety disorders, bipolar disorder, and the like. Typical insomnia is defined as lasting more than 3 months. There is a short-term specifier for insomnia lasting 1–3 months, and an atypical specifier for insomnia for presentations that don't fit those qualifications. Transient insomnia would be insomnia lasting less than a week, and temporary insomnia would be insomnia lasting a month. Therefore, unless your patient reports insomnia for more

TABLE 3–6.   **Cognitive and supportive approaches to the same problems**

Patient says…	CBT response	Supportive response
My life is over!	You're catastrophizing!	It's not that bad and we're here to help.
I'll die if I can't sleep!	No one dies from not sleeping.	We can help you to sleep. This has worked for the other people here.
I'll lose touch with my children	That's another error in thinking; they will remember you	Let's see how we can keep you in touch with them.
I lost my job.	It's not the end of the world. There are other jobs!	We can improve your job skills while you are here so you will be better able to get a job when you get out.
I am so depressed	Let's look at the cognitive errors that connect your thoughts to your depression.	Let's think of ways to improve your self-image, keep you busy, and cheer you up with activities.
I am a criminal.	Your choice of criminality shows errors that we will correct.	You have tried to meet your life goals in the wrong way, and we will teach you the right way.

than 1 month, his insomnia would be an atypical one, or what previous researchers called an "adjustment insomnia."

You probably know that it is part of correctional culture to discount the importance of insomnia. Although all the professional organizations state on paper that the standards for treating prisoners should be the community standards, correctional medical directors and prison administrators seem to endorse a major exception when it comes to insomnia and consider it, as we did above, as a kind of science fiction! Although European countries even use addictive medications for sleep, such use in this country is virtually anathema. Most medical directors even oppose the use of nonprescription medications (such as diphenhydramine, or brand name Benadryl) for sleep. It seems to be the dominant—even if unstated—belief that prisoners deserve to suffer as much as possible from their insomnia and that, after all, they'll probably get used to the noise and disruptions anyway. Although it is true that many prisoners do adjust in time, we disagree with attitudes that are insensitive, inhumane, and punitive.

There are understandable reasons to avoid the use of medications for sleep, the major one being the misuse and diversion of sedating medications. It is true that there is a high rate of requests, including those related to malingering, for medications to manage insomnia. Despite the admitted amount of malingering to obtain sedating medicines in prison, there is also a lot of genuine insomnia. Moreover, patients continue to get sedatives under other guises as anxiety or depression treatments. Some also malinger serious mental illness to get sedating antipsychotics when they can't get sleeping pills.

The authorities like to say that nobody ever died from lack of sleep. However, that is not true. Insomnia is an independent risk factor for suicide (Lin et al. 2018). Moreover, sleep disorders and psychiatric disorders interact mutually (Khurshid 2016). As Randall et al. (2019, p. 827) note, "Insomnia is a serious condition that affects over 60% of the prison population and has been associated with aggression, anger, impulsivity, suicidality, and increased prison health care use." And it now appears established truth that "[s]leep disturbances and depression are closely linked and share a bidirectional relationship....Insomnia is an established and modifiable risk factor for depression, the treatment of which offers the critical opportunity to prevent major depressive episodes, a paradigm-shifting model for psychiatry" (Plante 2021, p. 186). Finally, after some differences in research, it was most recently reported that sleeping pill treatment for severe insomnia reduces suicidal ideation (McCall et al. 2019).

Access to those pills being limited, you have the nonpharmacological techniques to put the patient, if not the problem, to bed. Adjustment insomnia, short-term insomnia, and even chronic insomnia can be treated successfully with single-session CBT and education. Randall et al. (2019) found a "one-shot" cognitive therapy quite effective for insomnia. It utilized a 60- to 70-minute session using a sleep log and an informational brochure. The CBT methods used for insomnia are called CBT-I. Many other methods and programs are also available. Since group therapy is much more efficient when the curriculum is fairly standard, group therapy is recommended. There are also extended forms of CBT-I delivered in four to eight sessions (more on this in a moment). For patients whose insomnia is dominated by nightmares, we have already recommended one particular 12-session treatment (which we have used) in Chapter 2. Nightmares that are a feature of PTSD can also be treated as part of the PTSD as we'll discuss in Chapter 6.

There are many effective interventions. *Sleep hygiene* helps to develop regular habits addressing the sleeping environment that improve the ability to fall asleep. It is often incorporated into CBT-I. We use our own sleep hygiene handout, and we have put our instructions in Table 3–7. You can make your own modifications. Our approach is to go over them with each person—that is, talk about mitigating the noise, not watching the clock, and not using the bed for anything other than sleep (although this is not always possible in a prison where the detainee may have to sit on the bed). Many instructional brochures are available on the internet. The usual brochure with the admonition to "use the bed only for sleep or sex" will of course inspire guffaws. Sleep diaries and brochures can be downloaded from government websites such as National Institutes of Health (2019). Also distribute earplugs whenever in whatever quantities allowed or advise patients to make them. Teach guided imagery and progressive relaxation. We are pleased that prisoners find the various sleep management techniques helpful, sometimes to their own surprise.

Having done what you can to treat the symptoms of insomnia, you should address the worries and life issues underlying it—also, because insomnia is a risk factor for dangerous or dysfunctional behaviors. See the talking points in Table 3–8. Discussing the reasons for insomnia can be very fruitful, as is using open-ended questions like "What's bothering you the most?" Presumably what keeps a patient from falling asleep is high on his or her list of worries, and these may help to form or revise the treatment plan. The most important worries are likely to be the new ones that were created by the incarceration. One sleep hygiene technique is for patients to create a worry book at the bedside in which they can list the things they think about instead of falling asleep.

If you do have time or do not have a group program, there is a multi-session *individual* therapy program for insomnia described in a detailed article with some actual session dialogues and sample psychotherapy instructions (Kaplan and Harvey 2014). Key aspects include:

TABLE 3–7.	**Sleeping better in jail or prison**

Practice sleep hygiene. Sleep hygiene doesn't mean just washing your face and brushing your teeth. It's about having good habits before going to sleep.

Plan to sleep whenever you lie down in your bunk.

Don't take long naps, especially not late in the day.

Associate the bed with sleep and only sleep. This is not always possible, but at least try to go to sleep when you lie down. If you are reading or talking to your cellie, sit up.

Try not to lie in bed for a long time. If you are not falling asleep, get up for a few minutes. Certainly, you should not be going to bed at 7 or 8 P.M. trying to sleep. Wait until you are really sleepy before you lie down.

Sit up if you can't sleep and do something else like reading.

If you don't fall asleep in 20 minutes, sit up or stretch for a few minutes.

Exercise and do so, if you can, as early in the day as possible.

If phone calls tend to get you upset, don't make calls just before bedtime.

Develop a bedtime ritual that relaxes you and gets your body into the habit of going to sleep. For example, try washing your face and hands, wiping your face with a washcloth, and so forth. This ritual should take you a few minutes and be something you always associate with going to sleep.

Don't watch the clock. That is, don't check the time in any way, and avoid looking at a clock if it is on the wall; clockwatching "trains" your brain to wake up and look at the clock, so it always makes the situation worse.

Put your worries aside. If your worries are keeping you up at night, it helps to write them down in a "worry book." That way you don't have to constantly think about the worry, but you know how to find it if you have to. Similarly, a "things to do list" by the bedside "offloads" your thought of what you have to do tomorrow and the rest of the week.

Avoid caffeine as much as possible late in the day; some people find that they need to avoid caffeine even after 2 P.M.

If you tend to get heartburn after meals, get it treated or don't eat just before you lie down.

If you have aches and pains that tend to wake you up at night, get them treated.

Be patient. If you are new to prison or there has been a change in your cell, it takes a few days to get used to the new circumstances.

Using what we call sleep restriction, schedule yourself to go to the bed a little later each day until you fall asleep right after you lie down.

Cut down the noise and light. Get a set of earplugs from medical or mental health or buy them in the commissary.

Cover your eyes with a paper towel or washcloth or whatever works to block the bright light, since lights at bedtime tend to reset our biological clocks to stay up later.

Develop a trust with cellmates so that you feel comfortable putting in your earplugs or towel face mask so you don't get paranoid. Tell them it is okay to wake you up if something happens that you need to know and that you won't be angry if they do. Promise the same for them.

Learn to relax. Your mental health counselor will teach you about progressive relaxation.

Go to a safe place—in your mind. Create an image of a pleasant, safe place where you can imagine yourself as you go to sleep. Maybe you are on the beach with the waves gently rolling in!

When you wake up, develop a ritual such as brushing your teeth, washing your face, or doing a little light exercise that gives you energy and that you associate with becoming active for the day. Talk to people, don't skip breakfast, and resist the urge to go back to bed until lunch.

Keep the same schedule every day, including weekends, and do not sleep late or take extra naps on days you do not work.

If there is a major change in your sleeping patterns or amount of sleep, tell your therapist about it.

TABLE 3–8.	Talking points: Discussing insomnia in individual sessions

1. (Unless the patient has clearly established chronic insomnia.) Insomnia is usually transient, so the best "treatment" is patience and reassurance that it will diminish in time.

2. It is possible to train yourself to wake up frequently, which is the opposite of what one wants to do. In other words, a person can learn "not to sleep." But the good news is that you can also learn "to sleep" through relaxation, guided imagery, and sleep hygiene.

3. It is natural to wake up a few times during the night.

4. There is no insomnia treatment, medicine or nonmedicine, that will "put you to sleep" for 8 or 10 hours.

5. If you want to sleep at night, avoid taking long naps, especially at the end of the day.

6. There is nothing magical about "needing 8 hours of sleep" at night. Most adults actually sleep less than that. If you do not fall asleep easily during the day, you are probably getting enough sleep during the night.

7. If you have issues other than your insomnia, let's discuss them. Did you get bad news from your attorney or from home? Have you been getting depressed or anxious? We can treat you with psychotherapy or, if the insomnia is bad enough, refer you for medicine.

8. (This is meant to address the issues of requesting sleeping pills and outright malingering for medicine.) We know it seems easier sometimes to want to "sleep the time away," but we are doing our best to keep you (men or women—individually or collectively) active during the day and not sleeping excessively. Please try not to ask for pills just to sleep the time away. If you are suicidal or depressed, we will deal with it (if you tell us!). But the insomnia will get better if you follow the principles of sleep hygiene.

- Educating the patient about the two-process model of sleep that involves circadian rhythms and sleep homeostasis (not a good word to use in prison; we use the terms "pressure" or "urge" to sleep). We explain how sleep restriction is desirable because it improves the urge to sleep.
- Discussing the deleterious effects of late-day naps on daily rhythms.
- Addressing the fundamental role of *worry* in initially preventing sleep and becoming a perpetuating factor of insomnia.
- Addressing dysfunctional beliefs about sleep, such as that one must have 8 hours of uninterrupted sleep to function the next day.
- For patients who believe that they have to "conserve energy" during the day, encouraging the experiment of resting for a few hours and then expending energy for a few hours; expending energy actually creates more energy and improves mood.
- Teaching them to develop a bedtime "wind-down" ritual and a wake-up routine.
- Setting reasonable goals such as falling asleep in 30 minutes and not awakening more than three times rather than falling asleep immediately and not waking up until morning.

We incorporated many of these ideas in Tables 3–7 and 3–8. If you are interested in doing the detailed step-by-step approach, consider the program of Perlis et al. (2008) or the self-help guide by Jacobs (2009).

If you are a gatekeeper to prescribers, you might have been told not to refer anyone for sleep medications. If your institution has the resources to treat insomnia nonpharmacologically, that might be reasonable. However, many institutions do not have the resources or expertise to treat all cases of insomnia without medications. Some cases will still have to be referred, and you should develop an understanding with your prescribing colleagues as to when and why you will be referring patients. Unless the sleep disturbance is severe, we suggest that patients not be referred after the first visit or even the first week, giving them a chance to fill out a sleep diary and try out the nonpharmacological methods. It is true that many will return and claim, "It didn't work," but some will not because they have learned to cope in their new environment.

Diagnostic Issues

We urge you to get to know your patient and not to diagnose excessively or prematurely. Diagnoses may create an obligation for certain "doses" of therapy. We suggest reviewing the Z codes in ICD-10 or DSM-5-TR. These codes refer to conditions that fall short of a full diagnosis because they refer to an examination, a facet of history, the psychosocial circumstances of the patient, or the health status of the patient. Examples include those for a family history of a mental or behavior disorder, a personal history of psychological trauma, or just for incarceration. A personal history of trauma should sensitize you to the possibility of another related diagnosis. See Chapter 6 for further discussion.

To Medicate or Meditate? Is That the Question?

In today's prisons, even with the expansion of prescribing responsibilities to nonphysicians, there is still a shortage of prescribing providers, who keep busy writing prescriptions for psychotropic medications and monitoring their patients. They cannot even do the latter by themselves, since monitoring requires ongoing observations by other staff for desired effects and undesired side effects. There are guidelines for prescribers who work with therapists, but we are looking at the other side of the coin now.

The first thing we can do is ask you to have a little sympathy for the prescriber. This may be hard to generate if you realize that the prescriber:

- Spends less time per session with the patient.
- Lacks the intense therapeutic relationships that develop.
- Probably gets paid more per hour.
- Has less social interaction with the institution.
- And despite all that, has a higher level of prestige!

But at least keep in mind that prescribers have a much higher level of liability. That includes the legal issues, side effects, and allegations of damage or death.

Having ourselves worked on both sides of that aisle, we realize that nonprescribers often have much jealousy and resentment toward the prescribers in their institutions. The feelings you have toward your prescribers might very well be justified, but we recommend that you don't let those feelings bias your care and management of patients. Prescribers are subject to malingering and manipulations and outright bullying and threats by prisoners to obtain medications unnecessarily. Excess medication may be desired to sleep away the time, to achieve psychiatric effects such as highs or lows, or to trade with others for privileges, food, or phone time. You should keep in mind the needs and values that you believe should be applicable to your patient. You should communicate (to both patient and prescriber) if you think the person is overmedicated. Perhaps you think prescribers ought to know better, but perhaps they do not, and you are improving your patient's treatment (or at least making it more fair) by telling them.

If you have quality concerns about prescribers, these should be reported through the usual channels for quality management, but not in ordinary progress notes. For example, if you think the prescriber is "overmedicating" the patient, you should not use that particular value-laden term in lieu of a more objective "appears sleeping late in the day" or "is walking unsteadily." Also take action on any dangerous side effects such as those that create a fall risk. *If you are willing to document it, you must be willing to deal with it.*

Differences in diagnoses are common among members of a multidisciplinary team and can be worked out in treatment planning. We have not had a problem with differences of opinion when different providers are actually treating different conditions. For example, the prescriber may consider it appropriate to treat a patient's depression and anxiety without drawing a firm conclusion as to whether the patient's symptoms meet all the criteria for PTSD.

As busy as you may be, there is much to be gained by reading the prescriber's notes. They may include a measurement of how depressed or psychotic the patient appears to be as well as an indication of the side effects that the prescriber notices. You might find yourself with a potential dialogue like the following:

> Mr. Smith, I noticed that you told Dr. Miller last week that you were feeling much worse, and then he increased your medication dosage. (You may get a response or not or may continue.) I'm surprised at reading that, because you told me last time you were doing quite well. Is there something more that I need to know? (This is of course the type of intervention known as a *confrontation*.)

Many nonprescribers feel obliged to follow the dictum "If any doubt, refer them out!" This is, sad to say, fairly good advice in today's correctional settings. But you do not have only the option of sending the patient for possible medication. Don't forget that you also have the option of second opinions from your colleagues and/or your department head.

And finally, here are the other things you should be doing rather than referring for medication:

- Assume that your patients will read your notes soon after you write them unless your state has a statute that prevents them from doing so. Even if they can't, it is easy for prisoners to get notes from their attorneys.
- Explain to patients that "we are never going to agree on everything" written in a note, perhaps not even the diagnosis.
- When you need to document in front of your patients, try going over what you are writing.
- If they have strong feelings about what they read in the notes (e.g., "Why did you say that I swore I was going to kill you?"), handle it on the spot.

- Refer patients to the medical records department for the legal methods they may employ of disagreeing with or "correcting" a mental health progress note.
- Use authoritative sources such as legitimate information on paranoia and ask them, "What do *you* mean by paranoia?" By redefining and reframing the term, you may get them to accept that they are paranoid.
- Discuss the advantages of having a diagnosis (e.g., living in the mental health unit). Explain to them that you and they may not like labels but that such labels are required for treatment.
- Discourage their use of your note as a "talking point" every time they see you. Point out that they are using this as a way of avoiding the real emotions of psychotherapy.

Self-Disclosure

We ourselves have advised judicious self-disclosure when working in supportive psychotherapy. This does not usually backfire in community mental health settings, but it does present problems in correctional settings. A big problem with self-disclosure is that you will not know when to stop, even though you think you know when you were going to stop when you started!

Case Vignette

> PATIENT: I always wanted to go to college, but I couldn't afford to.
> THERAPIST: You know, I didn't go to college right after high school, but I went back 4 years later.
> PATIENT: Oh, really, was it because you had kids to take care of?
> THERAPIST: Uh, yes, I have 4 kids.
> PATIENT: How old are they?
> THERAPIST: I've got a 14-year-old boy, an 11-year-old daughter, and 8-year-old twin boys.
> PATIENT: Wow! I'll bet you weren't planning to have two more when you had those last two!
> THERAPIST: You're right! We figured that three children would be perfect, but of course we love all four!
> PATIENT: Well, I'm sure you can afford to give them the things they like! I sure envy you for that! But what does your husband do?
> THERAPIST: Well, maybe that's enough about me…how are your kids doing? (the ones the patient abandoned when he went into prison…)

But of course, you know that everything you say will be shared with everyone else, including the antisocial predators, and your patients' families will check your Facebook page and Google you. Be careful what is shared and also what can be known about you (e.g., what is talked about in the hallways and what is seen in the parking lot).

What Do You Say After You Say Hello?

Such was the title of a popular self-improvement book (Berne 1977) about how people's lives and so-called life-scripts are determined by their interactions with others.

As a therapist, you have a lot of training that should make you comfortable in moving beyond the ordinary pleasantries of starting a conversation. Once you have engaged your patient in therapy, what is your agenda? We found an interesting compilation, based on a prison research project that was done during the time when research was telling people "nothing works" (the 1980s), that addresses the key discussion points (McGuire and Priestly 1985). These include:

- Re-creating their offense.
- Understanding the victim's perspective.
- Measuring the person's self-esteem.
- Learning social skills (e.g., resisting peer pressure to commit crimes).
- Learning self-control such as of precursors to violent behavior.
- Discussing the patient's impulsiveness and risk-taking behaviors.
- Dealing with boredom in the prison and using time for positive change.

The title of that book was *Offending Behaviour: Skills and Stratagems for Going Straight*. The subtitle obviously prompted a Google search to remind us of the difference between a "strategy" and a "stratagem." A *strategy* is an overall plan or agenda. A *stratagem* is a useful device or small-scale intervention to achieve the overall goal. Both are clearly necessary in supportive psychotherapy. You have got to have a plan for the therapy (your strategy) and a lot of interventions (your stratagems) for getting there.

Key Points

- Entering the institution can be an overwhelming experience, threatening the patient with unpleasant feelings and thoughts and you the therapist with TMI (too much information).

- Patients have strong reactions to incarceration that need to be addressed quickly.

- Methods of trauma-informed therapy in corrections should be employed at the start.

- You need to know the advantages and disadvantages of both group and individual psychotherapy.

- Prisoners do need to know the ground rules of psychotherapy, including what is or is not kept confidential.

- As far as what you write in the chart and what you disclose about yourself, you should apply the Miranda warning to yourself: "Everything you say can and will be held against you."

- Methods of cognitive therapy can help to defuse cognitive errors such as catastrophizing that occur upon admission.

- Insomnia is probably the number one problem reported by persons entering prison, yet there is opposition to treating it with medication. Psychoeducational methods, including sleep hygiene and cognitive-behavioral sessions, are worth promoting.

- Knowing when to refer to prescribers for a specific problem—and this applies not just to insomnia—can be difficult. Not everyone should be referred immediately for every problem. Have some faith in psychotherapy, psychoeducation, and even the "tincture of time" to resolve problems.

- You should not discuss quality assurance issues or air personal disagreements in the chart.

- We recommend some restraint or delay in ascribing significant diagnoses to patients.

- We advise against almost all therapist self-disclosure in these settings.

References

Albany Chesterton Society: Who are we? 2020. Available at: https://albanychesterton.wordpress.com/about. Accessed October 11, 2020.

Beck AT, Emery G (with Greenberg R): Anxiety Disorders and Phobias: A Cognitive Perspective. New York, Basic Books, 1985

Beck JS: Cognitive Behavior Therapy, 2nd Edition. New York, Guilford, 2011

Berne E: What Do You Say After You Say Hello? New York, Grove Press, 1977

Branch R, Willson R: Cognitive Behavioural Therapy Workbook for Dummies, 2nd Edition. Chichester, West Sussex, UK, Wiley, 2012

Burnett-Ziegler I: Commentary: How the Breonna Taylor decision traumatizes Black women. Chicago Tribune, October 2, 2020. Available at: www.chicagotribune.com/opinion/commentary/ct-opinion-breonna-taylor-black-women-trauma-20201002-zjytpdig6jddb-mvkmpey5lbxcu-story.html. Accessed October 4, 2020.

Columbia University: Columbia-Suicide Severity Rating Scale (C-SSRS): scoring and data analysis guide. 2020. Available at: https://cssrs.columbia.edu/wp-content/uploads/ScoringandDataAnalysisGuide-for-Clinical-Trials-1.pdf. Accessed July 9, 2020.

Dumond RW, Dumond DA: Mentally disabled inmates: concerns for correctional managers, in Managing Special Populations in Jails and Prisons, Vol II. Edited by Stojkovic S. Kingston, NJ, Civic Research Institute, 2010, pp 5-1–5-45

Freeman A: Cognitive therapy: an overview, in Cognitive Therapy: Applications in Psychiatric and Medical Settings. Edited by Freeman A, Greenwood VB. New York, Human Services Press, 1987, pp 19–35

Grayson B, Stein MI: Attracting assault: victims' nonverbal cues. Journal of Communication 31(1):68–75, 1981

Jacobs GD: Say Good Night to Insomnia: The Six-Week, Drug-Free Program Developed at Harvard Medical School, Revised Edition. New York, Holt, 2009

Kaplan KA, Harvey AG: Treatment of sleep disturbance, in Clinical Handbook of Psychological Disorders: A Step-by-Step Treatment Manual, 5th Edition. Edited by Barlow DH. New York, Guilford, 2014, pp 640–669

Khurshid KA: Bi-directional relationship between sleep problems and psychiatric disorders. Psychiatr Ann 46(7):385–387, 2016

Lin H, Lai C, Perng H, et al: Insomnia as an independent predictor of suicide attempts: a nationwide population-based retrospective cohort study. BMJ Psychiatry 18:117, 2018

McCall WV, Benca RM, Rosenquist PB, et al: Reducing Suicidal Ideation Through Insomnia Treatment (REST-IT): a randomized clinical trial. Am J Psychiatry 176(11):957–965, 2019 31537089

McGuire J, Priestly P: Offending Behaviour: Skills and Stratagems for Going Straight. London, BT Batsford, 1985

Miller NA, Najavits LM: Creating trauma-informed correctional care: a balance of goals and environment. Eur J Psychotraumatol 3:1–8, 2012 22893828

National Institutes of Health: Sleep diary and sleep brochure. NHLBI Publications and Resources. 2019. Available at: www.nhlbi.nih.gov/health-topics/all-publications-and-resources/sleep-diary and www.nhlbi.nih.gov/health-topics/all-publications-and-resources/sleep-brochure. Accessed October 18, 2019.

National Suicide Prevention Lifeline: Columbia-Suicide Severity Rating Scale (C-SSRS). 2020. Available at: https://suicidepreventionlifeline.org/wp-content/uploads/2016/09/Suicide-Risk-Assessment-C-SSRS-Lifeline-Version-2014.pdf. Accessed July 9, 2020.

Perlis ML, Jungquist C, Smith MT, Posner D: Cognitive Behavioral Treatment of Insomnia: A Step-by-Step Guide. New York, Springer, 2008

Phrases.org: Abandon all hope. 2020. Available at: https://www.phrases.org.uk/meanings/abandon-hope-all-ye-who-enter-here.html#:~:text=The%20expression%20%27abandon%20hope%20all%20ye%20who%20enter,used%20%27All%20hope%20abandon%20ye%20who%20enter%20here%27. Accessed July 7, 2020.

Pine F: Supportive psychotherapy: a psychoanalytical perspective. Psychiatr Ann 16:526–529, 1986

Plante DT: The evolving nexus of sleep and depression. Am J Psychiatry 178(10):186–902, 2021 34592843

Pollock JM: Counseling Women in Prison. Thousand Oaks, CA, Sage, 1998

Randall C, Nowakowski S, Ellis JG: Managing acute insomnia in prison: evaluation of a "one-shot" cognitive behavioral therapy for insomnia (CBT-I) intervention. Behav Sleep Med 17(6):827–836, 2019 30289290

White J: Tales of Sector General: The Galactic Gourmet, Final Diagnosis, Mind Changer. New York, SFBG Science Fiction, 1999

White J: Alien Emergencies: A Sector General Omnibus. New York, Tor Books, 2002

Whitten L: Trauma-informed correctional care: promising for prisoners and facilities. Corrections.com. April 28, 2014. Available at: www.corrections.com/news/article/35950-trauma-informed-correctional-care-promising-for-prisoners-and-facilities. Accessed August 12, 2020.

Wright JH, Brown GK, Thase ME, Basco MR: Learning Cognitive Behavioral-Therapy: An Illustrated Guide, 2nd Edition. Arlington, VA, American Psychiatric Association Publishing, 2017

4

Managing Therapy

Now that you are familiar with the challenges involved in engaging patients in therapy, we shall discuss how to establish a professional and supportive relationship with prisoners and how to deal with issues including transference, countertransference, resistance to therapy, and the therapist's risk of loss of efficacy and satisfaction called "burnout."

The Supportive Relationship

"Gabby" is a software program (not a person) that helps patients with chronic pain and depression. Two groups of patients are introduced to Gabby. One group is told that Gabby is an artificial intelligence program. The other group is told that Gabby is a person in the next room who is communicating with them in a way that preserves anonymity. Results: People who thought they were talking to a computer "were less fearful of self-disclosure and displayed more intense expressions of sadness compared with people who thought the conversational agent was controlled by a human" (Miner et al. 2017, p. 1217).

What does this tell us? Choose one or both of the following.

1. It is inhibiting for your patients to open up to you—a real person.
2. Some researchers think that artificial intelligence programs like Gabby, called *conversational agents*, can be used to save money in health care institutions.

Both are true. Research shows that it is more inhibiting to share one's feelings with a real person than with a computer. As for the second, conversational agents are already in use, and the authors of that study are concerned that appropriate evidence-based trials of effectiveness be conducted. But now that we have got you worried about job security, we will go back to the first point. You need to work initially and to help your patients overcome their inhibitions in talking to you and develop real rapport and a therapeutic relationship.

Depending on your own opinions about criminal behavior, you may believe that your patients made a series of choices that were "criminogenic" or that they perhaps had few real choices, and that the ones they did were based on their genetics, upbringing, community, educational and employment opportunities, and family environment, with elements expressing social injustice. And once they enter prison, your patients do not have many choices. They have probably not chosen to live in prison (although some do) and were not able to choose their cell, their neighbors, their clothes, or their therapists. Nevertheless, having a supportive relationship with them is important. A supportive relationship will keep them in therapy and help them to continue benefiting from it. It may also keep them be safer to others in the facility and safer to themselves.

The relationship between therapist and patient has three components:

- The real but professional relationship, which assists in the development of
- The working (or therapeutic) alliance, which creates
- The transferential relationship.

A supportive relationship is not a friendship, but it may involve elements found in a friendship. The classic description of this is Jerome Frank's paradigm of psychotherapy, in which he identifies four features common to all psychotherapies (Frank 1975, pp. 124–125):

1. A structured, "trusting, confiding, emotional" relationship that boosts the patient's morale
2. A treatment setting with an aura of safety and sanctuary
3. A conceptual scheme or explanatory model for the patient's problems that provides a rationale for the patient's treatment and relief
4. Therapeutic procedures consistent with the conceptual scheme that relieve the patient's anxiety and encourage new behaviors

The first two elements provide the basis for a supportive relationship by creating the emotional activation necessary for behavioral change and even straightforward learning. A supportive relationship may itself be therapeutic and also makes it possible to implement other techniques. However, there is a lot more that can be said about the role of a psychotherapist as a healer, comparing this role historically back to the roles of shamans in ancient societies and religious healers in modern ones. (For more, see Frank and Frank 1993; Nestler 2000.)

Desirable, possible, and nonsupportive elements of a supportive relationship are presented in Tables 4–1, 4–2, and 4–3, respectively. You should actively promote the development of the most desirable elements. For example, you might express concern for the patient rather than assume it is understood. This is an aspect of supportive therapy that creates uneasiness when working with some prisoners, especially criminals. We do not think it is required to "like" your patients using the normal meaning of the word. But it helps to be able to find something about your patients that you can relate to, a mutual respect for each other as human beings at least. There ought to be some healthy part of a patient that you have empathy with, or a weak part that you think deserves shoring up. In fact, classical therapists spoke of a "corrective emotional experience" (Alexander and French 1946) to explain the ability of supportive therapy to

TABLE 4–1.	Desirable elements of a supportive relationship

The setting allows for:

Mutual safety and security in a prison (e.g., visual oversight by or availability of correctional staff, panic button or devices)

A moderate to high level of activity in both participants

Therapeutic structure including reasonable comfort, quiet, and privacy (preferably no cell-side psychotherapy)

Two-way communication

Relative clear understandings of appointment times, frequency, and availability

Adjunctive use of other treatments and therapies including medication if needed

The therapist shows:

An involved, interested, active attitude in doing the therapy

Willingness to develop and contribute to a real but professional relationship

An attempt to develop a positive transference in the patient

An ability to manage a negative transference

Empathy and concern for the patient

Nonjudgmental acceptance or respectful tolerance of at least some aspects of the patient's self

Willingness to understand even a criminal's behavior (without condoning)

An attempt not to condemn or moralize about a criminal's failures to conform to the law but instead to maintain a constructive attitude to helping criminals change

Respect for the patient as a human being

Genuine interest in the patient's life activities and well-being

An attempt to find redeeming qualities in a criminal

Maximum allowance of the patient's autonomy to make treatment and life decisions

Commitment to work out a mutually acceptable treatment plan that addresses criminality and prevention of recidivism

The patient shows:

Respect for the therapeutic setting as nonviolent and mutually safe

Respect for and nonmanipulation of the therapist for criminal or nontherapeutic ends

Respect for the therapist's time and needs to see other patients

Willingness to speak honestly about life events without frequent misrepresentation or lies

Acceptance of the therapist's supportive role

Willingness to participate in the therapeutic program and adhere to the therapeutic structure

Willingness to develop meaningful treatment goals, including addressing criminal thinking styles, criminogenic elements in history, and prevention of recidivism

reparent patients who have had abusive childhoods. They elaborated the concept of a therapeutic (Zetzel 1956) or working alliance (Greenson 1967) to describe the shared agreement of patient and therapist working together.

Transference

Early on, Freud noticed that patients often began treating him like a parent. He described *transference* as the process in patients of developing attitudes and feelings that are "transferred" from their feelings toward parents or significant others in their ear-

TABLE 4–2. **Possible elements of a supportive relationship that must be very carefully controlled if present at all**

Maybe and "it depends" to:

Socialized and shared activities if therapeutic (Meals or "parties" on the mental health unit or therapeutic community might be part of the therapeutic program, or games or walks between offices, depending on level of patient's function, but these are not things you would do with most patients.)

Therapist's relationship to the patient's family (Can be a legitimate part of the therapy if allowed but can create splitting in the relationship with the patient.)

Therapist's self-disclosure (We recommend little to none.)

Humor (A touchy area; you have to know your patient well.)

Physical contact (In general, we avoid all physical contact, do not even shake hands, etc.; so no pats on the shoulder for either sex. But certain staff may have to touch patients involved in positioning, restraints, and so forth.)

Allowing some dependency (Only to the extent required or agreed upon in the treatment plan.)

---

lier life. He presented this as a mostly unconscious process. Supportive psychotherapists often take on the role of parental figures with persons who had poor, lacking, or abusive parenting in their own lives. Your patients may also be parents themselves and may be economically disadvantaged, be absent from their family, lack in parental skills, or even be abusive to their own children. You have an opportunity to be a model "good parent" to your patients. However, your therapy that reprises parent-child relationships can rekindle both good and bad aspects of those relationships. This can be dealt with if properly managed.

Freud knew that a positive transference can be erotically or emotionally dependent. In another of Kellerman's psychological thrillers, it is cutely called "inappropriate glomming," but that does convey the proper idea (Kellerman 2016, p. 22).

Positive or negative, you should stay aware of the transference, but that does not mean you should talk about it each time you recognize it. However, you frequently have to manage it to maintain what we call a *balanced transference* (see Table 4–4), including managing what our fictional doctor calls "inappropriate glomming." Extreme transferences can result in sexual obsessions or assault (possibly of you), displaced destruction of prison property, rejection dysphoria, or undue dependence on you. Or if a transference is mildly negative, you will want to use your alliance-building or rebuilding techniques to restore a positive relationship.

Just as motives attributed to oneself can be mistaken, attributions to others are frequently distorted, often because of the transference. A patient may attribute motives to the therapist that are blatantly irrational but powerfully felt. For example, the patient may feel that the therapist is sexually interested in him if the therapist criticizes the patient's spouse. If the therapist has to leave a session early, the patient may think the therapist was bored. Whenever the therapist observes an attribution of motives to self or others (including the therapist), he has the opportunity to help the patient correct any distortion of reality by offering better explanations.

Prisons raise special transference issues. Your patient can't leave. As far as therapists are concerned, usually it's you or the road. Well, not the road—it's you or the yard. They may or may not be able to change therapists. They may need you for favors or

TABLE 4–3.	Nonsupportive elements in a relationship

No to the following:

Just sitting there

Creating long silences

Verbally demeaning or abusing the patient

Becoming inappropriately involved (not necessarily romantically but too close)

Establishing real friendship or romantic or sexual involvement

Pitying

Forming a true peer relationship

Humoring, making fun of, talking down to the patient

Tacitly colluding about or mutually avoiding areas that need to be explored ("pseudomutuality")

Receiving or giving gratifications (e.g., telling jokes) that do not serve a therapeutic purpose

Accepting any sort of "gift" unless it is really not a gift but an item of therapy (e.g., a journal, a homework assignment) or something that can be put on the chart (e.g., a drawing should not be kept but can be charted as a therapeutic item)

Behaving in ways that are ethical violations or violations of institutional rules or law (Applies to therapist and patient.)

Buying into a criminal's justification for crime

Accepting a criminal's psychological defenses such as rationalizations and externalization of blame

Uncritically agreeing with any patient's view of himself or herself

Agreeing with a patient's delusions

---

privileges. This may lead to mixed feelings such as those that children have toward abusive parents: they need them but they can't love them. Prisons are like a new family to many residents, consistent with the Latin phrase (often used for colleges or residential institutions) of being *in loco parentis* (in the role of a parent). So pardon us for mixing three languages, but consider this:

> Prisons are *in loco parentis*,
> They're like crazy parents,
> And they're overcrowded
> Like the first line of "La Bamba"…

Even if the patient's family of origin was positive and nurturing, prisons can reverse that role, which is why we likened them to "crazy parents" above. Crazy, arbitrary, oppressive, or downright abusive. And the prisoners must dance to them, but definitely not in the happy dance of "La Bamba." The criminal justice system, the state, the society as a whole, and people not of one's social group or race all represent sources of negative transference that can be reflected in angry feelings toward the therapist. So it is that you may discover that your patient's negative transference reflects not anger at his family but anger at his cellmates. This calls for explanation. Knowing that you are also trapped and unable to "fire" them, patients may also vituperate against you or devalue you in the therapy. "What good are you? You can't do anything for me! You can't get me released, and you won't even write me a letter of recommendation!"

TABLE 4–4.	Balancing or managing the transference

Address mildly or strongly negative transferences.

Quickly address serious "therapeutic ruptures" and admit mistakes if they hurt the therapy.

Leave alone mild and harmlessly positive transferences.

Address to weaken erotic feelings.

To weaken the transference, make meetings shorter and less frequent.

To strengthen the transference, make meetings longer and more frequent.

Without explaining, ask the patient what he or she believes.

Correct mistaken beliefs in a matter-of-fact manner.

Always keep yourself safe.

Let's Hear It for the Boy

Since most of those in prison are male, effective engagement in therapy requires understanding of male development, and especially the developments that lead certain men to criminality or violence. An account of men's development, written during the period in the United States of the various men's movements, asks us to consider the male peer influences toward self-reliance, superiority, and violence (Glicken 2005). Many male prisoners are fearful of the personal revelations they think will be necessary in therapy. Glicken recommends that therapists:

- Give patients adequate time to develop trust.
- Structure therapy (rules create less anxiety than open-ended activities).
- Use metaphors and stories (as mentioned in Chapter 2).
- Let them draw their own conclusions from the lessons of therapy rather than give them the whole answer (which can be embarrassing to them).
- Help them work through their parenting issues of their mother and possibly absent or abusive fathers (whom they may have modeled themselves after).
- Help them to undo their inappropriate conceptions of relationships to women.
- Work through their false assumptions of the relationship between masculinity, criminality, and violence.

Negative Therapeutic Reactions

Some patients seem to worsen with therapy. Freud pondered this issue throughout his career and thought that it might have to do with guilt at getting better. One of Freud's patients, Joan Riviere, became an analyst herself and concluded that the negative therapeutic reaction reflects a desire to spite the therapist or prove that they are not so good as they think they are (Wikipedia 2020a). Or it may reflect envy of the therapist's power.

Case Vignette

The therapist was working with a young woman with borderline personality disorder who occasionally did cut herself; however, she had not done so for several months. They had just spent some extra time discussing her father's coldness and unavailability.

The session had apparently gone well, and the patient left seemingly happy. Five minutes later, the staff called the therapist and reported that the patient had (deliberately to all appearances) badly jammed her thumb in the cell door as the officers were closing it. The patient was treated and brought back. The therapist wondered if the patient's behavior had the meaning that Freud originally ascribed to it, that of feeling guilty at getting better? The therapist wondered if the behavior was a transference reaction. Was the patient trying to "prove" that the therapist could not cure her and that the extra time was not worth the effort? What happened is that the patient, thinking primitively, identified the therapist with her father and declared "My father never did anything good for me."

High-Profile Patients

They may be movie stars, mafia dons, or dishonest CEOs. Most high-profile patients do quite well and rarely have institutional problems. Rather, they develop a sycophantic following since their power is naturally attractive to low-status prisoners and, as for immediate satisfactions, it's possible to "feed" the commissary accounts of just about anybody using the proper procedures even if it violates institutional rules. However, if you do see a high-profile patient, you may find yourself enjoying it more than you should as you bask in his shadow and imbibe the little secrets in his life. Please pay attention to the effect it has on your judgment.

Psychopathic Patients

We discuss psychopathy in Chapter 10. You will work with psychopathic patients, although many psychopaths may be "white collar psychopaths" or high-profile patients who do not want or need services. However, if you do work with a psychopathic patient, you must constantly be wary of manipulation. The psychopath may have all the time in the world to warm you up to him. He may be willing to wait 10 years before he asks you for your cell phone.

Something you should assess in the high functional criminal, including the psychopathic one, is general intelligence. Although criminality does have an association with low intelligence, there is a small group of highly intelligent psychopaths (as in Sherlock Holmes' nemesis Professor Moriarty or Hannibal Lecter in *The Silence of the Lambs*—a psychiatrist but fortunately a fictional one) who have "overcome" the normal protective factors that intelligence provides of social commitment, attachment, and involvement. Such persons, if properly assessed and treated, have good outcomes in therapy because of their intelligence, but if wrongly treated they can be especially dangerous criminals (Oleson 2016a, 2016b).

One risk of working with psychopaths is the development of *pseudomutuality* in therapy sessions. This term refers to pathological characteristics in families who appear to be congenial and get along while disregarding the animosity between members. You can find yourself developing a kind of tacit agreement with them, talking along merrily while failing to address the real issues. So be warned: "Psychopathic individuals who establish a pattern of pseudomutuality in the therapeutic relationship either quickly understand the lack of opportunity for real gratification and drop out of treatment or become focused on attempting to use the relationship to inappropriately gratify real or imagined needs. In the latter case, in order to elicit the therapist's good will and expected personal gain, the patient may come across as increasingly needy or may become coercive" (Winston et al. 2020, p. 94).

Mismanaged Empathy, or "How Do You Solve a Problem Like Prilicla?"

The problem that arises with the above pseudomutuality is mismanagement of empathy. In order to sit and simply spend time with somebody, you have to have some type of feeling within yourself that sustains the relationship. Once more, there is a lesson to be learned from the world of Sector General Hospital. Prilicla is a delicate, insectlike alien with two problems. The first is its tongue-twister name. (The custom in Sector General is to avoid sexism by referring to aliens as neuter.) The second is the fact that it is an empath, that type of being made popular in various episodes of *Star Trek* such as counselor Deanna Troi. But the problem for Prilicla of being an empath is that it can't turn off its empathy. Any negative emotions, including those it creates in its conversations with others, are reflected back to it and palpably hurt it. And Prilicla is really quite delicate—if one of its wings flutters too much it will fall to the floor and one of the humongous aliens in the hospital will probably stomp on it by mistake! The solution: It has to kind of stretch the truth a lot and constantly smooth things over so that it doesn't absorb negative emotions from its companions (White 2001, p. 371).

A distinction is made between empathy and sympathy. Empathy is a type of understanding, while sympathy is more of a feeling (Merriam-Webster 2020). Empathy is a newer word and fills the niche for a type of objective and separate understanding rather than just feeling what someone else feels. It is an attunement that comes from putting yourself in the patient's place, to understand how she got to be where or what she is today. This is distinct from sympathy, which consists of feeling what she feels. Sympathy is what you feel for a relative who lost someone to COVID-19. Empathy does not require sympathy. It is better to "have" rather than to feel empathy for your patients. Empathy is compatible with professional detachment.

Certainly, it's possible, with presumed professional detachment, to feel so superior to your patients that you can profess sympathy without actually having it. In fact, there is another alien in our sci-fi hospital who is so above it all that he humblebrags that he has such a high intelligence, generous personality, and exalted ethical values that he can forgive the wrongs, shortcomings, and shallow thinking of the human beings he encounters. After all, he implies, it's the least he can do, for he is far above getting angry or irritated by his encounters with mere humans (White 2001, pp. 451, 458)!

At the opposite end of the spectrum, it is common to develop an absolute dread of seeing certain patients. For example, the patient may have the characteristics of a predator, narcissist, antisocial personality, psychopath, or all four. Or he may be a depressed lifer who overwhelms you with his hopelessness. Or be someone who just annoys you for reasons from your past which you do not fully understand. Some combinations, such as the male predator/young woman therapist, can be particularly toxic. You put up with an awful lot to do your good in a prison, but sometimes it is just too much. Don't overestimate yourself, don't get manipulated, and declare your limits.

Therapists also need to be aware of the difficulties and misconceptions involved in working with persons who are habitual criminals (i.e., persons with a long and established criminal lifestyle, not just persons who have committed one or several crimes). Criminals have serious issues of trust. They will accuse you of not trusting them and will often pressure you into saying something that you do not feel, namely, that you trust them. Boyd Sharp, the program administrator whom we quoted in Chapter 2, tells us that a relationship with criminals is built on "expectation, accountability and responsibility." These criminals (and we are talking about people with established criminal lifestyles, not just persons who have been convicted of one or several crimes), typically complain that therapists do not trust them. However, they have a shallow concept of trust, and when it is pointed out that they cannot be trusted, they are really bothered by the fact that the therapist does not take their lies at face value and cannot be manipulated (Sharp 2006, p. 115).

Managing the Transference

Managing the transference means maintaining a balance by addressing the extremes of positive and negative transference. For example, you can explain a potentially erotic transference as a good thing that the patient likes you, but that's something that cannot be carried too far. You do not need to relate the patient's feelings to unconscious components. You can leave alone a mildly positive transference, but you will usually need to address a mildly negative one. Without offering explanations initially, pay attention to your patient's beliefs and what it is about them that leads your patient to have transferential feelings about you.

Although it is not always possible due to session requirements, you can try to change the frequency of meetings and the duration of sessions. You should also avoid generating expectations of gratifications and then failing to follow up on them. If you say, "I'll always be available when you need me," and then refuse to answer the patient's request for an extra session, you may expect his wrath to descend upon you in the next one.

Psychotic Transference

Psychotic patients can become delusional about you. This is referred to as a *psychotic transference*, and it can create disruption and danger in the therapy. Sometimes the patient comes to believe that you resemble some other significant person in her life, such as a previous doctor. Perhaps they recall a good relationship or a bad one. If the psychosis attached to the transference is fairly weak, you can usually defuse it with a little reality testing. You might say, "Oh, maybe I look like your previous doctor, but I was not working in the prison last year (or wherever they say about their previous doctor). Do you want to tell me about him?" We assume that the development of a psychotic transference expresses a wish or fear about your patient's current treatment. If the transference is potentially negative or dangerous, you may want to distance yourself somewhat from the patient and minimize the sessions until you can work through the psychosis. Later, when the psychosis is resolved, you can talk about it more.

Institutional Transference

Institutional transference in a criminal justice system consists of a prisoner's transference to the treating institution or the system taken as a whole. It involves a parental personalization of the institution, and like other transferences, it may be positive or negative. Institutional transferences to prisons are often negative, but some prisoners can develop a positive institutional transference even if they have difficulty relating to people. Negative transference about the prison (or other treatment staff) may represent splitting or a safer displacement of negative attitudes about you onto others in the clinic. Given the obvious dangers of a negative transference to the therapist, it may be best to leave negative *institutional* transference uninterpreted. Negative transference to specific staff, however, may need to be explored because it can represent potential danger. For example, what do they mean when they say, "Some of the staff here treat you like sh--!" Are you one of the "some"? (And we have sometimes heard such statements directed at us but made in the third person, haven't you?)

We do find it doesn't hurt to poke fun at the institution's little foibles in order to side with a patient. For example, you can joke about the loud noises, limited choices of Ramen noodles in the commissary, and expense of the phone calls. You can say that "I realize I can go home at night and you're already home." Or "Some of the COs [corrections officers] can be really tough, although I do think most of them are fair…but you know, people are different…not everybody is the same…you've got to expect some differences…and you guys always talk about the differences between the COs, so you know that already, don't you?"

A patient's perception of the institution as almost omnipotent but impersonal can be beneficial for grandiose patients who identify with sources of power, as well as those who cannot acknowledge dependence on an individual therapist (Safirstein 1968). The stability of care in the prison system can also be emphasized when therapy with an individual therapist ends.

Funny or Not? You Make the Call!

Some therapists warn against any humor at all in therapy, and we can respect that position since humor can be taken the wrong way, especially by prisoners with severe personality disorders and mental illness. If the patient has neither, then perhaps you can use humor in the normal way.

Over the years, we had the occasion to see one of those annual training videos about sexual harassment called, appropriately, "Sexual Harassment: You Make the Call!" (Coastal 2000). What we found interesting about the video (other than seeing it 10 times) was that some of the decisions they ask you to make are quite difficult. For example, to know if an action constitutes harassment, you need to understand what is called the reasonable personal standard. Would there be something different called a "reasonable patient standard" for using humor with prisoners? Some guidelines:

- Many patients, even some who are paranoid, have excellent senses of humor, and you can sometimes "side with them" about the way that staff members mistreat them.
- Some other patients have no sense of humor at all and cannot even tell if you are making a joke or being sarcastic.
- Still other patients will misunderstand your neutral or innocuous statements and make accusations against you "out of the blue."

Case Vignette

A Latino therapist works with a Latino patient and talks about the jokes that have been made about Latinos (Ramirez 2014). The patient is offended and files a grievance.

There is not enough information here to conclude that the therapist made a mistake, but it is likely that he misread something about their therapeutic alliance. A lesser reaction on the patient's part could have been, "Oh, no, that's really offensive, I'm really sensitive to things like that because of the way I've been treated...," but not filing a grievance.

Dependency and Entitlement

Dependency and entitlement occur in all forms of psychotherapy and can be problematic. Dependency is less objectionable than entitlement and may be unavoidable and indefinite, as in a patient with schizophrenia serving a long sentence who requires indefinite therapy. Entitlement, on the other hand, connotes the expectation of attention and services that are inappropriate. Not all dependency, however, turns into entitlement. Indeed, patients, like children, may require nurturance at appropriate times in order to grow up or out of therapy. Therefore, you should expect to regulate the amount of dependency or what you might call "entitled expectations" as the patient progresses through therapy.

Resistance Is Futile (If You Know How to Deal With It!)

Although prisoners abide by their Convict Code of sticking together and not ratting anyone out, a good way to describe many prisoners' attitudes is Walt Whitman's "Resist much, obey little." This was a political message to states and cities about freedom, and although not intended for prisoners, it does a good job of expressing the prisoner's philosophy of opposing the government's attempt to control him. For some prisoners, whatever they can oppose, they will oppose. Perhaps this makes sense as an attitude to take toward the prison, but psychotherapy is supposed to be a shared enterprise with shared goals. It may "make sense" for a prisoner to oppose a goal of becoming a noncriminal, but there may be other goals, such as lifting his depression, that he wholeheartedly embraces.

The culture of men's prisons has been described as that of "toxic masculinity" (Kupers 2005), which, in conjunction with the Convict Code, is a major source of treatment resistance. We discuss this in Chapter 12, but here we discuss some of the individual forms that resistance takes.

Whether it is in their personal interest or not, many patients show resistance to therapy. Resistance consists of factors that slow down, defeat, distract, divert, or terminate the therapy because your patient does not want to learn or gain insight in the direction that helps his progress toward his treatment goals. Resistance can be obvious, as in "I don't want to see you anymore. Goodbye." It can show itself in prolonged silences. Therapists doing motivational interviewing formerly had a concept of "rolling with resistance" but now have redefined that concept in other terms as a patient is deemed to be engaging in "sustain talk" (Miller and Rollnick 2013). Resistance can also be reframed as a strength or feisty spirit. "When you don't want to see me, you stay away for a month, don't you?" However, we still consider resistance to be a real factor that can block or slow down therapy, and we are not yet convinced that it is clinically (or politically) incorrect to use the term, especially when the patient is persistent in maintaining criminal thinking patterns. When you tell your patient about resistance, however, you can describe it differently. We do not go so far as to call it "sustain talk," but we do refer to "reluctance" (e.g., reluctance to speak freely about one's past, reluctance to change one's lifestyle). Sometimes there is resistance just in getting started. This is a particular problem in patients who must be seen according to various mental health protocols, and also those referred by other sources for therapy because of a concern about their behavior.

How do you deal with silence? You can explain it directly as "It seems like you don't want to talk about (your crime, your mother, your significant other)?" In the world outside, patients who pay for timed psychotherapy sessions will be allowed to stay through silence. In psychoanalysis, the analyst may conduct (if you want to call it that—could a conductor conduct a symphony of 45-minute silence?) a silent therapy session or even issue periodic interpretations of the patient's silence. Not in a prison, where they do not say it best when they say nothing at all. In our methods of "triaged" supportive psychotherapy, we may vary the time of each session based on need. If there is a prolonged silence, we do have to make sure we don't have a psychotic patient who is about to become violent, but do have just a bored or sullen patient who was awakened to come to the therapy session. If the latter, we issue a fairly neutral opinion (rather than a hostile one explaining their resistance) such as "It seems like we have covered what you *want* to talk about, so I guess we're good until next time." In the next session, the silence is a good subject to begin with. "I remember that last time, you were quiet, so are you able to tell me more about that?" You are following the principle of "strike while the iron is cold"—that is, you are asking about an issue after it has cooled off.

Prisoners can be no-shows through no fault of their own, such as lockdowns, conflicting appointments, attorney visits, outside appointments, or mistakes in the pull list. Your makeup policy should be clear in advance. Deliberate no-shows are still possible since the patient can simply refuse to come. In some places, patients can be written up for disobeying an order. In some cases, when patients are particularly paranoid or have severe mental illness, we make special arrangements to see them in the dormitory or have them brought individually to the clinic so that they do not have to sit with others in the waiting room. If someone else notices the arrangement and asks for it himself or herself, we say: "Everybody is different, and everybody gets the kind of program that they need. You don't need to come individually to the office. You are sociable and sit around and talk with your friends, so you don't need a special arrangement."

Experts who deal with involuntary clients have considered what works and does not work in therapy. One admonition that goes against the grain of many is "Don't ask questions!" (Brodsky 2011, p. 47). Brodsky, who earned his keep treating military prisoners at Fort Leavenworth, urges therapists with coerced clients to avoid the standard questions that tend to produce instant resistance and if anything, the wrong answers. Examples (modified from Brodsky 2011, p. 71) are:

- Why do you keep getting into trouble?
- Why do you use those drugs when you ought to know better?
- Why do you have such an anger problem?
- Why can't you just stop hitting people?
- Why do you keep on abusing your partner?

These are questions that we hope will be answered in therapy, but they can easily turn off a reluctant patient who wants treatment for his distress but not the "trouble" he gets into. In time, he may realize that his "trouble" is the major cause of his distress, but not yet. Brodsky provides guidance on how to do therapy with reflections and re-statements and redirection but sans questions. For example, instead of a question about anger, the therapist observes that anger has gotten the patient into trouble and gets in the way of other things he wants in life.

Brodsky thinks asking "why" questions presumes that there is a certain kind of in-sight that is necessary for personal change—hence the questions that attempt to engen-der such insight. He reminds us that offenders associate the questioning of therapists with the interrogations of law enforcement and the presumption (which many never admit) of guilt for the crime. However, eventually, in many schools of therapy, it is considered important to answer the "don't ask" questions, since the causes of dysfunc-tional behavior need to be understood. For example, in CBT or dialectical behavior ther-apy, the therapist and patient may develop a "chain analysis" of events leading to problem behaviors. But on the assumption that some questions are necessary with re-luctant or resistant clients, we think it is less threatening to ask them in a certain man-ner (based on Harris 1995, pp. 35–36):

- Do you have any questions about why exactly you are here?
- What were your thoughts in coming here?
- In the past did you ever find it helpful to talk to a teacher, counselor, clergyman?
- What do you think will happen if you don't come to this office?
- If you weren't angry about coming here, what would you want to talk about?
- When people make you do things, what negative feelings do you have?
- When you are forced to do something, do you think you are more resentful or less resentful than other people?
- Are you angry at me because you think I am forcing you to be here?

It is okay to encourage patients to be the ones asking the questions, since this takes them out of their "Resist much, obey little" mode. This does not require you to have answers, nor allow the patient to derail the therapy with questions about their prog-nosis or when they will be getting well and completing their therapy, if these things are not known at the time of the questioning. The answer to those questions may be: "I don't know now. We'll probably know eventually."

Resistance to change may occur because of gang membership. Much is being done these days to help gang members "get out and stay out," yet gangs exert pervasive influence both inside and outside prisons. This topic is addressed at greater length in Chapter 12.

Those persons we called "criminals" are particularly good at resisting change in psychotherapy. Many of them know they are spouting "baloney and fleeing [you] the slicer" (a phrase from a 1967 political discourse, when conservative William F. Buck-ley Jr. sarcastically said why Robert F. Kennedy refused his interview; Popik 2011). Gathering from a number of sources and adding a few funny names, we compiled, in Table 4–5, strategies of resistance with hints at how to overcome them. Keep in mind that these are behaviors in really resistant persons and may not describe the majority of your patients. For example, patients who try to derail the therapy with long stories can be told, "I hear you, but let's get back to the question" or simply "Uh-huh, but what about the questions I asked you?—what about the crime, your marriage, or the daughter who says you abused her?"

A well-known program targeting criminal and addictive thinking tackles the avoidance, diversionary, and disruptive tactics that criminals use to disrupt their therapy and avoid confrontation with their personal criminal behaviors (Collaboration of Chemical Dependency Professionals 2002). These include:

- Lying in any number of ways: by commission, by omission, by being vague, being silent, or selectively remembering or being forgetful.
- Creating diversions such as accusing others, arguing over words, shaming oneself to get sympathy, and speaking fast or slow to annoy others or get them off the track.
- Creating chaos: disrupting the unit, accusing others of misunderstanding them, changing the story, and constantly demanding their rights.
- Seeking attention: doing things to disrupt the group; arguing with and aggressively opposing staff.
- Splitting staff, including spreading rumors about them.
- Using sarcasm, teasing, and threats.

It is gratifying to overcome a patient's initial resistance or hostility, but keeping patients coming back requires attention. Elliott (2002) has described strategies for doing so, including:

- Avoid extended debates, because criminals need to save face and will switch to a strategy of "win at all costs."
- When using confrontations, make them appear as constructive criticism.
- Redirect disruptive patients back to the issue and away from their distraction ("Let's talk about what's going on with you now, not what happened in the past").
- Reverse patients' attribution of responsibility when they blame someone else for their situation. For example:
  - "So you're saying you have such little self-control that you blame other people for your lack of self control?"
  - "So you're saying that you're incapable of self-reliance?"
  - "So you say that one good deed makes up for all the pain and suffering you have caused other people?"
  - "So you're saying that this counseling is not worth it? Does that mean that everything about you has been fixed?"
  - "Have you given half as much to other people as you have expected them to give to you?"
  - "You keep saying that respect is very important to you. How much respect are you giving (me, your family, your cellmates) now?"

Other suggestions (based on Harris 1995) are to:

- Create some kind of early success for your patients, such as in an easy but gratifying homework assignment.
- Ask patients what they perceive as the roadblocks to the therapy.

TABLE 4–5. **Strategies of resistance and their counters**

Resistance strategy	Example	Countering tactic
I shall deny, Vy	Denying the crime or issue	"Just say no" didn't work for drugs, either. Denial being one of the basic defense mechanisms, explain this to them as being part of criminal thinking styles.
Let's be fuzzy, Ozzie	Being vague in answering your questions	Ask them for details; confront unnecessary vagueness.
Let's not talk about that, Matt	Defocusing onto some safe topic	Investigate their avoidance and fears if genuine.
I'm just a rambling boy, Joy	Rambling on but in actuality avoiding the question	Point out that they are normally quite precise and put the session back on track.
I think I'll lie, Cy	Telling you outright lies that you can easily check	Confront them about the value of chronic lying in their lifestyle.
Let's put that off, Geoff	Not wanting to talk about it now	Ask: If not now, when? Schedule a time to talk about it.
Here's what you want to know, Joe	Telling you the party line as if they mean it ("I'll never use drugs again, it's not a problem anymore")	Confront them about the unrealistic aspect of absolutes and their sincerity in making such absolute predictions of their behavior.
Maybe, Baby	Making noncommittal statements like "I guess I could do that, maybe I could do that, I think"	Ask them why they cannot use the language of commitment. A commitment is not a prediction of success but a determination that they should be able to express. Compared with previous item, commitment would be "I want to stop using drugs."
Let's go for a spin, Min	"Spin the therapist": a common criminal game in which they get you (and their other providers) running around working on solving a problem that should not be solved because they have already heard it will not be given to them	Review their efforts and "spinning" and how they have (temporarily at least) lost the right to ask for special favors involving you making "asks" of others in the institution.
If at first you don't succeed, try it again, Reed	Asking again and again for the same thing: we consider this a variant of "spin the therapist"; they ask you to try it again even though your efforts failed the last time; often this relies on their assumption that you do not share information with other providers	Point out that the various providers do confer with each other and that one of them cannot be "worked" to accomplish something at cross-purposes with the others.

TABLE 4–5.   **Strategies of resistance and their counters** *(continued)*

Resistance strategy	Example	Countering tactic
Don't hurt poor old me, Dee	Portraying themselves as victims rather than perpetrators	Explain and dissolve claims of victimhood as part of criminal lifestyle.
How about some snark, Mark?	Using sarcastic humor to demean you or the institution.	You should advise them to park the snark when it's about you but you may have to tolerate some negative institutional transference.
Let's get sexy, Lexi	Making sexual comments that you have to deal with	Call out, set limits to that type of behavior or discipline.
It's about race, Stace	Blaming you or society for racism	Of course this must be taken seriously and be discussed but personal components of responsibility have to be acknowledged.
I'll give you some flak, Jack	Insulting or demeaning the therapist to draw attention away from themselves	Discuss zero tolerance for abuse of therapist. They can question and complain but they cannot insult you.
And I won't come back, Mac	Staying away from the session	Explain their avoidance and what they are missing in their progress in treatment.
Get on my (not your) train, Jane	Hijacking the whole train by asking for some special favor today ("I need this from you, Doc")	Understand their needs may be important, but determine if the session should be addressed to those needs.
I've found God, Todd	Using references to God as taking care of all problems, but not making any personal commitments	Faith-based coping is great, but ask them to explain HOW, not THAT, God has taken care of their problems.
Forget the plan, Stan	Introducing new or numerous goals not relevant to their criminological or mental health needs	Redirect back to the treatment plan.
I like you, Ike	Using blandishments to distract from therapeutic material	Call them out on the strategy and clarify the professional therapeutic alliance.
You want to be hit, Mitt?	Becoming combative or assaultive in the session	End session and impose discipline.
Let's get mad, Tad	Having false fits of crying, fake rage, and ventilation to avoid confronting a topic	Give time to cool off and call them out about their histrionic behavior.

- Get buy-in on a problem they want to work on.
- Develop the treatment plan with them.
- Rather than disagree with their beliefs, ask patients to tell you the evidence for their beliefs.

Countertransference

In psychoanalytic theory, *countertransference* referred to a therapist's projections onto the patient of unconscious attitudes and feelings. However, in its common, broad definition today, it denotes all the therapist's feelings toward a patient. Your feelings can help you to understand a lot about your patient's pathology, as well as about yourself. Some of this is obvious: it is natural for you to feel sadness when you work with a depressed patient, or to feel disgust or repulsion when encountering a person who has done sadistic things. And feeling manipulated may mean that your patient has an antisocial personality disorder. Countertransference reactions can include (categories from Knoll [2009], mostly our own elaborations):

- Isolation of affect—the therapist isolates his feeling of being horrified, working in a distant, ritualistic way and going through the motions.
- Therapeutic nihilism—the therapist gives up on the patient.
- Malignant pseudo-identification—the patient emulates the therapist's characteristics, leading to inappropriate closeness and favoritism in the relationship; compare this with the "pseudomutuality" we previously discussed.
- Assumption of similarity—the therapist should not assume that the patient operates from desires or motives similar to the way the therapist operates.
- Fear—some forensic psychiatrists point out the fear is probably a normal reaction to being in the presence of a predator.
- Disgust—similar to fear, disgust is an "animal" reaction that is hard wired in our emotional system (the mental analogue to rejecting poisonous food).
- Counterphobic denial—a blind spot in defenses or a feeling of invulnerability can lead the therapist to take risks in working alone or in isolation with predators.
- Self-devaluation: the therapist devalues himself because of his inability to treat or cure; this may also involve the feeling one gets from the self-assured, haughty superiority of the psychopathic patient.
- Hatred, desire to punish or destroy—it is understandable when the therapist has such reactions, but they need to be kept in check.

Pay attention to how you perceive your status in the therapy situation. Perhaps you became a therapist out of desire to help people, or perhaps you felt a need to have a high-status occupation. Perhaps you feel like Albert Camus' Dr. Bernard Rieux in *The Plague*, who says he doesn't know what is in store for him, but all he knows is that there are sick people to cure (Camus 1947/1991, p. 127). Camus never caught the plague, but from the age of 17 he did suffer from tuberculosis, of which we shall say more along the way (Earle 2020). Perhaps curing disease is like investigating a mystery. Our fictional Master Chef of the Introduction, Gurronsevas, also tries to find the cause of an epidemic—possibly a virus, possibly food poisoning—that is making the doctors in his hospital delirious. (Gurronsevas would make an excellent private eye—or eyes, since he has four of them, or a gumshoe, since he has six feet. Oddly though, for a ga-lactic gourmet, he has only one mouth.)

Countertransference feelings are relational, but they can be divided into those pre-dominantly caused by factors in the therapist, in the patient, or in the therapy itself (see Table 4–6). This includes rational reactions such as fear when a patient becomes threat-ening, or satisfaction when a patient gets his parole. Important countertransference reactions may warn of danger, but sometimes a therapist may be unaware of the dan-ger. According to Schwartz (2003, p. 3-9), while mental health professionals are paid to deal with challenging behaviors and put up with all sorts of people, one has to won-der if a therapist who falls in love with a serial killer and throws away her career is responding to something within the prisoner or something within herself that the in-mate has tapped into. It's difficult, of course, to appreciate such unconscious evoca-tions. However, noticing your behavior toward patients will bring many such patterns to light, as when you find that you're replaying patterns of juvenile competition with your siblings. If there is trauma or victimization in your own history, dealing with abusers and predators may bring up strong feelings that the patient will perceive. These feelings can be triggered by characteristics such as physical traits or behaviors, linguistic characteristics, or similar aspects of their lifestyle or history (Schwartz 2003, p. 3-10).

In prison we expect to work with patients who have low frustration tolerance, poor coping skills, and anger control issues. Nevertheless, we have our own low threshold when encountering threatening and potentially violent behaviors. If you feel the in-terview setting has become unsafe, immediately call for help and/or terminate the in-terview. If you are getting the feeling that a patient is "grooming you" for an assault, develop a plan to change therapists or provide other safety factors. Prisoners may also become possessive of you and jealous of others' access to you, creating assaults and hos-tility among the prisoners themselves.

A less-threatening affect, boredom, arises frequently in all types of therapy, but the supportive psychotherapist might be tempted to attribute it to the supposedly mun-dane or prosaic nature of the work. Rarely is this the case. Often boredom is generated because the patient is avoiding productive therapeutic work and/or obscuring feel-ings in a wealth of detail. Or the therapist may be bored because she cannot move the therapy onward.

Think about your attitudes toward your work and the institution. These could be described as your own "institutional transference." For example, Gould (2003) has written a detailed analysis of power relationships in correctional institutions. Psychol-ogists can be drawn to extremes of tough and soft stances toward patients. The tough stance makes psychologists similar to correctional officers. The weak stance makes them vulnerable to manipulation. The alternative is a professional, neutral stance in which the psychologist "advocates for what is fair and humane....It is important to be fair, upfront, and consistent with inmates" (Gould 2003, p. 1-24). According to Gould's analysis, there are major differences between traditional mental health treatment and correctional psychology. We have adapted some of his comparisons in Table 4–7. Per-haps you will feel that your training makes you tend to work on the left side of the table but that your work experience moves you toward the right. In doing supportive work, we do think you can often (but not always) work successfully on the left side of the table.

TABLE 4–6.   **Causes of countertransference**

Within the therapist

Different racial/cultural/ethnic background from patient

Mutual blind spots shared with the patient (arising from similar personal or cultural assumptions)

Avoidance of important issues ("pseudomutuality")

Assumptions (often unconscious) about prisoners or criminals

Idealized perception of role as healer and helper

Personal "gut" response to knowledge of patient's crimes (e.g., therapist was a victim of violence and patient committed a similar crime)

Personal reaction to patient's style of talking or complaining

Inadequate understanding of the patient's mental illness

Transferential elements in therapist's past (patient evokes relationship with significant others in therapist's past, both positive or negative, such as a benevolent father or an abusive one)

Pity

Unresolved issues in the therapist's life

Overidentification and sympathy in place of empathy

Admiration and identification with a high-profile patient

Within the patient

Criminal lifestyle issues (see maneuvers illustrated in Table 4–9)

Splitting

Pathological lying

Psychopathy

Symptomatic behavior

Primitive affect

Poor hygiene and self-care

Lack of insight

Repetitive failures in coping

Intelligence and verbal ability different from the therapist's

Lack of motivation

Nonadherence with medication regimen

Nonadherence with other prescribed therapies

Failure to follow the therapist's advice

Hurtful behavior toward family members

Dependent traits (see below)

Within the therapy

Real relationship too intense

Dependency on the therapist

Anger and/or hostility toward the therapist

Paranoid or threatening behavior

Manipulation

Persistent suicidality or creation of emergencies

"Acting out" in the therapy

"Acting out" outside the therapy

Time demands on the therapist (e.g., the "difficult" patient)

Stress in the therapeutic session

TABLE 4–7.   **Differences between mental health training and correctional psychology demands**

Traditional mental health treatment	Correctional psychology
Follows medical model; patient not to blame for illness and not responsible	Follows moral model; holds that criminal is responsible for criminality
Supports patient's strengths	Shows patient to be using dysfunctional defenses and criminal thinking
Generally trusts and believes patient	Is wary of trusting prisoners and expects that there will be lying and criminal maneuvers to defeat or impair therapy
Allows patient to lead the therapy (e.g., rideshare client sets destination with rideshare driver)	Expects the therapist to drive (patient is picked up by a car with a set destination)
Follows patient's values	Expects the therapist to teach prosocial values
Has as its goals the alleviation of negative feelings and improvement of self-esteem	Has as its goal to teach critical and moral attitudes toward behavior
Concerns itself first with patient welfare	Concerns itself first with the safety of others (e.g., potential victims) and the public
Works to alleviate guilt	Works to induce guilt
Concerns itself with how the patient feels	Concerns itself with how the person acts
Holds that the patient is accountable to self	Holds that prisoner is accountable to society
Maintains reasonable confidentiality (with the usual exceptions)	Maintains limited confidentiality
Relies on clinical judgment	Relies on team decisions or administrative orders

Source.   Partly based on Gould 2003, p. 1-23.

Can a Tiger Lose Its Stripes?

The above is a question that you, throughout your career, must answer, or at least try to answer—perhaps differently at different times. That is: Will criminals always be criminals? Will those bad boys always be bad boys? Or can they change? Your attitude toward this (a form of countertransference) affects your therapy.

Are criminals intrinsically or genetically different from other people? There is still a lot of speculation about these issues. Can criminals be reborn? Does this require a religious conversion or rebirth, or is there some other way they can be "reborn" and rise from the ashes of their past lives and become lawful citizens? Is this possibility merely a science fiction or fantasy believed only by prison reformers? Like a recovered coronavirus victim, can a reformed prisoner be "reinfected" with the "illness" of criminality, or will he be free of reinfection for life? Is there some way we can "immunize" our young people against the scourge of criminality? What does that take? Healthier families, schools, neighborhoods, and jobs? The slow and painful correction of systemic racism and social injustice?

We will elucidate this issue with a true story.

For many years, the Las Vegas strip was dominated by the famous animal act of Siegfried (Fischbacher) and Roy (Horn). Siegfried and Roy trained wild animals and showed them off spectacularly on stage. They performed 5,000 shows. They were also famous for saving tigers and lions from extinction. But the show ended abruptly in 2003, on Roy's 59th birthday, when his starring beautiful tiger, Mantacore, attacked him on the neck. Roy Horn recovered slowly, painfully, and partially from that attack, and lived on much longer until he was finally attacked and killed by the coronavirus. His name lives on in the memory of Las Vegans and on one of their thoroughfares ("Roy Horn of Siegfried and Roy Dies From Coronavirus at 75" 2020). (Siegfried also died, at the beginning of 2021, not from COVID-19 but from cancer.)

There were some jaded folks in the entertainment industry who reacted to Roy's tragic accident with the comments, "What did you expect? Despite all that training, a tiger is still a tiger. A tiger never loses its stripes." In fact, there was some disagreement about what had happened. Some people said that Roy had made a mistake in departing from his usual routine. Some said that a person in the audience with a wild hairdo had upset the animal. Roy himself proposed the theory that Mantacore was trying to save him. Roy said he was feeling dizzy and fainted, and Mantacore dragged him off the stage to protect him from the crowds. The U.S. Department of Agriculture even investigated the incident but came to no conclusion.

So, what is the upshot? You shouldn't be surprised by a tiger being a tiger, and you shouldn't be surprised when a criminal behaves like a criminal? Don't take those criminals personally. Don't fault a criminal for being a criminal. They're going to think and behave like criminals, and it's not your fault if they cannot change. As we mentioned earlier, Sharp (2006) says that criminals choose 100% of the time to be criminals but that they can be changed by cognitive restructuring. To us, this appears to be a challenge. Is this "cognitive restructuring" a way to teach them the "cognitive" error of their ways? How simple! Why didn't anyone think of this before? Sharp's work is based on the criminology theories of Yochelson and Samenow (1976) and the criminal thinking styles similar to those we introduced from Walters.

Or would you take Roy's position and believe the best of Mantacore—that Mantacore had acted out of benevolence and had not reverted to his original violent nature? In other words, even after you get bitten in the neck (figuratively, we hope) by one of your patients, do you still attribute the best of motives? Or the worst? Can you *blame* them for being criminals or *forgive* them for being criminals because of why they became criminals?

If we were to ask you if you believed either of the following statements, would you find these to represent the extremes?

- Everyone consciously chooses everything they do in life.
- No one should be held responsible for anything they do.

Surely the latter must be false, or why would we be responsible, moral, human beings? But the first statement must be also false, if only because Freud convinced us that some of our motives and knowledge are not consciously known. Most theories of criminology take a stand on how much of criminal behavior is the responsibility of the criminals themselves. And from that seem to derive the various agendas of what should be done in criminal justice systems.

Know yourself (as Socrates said) and where you stand on this issue. We are not telling you *where* you should stand. Rather, we ask you to *know where* you stand. Can a prisoner ever shed his stripes for good? When it comes down to the crunch, will the criminal show his true nature? Are you disappointed when they trick you, cheat you, or sue you? Will criminals always be criminals? Is it foolish to label criminals "criminals" because it is a self-fulfilling prophecy? Will a lying liar always lie? Or can some criminals change in some degree, in partnership in psychotherapy? Your therapy is affected by your attitude toward these issues. And to end on a more somber note (this one about leopards, or perhaps "Spots and Stripes Forever"), a longitudinal study concluded that "no evidence has been produced to indicate that policies that have increased the probability of arrest, punishment severity, and average length of sentence have significantly deterred the likelihood of subsequent criminal behavior" (Ezell and Cohen 2002). But could that be because none of those policies directly address the social injustices that contribute to crime?

In the wake of the many mass shootings in the United States, forensic psychiatrists reminded us that it is comforting, and a temptation (but not true), to assume violence (e.g., of mass shooting) arises from some sort of mental aberration or illness (Knoll and Pies 2020). So we urge you to avoid a "rush to diagnose" persons with bizarre or cruel or unthinkable behaviors or crimes. The rush to diagnose may just be a countertransference reaction that somebody who is "so bad" must be mentally ill.

Burnout

Job stress refers to the psychological reactions of tension, anxiety, frustration, and worry that are caused by work (Lambert and Hogan 2018). *Burnout* is farther along the scale. You can get burnt out by caring too much, working too hard, or having a sense that you can never do enough. "Burnout is an umbrella term for a wide range of experiences with similarities and significant differences" (Summers 2020, p. 898). For example, you might think that you can never work hard enough and that people will die if you don't do everything yourself (Van Dernoot Lipsky and Burk 2009, p. 59, talking about an attorney for people sentenced to capital punishment). Admirable, but there is a risk of overcommitment. Another person says that the pressure is phenomenal and he needs to have 10 copies of himself to get the work done because "extinction is forever" (Van Dernoot Lipsky and Burk 2009, p. 58). This is from a researcher attempting to prevent the extinction of frogs. Also admirable, and we would hate to live in a world where Kermit was the only representative of a previously living species, but there is a limit to what one individual can do, and in fact acknowledging the importance of collaborative care is one means of preventing burnout (Kern 2018). Van Dernoot Lipsky and Burk do think that the animal researcher has succumbed to some grandiosity, or an inflated sense of importance related to his work.

Burnout can affect all workers in the helping professions. There was a resurgence of interest in it when health care systems were overwhelmed with coronavirus patients. Prisoners who never imagined being released were suddenly infused with (often false) hope. In the systems that we worked in, our existing patients worried about catching the illness, and others who would not normally be patients developed anxiety disorders. For months we listened to complaints about the disinfectant spray that was being used to sanitize the facility. The usual bunch of prisoners started complaining about the violations of their rights, and some said they were suicidal. It was not an easy year facing genuine and feigned illness, or genuine and mock outrage.

The fundamental features of burnout are exhaustion, cynicism, and a sense of in-effectiveness in one's work (Moffic et al. 2020). Exhaustion is a basic feature, and disengagement a coping response. Depression often occurs and should be treated, and depressogenic work factors should be addressed such as by maximizing autonomy (Summers et al. 2020, 2021). Debate continues about whether calling the condition "burnout" is a way that mental health practitioners want to avoid considering themselves to have a mental illness themselves (Badre 2020). Other features noted years ago were fatigue, irritability, gastrointestinal upset, insomnia, dysphoria, anxiety, and lack of curiosity (Caton 1984). Burnout per se is not listed in DSM-5 or DSM-5-TR but is coded in ICD-10. Burnout is an issue for all clinicians, including nurses and physicians, whose burnout rate is twice as high as that of other professions (Babyar 2017). Some widely used instruments to measure burnout are the Maslach Burnout Inventory (Maslach and Jackson 2020) and the Oldenburg Burnout Inventory (Reis et al. 2015).

There are many studies of burnout in the correctional occupations, including among correctional psychologists. Some staff claim burnout but use it as an excuse for failure to address possible avenues of change. Associating with defeated and unhappy staff, including overworked correctional officers, can easily defeat your enthusiasm. Morgan (2010) surveyed levels of burnout of psychologists in university counseling centers, VA facilities, public psychiatric hospitals, and correctional facilities. Correctional psychologists fared poorly in job burnout but better in life satisfaction, and the author concluded that the remedies for burnout should include improving professional identity.

Burnout and its causes appear to reside in broad system factors that influence both physician wellness and patient care (Pollock 2018). Using a model comparing the job demands and job resources enables researchers to understand how to bring those two closer together so the discrepancy does not create job stress. On the side of the individual worker are role stressors (role conflict, role ambiguity, and role overload), work-family conflict, and perception of danger or fear of victimization. The job resource side includes input into decision-making, instrumental communication, and quality supervision that is supportive and considerate. Interventions include those that reduce fear of victimization, improve input in the organization's decisions, and bolster the sense of procedural justice in the workplace, and training to reduce conflict at work and home (Lambert and Hogan 2018). These include employee assistance programs, peer support groups, social activities, and training in relaxation.

In another article, which notes that there have been more than 6,000 studies on burnout (Lambert et al. 2015, citing Schaufeli et al. 2009), the observation is made that correctional staff believe in both support for punishment and support for treatment. As a staff person "burns out," there is a shift from supporting treatment to supporting punishment. The authors conclude, "Emotional burnout can take its toll psychologically on a person, which could result in a person developing unfavorable views toward inmates. Staff suffering from high levels of burnout may take their frustration out on inmates through reduced support for treatment and increased desire for punishment" (Lambert et al. 2015, p. 4).

Table 4–8 presents what we think are important causes of burnout related to countertransference. Professional organizations recognize the risk of burnout. For example, the American Psychiatric Association (2021) and the American Psychological Association (Clay 2018) both have resources. Recommendations include:

- Access your self-care resources, including a new self-care assessment for psychologists (Dorociak et al. 2017).
- Try mindfulness.
- Change the way you think about your work.
- Get moving. Both cardiovascular and resistance training seem to help.
- Get political. Listen to those podcasts you like and seek social justice. For example, consider how to advocate for social justice (Jacobs and Vance 2020) and how to address racism in the correctional setting (El-Amin and Sufrin 2020).
- Unplug during nonwork hours both technologically and mentally.

You Are in Control

When you are managing therapy, it is a good idea to remember that in the end, as much as you may have ceded the therapy session to the patient for the duration, you remain in control. And we all know what "control" means, since it the central office that controls and announces movements through the facility. *The Outer Limits*, the legendary 1963 TV series, began with a picture of an oscilloscope and a "control voice" that intoned:

> There is nothing wrong with your television set. Do not attempt to adjust the picture. We are controlling transmission. If we wish to make it louder, we will bring up the volume. If we wish to make it softer, we will tune it to a whisper. We will control the horizontal. We will control the vertical. We can roll the image, make it flutter. We can change the focus to a soft blur, or sharpen it to crystal clarity. For the next hour, sit quietly and we will control all that you see and hear. We repeat: There is nothing wrong with your television set. You are about to participate in a great adventure. You are about to experience the awe and mystery which reaches from the inner mind to… (Wikipedia 2020b)

No, we are not suggesting that you emulate the control voice of *The Outer Limits*. This is not exactly an egalitarian view of psychotherapy, but it is a reminder that ultimately the control of the session is up to you. Most of the time, you and your patient may be partners or co-creators, but there are many times that you can or must assume control. You can tone down, slow down, or moderate your patient's anger. You can rewind, pause, or repeat the production in slow motion. Do not let your patient hijack the therapy with boring or worthless details or dangerous escalation to violence. You need to know that you are in control. If not, we suggest you take a safe break. Do not let your patients destroy you. And if you let them, some of them can do that.

Engagement in Therapy

In the outside world, engagement precedes marriage, but in prison, a lot of things are topsy-turvy. Prisoners may be wedded to the institution, but they may not yet be engaged in treatment. Newly admitted individuals may be fearful of asking for help. Younger males have many concerns about seeking mental health services, as in most prisons they perceive the services as stigmatizing from their peers, a sign of weakness or of being "crazy," and isolating (i.e., resulting in social isolation or physical assignment to a different yard or unit) (Morgan et al. 2004). Suicidal inmates may be reluctant to seek care because of their fear of losing access to property, being forced to move to restrictive housing or infirmary, and experiencing a loss of privacy by monitoring (see, e.g., Bauer et al. 2011). You will become used to this "paradox." The patient admits he is suicidal but begs

TABLE 4–8.   **Avoiding countertransference burnout**

Attitude	Approach to solution
"I must personally cure my patient."	Many patients in corrections, whether criminals or not, have too much history to be 100% curable in any sense of that word. Moreover, patients in these systems are treated in a team and with team responsibility. You should accept your role on a treatment team offering long-term interventions, but you can still enjoy the successes (balanced by some setbacks) that you will see in therapy.
"My mentally ill patients do not appreciate me."	Patients with serious mental illness (SMI) have their ups and downs, but most of the time they do appreciate your supportive role in their care. There are many satisfactions in helping seriously mentally ill patients.
"I don't know what to do."	Learn from your colleagues and professional meetings. Your colleagues are a great resource. There is also a vast research and technical literature (and to a lesser extent, the funding to implement it) in correctional treatment. Make use of it.
"It's depressing to deal with all these hopeless prisoners all day."	You do have to be realistic with what you can do, given the abuse and disadvantage that many of your patients have experienced. Look at your treatment plans and find some small areas where you can make progress.
"Criminals do not want to change."	It depends on the criminal. There is a body of published data that shows that they can change, but effecting change often requires intensive programming.

you not to take him out of his cell, and you reluctantly tell him that you must. But you wonder what is going to happen the next time. Will he tell—or just make the attempt?

Triage and Supportive Psychotherapy

Your time is limited. Patients with severe mental illness may require a certain number of sessions or time, whether that really benefits them or not. You have other commitments, such as to the groups that you do and your department meetings. There are patients in crisis, patients in the infirmary, lockdowns, and so forth, possibly resulting in your having to cancel some of your other sessions with existing patients. But within those, try to control your time and to the extent that your patients need it. Possibly there will be some patients who are easier to spend time with or more interesting than the others or simply less threatening. It is a small indulgence to your countertransference, to spend your time with them. But you need to distinguish between a small indulgence and unfairness to the others.

There are "therapy junkies" inside prison just as well as outside. You will hear the cries of "I need more time" and "I need an extra session now!" Requests of this sort may be justified but should only be considered based on the concept of triage: the people who need it should get it, and the people who don't need it should not get it. Mention that frequent "cries of wolf" will eventually fall on deaf ears. Yes, there are patients in perpetual crisis and the usual "frequent fliers" to the infirmary, but eventually you will find the proper methods for dealing with them. Many patients want to show that they are particularly likeable (or good) so as to deserve the extra time. You are usually better off explaining what you are doing when you do it. You are giving them extra time, which is what you would do for anybody in the same position. Everybody gets what they need. Everybody is special, but nobody is more special than anybody else. "No one has to think they win favors from me." You must be prepared to be told that they have seen you are giving an extra session to some other specified person. Your answer will be, "If they got it, they needed it. But thank you for mentioning it, because I wouldn't want you to be bothered by the thought that I play favorites."

Treatment Planning

Treatment planning can be challenging. Collaboration with other staff may be limited. Long-term treatment and planning may be interrupted by unpredictable transfers or expiration of sentences, limited movement, attorney visits and court dates, and disciplinary actions.

Many good treatment planning guides are available. The well-known series by Jongsma and associates has one about parole and probation but not specifically for prisons (Bogue et al. 2012). The manualized programs that we discuss throughout this book have great strengths and suggest success on many fronts, but they are not universally adapted by prison systems, dropout rates are high, and a program may be a one-size-fits-all for the participants. Moreover, such programs are oriented at behaviors and attitudes, not necessarily the mental health of incarcerated people. To date, the research on the effectiveness of these programs has been focused mainly on recidivism as a measure of success. Most are group programs that leave little room for adaptation for mental illness. However, within those guides, there are excellent suggestions for individual activities and topics for psychotherapy patients (see, e.g., Berman 2015; Mariush 2002; Tafrate et al. 2018; Wanberg and Milkman 2008).

Figure 4–1 is a treatment plan modeled after ones we have used. We still like the venerable problem-oriented treatment record originated by Lawrence Weed (1969) (see also Ryback et al. 1981); you start with a patient problem list, linking it to goals of treatment and specific interventions to meet those goals.

Another concept is the SMART acronym—Specific, Measurable, Achievable, Relevant, and Time-Bound—which originated in the business (not medical) sector in 1981 (Doran 1981). However, a short trip through the blogosphere shows that Doran himself did not think that every goal could be assigned all five criteria, and many who follow the SMART model admit that not all worthwhile goals may be measurable. But SMART is still useful as a general guide, and it is easy to find ways to measure things once you get the hang of it. For example, most feelings, moods, or urges can be reported using numerical scales, and there are published scales for nearly everything. An example is the Brief Psychiatric Rating Scale (BPRS; Overall and Gorham 1962), another standby in the mental health field, and the original version is in the public domain. The original assesses 18 items— and later versions do 24—on a 7-point scale. Items include anxiety, depression, guilt, and hallucinations. A search will yield numerous links to the instrument itself. But you do not have to use the whole instrument. You can measure a patient's rating on an individual item (e.g., "Patient's depression is rated as less than 3 on the BPRS 7-point scale").

One link in our neck of the woods we found at San Mateo County Health (2020). Or you can simply report the number of days per week or month that a patient has delusions or hallucinations. The Patient Health Questionnaire–9 (PHQ-9; Kroenke et al. 2001) developed by Robert Spitzer and others is also unrestricted and can be used to measure progress in therapy (American Psychological Association 2020). However, see the caveat in Chapter 9 about using it to measure absolute severity of depression.

Our approach is modular and concise. Call it the "KISS" method—no, not in recognition of the rock group, but for the acronym "Keep It Simple and Supportive." That means, according to Ward et al. (2006):

- Foster patient participation and buy-in.
- Maximize patient autonomy despite the correctional environment.
- When it doesn't conflict with prosocial goals, address patient self-esteem issues.
- Aim for approach goals rather than avoidance goals (a technique used in the Good Lives Model of treatment that is discussed in Chapter 13).

In addition to the scales mentioned above, you can use the Rosenberg Self Esteem Scale (Rosenberg 2021).

We don't try for more than five problems or objectives on a treatment plan, and we preface it with a short blurb, not a five-page psychodynamic case formulation. It is easy to update and extend your blurb each time you update the plan. As each objective is reached, a new one is developed. Some objectives will be physical, such as addressing sleep problems, medicine side effects, and appetite; others will be related specifically to the mental distress or illness presented and include activities that are designed to help. Developing a treatment plan in prisons and jails, as in other settings, should begin collaboratively with the patient. Ownership of the plan is key to encouraging your patient to adhere to it.

Treatment planning makes it possible for staff to work together:

- To develop and establish plans for the therapy.
- To make sense of the process and be able to measure progress.
- To give therapist and patient an understanding of the problems and the process for improving the patient's mental health.
- To coordinate care across therapy sessions, groups, psychoeducational activities, and medication.
- To provide information to the nonmedical staff in the event of disciplinary actions.
- To identify goals and progress made for both the staff and the patient and to have information in modifying the activities and goals as therapy proceeds.
- To provide a record of the therapy for future placement of the individual in programs within the institution, in transfers from one institution to another, and in providing information to agencies outside the institution once the prisoner is eligible for release.

Treatment planning helps the therapist:

- To provide a pathway for the patient to learn to identify and manage symptoms and progress.

Brief History

Mr. Jones is a 35-year-old single man who has been struggling with a psychotic mental illness for 15 years. Now he is in prison for the third time for possession with intent to sell methamphetamine. He has had three previous inpatient psychiatric hospitalizations, the latest in 2019, which lasted for 2 weeks. He has previous convictions for assault with a deadly weapon and a DUI. He has two sons by his previous marriage. He has never gotten his GED. He has been in the county mental health clinics, but he never seems to stick with his medicines. We've got a lot of issues to tackle with this patient, but no one seems to be able to turn around his mental health conditions or his criminal behaviors. He could probably be a better father, too.

DSM-5 Diagnoses

Methamphetamine use disorder, severe; alcohol use disorder, severe

Schizophrenia

Adult antisocial behavior (but we do not think he is a lifestyle criminal)

Problem List

Patient has a history of suicide attempts (a priority safety issue)

He gets into fights frequently (and he does that when he is in jail or prison) (interpersonal issue)

He was using methamphetamine (substance issues and alcohol)

He hears voices (mental health issue); we may not be able to fit every single problem on the treatment plan, but these might be the ones to target in the initial plan

Long-Term Goals   Target Date: 6 months

Get his GED

No suicide attempts in 6 months or tells therapist prior to considering an attempt

No institutional discipline for at least 6 months

Complete his co-occurring disorders classes

Current Objectives (Short-Term Goals)   Target Date: 90 days

State he is hearing hallucinations less than one day a week

Attend all his group meetings

Attend 90% of his medical management and adhere to his mutually agreed-on treatment plan

Attend 90% of his psychotherapy sessions

Make at least a monthly contact with his two sons

FIGURE 4–1. Sample treatment plan.

Interventions

Psychotherapy every 2 weeks by Dr. Able
Medication management monthly by Dr. Baker
Exercise in the yard (daily, self-directed); Diet for Health
Written assignment at every therapist meeting
Coping skills review and repetition at every therapist meeting
Controlled breathing and mindfulness taught once and review in 2 months
Co-occurring disorders group twice a week
Attendance at his substance user group
GED classes

Follow-up and Review Date(s)

3 months
6 months

Signatures and Dates

Therapist/Case Manager

_____Date_____

Prescribing Provider

_____Date_____

Social Worker

_____Date_____

Patient (I agree with this treatment)

_____Date_____

Patient (I DO NOT AGREE with this treatment plan)

_____Date_____

Reasons_____

FIGURE 4–1. Sample treatment plan. (*continued*)

- To help the patient develop skills in formulating goals and learning the steps needed to attain them.
- To identify problems that can be addressed in therapy and other interventions such as social, vocational, or academic training.
- To individualize the goals for the patient.
- To encourage adherence to the plan and participation in the success of therapy.
- To identify any changes and adapt the treatment to new or newly identified problems.

Treatment plans should take into account the assessments performed in admitting the person to the facility as well as any history of treatment prior to admission. Plans should be individualized, with the patient and the therapist identifying problems and possible solutions, ways to measure progress, and aspects that lend themselves to adjustments as therapy progresses (Makover 2016; Novalis et al. 2020). Treatment actions should be usually phased in to streamline the process for the patient and avoid overwhelming him with too many concepts at once. Changes should be gradual across the therapy as appropriate to the individual (Yee 1989). Participation in developing the plan and monitoring its success will give the patient a sense of control and accomplishment as well as teaching him self-management. It is important to communicate the treatment plan both verbally and in writing, since a large proportion of prisoners have limited reading skills, and repetition is necessary as well. Homework assignments should be behavioral for the most part and tailored to your patients' educational levels as well as their mental health needs (Aufderheide 2013).

Techniques to Make Treatment More Effective

Treatment plans are made more effective by effective therapy. In the next few pages, we will discuss a variety of techniques.

Generating and Conveying Empathy

There is something primal and noncerebral in establishing a relationship with another person, especially a prisoner who may have had a life of abuse from trusted others. One psychologist working in jail says that therapists bring to the therapy something that is decidedly animalistic or mammalian in nature that patients do not even experience in childhood because it is a basic animal function that is adaptive in the way that fear and aggression are. He likens this quality to the nurturing features experienced with attachment, safety, connections, or even love (Rajagopal 2016).

Earlier, we noted the difference between empathy and sympathy. Experienced therapists have a repertory of empathic statements. These can be the simply echoing back of things the patients have said. A classic therapist, Leston Havens, recommended "simple empathic statements" like "How awful," "It must have hurt," and "You wanted to be loved," which often extrapolate slightly from the patient's own statements to show that the therapist has been listening closely (Havens 1978). More complex empathic statements begin with the recognition of the patient's isolation ("No one understands you") and the validation of the patient's responses to experience ("No wonder you were frightened") (Havens 1979).

Many other supportive techniques can be used, frequently several in one therapy session. You can tell a woman who has had a succession of abusive partners, "You seem to be a loyal and loving person. You fall in love with people who seem needy and you try to help them, but they need too much, maybe too much. You are caring and you want to save people, maybe in the way you tried to save your alcoholic father. Now we see that you probably need to choose a more reliable partner, or find a way to go it alone, but not to allow yourself to fall into an abused situation." Here you are reflecting (on her history of abuse), reframing (her loyalty and not poor judgment was partially responsible for her victimization), emphasizing her strengths (caring, helping), empowering her to avoid victimization in the future, and instilling hope (see below).

Instilling Hope

The meme "Hope is not a strategy" has been batted or bruited about for years in politics (both sides of the aisle), the military, and the world of sales and investment (see Your Dictionary 2020). We also chanced to read about another "Gray Man" (i.e., a prisoner), a fictional anti-hero former CIA operative trying to get himself back on the right side of the law or get killed in the process. At the beginning of the book, he reflects on the fact that his trainer imbued him with that advice and says he agrees with it, but by the end of the book, he decides it conveys a pragmatic truth (Greaney 2020, p. 4). But references to the value of hope abound in literature, and as in our previously quoted psychologist/detective series, it is said that there is nothing without hope (Kellerman 1995, p. 145). There is a value to instilling hope in people who lack it. Some prisoners are so bad off that you may feel you are lying to express any hope for them at all. But you may have to nurture some kind of hope even if you expect your nose to grow like Pinocchio's. Perhaps they won't believe it, but there is at least one case in which you may need to cross your fingers and offer it: When you are dealing with an acute suicidal crisis. Is it a lie to say, "You'll get through this. You'll feel better soon"? Would you rather tell them that you think they are hopeless and that they will probably be dead in a year? Of course, we also warned you some time back against offering false reassurances. We do mean that—*in general*. Don't promise something you can't deliver (like a trip home), but do promise something you can (your hope for their future). An expectation to get well in other contexts has been called a *placebo effect*. Studies show that "expectancy or placebo effects account for 15% of the variance in positive client outcomes" (Scott 2008, p. 39, citing Asay and Lambert 1999). And while we're at it, the same source asserts that "the quality of the therapeutic relationship accounts for 30% of the change that clients experience in treatment." (Scott 2008, p. 37). Not just fictional characters but practicing clinicians emphasize the value of hope in psychotherapy (Benabio 2019).

Reframing

You can reframe just about anything, and do it many times, although if you reframe a physical picture, it would surely fall apart eventually. Reframing is a well-known and perhaps well-worn technique in which the meaning or purpose of a puzzling or misunderstood behavior is reexplained in a positive manner. You are used to our caveats by now, so it should be no surprise when we say that there is potential danger in normalizing criminal behavior by reframing; both reframing and normalizing criminal behavior must be done with caution. We do reframe behaviors of seeking out abusive partners and well-meaning but misguided attempts to save one's abusive parents. You have to point out that it is not "stupid" to find such a partner but that it might be an attempt to save the mother or father you could not save and is just unlikely to succeed. Similar reframes can also be used when a person tends to become codependent to drug abusers in an apparent attempt to save them.

Adjusting the Therapy to the Patient (One Size Does Not Fit All)

"Sicker" does not necessarily translate into "more therapy." For example, stable patients with schizophrenia may not have much to say and merely need to touch base with you occasionally and briefly. Patients in the infirmary may need a session of variable length daily or twice daily. You can start with a trial and see if therapy benefits the patient. You can try short sessions and see if they should be made longer, but make sure you explain this in advance so your patients do not feel you are cutting them short. Some brief in-office checks can be done in a few minutes. (We are not referring to the brief cell-side safety and wellness checks, which are not psychotherapy.) Medical practitioners in most settings are used to task-driven rather than time-driven endpoints for services, but the traditional payment systems for psychotherapy are time-based. Except as required by your documentation system, you have considerable control over the time you spend with patients.

Reacting and Adjusting to Your Patient's Style

Monitor the pace and content of therapy and adjust it as necessary. If the patient is getting too emotional, interrupt in a caring way with a desire for details. "Whoa there, I'm lost. Who did this to you and when? What year did this happen? Tell me his name, so I can separate him out from your other brothers." And so forth. Of course, many patients have a lot to unload in the first session. Crying does not mean they will cry for the rest of the afternoon, but you should monitor strong emotions and moderate them as well. "Okay now, slow down, calm down." You will be using your voice to teach guided imagery, meditation, and progressive relaxation.

Developing Your Own Impression

Diagnoses change, and you should avoid locking into a diagnosis and formulation within the first hours. Compare your diagnosis to the record, but don't automatically let the record prevail. Cultivate a flexible style that is in many aspects matched to the patient's own style of perceiving or communicating. For example, an overly intellectual patient may do best with intellectual explanations (Dewald 1971, p. 105). Pay attention to the patient's preferred sensory modality (e.g., visual, auditory, tactile), his rate and style of speech, or the type of metaphors he uses.

Also, as you home in on your patient's style, keep in mind that your patient is reading you like a book. He is picking up your intonations and your nonverbal behavior, including facial expressions, gestures, and body language. Psychotic patients are actually quite adept at that because they tend to discount words and go directly to your emotional expression.

Case Vignette

The therapist began interviewing a floridly manic young woman who had just been brought into the office by her CO. Certainly, there was no reason to think she would be assaultive, and there were plenty of other people around who would intervene if that happened. After a few minutes, she announced: "You're really afraid of me, aren't you? Do you think I'm going to hit you? I'm not going to hit you…I'm not going to hit you!" The therapist admitted she was right, but added: "It's not that I really think you would hit me, but that's the emotional reaction you generated in me. And I'm a therapist. Do you realize what kind of a reaction you are creating in your cellmates and in your CO who brought you in here? What should we do about it?" The patient agreed to treatment.

You will develop your own styles or even stylistic quirks. One of the things we struggle with ourselves is what is called "the editorial we," that is, the use of "we" to refer to oneself. In psychotherapy, it is indeed helpful to refer to the "we" or "us" that is the two of you, as in "What did we talk about yesterday?" This use is a normal way (sometimes called "joining") to maintain a therapeutic alliance. We also described confrontations as "a looking at together" rather than a "face-off" off between you and your patient. You can say, possibly a little sardonically, "We just can't have you quitting your job, can we?" However, we do not use "we" exclusively, and we avoid it when it seems patronizing. We prefer to use "I" when we are emphasizing a personal concern, such as in "I am worried about that cut on your arm. How did that happen?"

Asking Permission

There is also nothing wrong with asking permission. "Are you ready to talk about your father? I still have a few questions about him." You will develop your stylistic opening sentences. It depends on what works for you and them.

Exploring Surface Issues

A therapist begins in a matter-of-fact but empathic way to explore surface issues. "This has been a difficult time of your life." The explorations become deeper as they turn to the patient's feelings about events in his life. "You seem to be worried about the financial burdens your imprisonment is putting on your family." Or "You've told me that the voices you hear have been bothering you less since you started taking medicine." Summaries can be made which are an extension of the patient's chief complaint. "It seems that your most important concern is having a place to stay when your sentence expires."

Making "Happy Talk"

"Happy Talk" was a song from the 1949 Rodgers and Hammerstein musical *South Pacific*. In it, Bloody Mary sings about her dreams for the future. It has had some famous covers, such as Ella Fitzgerald's, although the original song has been considered racist because of its artificial pidgin language. However, the term "happy talk" is now given to the friendly banter between newscasters, such as when there is a transition between segments, and we have recently heard it used to mean the overly optimistic talk of some politicians. Any of these meanings can be put to use in your sessions—that is, talk of hopes and dreams, bantering or friendly filler talk, and perhaps a little overly optimistic talk. Just be aware of what you say and why you say it. You are trying to show empathy, build rapport, develop a positive transference, and so on.

Some part of a therapy session should focus on immediate goals. "Just talking" is not forbidden, as long as *you* know that "just talking" is not what the patient might mean by "two friends just having a conversation." It should also not be allowed to become an abusive harangue as we previously suggested can happen when a patient "hijacks" control of the session. But you can also start with "What shall we accomplish *today*?" or "How would you like to be improved when you walk out of here?" Sharing their lives is an important part of supportive psychotherapy for most people, so you need not feel obliged to interrupt a long conversation as long as it does not serve as resistance or a defense against talking about more sensitive matters that need to be addressed immediately. If it is an avoidance of an issue—a frequent one we find is that the patient has just been sanctioned for a fight, harboring contraband, or so forth—then the conversation should be diverted.

Correcting Early Problems

Dealing with problematic feelings early correlates with success in therapy. As Foreman and Marmar (1985) recommend:

- Examine your countertransference such as your feelings of boredom or being entertained or being threatened.
- Watch the patient: Does she seem bored? Does she seem anxious to end the session?
- Bring up the treatment plan and mutually decide if you are achieving its goals; if not, what next? Change the plan or change the therapy.
- Remember that it is okay to ask for feedback.
- Look for "acting out," such as getting into fights after a therapy session. Is the patient really displacing the anger he has at you?
- Don't assume that every behavior has a purpose. Many therapists believe that every behavior has a purpose, and Freud even thought that many behaviors are overdetermined. But we disagree. *Ipso facto*, every behavior has a cause but not necessarily a purpose, if by purpose you mean some conscious, stated purpose of the actor. Some behaviors are like leftover random habits, or they can reflect the repetition compulsions that Freud described.
- Try this: "I recognize what you are trying to do, but you are not going about it in the best way."
- Confront threatening and abusive patients.

Generating an Expectation of Realistic Gains

Psychotherapies may be effective because they generate an expectation of success. For example, a patient may talk in a second session of getting her "first good night's sleep" after the first session. Although it serves little purpose to *tell* prisoners that you will be a warm, supportive force in their lives who will lighten their burdens and lift their spirits, it does help to try to foster positive expectations and minimize negative ones by the encounter itself, its emotional subtleties and understatements, and the maturation of trust.

Continuing Working on Issues That Are Likely to Be Ongoing

Ongoing issues are those that you want to address after you have established rapport and developed the supportive relationship and alliances. These may include recovery and empowerment from past trauma, amelioration of mental distress, development of a relationship to family members, and reintegration into the community. Some guidelines:

- Ask your patient to write down three things he has learned from therapy.
- And three things he wants to accomplish in future sessions.
- Ask the patient what he wished you had covered already.
- Revise your treatment plan accordingly.
- If your patient has criminogenic needs, begin to address them at the level of detail we discuss below.
- Generate positive expectations. If you have hit a rough spot in the therapy, point out that both of you were able to work through these problems in the past and move on.

Addressing Criminogenic Factors

In therapy you choose interventions based on your mutual goals of lessening future criminal behavior and recidivism. These goals may not be important for a particular patient. But if and when they become important, recall the eight criminogenic factors from Chapter 2. Table 4–9 provides strategies for countering these criminogenic thinking styles. (We defined this "gang of eight" back in Table 2–5.) In addition to the eight criminogenic risk factors, you can ask about four behavioral dimensions of a criminal lifestyle (Walters 2001): irresponsibility, self-indulgence, interpersonal intrusiveness, and social rule breaking. Although there are structured programs to teach persons with a criminal history to think in new ways, there are also individual interventions (Walters 2012, p. 123):

- Tell me about your life before crime, your initiation into crime, and how you became committed to a criminal lifestyle.
- What kept you involved in criminal activities?
- What is there that will discourage you from continued involvement in a criminal lifestyle?
- What is your view of schools, society, and work?
- How do you rate yourself on the (eight) thinking styles and (four) behavioral styles of a criminal lifestyle?
- If you were to abandon the lifestyle today, what would you miss most?
- How do you see your future?

Walters also gives general strategies to be used in therapy based on the well-known finding that many alcoholics as well as criminals naturally—that is, on their own

TABLE 4–9.   **Countering criminogenic thinking styles**

Thinking style	Description	Countering strategies
Mollification	Criminals may use false justifications to blame the victim or the injustices of society for their actions.	This is a good place to start, since there may be partial truth in the causal factors leading to their lack of opportunity in society. But while you may express some empathy with their position, you begin to point out that being poor does not justify assaulting and robbing an elderly person, stealing money from their employer of 10 years, and so forth.
Cutoff (implosion)	Criminals cut off their moral thinking using mental "memes" or "tropes" like "What the hell" or "No point thinking about it— just do it," and they also use substances to impair their judgment; many criminals report breaking the law while under the influence of substances.	This is one of the easier ones to describe but the hardest for patients to address. The strategy for countering this thinking style involves helping them to avoid the use of substances to cut off their moral thinking and the verbal or mental tricks they use for doing criminal things. Also, it involves teaching them self-control.
Entitlement	Criminals think they are unique or special and don't have to follow the rules of society (here, we see the traits of narcissistic personality disorder).	You can tell patients, as Walters (2001) does, that they misidentify wants as needs. Society is a place where people need to earn money and privileges legitimately, and criminal shortcuts do not prove one's worth. You can also explain narcissism, employing treatment strategies used by experienced therapists.
Power orientation	Criminals experience lack of power as a "zero state" that they must counteract by having power and controlling others (Walters 2001).	We want to help patients to understand their inherent sense of deficiency and deal with it, but not by grandiose attempts to exert power over others. As in the preceding category, this can require long-term therapy.
Sentimentality	Criminals think they are "good people." They give money to charity, get sentimental about pets, and support popular causes that good people support, and will point to these examples of their goodness.	You can point out that isolated instances don't make for the central elements of their lifestyle that are damaging to others and that, frankly, their "random acts of kindness" don't fool anybody.
Superoptimism	Criminals believe they won't be found out and won't be caught, and in general they are not caught (other than in that one instance that got them into prison).	You can point out the consequences of their latest crime and how any prison is full of people who were sure they would not be caught; you can also explain that their superoptimism is unrealistic and immature and will eventually deprive them of a normal life.

TABLE 4–9.   **Countering criminogenic thinking styles** *(continued)*

Thinking style	Description	Countering strategies
Cognitive indolence	Criminal reasoning is full of major gaps and flaws; they do not follow ordinary laws of logic in drawing conclusions about the world or other people.	You will have frequent opportunity to say, "Whoa, what are you saying? How in the world did you arrive at that conclusion?" Don't be too harsh at first.
Discontinuity	Unlike law-abiding people, criminals switch styles and personalities, becoming risk-taking and exhibiting criminal behavior without an awareness of the contradictions in their values.	You can point out patients' Jekyll and Hyde personalities: e.g., how they are calm in an interview but exploded and assaulted a police officer in the community. Self-control is erratic.

Source.   Suggested by and partly based on Walters 2001, but we drew the examples from multiple sources consistent with his writings.

without specific professional help—stop drinking or stop committing crimes (Walters 2002). Try these:

- Emphasize role conflicts. For example, a father is made aware that his criminal style conflicts with his desire to be a good father, husband, provider, and worker in business.
- Find substitutes for criminal behaviors, such as in work, hobbies, activities with family, and sports.
- Help patients to change their identity. We have spoken elsewhere of the use of the term "criminal." Whether or not we want to apply this label to the patient depends on the use of that term "criminal" in describing the patient's identity to her or asking her to change it. A person is told "your crimes do not make you a criminal for life, and you need to tell your friends that you are no longer a criminal, either."
- Create incongruence between patients' goals in life and their criminal lifestyle. Walters (2002) points out that criminals satisfy a certain type of need, best called "visceral," which involves immediate satisfaction and feeling. But there are also social, work, and intellectual needs. These include the desire for education, family love and attachments, and satisfactions from work. Create discrepancies between criminal goals and other goals.
- Do not assume that offenders are unmotivated in general. Rather, they may be unmotivated to do certain things and motivated to do others. For example, a patient may have a strong desire to get his college degree, not to stop robbing people.
- Address (with the appropriate level of confrontation) the externalization of blame that is heard in habitual criminal thinking. You may find that repeat offenders or lifestyle criminals blame everything except the sun and gravity for specific crimes (Sharp 2006, pp. 96–97). They blame their "wants" for drugs or money, their gang membership, or the pressures of a boyfriend or girlfriend. They will reflect, redirect, and redefine your questions. They will ask you, "Didn't you ever drink and drive, Doc?" "Didn't you ever hit your wife, Doc?" and so on.
- Help patients to find meaning in life. The psychiatrist and existential philosopher Viktor Frankl gave a name to the emptiness in people's lives that they felt between work weeks. He called it "Sunday neurosis." This meme has found its way through-

out the web, but the original, from *Man's Search for Meaning*, published in 1946 and much reprinted, is still worth reading, since Frankl's philosophy is the one about finding meaning even while imprisoned (he lost most of his family but survived being in a concentration camp). He believed that a person can survive anything if he has a meaning to live for. Frankl's writings and philosophy have been studied by prisoners, although not as widely as we would have thought. We found an interesting blog from a lawyer who fell into bad times and prison and was inspired by Frankl to become a minister (Grant 2014).

Shampoo, Rinse, Repeat: Making Use of Repetition

Therapists have always appreciated the value of repetition. If the shampoo reflects the basic explanation you intended to give in the session, the rinse represents the in-session follow-up to allow some time to wind-down and let them go back to the dorm. The "repeat" is the need to repeat the process more than once to learn the intervention permanently. Keep in mind that most of your patients are not psychologically minded. They may not even understand explanations of psychological causality. Put pithily, "They're a stranger in the land of their mind" (Battaglia 2019, p. 73).

Educational interventions should "tell 'em what you're gonna tell 'em, tell 'em, then tell 'em what you told 'em." (This has several versions, of which the earliest seems to be a from a preacher named Jowett in 1908.) Similarly, a prominent motivational writer (Lewis 2008, pp. 120–121) talks of "verbal flagging" and "call-to-action" statements to highlight advice in advance with phrases like "Here's something worth remembering," including an injunction to write it down (and as with safety plans, which we discuss in subsequent chapters, the patient—not you—should do the writing).

Hitting the Pause Button

The remote control for your cable TV probably has a button that pauses your program. Plan to do the same once in a while in therapy. If your patient is overly emotional (as often happens in an early session), learn how to hit the pause button without angering or alienating him, have him rewind a bit, repeat something again, and so forth. A common question at this stage is "Are we making progress?" Progress may be seen in words or deeds reported or deeds seen (see below). You may pick up that the patient is less distressed or disabled by his symptoms. However, if you conclude that progress is less than expected, consider the possible causes of therapeutic slow-down or stalemate in Table 4–10.

Directing the Content

Sure, there is room for a little bit of "happy talk." But general interest or sociability is not sufficient to "fill the hour" with conversation. You must usually be directive of content, especially if you are meeting with the patient as infrequently as once a month. In insight-oriented therapy, a therapist often listens to a variety of topics and finds a central theme running through them all. In the previous chapter, we called this the "red thread." In supportive therapy, the therapist does more than locate or comment on

---

TABLE 4–10.   **Causes of therapeutic slowdown**

Causes primarily in the therapeutic relationship

Transference "unbalanced" (not managed in the ways we describe)

Seriously disturbed transference (either addressed or unaddressed)

    Erotic (genuinely so or due to patient's efforts to sexualize the transference)

    Hostile (e.g., due to patient's poor parenting)

    Psychotic

Lack of relationship or therapeutic alliance (patient is not meaningfully engaged in the supportive relationship with the therapist)

Absence of transference

Causes primarily in the patient

Absence from therapy (unless caused by therapist's poor technique)

Deflation of initially high expectations

    From the therapy

    From the therapist

    From the prison mental health department

Anxiety too high from therapist's confrontations (e.g., of patient's criminal thinking styles)

Weakening of patient's defenses (e.g., inability to externalize cause of his or her failures)

Patient's feeling of being manipulated

Worsening of patient's underlying biological condition (progression or exacerbation of disease)

Change in patient's circumstances (e.g., relationships, financial, job, educational)

Negative therapeutic reactions

Causes primarily in the therapist

Countertransference reactions (does not like character or personality of person who commits crimes)

Difficulty in relating to patient with empathy (when patient is accessible)

Explanations incorrect or not comprehensible to patient (e.g., do not match the patient's ability to understand explanations)

Therapist burnout (loss of efficacy and/or satisfaction in the work)

---

these veins of thought; she must do more active data collection by taking a more directive stance.

Updating

There may be a yard and not much else of an "outside" for your patients, but there is also an outside family and community, and possibly some legal developments. We always seek continuity with "problems and promises" left over from the last session. You've got your notes to remind you, and your patient may even have forgotten what you promised to talk about in this session. It strengthens your alliance to show that you remember and you care. It also helps if you do not pause for a long time while you look up your notes, thus making it obvious that you did *not* remember.

In follow-up visits, we suggest you start with a subjective assessment (the "S" part of the classical SOAP note: subjective, objective, assessment, plan—sometimes followed by an E for education) but add what is called an "interval history" up front, and then a mental status and a suicide risk assessment, and of course complete your initial assessment and make future plans. If possible, a therapy note should discuss the interventions during the session and how they relate to the treatment plan and then relate the patient's response to the interventions or any problems that were encountered. While you are writing, ask yourself:

- Do I know what has happened in my patient's life since the last session? Can I independently verify it rather than just rely on his account?
- Is the patient relating material relevant to the treatment plan? Or does the treatment plan need revision?
- How are the transference and countertransference going?
- What is the patient's current level of function, work, and discipline?
- Has the mental status (above) changed to suggest a change in treatment needs?
- Do I need to review the history again?
- Do I need to "lay off" the more anxiety-provoking work because the patient needs more support at this time?

Normalizing

Normalizing is a technique that can be used to improve self-esteem or reduce concern over symptoms or dysfunction. We will also discuss normalizing when we talk about hallucinations in Chapter 8. For example, if a patient grieves the separation from her children, you can certainly say, "It's normal to be worried since you've never been away from your children in the past." But be careful not to normalize habitual criminal behavior. Persons with criminal lifestyles normalize (using the defense of rationalization) their criminal behaviors. Despite what they may imply or even argue to your face, criminal behavior is not the "new normal." Maybe social distancing, but not criminal activity. They may believe that "everybody steals" and "everybody uses drugs." Persons in organized crime find what they do to be entirely normal with their peer group, but they are well aware that they are not normal citizens.

Isolated offenses can be dealt with sensitively without wholesale approval. If you deal with a mother who cashed a bogus check to feed her family, do you say, "It is normal to commit a nonviolent crime to feed your children"? If so, we understand your intention, but we think you're using the wrong word. Perhaps it is "common" or "understandable" or "forgivable."

Focusing on Specific Issues

You can spend a session on a single topic or a few related topics such as family issues. Brief psychotherapy does this all the time. Some of your patients will be able to choose their own focus, but others will focus on something that is a total waste of time or deliberate diversion. The latter, like a loose lens, need constant refocusing! However, sometimes it is you who have to do some jumping around in order to cover multiple issues going on (e.g., family, legal, discipline) or some serious issue that you believe needs immediate attention (e.g., possibly suicidal statements). This is a time-honored way of doing therapy called "distributive psychotherapy" (Holmes 1988). The techniques in Chapter 2, such as restating, echoing, and tracking, can be used to reinforce areas of the conversation that you want to explore. You may sometimes have to call a dead stop, as with a prisoner who spends the first half of the session complaining about the CO who tosses her cell more frequently out of some personal animosity. "We have dealt with that (or will deal with that), but don't think we are making progress if we continue to talk about that problem. Maybe we should move on to (you name the problem)." At other times, you may want to delve into the patient's tendency to repeat certain stories and items and never resolve them ("repetition without resolution").

Noticing Discrepancies

Become familiar with the differences between behaviors in the office and behaviors on the cell block. COs and other prisoners will frequently paint a picture of the patient that is at complete variance from the one that would be painted based on the patient's in-office behavior. You yourself will often see your patient on the unit or in casual interactions with officers or other prisoners or with other providers. Make use of all your sources of information. Sometimes you will have to use them in confrontations or at least in pointing out discrepancies.

Noticing Unusual Behaviors

Unusual behaviors deserve comment. If the patient can't sit still and paces around the room, is she in a serious crisis, or is she showing the restlessness that can come from antipsychotic medications? Does the patient start filing her nails? Are you going to comment on that?

Avoiding Gifts and Gift Giving

In the prison setting, there are no gifts. Anything you give a patient, such as a handout or pages for journaling, should be part of the therapy. Anything a patient gives you, such as a drawing, can be appreciated and explained ("Did you feel you had to give me a gift?") but should be either returned or added to the patient document section of the chart. We know people who do not follow the recommendations, but we think they disregard them at their own peril (e.g., keeping portraits from a patient who is an artist).

Working With the Good Patient

Some patients seem to do everything you ask and beyond. They work all the programs, never get into discipline, and have good relationships with both staff and other prisoners. Are these patients too good to be true? Are they grooming you for a favor? The phenomenon of "institutional insight" (Weiner 1982) does apply to mentally ill patients, and another known behavior is "faking good." So it could just be that a patient with mental illness is trying to please you, but there could be ulterior motives at work. However, sometimes we do find that superficially "good" patients find that it feels good to behave as if they were good (e.g., they are not getting into discipline).

Learning About Trauma

All treatment needs to be trauma informed, and we talk about this in several other places. Learn how to elicit histories of trauma in reluctant patients at different times or when the time is right. However, we find that negative answers are sometimes understated or downright untrue. Sometimes you can get at a trauma history by asking how a patient was punished as a child.

Some patients put themselves into situations where they are likely to be retraumatized, as if they are repeating situations in which they were abused in order to change their response or "cure" the abuser. Perhaps this is one of those Freudian "repetition compulsions" that we mentioned earlier. The full understanding of these is beyond our scope, but you can use that as an explanation that gets the patient's attention and gives the behavior a name. "Let's name it so that you recognize and don't repeat it." This is a salutary use of labeling.

We have summarized some hidden issues in Table 4–11. Some of these will become obvious to you even though your patient thinks they have concealed them. An analogy (courtesy of another mystery writer) is that they are like a little treasure that a child seeks to conceal in her hand in a way that draws attention to it (Christie 1974, p. 47).

Judging the Effectiveness of Interventions

When an intervention is effective, you should expect to see changes, ranging from verbal to reported behavior to actual behavior you observe in the prison. Often, a patient should show avoidance of typical criminal excuses for behavior and increased personal responsibility incorporating more mature defenses and coping strategies.

1. Initially, a patient may seem to understand your intervention but throw it back in your face and tell you it failed. "I tried to tell the CO I had been hit, and he didn't listen to me."
2. The next stage may consist of remembering and echoing back what you said, or making a commitment to implement the intervention.
3. The next stage may show that he used the intervention and it worked. "I did what you said, I didn't hit back. I dodged him. The officer saw what happened, and he wrote up the other guy, not me!" You should reinforce such behaviors. While we said that a rule of explanation of unpleasant items is to strike while the iron is cold, a rule for reinforcement of good behaviors is to praise while the iron is still hot! "Great job. You did well!"

Being Dynamic

Finally: Session management is dynamic. It requires adjustment within each session and modification of your strategy between sessions. We also hope that you are a dynamic person, because it takes a lot of energy to do therapy in these settings!

Ending Therapy

Supportive psychotherapy can be given briefly for crisis or indefinitely for chronic illness or personal deficiencies. You can change parameters with a particular patient, varying the frequency or duration of the sessions. Depending on the mental health category of the patient, you might also be able to stop the therapy entirely. Or there may be reasons why the patient changes therapists. A planned termination also occurs when the patient leaves the institution. Each person you work with knows the grief

---

TABLE 4–11.   **Hidden issues: or, what you don't hear about can hurt the therapy**

A. Recent experiences that prisoners may not report to you
    1. Recent fight or discipline they don't want you to know about
    2. PREA incident or activity
    3. Substance use on unit
    4. Problems at home
    5. Legal developments in the case (may be positive or negative)
    6. Abuse or bullying on the unit (by staff or prisoners)
    7. Suicidal thinking
    8. Other but nonsuicidal symptoms (e.g., not talking about hallucinations)
    9. Change in job or education status (quit their job or dropped out of GED program)
B. Past history/unknown future
    1. Abuse (of them or of others)
    2. Criminal acts not reported in their records
    3. Previous losses they have not talked about
    4. Their plans for future crimes
C. Education and vocational needs you have not discussed with them
    1. Need to read patient's record and assess their capacity to learn and determine whether there are learning disabilities
    2. Need for therapeutic interventions to take intelligence and education level into account
D. Wishes, needs, and psychological defenses that the patient is expressing in the therapeutic relationship
    1. Need to be sick and play dependent role
    2. Fear of losing the therapist if the patient gets well
    3. Avoiding issues that will place them in a bad light (criminal wants to appear as good person)
    4. Playing or manipulating you for the fun of it ("duping delight")

Note.   PREA=Prison Rape Elimination Act.

---

of leaving friends and family behind when he or she came into the prison, so leaving you behind is not going to destroy him or her. Because of the uncertainties in timing, you must be prepared for terminations. For most, getting out has a positive expectation and is a true celebration. Other times, such as when a presentence jail detainee loses his case, the effect may be catastrophic. If it is you who are leaving, the change can be difficult. We know of some such partings where the therapist just left and told nobody. But we think that you should do some termination work in consideration of your colleagues as well as your patient.

Key Points

- A supportive relationship is not a friendship but has some elements found in a friendship.

- A supportive relationship has a real aspect, a working alliance, and a transferential aspect.

- The concept of transference (including institutional transference) refers to the patient's attitudes toward the therapist or confining institution. Supportive psychotherapy encourages a positive transference and attempts to lessen a negative one.

- Many patients, especially those with established criminal lifestyles, can impede psychotherapy through strategies of resistance that can distract, divert, or literally destroy the effectiveness of the psychotherapy. Counter strategies are suggested.

- Countertransference refers to the therapist's reactions and feelings toward the patient and needs to be understood as an aid in understanding the patient and performing therapy.

- At some point (or point in their careers), therapists must consider their attitudes toward criminals and whether criminals can change or reform.

- Burnout is a common problem when therapists lose their enthusiasm, efficiency, and ability to cope with the requirements and stresses of performing psychotherapy.

- Treatment plans should have behavioral and measurable goals and should be individualized and phased in.

- It is important to recognize that you are ultimately in control of the therapy session.

- Gifts are generally forbidden in this type of setting.

- Individual techniques such as conveying empathy and hope, normalizing, reframing, and even making "happy talk" (positive and alliance-building efforts) can be useful.

- You need to be ready to pause, rewind, repeat, update, and refocus the therapy as needed.

- Even with a trauma-informed history, you may have to work hard to excavate trauma-related hidden issues.

- You should be dynamic and willing to change during and between therapy sessions.

References

Alexander F, French TM: Psychoanalytic Therapy: Principles and Applications. New York, Ronald Press, 1946

American Psychiatric Association: Well-being and burnout. 2021. Available at: www.psychiatry.org/psychiatrists/practice/well-being-and-burnout. Accessed October 10, 2021.

American Psychological Association: Patient Health Questionnaire–9 (PHQ-9). 2020. Available at: www.apa.org/depression-guideline/patient-health-questionnaire.pdf. Accessed December 28, 2020.

Asay TP, Lambert MJ: The empirical case for the common factors in therapy: quantitative findings, in The Heart and Soul of Change: What Works in Therapy. Edited by Hubble MA, Duncan BL, Miller SD. Washington, DC, American Psychological Association, 1999, pp 33–56

Aufderheide D: Mental illness in administrative segregation: how to bullet-proof your program against litigation. Correctcare 23:14–16, 2013

Babyar JC: They did not start the fire: reviewing and resolving the issue of physician stress and burnout. J Health Organ Manag 31(4):410–417, 2017 28877620

Badre NM: Burnout: a condition that rebrands mental illness for professionals. Clinical Psychiatry News 48(4):13, April 2020

Battaglia J: Doing Supportive Psychotherapy. Washington, DC, American Psychiatric Association Publishing, 2019

Bauer RL, Morgan RD, Mandracchia JT: Offenders with severe and persistent mental illness, in Correctional Mental Health: From Theory to Best Practice. Edited by Fagan TJ, Ax RK. Thousand Oaks, CA, Sage, 2011, pp 189–212

Benabio J: Hope is one of our most important gifts to patients. Clinical Psychiatry News 47(4):10, April 2019

Berman PS: Case Conceptualization and Treatment Planning: Integrating Theory With Clinical Practice, 3rd Edition. Thousand Oaks, CA, Sage, 2015

Bogue BM, Nandi A, Jongsma AE: The Parole and Probation Treatment Planner. New York, Wiley, 2012

Brodsky SL: Therapy With Coerced and Reluctant Clients. Washington, DC, American Psychological Association, 2011

Camus A: The Plague (1947). Translated by Stuart Gilbert. New York, Vintage Books, 1991

Caton CLM: Management of Chronic Schizophrenia. New York, Oxford University Press, 1984

Christie A: Towards Zero. New York, Pocket Books, 1974

Clay RA: "Are you burned out?" Here are signs and what to do about them. American Psychological Association Monitor 49(2):30, February 2018. Available at: www.apa.org/monitor/2018/02/ce-corner. Accessed July 5, 2020.

Coastal: Sexual harassment: you make the call. 2000. Available at: www.atlantictraining.com/shop/sexual-harassment-you-make-the-call-for-office-training-video-program.html. Accessed May 24, 2020.

Collaboration of Chemical Dependency Professionals from the Minnesota Department of Corrections and the Hazelden Foundation: Criminal and Addictive Thinking Workbook: Mapping a Life of Recovery and Freedom for Chemically Dependent Criminal Offenders. Center City, MN, Hazelden Foundation, 2002

Dewald PE: Psychotherapy: A Dynamic Approach, 2nd Edition. New York, Basic Books, 1971

Doran GT: There's a S.M.A.R.T. way to write management's goals and objectives. Manage Rev 70(11):35–36, 1981

Dorociak KE, Rupert PA, Bryant FB, Zahniser E: Development of the Professional Self-Care Scale. J Couns Psychol 64(3):325–334, 2017 28277686

Earle S: How Albert Camus's The Plague became the defining book of the coronavirus crisis. The New Statesman, May 27, 2020. Available at: www.newstatesman.com/the-plague-albert-camus-coronavirus-resurgence. Accessed November 8, 2020.

El-Amin WW, Sufrin C: Addressing racism in correctional health care. CorrectCare: The Magazine of the National Commission on Correctional Health Care 34(3):5, 14, Summer 2020

Elliott WN: Managing offender resistance to counseling—The"3R's." Fed Probat 66(3):43–49, 2002

Ezell ME, Cohen ME: Can a leopard change its spots? Continuity and change in criminal offending patterns among three samples of serious chronic offenders. NCJRS Abstract NCJ 213005. Washington, DC, U.S. Department of Justice, Office of Justice Programs, October 2002. Available at: www.ncjrs.gov/App/Publications/abstract.aspx?ID=234498. Accessed December 25, 2020.

Foreman SA, Marmar CR: Therapist actions that address initially poor therapeutic alliances in psychotherapy. Am J Psychiatry 142(8):922–926, 1985 4025587

Frank JD: General psychotherapy: the restoration of morale, in American Handbook of Psychiatry, 2nd Edition, Vol 5: Treatment. Edited by Freedman DX, Dyrud JE (Arieti S, editor-in-chief). New York, Basic Books, 1975, pp 117–132

Frank JD, Frank JP: Persuasion and Healing: A Comparative Study of Psychotherapy, 3rd Edition. Baltimore, MD, Johns Hopkins University Press, 1993

Glicken MD: Working With Troubled Men: A Contemporary Practitioner's Guide. Mahwah, NJ, Lawrence Erlbaum, 2005

Gould MA: Issues of power and oppression, in Correctional Psychology: Practice, Programming, and Administration. Edited by Schwartz BK. Kingston, NJ, Civic Research Institute, 2003, pp 1-1–1-30

Grant J: Viktor Frankl & me. Criminal justice insider podcast with Babz Rawls Ivy and Jeff Grant, January 12, 2014. Available at: https://criminaljusticeinsider.com/viktor-frankl-me-by-jeff-grant. Accessed September 13, 2020.

Greaney M: One Minute Out: A Gray Man Novel. New York, Berkeley, 2020

Greenson RR: The Technique and Practice of Psychoanalysis, Vol 1. New York, International Universities Press, 1967

Harris GA: Overcoming Resistance: Success in Counseling Men. Lanham, MD, American Correctional Association, 1995

Havens L: Explorations in the uses of language in psychotherapy: simple empathic statements. Psychiatry 41(4):336–345, 1978 715094

Havens L: Explorations in the uses of language in psychotherapy: complex empathic statements. Psychiatry 42(1):40–48, 1979 760133

Holmes J: Supportive analytical psychotherapy. An account of two cases. Br J Psychiatry 152:824–829, 1988 3167469

Jacobs J, Vance M: Advocacy as antidote to burnout: perspectives from intern year. Psychiatric News 55(16):9, August 21, 2020

Jowett JH (attributed to): Three Parts of a Sermon. Northern Daily Mail (Hartlepool Northern Daily Mail). August 13, 1908, Quote Page 3, Column 4, Durham, England. (British Newspaper Archive). Available at: https://quoteinvestigator.com/2017/08/15/tell-em/#note-16654-1. Accessed May 9, 2020.

Kellerman J: The Web. New York, Bantam Books, 1995

Kellerman J: Breakdown: An Alex Delaware Novel. New York, Ballantine Books, 2016

Kern J: Collaborative care as a way to stave off burnout. Psychiatric News 53(14):6–7, July 20, 2018

Knoll JL IV: Treating the morally objectionable patient: countertransference reactions. Psychiatric Times, April 13, 2009. Available at: www.psychiatrictimes.com/view/treating-morally-objectionable-patient-countertransference-reactions. Accessed July 16, 2020.

Knoll JL IV, Pies RW: Cruel, immoral behavior is not mental illness. Psychiatric Times 37(2): 2020. www.psychiatrictimes.com/view/cruel-immoral-behavior-not-mental-illness. Accessed January 18, 2021.

Kroenke K, Spitzer RL, Williams JB: The PHQ-9: validity of a brief depression severity measure. J Gen Intern Med 16(9):606–613, 2001 11556941

Kupers TA: Toxic masculinity as a barrier to mental health treatment in prison. J Clin Psychol 61(6):713–724, 2005 15732090

Lambert EG, Hogan NL: Correctional staff: the issue of job stress, in The Practice of Correctional Psychology. Edited by Ternes M, Magaletta PR, Patry MW. Cham, Switzerland, Springer, 2018, pp 259–281

Lambert EG, Barton-Bellessa SM, Hogan NL: The consequences of emotional burnout among correctional staff. SAGE Open April–June 2015. Available at: https://journals.sagepub.com/doi/pdf/10.1177/2158244015590444. Accessed August 20, 2020.

Lewis A: The 7 Minute Difference: Small Steps to Big Changes. New York, Kaplan Publishing, 2008

Makover RB: Treatment Planning for Psychotherapists: A Practical Guide to Better Outcomes, 3rd Edition. Arlington, VA, American Psychiatric Publishing, 2016

Mariush ME: Essentials of Treatment Planning. New York, Wiley, 2002

Maslach C, Jackson SE: Maslach Burnout Inventory. 2020. Available at: www.mindgarden.com/315-mbi-human-services-survey-medical-personnel#horizontalTab2. Accessed July 5, 2020.

Merriam-Webster: What's the difference between sympathy and empathy? Though the words appear in similar contexts, they have different meanings. Available at: www.merriam-webster.com/words-at-play/sympathy-empathy-difference. Accessed December 13, 2020.

Miller WR, Rollnick S: Motivational Interviewing: Helping People Change, 3rd Edition. New York, Guilford, 2013

Miner AS, Milstein A, Hancock JT: Talking to machines about personal mental health problems. JAMA 318(13):1217–1218, 2017 28973225

Moffic HS, Levin RM, Rouse H: The history of burnout in society, medicine, and psychiatry, in Combating Physician Burnout: A Guide for Psychiatrists. Edited by Loboprabhu S, Summers RF, Moffic HS. Washington, DC, American Psychiatric Association Publishing, 2020, pp 3–26

Morgan RD, Rozycki A, Wilson S: Inmate perception of mental health services. Prof Psychol Res Pr 35:389–396, 2004

Morgan RD: Correctional psychologist burnout, job satisfaction, and life satisfaction. Psychol Serv 7(3):190–201, 2010

Nestler E: Jerome Frank: reconsidering a classic on healing in secular and religious contexts. Arch Psychol Relig 23:123–131, 2000

Novalis PN, Singer V, Peele R: Clinical Manual of Supportive Psychotherapy, 2nd Edition. Washington, DC, American Psychiatric Association Publishing, 2020

Oleson JC: Criminal Genius: A Portrait of High-IQ Offenders. Oakland, University of California Press, 2016a

Oleson JC: High-IQ offenders: too much of a good thing. American Academy of Psychiatry and the Law Newsletter 41(3):10, 30, September 2016b

Overall JE, Gorham DR: The Brief Psychiatric Rating Scale. Psychol Rep 10: 799–812, 1962

Pollock D: Broad system factors influence physician wellness, patient care. Psychiatr News 53(6):4–5, 2018

Popik B: "Why does the baloney fear the slicer?" (politician avoiding a tough interview/debate). Blog entry from September 1, 2011. Available at: www.barrypopik.com/index.php/new_york_city/entry/why_does_the_baloney_fear_the_slicer_politician_avoiding_a_tough_interview. Accessed July 9, 2021.

Rajagopal S: The imprisoned brain: psychotherapy with inmates in jail. Psychotherapy.net 2016. Available at: www.psychotherapy.net/article/psychotherapy-prisons. Accessed July 17, 2020.

Ramirez T: 14 of the worst Latino e-cards: not amusing, not at all. Cosmopolitan, January 29, 2014. Available at: www.cosmopolitan.com/entertainment/news/a19477/offensive-latino-ecards. Accessed July 5, 2020.

Reis D, Xanthopoulo D, Tsaousis I: Measuring job and academic burnout with the Oldenburg Burnout Inventory (OLBI): factorial invariance across samples and countries. Burn Res 2(1):8–18, 2015

Rosenberg M: Rosenberg Self Esteem Scale. College Park, University of Maryland, Department of Sociology, 2021. Available at: https://socy.umd.edu/about-us/rosenberg-self-esteem-scale. Accessed June 20, 2021.

Roy Horn of Siegfried and Roy Dies From Coronavirus at 75. New York Times, May 8, 2020. Available at: www.nytimes.com/aponline/2020/05/08/us/ap-us-obit-roy-horn.html. Accessed May 15, 2020.

Ryback RS, Longabaugh R, Fowler DR: The Problem Oriented Record in Psychiatry and Mental Health Care, Revised Edition. New York, Grune & Stratton, 1981

Safirstein SL: Psychiatric aftercare in a general hospital. A system of prevention in the community. Psychother Psychosom 16(1):17–22, 1968 4304940

San Mateo County Health: Brief Psychiatric Rating Scale. 2020. Available at: www.smchealth.org/sites/main/files/file-attachments/bprsform.pdf. Accessed December 28, 2020.

Schaufeli W, Leiter M, Maslach C: Burnout: 35 years of research and practice. Career Development International 14:204–220, 2009

Schwartz BK: Establishing a mental health unit within an institution, in Correctional Psychology: Practice, Programming, and Administration. Edited by Schwartz BK. Kingston, NJ, Civic Research Institute, 2003, pp 3-1–3-22

Scott W; Crime and Justice Institute: Effective Clinical Practices in Treating Clients in the Criminal Justice System. Washington, DC, U.S. Department of Justice, National Institute of Corrections, 2008

Sharp BD: Changing Criminal Thinking: A Treatment Program, 2nd Edition. Alexandria, VA, American Correctional Association, 2006

Summers RF: The elephant in the room: what burnout is and what it is not. Am J Psychiatry 177(10):898–899, 2020 32660298

Summers RF, Gorrindo T, Hwang S, et al: Well-being, burnout, and depression among North American psychiatrists: the state of our profession. Am J Psychiatry 177(10):955–964, 2020 32660300

Summers RF, Gorrindo T, Hwang S, et al: Psychiatrist burnout (letter). Am J Psychiatry 178(2):204–205, 2021 33517753

Tafrate RC, Mitchell D, Simourd DJ: CBT With Justice-Involved Clients: Interventions for Antisocial and Self-Destructive Behaviors. New York, Guilford, 2018

Van Dernoot Lipsky L, Burk C: Trauma Stewardship: An Everyday Guide to Caring for Self While Caring for Others. Oakland, CA, Berrett-Koehler Publishers, 2009

Walters GD: Overcoming offender resistance to abandoning a criminal lifestyle, in Tough Customers: Counseling Unwilling Clients, 2nd Edition. Edited by Welo BK. Lanham, MD, American Correctional Association, 2001, pp. 77–97

Walters GD: Maintaining motivation for change using resources available in an offender's natural environment, in Motivating Offenders to Change: A Guide to Enhancing Engagement in Therapy. Edited by McMurran M. Chichester, West Sussex, UK, Wiley, 2002, pp 122–135

Walters GD: Crime in a Psychological Context: From Career Criminals to Criminal Careers. Thousand Oaks, CA, Sage, 2012

Wanberg KW, Milkman HB: Criminal Conduct & Substance Abuse Treatment: The Providers Guide, 2nd Edition. Thousand Oaks, CA, Sage, 2008

Ward T, Vess J, Collie RM, Gannon TA: Risk management or goods promotion: the relationship between approach and avoidance goals in treatment for sex offenders. NCJ 214944. Aggression and Violent Behavior 11(4):378–393, July–August 2006

Weed LL: Medical Records, Medical Education and Patient Care. Cleveland, OH, Case-Western Reserve University Press, 1969

Weiner MF: The Psychotherapeutic Impasse. New York, Free Press, 1982

White J: Beginning Operations: A Sector General Omnibus. New York, Tor Books, 2001

Wikipedia: "Joan Riviere." 2020a. Available at: https://en.wikipedia.org/wiki/Joan_Riviere. Accessed July 10, 2020.

Wikipedia: "Outer Limits." 2020b. Available at: https://en.wikipedia.org/wiki/The_Outer_Limits_%281963_TV_series%29. Accessed July 5, 2020.

Winston A, Rosenthal RN, Roberts LW: Learning Supportive Psychotherapy: An Illustrated Guide, 2nd Edition. Washington, DC, American Psychiatric Association Publishing, 2020

Yee WK: Psychiatric aspects of psychoeducational family therapy. Psychiatric Annals 19:27–34, 1989

Yochelson S, Samenow SE: The Criminal Personality. 3 Volumes. New York, Jason Aronson, 1976

Your Dictionary: Who said "Hope is not a strategy?" 2020. Available at: https://quotes.yourdictionary.com/articles/who-said-hope-is-not-strategy.html. Accessed November 14, 2020.

Zetzel ER: Current concepts of transference. Int J Psychoanal 37(4-5):369–376, 1956 13366506

PART II

Core Issues

5

Crisis, Self-Harm, and Suicidal Behavior

In this chapter we discuss the prevalence and prevention of suicides in jails and prisons, the reasons for the high risk of suicide, the challenges of assessing suicide risks, and the fundamental tasks of providing psychotherapy to prisoners who are at risk for suicide or self-injury. We do so using a broad-brush approach that relates suicide prevention to the management of other crises, including the management of grief. We also discuss the management of chronically suicidal patients and the relationship of nonsuicidal self-injurious behavior to suicidal behaviors.

Crisis and Grief Counseling

In Chapter 3 we recognized that entry into a prison can create a crisis and sometimes a suicidal one. Suicide risk is increased during the first week (often 24–72 hours) after jail entry, after court conviction, and during subsequent jail-to-prison transitions (where the risk is high for the first year), as well as upon release back into the community. Stressors upon prison entry include:

- The conviction and legal setbacks.
- Separation or divorce or loss of child custody.
- Loss of what the individual had in the community.
- The development or exacerbation of mental illness.
- Trauma or violence (physical, verbal, sexual) inflicted upon the prisoner or by the prisoner upon someone else (i.e., stressful for the offender as well as the victim).
- Stress in new relationships (e.g., an abusive relationship).
- Changes in prison situation (the best-known being placement in disciplinary segregation).
- Health-related issues (e.g., diagnosis of debilitating or terminal illness).
- Substance-related issues (e.g., intoxication upon entry, use of drugs within prison, withdrawal, or prolonged cravings).

- Grief related to deaths in the outside world and inability to process it in the usual ways.
- Grief related to other losses (e.g., pets, finances, home, friends, relationships, break-ups, loss of future aspects of the self, lost opportunities for education, employment, future relationships, and the future perspective itself). We discuss these later as examples of *disenfranchised grief.*

A *crisis* is a situation in which a number of factors (sometimes but not always including a single precipitating factor such as incarceration) overwhelm (or are perceived to overwhelm) a person's capacity or resources to cope with them. A crisis is time limited, although those limits have sometimes been turned into years, as in crises of immigration, violent crime, coronavirus, climate change, and the like. A crisis may be a disaster for a person, family, community, nation, or the planet. For patients, a crisis may *develop in* and/or *last for* minutes, hours, days, or weeks.

A crisis can result in permanent impairment or violence against oneself or others, including death, such as from suicide. The person in crisis may emerge from it in a weakened and traumatized state and even more vulnerable to further crises. On the other hand, he could also emerge from the crisis no worse off or even improved in his situation, since some or all of the issues raised by the crisis may have been resolved or the experience may have led to improved personal resilience and coping capacity.

Given our definition, a crisis can be resolved in a number of ways:

- The precipitating factors can be removed or modified.
- The person's coping skills can be improved so that he is able to cope with the crisis.
- The person's resources to combat the crisis may be augmented so that he can overcome the crisis in that way.
- Another person or persons can help the person in crisis to get through it, through their support or use of their own resources.
- Since sometimes a crisis "exists in the eye of the beholder," the person's perception of the crisis might be changed so that he no longer perceives it as overwhelming.

The use of supportive methods in crisis situations is fairly standard. There are many books on crisis management, and the audience for them is wide-ranging, from unlicensed disaster aid workers to licensed doctoral level therapists. So you may read that "crisis counseling is not psychotherapy." This admonition is meant to advise readers that they may not be licensed to diagnose and treat mental illnesses. Also, it is sometimes assumed that psychotherapy is a confrontational, anxiety-provoking experience or fosters uncovering of unconsciousness material and that such therapy should not be attempted during a crisis. All that may be true, but you (yes, this means *you*) are able to do psychotherapy in a crisis setting, especially if it is supportive psychotherapy. A crisis is not the time to address a patient's criminogenic tendencies. Maybe later, though not now! But it may be a time to improve emotional regulation and social skills. Some books still espouse Rogerian concepts such as having an "unconditional positive regard" for your client. We think this is overstated, and what the therapeutic alliance requires is professional respect and some personal warmth. You do not need unconditional positive regard for a sadistic psychopath—not even for a sad one as opposed to a sadistic one. In addition, unlike in crisis work, your interventions with prisoners do not have to be time-limited. True, you will probably need to manage the crisis in a finite manner, but you won't be going away, and you may be continuing as the patient's therapist indefinitely.

Most texts use a "stagecoach" theory of crisis therapy. That is, they tell you the *stages* of a crisis and show you how to *coach* your patient through them. Sometimes they tell you that the stages can be somewhat mixed together and are not meant to be approached inflexibly. We discussed several staged approaches in our previous book (Novalis et al. 2020). There is a much similarity in crisis therapy approaches, and (with a few exceptions) you can probably pick any popular one (e.g., Kanel 2012). However, we recently found a "task model" of crisis management that recognizes that tasks may not necessarily be sequential and may need to be repeated or done in different orders. A review of the leading crisis therapy textbooks showed that there are variations around three continuous tasks (assessment, safety, and support) and four focused tasks (contact, reestablishment of control, problem-solving, and follow-up) (Myer et al. 2013). These tasks are familiar to most therapists. However, the task with the most immediacy is reestablishing control, and that is what we would consider the central task of crisis management.

It has been a meme of counseling that the Chinese word for "crisis" is a combination of the words for "danger" and "opportunity." However, a closer look shows this to be based on misunderstanding. The Chinese word for crisis (simplified Chinese: [危机]; traditional Chinese: [危機]; pinyin: wēijī, wéijī) is a combination of the characters for "danger" and "decision point," but the meme that the second character means "opportunity" is based on a linguistic confusion that was popularized by President John F. Kennedy in a series of campaign speeches in 1959 to 1960 (Wikipedia 2020a). Somewhat later, during 13 agonizing days in October 1962, President Kennedy had his own crisis (the Cuban Missile Crisis) that brought the United States and the Soviet Union to the brink of nuclear war. It's unclear whether that crisis directly created any opportunities, although it was followed by a nuclear arms treaty and a hotline between the two countries (History.com Editors 2019). This is not a story you need to tell your patients, however. They already know that their crisis is a bad thing, so you should not use a historically incorrect meme to reframe it as heart-warming opportunity for growth. True, the crisis of entering a prison can be reframed for women as an opportunity for safety from community and intimate partner violence, a drug and alcohol-free environment, food and board, and medical and mental health and substance use disorder treatment. For men, the environment is more dangerous. But there is one definite opportunity in the crisis. It is an opportunity to establish a positive therapeutic alliance with your patients. In other words, their needs in the face of crisis can assist the ability to develop a positive bond with you for their current and future therapy. You can even tell them about what kind of communication "hotline" they will have to reach you.

It is further (and historically) correct to say that a crisis is a decision point or inflection point at which their life can change depending on the proper decisions that you will support them in making. Criminologist Glenn D. Walters, whom we introduced in Chapter 1, views a crisis as the starting point of "arresting" (his word) the criminal lifestyle (Walters 1998). Classifying crises by sources (internal vs. external) and motives (approach vs. avoidance-oriented), there are four kinds of crisis, each of which can play a role in a person's life to develop new commitments and consider new options compatible with a noncriminal lifestyle.

Grief

Grief "describes the emotional, cognitive, functional, and behavioral responses to a meaningful loss" (Zisook et al. 2020, p. 557). *Bereavement* is "the death of someone close. Bereavement is a nearly universal phenomenon that may be experienced many times by those living long enough to lose loved ones" (Zisook et al. 2020, p. 557). *Mourning* is the process of adapting to that loss, and for most persons is eventually successful in transforming acute grief into *integrated grief* in which the bereaved person gets on reasonably well with her life. This requires adaptation to the death with changes, some obvious and some not so obvious, in one's daily activities and self-concept to take into account the absence of the bereaved person.

Because of their many losses, prisoners are often "stuck" in a prolonged state of grief. This probably is related to the phenomenon that prison imposes a psychological "deep freeze" on personal development, and prisoners are stuck at a level of psychological development years younger than their physical age, which is actually accelerated. Failure to integrate grief results in *complicated grief*, a condition in which the bereaved remains dysfunctional and preoccupied with the memories of and yearning for the deceased. Prisons foster complicated grief because the prisoner is unable to mourn a loss in the normal way (e.g., not being allowed to mourn with family or go to the funeral) (Schetky 1998). In many intakes, we hear that the patient is still suffering from loss of a child or spouse that occurred 5 or 10 years ago. There is also a type of grief called *disenfranchised grief*, in which the situation is not one normally recognized by society as one that involves grieving. This can include death but may also involve many other losses of the type that prisoners experience, such as loss of home, finances, or connection to family.

Acute grief is a well-known syndrome consisting of the following (Zisook et al. 2020, pp. 558–559):

- A sense of disbelief
- Frequent strong feelings of yearning and sorrow
- Feelings of insecurity, emptiness, and loss
- A mixture of other feelings
- Persistent thoughts and images focused on the deceased
- Loss of interest in ongoing life

Many people are familiar with the five stages of grief proposed by Elisabeth Kübler-Ross: denial, anger, bargaining, depression, and acceptance. Lately, these are not used as the inevitable paradigm, and as we mentioned, there are now task-based rather than stage theories of grief as there are for crises in general. For example, Worden (2018) presents the following tasks for grieving: accepting the reality of the loss, processing the pain of the loss, adjusting to the new environment without the deceased person, and remembering the deceased while getting one with one's life. The general rule for duration of acute grief is 6–12 months. Holidays and anniversaries can trigger memories that bring back the sadness from an earlier time. However, we would like to make one point about ordinary grief due to the death of a family member or friend. The occurrence of a death does not automatically warrant referral to a grief group (even if you have one available). In fact, if a person does not need a grief group, his mental health symptoms (including those related to grief) may be worsened by attending a grief group.

So what is the third question you should be asking a bereaved prisoner?

1. I hear you've had a death in the family. How are you?
2. Do you feel like hurting yourself in any way?
3. Would you like to talk about this some more?

In ordinary circumstances (typical and nontraumatic situations): "In grief treatment, there really isn't a positive effect overall, and more than one-third of people get worse" according to one of the top researchers, George Bonanno (quoted in Campbell 2016; also see Bonanno 2019). So that is why your third question (after making a general inquiry and ruling out suicidal ideation) should be to ask patients what they want. If there is no wish to talk, do a follow-up wellness check but do not create a series of grief counseling sessions they do not need. Sadly enough, losses are so common in our prison population that even if prisoners have just entered our adult system at the age of 18, they have often suffered more losses than we have in our lifetimes. They have their way of dealing with loss, and it may not involve us. However, we do emphasize that the "no therapy" option applies to ordinary loss. The amount of traumatic and unexpected loss in our population is excessive, and the need for therapy should be assessed on a case-by-case basis.

Grief counseling can be slow, and you may have to set time limits for your sessions. Do not be surprised at the different reactions you encounter, and recognize that there are different ways that people handle grief. Offer practical and emotional support and encourage healthy outlets for the expression of grief (e.g., writing, drawing, physical activity). Do not hesitate to seek advice from a colleague. Tips for providing grief counseling for typical or normal grief situations are provided in Table 5–1.

Complicated Grief

"Persistent complex bereavement disorder" was a DSM-5 Condition for Further Study, and "prolonged grief disorder" became a mental disorder in DSM-5-TR. These two terms appear to be equivalent, although we have read that they are not equivalent to "complicated grief disorder" because of the latter's vagueness and lack of diagnostic validity (Maciejewski et al. 2016). However, because of the newness of the DSM-5-TR terminology, most of the literature we researched used the term "complicated grief," and we shall do so here. The new criteria, of course, are in DSM-5-TR. The 11th revision of the International Classification of Diseases (ICD-11) (Eisma et al. 2020) also has specific criteria. Complicated grief develops when a person struggles with accepting his loss and has reactions outside the typical grief reactions. According to some researchers, if the grief intensifies or persists for more than 6 months, complicated grief may develop (Bridges to Recovery 2020; Schwartz 2021). However, the DSM-5-TR criteria specify 12 months. Early treatment (if needed) of acute grief reduces the risk of complicated grief (Therivel and Kornusky 2018). Simon (2013) describes bereavement as a trauma to the attachment system, which, when it develops into complicated grief, can lead to "initial symptoms of traumatic distress, separation distress, care-giver self-blame (with survivor guilt), and decreased engagement in life" (p. 417).

TABLE 5–1.	"Normal grief" therapy tips

Encourage healthy outlets to express.

Offer emotional support.

Set time limits if needed.

Assess for suicidal ideation.

Recognize disenfranchised sources of grief.

Encourage timely expression of emotions.

Provide psychoeducational information.

Listen without judging.

Use active listening.

Use a collaborative approach.

Ask clarifying questions.

The message in treating complicated grief is not to "forget it and move on" but to include the loss and its influences on the individual's functioning without the negative effects. The goal of therapy is to help your patient to accept the loss, integrate it into his life, and learn to function in a healthy manner (Therivel and Kornusky 2018). Shear et al. (2020) report on several programs specifically tailored for bereavement for a loss through suicide (Jordan 2017) or persons who have lost someone because of violence. Also see the articles by Rynearson (1994) and Smid et al. (2015).

Complicated grief can occur when the normal adaptations to acute grief are blocked by:

- Dysfunctional thinking.
- Maladaptive behaviors.
- Difficulties with emotional regulation.
- Overwhelming social or environmental problems.

These issues obviously make prisoners particularly vulnerable to complicated grief.

Shear et al. (2020) and Iglewicz et al. (2020) describe *complicated grief treatment* (CGT), a hybrid that draws from attachment theory, cognitive-behavioral therapy (CBT), interpersonal psychotherapy (IPT), motivational interviewing, and psychodynamic psychotherapy. It uses concepts of prolonged exposure and an emphasis on personal goals and relationships. The CBT techniques address symptoms of painful intrusive memories and behavioral avoidance. The IPT features focus on reestablishing social interactions and connection with goals (Wetherell 2012). CGT can be administered in varied settings and assists the individual with the acceptance of the loss and adaptation to life without the deceased loved one (Iglewicz et al. 2020). Individuals suffering from complicated grief need structured and methodical interventions. Iglewicz describes seven core themes of treatment (Iglewicz et al. 2020). Since these methods were not specific to prisons, we will elaborate them now with emphasis on issues that apply to prisoners.

1. *Understanding and accepting grief.* Provide the patient with information to help her understand and accept grief, including the various aspects of "normal grief," what is involved with adapting to loss, things that could interfere with the grief process,

what complicated grief is, and the therapist's role in assisting her. In prison, normal ways of expressing grief may not be available. Encourage the patient to comment and ask questions as the grief process is explained. What appears as a disorganized world to the prisoner can be helped with some structure. Of course, it is particularly easy to normalize grief for prisoners and let them know that others have had their experience and coped with it. Those suffering from complicated grief will often have a sense of relief and renewed hope when they are given a diagnosis and a treatment plan.

2. *Managing emotional pain.* Accepting grief includes acknowledging and managing the associated painful emotions. Ask your patient to monitor his grief and measure when it is most acute and when he feels more relief and ask for an overall rating for the day. The monitoring is often helpful and involves little time and discussion. At the next session, discuss the circumstances around these mood swings and discuss how you can incorporate the findings into developing strategies for coping.

3. *Thinking about the future.* It is difficult for those with complicated grief to imagine a promising future. Starting in the second session, ask your patient to imagine that her grief is manageable and imagine what she wants for her life, and then working together, explore ways to work toward achieving these goals. Assess how serious she is about this plan and what would be entailed in achieving the goals and where to get help. The goals should be appealing and gratifying. Some people will struggle with this and may have to start with a simple task such as learning a new skill, finding a creative outlet, or beginning an exercise program. Set aside a few minutes at each subsequent visit to discuss and develop the plan.

4. *Strengthening ongoing relationships.* Encourage the individual to identify at least one person in whom he can confide, whether his cellie or a friend in the prison, a staff member, or someone in his family. If he has gotten a lay-in from work or kept to his cell, encourage him to get back to a daily routine. If it helps to start sharing activities with others in the unit, encourage him to do so.

5. *Telling the story of the death.* For the individual to accept the painful reality of the death being mourned, it is important for her to tell the story of the person, the death, and her reactions to the loss. Prompt the patient to verbalize what happened, starting with first learning of the death. Approach the telling in stages and help the patient to regulate her emotions, recap the story at each session, and then put it away and plan some activity that is meaningful or rewarding. As the sessions progress, this retelling will help her to fill in details and grasp the meaning of the of the story to herself.

6. *Living with reminders.* Many with complicated grief avoid speaking of the death and the deceased for fear that the reminders will trigger more pain. However, avoiding reminders will narrow and confine the lives of those with complicated grief. Encourage the patient to revisit the reminders and develop an acceptance of the grief as normal. As he does, he will come to remember the deceased with both sadness and appreciation of the role of that person and the grief in his life.

7. *Connecting with memories.* Educate the patient on how memories are an important part of connecting with loved ones. You can provide her with a series of questionnaires after she has told the story of the death several times. You can create your own questionnaires or access them from the Columbia University complicated grief website (Center for Complicated Grief 2020).

It is of interest that there was a study involving citalopram (an antidepressant), in which the "use of citalopram or placebo with supportive management did result in a moderate response, so this may be a reasonable approach if grief-targeted psychotherapy is not available" (Shear et al. 2020, p. 579). In other words, what was as an extremely minimal supportive therapy (performed by the pharmacist) had moderate effectiveness. That is a remarkable result, given what a real supportive psychotherapist can do! Conclusion (theirs as well as ours): Knowledgeable supportive psychotherapy, even without the full CGT program, would be expected to be moderately effective in treating complicated grief. So even if you do not implement the full CGT curriculum, you can effectively treat complicated grief by educating patients about their conditions and encouraging them to resume normal life activities.

Since there are some features in grief that also occur in PTSD, such as recurrent memories of the deceased, these conditions can appear to be similar if one considers the activating trauma to be the death of the relative or friend. (But PTSD experts seem to require that the death be sudden or unexpected to consider it to be a qualifying traumatic event.) However, flashbacks in PTSD are of fearful situations and not sad ones. The alterations in self-concept that suggest PTSD can also occur in major depression, which needs to be in the differential diagnosis. Suicidal behavior is another problem for people with complicated grief as they wonder if it would be better if they joined the deceased. Indeed, as we mentioned above, grief is caused by a traumatic separation, so the stressors are there (Simon 2013).

Grief and major depressive disorder may have some overlapping symptoms, and the therapist needs to consider that an individual can experience both grief and depression at the same time. But there are some important differences. With grief, there is a known loss and the person's focus is on that loss. With depression, a loss may or may not be known and the person's focus is on self. There will be fluctuating feelings of pleasure and fluctuating physical symptoms with grief; with depression, there is an inability to feel pleasure and prolonged functional impairment. Among others, the overlapping symptoms will include sadness, decreased energy and focus, anxiety, anger, isolation, and fear. Paying attention to the individual's wording will help you to differentiate between grief and major depressive disorder. For example, when discussing grief, does he focus on himself with talk of self-blame? Does he verbalize a sense of overwhelming guilt and increased hopelessness? These elements are more indicative of depression than grief (Ferszt and Leveillee 2009; Pritchard 2021) (see Table 5–2).

Disenfranchised Grief

Disenfranchised grief is a term used to recognize a response to loss that is not recognized openly by society or publicly mourned. If the grief is related to a death, it may relate to homicide or another type of death that is not natural or anticipated. The grief may have nothing to do with a death; it may instead have to do with some other type of loss or losses that are typical of what prisoners incur when they lose multiple aspects of their lives upon entry into prison. Disenfranchisement may occur because the relationship to the griever is not recognized, the type of death is not recognized, the loss is not recognized, or the griever is not recognized (Doka 1989, 2001; Doka and Tucci 2002; Kramer-Howe 2013; Zoll 2021). Grief may be marginalized for those suffering because the disenfranchised grief falls outside the lines of societal grieving

TABLE 5–2.   Grief, complicated grief, and major depressive disorder

Grief	Complicated grief	Major depressive disorder
Sadness, mourning	Obsession with the deceased person	Feelings of worthlessness
Low energy		Exaggerated guilt
Tearful	Deep unbearable sadness	Suicidal ideation
Poor sleep	Verbalizing "doom and gloom"	Helplessness
Decreased appetite	Irritability and quick to anger	Agitation
Poor concentration	Isolating to home	Loss of interest in pleasurable activities
Happy and sad memories	Lack of attention to grooming	
Mild feelings of guilt	Reckless, impulsive, and self-destructive behaviors	Exaggerated fatigue
		Low self-esteem
	Strong attachments to reminders of the deceased, or a strong aversion to reminders	

rules. In prisoners there are many examples, starting with the loss of friends and intimate relationships, family contacts, job, business associates, home, neighbors, and pets upon incarceration. The loss of one's normal daytime routine of having breakfast in the kitchen may be significant. Many others come to mind.

Suicide in Jails and Prisons

In our much-referenced sci-fi saga, empath Prilicla discusses the obligation to help some stranded fellow spacemen who seem reluctant or ambivalent about protecting themselves from the risk of exposure to radiation. It (remember that Prilicla is referred to as "it") suggests that the fact that the spacemen thought to don their spacesuits suggests that they do want to live, but even if not, Prilicla feels an obligation to save them. Prilicla's colleague, Dr. Fletcher, agrees that there is an obligation to prevent suicide, but adds that the obligation probably arises because no rational person can fully understand the motives of a suicidal person (White 1999, p. 32).

It's a rough analogy, and James White presumably did not feel the urge to digress about cases of legal provider-assisted suicide, but the analogy does suggest that suicide risks can come from a person's inner and outer space, and the spacesuits would seem to be a good representation of what we will call the protective factors to suicidal behavior. Moreover, the opinion is mooted that prevention of suicide is a transcultural value, an issue that we discuss in Chapter 13.

The number of suicides has increased, as has the rate, in the United States over the last 20 years. The rate increased 35% between 1999 and 2018, from 10.5 per 100,000 to 14. It increased approximately 1% per year from 1999 to 2006 and 2% per year from 2006 through 2018. In 2018, the suicide rate for males was 3.7 times the rate for females (22.8 and 6.2, respectively) (Hedegaard et al. 2020).

The prevention of suicide in jails and prisons requires the multidisciplinary team effort of administrative staff, correctional officers, medical staff, family members, and social workers. Suicide rates in state prisons are higher than those in the community, and suicide has been the leading cause of death in jails since 2000 (Mumola and Noonan 2010). Outside of jails and prisons, suicide is the 10th leading cause of death (Stone et al. 2018). The annual average rate of suicide from 2001 to 2016 was 17 deaths per 100,000 male state prisoners and 13 deaths per 100,000 female state prisoners. Because of the preponderance of men, the overall rate was 16 for state prisons and 10 in federal. The rates were much higher in the 1980s and 1990s and were stable for several years after that, but they have gone up in the last few years, as reported by Carson and Cowhig (2020). However, there is consensus that suicide prevention measures have been effective in prisons and especially in jails.

In 2002 the suicide rate in local jails (47 per 100,000 prisoners) was over three times the rate in state prisons (14 per 100,000 prisoners). Suicide rates among violent people in both local jails (92 per 100,000) and state prisons (19 per 100,000) were more than twice as high as those among nonviolent prisoners (31 and 9 per 100,000, respectively) (Mumola and Noonan 2010).

Criminal history is one of multiple factors that affects the suicide risk. Factors that ought to decrease the risk include the unavailability of firearms and the presence of close observation, but stress and mental illness increase the risk. We all know of the increased risk for suicide after sentencing and in newly admitted prisoners. Various statistical studies have shown, for example, that a third of suicides take place within 48 hours (Hayes 2010a) or 7 days of incarceration in jail (Gallagher 2018), or that in state prisons the risk is higher for the first year. In addition to the other diagnosis-related risk factors noted, we also point out that the presence of an adjustment disorder, though usually associated with a favorable outcome, should not be underrated as a suicide risk factor (Casey 2018). There are many other causes for an increased risk for suicide among the incarcerated compared with the general population. Higher rates of mental illness, lack of a support system, confinement, and the stress associated with incarceration all contribute to the increased risk (Hughes and Metzner 2015). Hanging is the most common method in jails—so common that all corrections officers have cutdown tools as well as handcuffs (Hayes 2010b; Roth 2018).

Jail suicide rates are higher than in prison and have that initial peak partially because of the trauma of incarceration, loss of employment and community, and loss of normal lifestyle. Persons entering jail may also be intoxicated, be undergoing withdrawal, or have serious mental illness (SMI) (Meagher and Chammah 2015; Tartaro 2019; Torrey et al. 2010).

Risk Factors

Entry into prison can also create a crisis and continued increased risk for suicide. Based on research by the World Health Organization, two clinical profiles were proposed for prison suicide. One is for pretrial detainees, who tend to be young and unmarried and arrested for the first time for minor or substance-related crimes. They are at highest risk after arrest and around the time of court appearances. No surprises there. The second is a group of persons incarcerated for violent crimes and with long sentences who have been in custody for 4–5 years. Their risk increases with time even though the overall burden of problems is low or moderate but not high. Attempts are being made to predict their risk based on their life trajectory (Kaster et al. 2017).

Prisoner suicide has many risk factors. Institutional risk factors might include overcrowding and lack of mental health services. A history of violent crimes and the presence of mental illness are risk factors associated with individuals. Other risk factors are a history of self-harm or suicide attempts, previous psychiatric treatment, a family history of suicide, prior prison stays, adverse life events, current mental health problems, major depressive disorder, anxiety, and psychosis, and severe personality disorders. Researchers continue to work on these issues and recommend an evidence-based nationwide approach to prevent suicide addressing both individual-level and facility-level components (Ramesh 2018). Extensive lists of risk factors and programmatic requirements are widely available (for example, see Knoll and Kaufman 2017). One caveat is that current models (in an outpatient study of millions of visits) appear to underpredict the suicide risk for Blacks, American Indians, and Alaskan natives (Coley et al. 2021). We will focus on issues that we think are of greatest importance to psychotherapists.

Specific situations of risk other than the incarceration itself include conflict with other prisoners, threat of rape or incident of rape, segregation, upcoming or recent court dates (especially 2 days before or after), family-related anniversary dates, impending release (a time of stress and fear for those with no support system), and upsetting visits or phone calls (Chamberlain 2019). According to Gold (2020), personal factors include substance use disorder, feelings of hopelessness, borderline and antisocial personality features, and a history of poor impulse control. Gold cautions to not rely solely on clinical impressions or self-reporting from patients, because they may not be forthcoming about suicidal ideation and clinical impressions are susceptible to error. For a summary of risk factors, see Table 5–3.

The CDC's National Center for Injury Prevention and Control has issued recommendations for uniform terminologies in reporting suicidal and self-harm events (Crosby et al. 2011). These include making a distinction among intent to harm self, intent to die, and a third category, "to escape" or some other reason. In addition, they suggest some standard questions when asking about such historical attempts (Crosby et al. 2011, p. 68):

- "What were you doing at the time of the incident?"
- "What were you feeling emotionally at the time of the incident?"
- "What were you expecting to happen as a result of your action?"
- "How did it happen?"
- "How did you hurt yourself?"
- "Who discovered what happened?"
- "How did you get help?"

There are certain terms that have become "unacceptable" because of their connotations or vagueness or for other reasons. Terms to be avoided include "completed suicide" or "successful suicide" or "failed attempt," which imply a desired outcome. They do not like the term "parasuicide," which should be replaced by the more specific "nonsuicidal self-directed violence" or "suicidal self-directed violence." The experts seem to want to assign the classification of such behaviors into a category of dangerousness, but we would assume you can still historically refer to behaviors as reckless rather than calling them parasuicidal. The term "suicidality" should also be further specified as either suicidal thoughts or suicidal behavior. So we have usually tried to avoid "suicidality" in lieu of the more specific terms. These recommendations do not seem to be an issue of political correctness; rather, they reflect the desire on the part of research-

TABLE 5–3.   A reminder of suicide risk factors

Mostly static and unchangeable	Subject to some modification by a therapist	Dynamic with the circumstances
History of mental health treatment; history of borderline personality or antisocial personality disorder features; chronic physical illness	Prison overcrowding (therapist can affect a cell assignment)	Adverse life events—starting from the day of entry, separation, divorce, loss of custody, financial loss or complete ruin, loss of profession or other sources of identity
Prior personal and/or family history of self-harm and/or suicide attempts, especially violent ones; rate for frequency, recency, risk/rescue ratio, outcome (e.g., hospitalization or not), followed up or not, etc.; nature of intent (e.g., to die, not to die, to escape, undetermined (see text and Crosby et al. 2011)	Current mental illness, especially serious mental illness or borderline/antisocial personality disorders or traits	Changes in or new mental health symptoms warranting therapy, including possible acute medication management; includes patient's report of being/becoming suicidal (but such reports not always reliable) (see text); includes reports/referrals by other prisoners or staff; active suicidal thinking, anticipatory acts, preparation or rehearsal; global insomnia
	Cravings or withdrawal associated with the substance use history	Severe guilt or shame
	Significant medical health problem or unaddressed issues (e.g., pain)	Impulsivity
	Obsession with death (may be chronic [see text] or of new onset)	Anxiety
Substance use disorder (including, but not limited to, increased risk from withdrawal from or craving substances)	Recent or chronic grief issues	Agitation, irritation, rage
	Solitary confinement—issues with recent or continued placement	Hopelessness
Receiving a long sentence (including in some cases the death penalty and time on death row) (some possibility of modification); also, a first incarceration	Refusal to take prescribed medications; help rejecting	Continued grief (includes complicated/persistent or disenfranchised)
		Being bullied
History of violent crimes and (to lesser extent) prior prison stay; severe personality disorder		Interpersonal conflict: with family, friends, officers, other prisoners; negative therapeutic reactions; sequelae of violent or sexual assault(s) or threat(s) of it
Upcoming release (date could change for better or for worse)		Changes in levels of personal characteristics (e.g., agitation, impulsivity, isolation, appetite) and cardinal symptoms of depression (e.g., hopelessness)
History of abuse as a child or adult—physical, sexual, domestic, emotional		Fearful of impending release (change the response to the anticipation)
Demographic factors associated with higher risk (e.g., older nonreligious male, but not necessarily white; some risk in juveniles as well		Lack of reasons for living (discussed later as part of crisis response safety plan)
LGBTQ identifications; other characteristics that make a person vulnerable to being a victim or subject of bullying in jail or prison		Loneliness
		Thwarted belongingness and perceived burdensomeness (see Mandracchia and Smith 2015)

Source.   Gold 2020; Gold and Joshi 2018; Knoll and Kaufman 2017; among others.

ers to have more specific categories when data are collected. Finally, the CDC paper objects to the value judgments implied in the terms "suicidal gesture," "manipulative act," and "suicidal threat." They prefer the objectivity of "nonsuicidal, self-directed violence," or "suicidal, self-directed violence," but they seem to offer no alternative for what we would call a manipulative verbal threat. Elsewhere, however, we have seen recommendations to use "suicide-related notification" or "conditional suicide-related communication" and variations thereof (Frey et al. 2020). We use "statement of contingent suicidal thinking or behavior" for the all-too-common statement of "If you put me into restrictive housing, I will become suicidal." Other classifications retain the term "suicidal threats" but classify such threats further based on whether there is a suicidal intent associated with them (Silverman et al. 2007). We are still going to use the somewhat qualified terminology of threats.

Protective Factors

Assessment is incomplete if it only looks at risk factors. Without an assessment of protective factors, the suicide risk may be rated too high and patient care made too restrictive (Simon 2011a). Protective factors (like a "spacesuit" against the toxic substances from outer space or toxic thoughts from inner space!) include the facility's resources and an individual's characteristics, respectively (Suicide Prevention Resource Center 2022). Multiple risk factors may place someone in the high-risk category. Comparatively, the more protective factors there are, the lower the risk (Suicide Prevention Resource Center 2022). The enhancement of protective factors will help to decrease the risks. This process must be long-term because the positive gains are not permanent (Western Michigan University Suicide Prevention Program 2020). According to Simon (2011b), protective factors are less complicated for patients to discuss than risk factors, but he cautions that the protective factors therefore tend to be overvalued. Table 5–4 should serve as a reminder of protective factors, many of which you can enhance in psychotherapy.

Assessment and Management of Suicide Risk

In legal settings, the standard of care for suicide risk assessment may invoke the concept of what acts a reasonable clinician should perform. The minimum activities involved would appear to be gathering information from the patient, gathering information from other sources, estimating suicide risk, treatment planning, providing documentation, and monitoring (Obegi 2017). Most institutions have policies and assessment instruments for suicide risk assessment and management, and we do not intend to advocate for a system that replaces your existing one. However, we have some guidelines for conducting assessments that would give you the opportunity to supplement your existing policies and instruments. First of all, keep in mind that screening and assessment for suicide are not the same. Screening is typically a one-time task and take places during intake. Screenings are brief and often administered by medical but not mental health staff, and questions may require only "yes/no" answers. Screening answers do not provide enough information for diagnosis but can provide enough information for further evaluation or interventions. Assessment is not a single event but ongoing and involves more frequent and extensive evaluations. There should also be

TABLE 5–4.   **Protective factors in suicide risk**

Individual	Institutional
Problem-solving skills; personal resiliency	Trained and observant staff
Spiritual/faith	Intake screening and assessment
Peer/family support (e.g., family visits)	Supportive housing situations (e.g., not segregated or restrictive)
Self-esteem	Communication between disciplines
Sobriety	Levels of observation
Impulse control	Staff attitudes
Receiving (and accepting) treatment for one's mental illness or other issues	Programs that identify and treat mental illness
Hope for the future	Institution-wide, multidisciplinary suicide assessment and prevention programs
Purposive activity (e.g., work, hobby, correspondence, peer groups [e.g., Bible study])	
Reasons for living (part of a crisis response safety plan)	
Therapeutic alliance with therapist	
Stable mood, minimal symptoms	

Source.   Knoll and Kaufman 2017, p. 583, among others.

treatment of substance use disorders, which reduces suicide risk during incarceration and immediately after release (Daniel 2006).

Actively suicidal persons usually require a one-to-one constant watch, while those who have some suicidal ideation but no specific plan may be safe with a 10- to 15-minute watch. Protocols also dictate the daily evaluations and progressive evaluations, stepdowns, and eventual discharge from a suicide watch, often to a lower-level but closely observed care called *psychological observation*. Discharge may involve further stepdowns to camera rooms or closely observed restrictive housing, but the negative influences of restrictive housing are described below. Anyone who has been on a suicide watch should be seen frequently after returning to the general population, usually at 1, 3, 5, and 7 days.

An interview with a patient on a suicide watch is not the best time to do a thorough assessment. When possible, assessments should take place in a location that offers privacy, confidentiality, and comfort. A complete assessment requires information from multiple sources, including any documents about the patient's past, recent, and present suicidal ideation and behaviors. The assessment should include a review of the person's mental health history, current behaviors, suicide risk, protective factors, and justification for interventions to reduce risk.

Obtain a history of trauma and abuse, family mental health history, and note any history of traumatic brain injury. Know the lethality of planned attempts. Assess for feelings of helplessness, hopelessness, and of being "trapped." Ask questions nonjudgmentally in a direct and matter-of-fact tone (National Commission on Correctional Health Care and American Foundation for Suicide Prevention 2019). Reflect an understanding of the patient's wanting to die to relieve what is frequently considered to be psychic pain. Psychic pain is a concept that has been related to suicide risk for many years, developed by Shneidman (1998), and its relevance to suicide risk been shown in a recent meta-analysis (Ducasse et al. 2018). Psychic pain involves three components: "an unpleasant feeling (which might include suffering), appraisal of an inability or discrepancy (e.g., between what is desired and what is achievable), and unsustainability (an unbearable, destructive situation that demands resolution)" (Yager 2015, p. 940). You may also find of interest the concept that suicidality involves three similar elements that the clinician calls the "three I's": inescapable, interminable, and intolerable (Chiles 2019, p. 22; see also Chiles 2018).

Some tips for conducting an effective assessment are shown in Table 5–5.

Challenges of Assessing and Treating Suicidal Behavior in Corrections

The complexity of correctional facilities creates challenges for assessing and treating suicidal patients (Table 5–6). One impediment is the differing viewpoints between the corrections staff and mental health providers. Corrections officers are wary of manipulative behaviors, and mental health providers are concerned with risk and prevention of suicide. Corrections staff may be mistrustful of reports of suicidal ideation and be more focused on maintaining order, whereas the mental health professionals recognize that some behaviors are not under the patient's control and that these behaviors may be intensified by the stress of being incarcerated.

Efforts to reduce suicides are complicated by those contingent statements or threats of manipulative threats of suicide mentioned above, and it may be difficult to distinguish among suicidal statements with no suicidal intent, nonsuicidal pleas for help by claiming suicidal ideation, and genuine suicidal ideation with a high risk of completing the suicide. Policies for management of suicidal patients (e.g., a single cell, suicide blanket, no visitors, finger foods) are meant to address safety but can be seen by patients as demeaning and punitive (Crumlish 2020), and they may avoid talking about suicide because they do not want to be restricted.

Most policies, of course, involve the transfer of suicidal patients into a higher level of care such as a suicide watch. It all depends on what is considered suicidal thinking (also called *suicidal ideation*) or suicidal behavior. Suicidal thinking can range from what is often called *passive ideation* (e.g., a wish to be dead, a wish that one didn't wake up in the morning), to nonspecific thoughts of suicide but no plan, to having a plan and an intent to carry out the act, to the act itself. We recommend a formal assessment instrument, as described in Chapter 3, such as the Columbia-Suicide Severity Rating Scale (Columbia University 2013). The following piece of advice is especially applicable to correctional settings, so we will quote it exactly: "Nonspecific suicidal thoughts that have no associated subjective or objective intent and that are fleeting or of short duration are not evidence of risk escalation beyond an individual's chronic baseline level" (Gold and Joshi 2018, p. 407, also citing Rudd 2014). And from another source (but the same volume): "Moreover, although several different terms have been used to refer to passive ideation (e.g., 'better off dead,' 'thoughts of my own death'), it is only a 'wish to die' that has been consistently associated with significantly increased risk, therefore eliminating other types of passive thoughts from the spectrum of suicidal ideation" (Posner et al. 2014, p. 19).

TABLE 5–5.	**Tips for assessing suicide risk**

Remember that screening and assessment are not the same.

Keep in mind that assessment is an ongoing process.

Include discussion of coping skills.

Ask direct questions in a matter-of-fact tone.

Avoid blanket questions.

Ask about specific behaviors.

Do not rely solely on self-report.

Include discussion of coping methods.

Reflect empathy and understanding of their pain.

Ensure privacy during assessment process.

Probe for suicidal desire, capability, intent, and mitigating buffers.

Determine how quickly suicidal thinking developed after a nonsuicidal period of thinking or feeling.

Determine what coping skills the patient used, what worked, and what didn't.

Determine intent to die or to self-harm or escape or other intent.

Assess for lethality of thinking and behaviors.

Assess for agitation/rage.

Assess for feelings of hopelessness and helplessness.

Compile history of current or past violent acts.

Assess for substance use disorders.

Refer to other professionals when appropriate.

Similarly, in people with chronic suicidal ideation and multiple attempts, the report of suicidal thoughts is not a helpful indicator of an escalation of risk (Gold and Joshi 2018; Posner et al. 2014). Thus (and something we have frequently heard in two-tiered institutions), a patient's report that "sometimes things are so bad that I think of jumping off the tier" is not an admissions ticket to a suicide watch. The chronically suicidal patient will be discussed in more detail below.

Therapeutic Interventions for the Patient With Suicidal Ideation

A patient on suicide watch is often not in a therapeutic environment. If you can, have the patient brought to you in a more officelike setting. A helpful guideline for conceptualizing a meeting with a prisoner who is suicidal is to see if the incident can or should be managed as a *crisis*. What makes an incident a crisis is that it often represents a confluence of influences or a "straw that broke the camel's back" in which an individual's coping capacity is overwhelmed and the individual sees suicide as the only solution at that moment because of a failure to cope or an inability to see another way out through forward thinking or problem solving. We believe this is the concept that clinicians are trying to capture when they characterize psychic pain as we described it previously. A crisis is by its nature a *transient* or *time-limited* event that is resolved by the individual's application of problem-solving skills, marshaling of resources and support systems, and the like. So you need to find out what brought about the crisis, then

TABLE 5–6.	Challenges of assessing and treating suicidal thinking in correctional facilities

Increased suicide rates

Higher rate of mental health issues in jails and prison compared with the general population

Challenge of assessing for actual suicidal thinking vs. claimed or contingent suicidal thinking

Frequent transfers out of the facilities

Disciplinary vs. therapeutic environment

Denial of suicidal ideation to effect release back into the general prison population

Difficulty of follow-up screening

Limited resources to provide treatment

Short-term stays

resolve it and reduce the suicide risk to a level that can be managed outside of the infirmary, and improve the long-term management of the patient's suicidal thinking.

The first session may include listening to the patient relaying his account of the most recent episode of suicidal ideation and/or behaviors. This disclosure will function as a foundation for treatment planning and a model for understanding how to halt the patient's desire to die. Therapeutic interventions include keeping the focus on managing the suicidal thoughts, instructing the patient on distraction techniques and coping strategies, physical activities, and techniques for requesting support. In addition to changing the perspective of negative thoughts and learning new coping skills, try to assist the patient to control impulsive behaviors and affective dysregulation. Goals include minimizing crisis states and establishing adaptive behavioral options to sustain a stable mood. By developing and broadening coping skills, suicidal persons gain more control over their self-destructive behaviors and the emotional destress that triggers them (Aviram et al. 2004). The treatment plan should be reviewed at every session and updated as needed.

Administrators can take actions to minimize bullying and other violence and to improve supportive interactions between prisoners and staff (World Health Organization and International Association for Suicide Prevention 2007) (see Tables 5–7 and 5–8).

Crisis Response Safety Plans

At some time before the patient is taken off a suicide watch, many facilities develop a crisis response safety plan (CRSP) with the patient in a cooperative effort (or revise an existing plan if there is one). It is important to note that a CRSP is not a "no suicide contract." No-suicide contracts are not recommended because they ask for a commitment to stay alive but without directions on how to do so (National Commission on Correctional Health Care and American Foundation for Suicide Prevention 2019). Research has not supported the effectiveness of no-suicide contracts. There appears to be more encouraging research for CRSPs, although we have also seen some criticism of effectiveness in the research base, so we would still not advise total reliance on any one method or intervention for suicide prevention.

Formats for CRSPs are available from many mental health organizations. For example, there is one with a detailed filled-in example for mental health consumers from the Maine Department of Health and Human Services (2021). Other examples

TABLE 5–7.	**Basics of managing suicidal patients**

Remove all sharps and other potentially dangerous objects.

Remain nonjudgmental and empathic.

Do not rush; allow time to discuss the issues.

Validate feelings.

Ask about suicidal ideation.

If the patient is at high risk, do not leave him or her alone.

Assess for plan and lethality.

Coordinate approach with patient and other staff.

Provide psychosocial education, including coping skills and goal-setting.

Set limits to ensure safe behaviors.

Focus on direct management of suicidal ideation and behaviors.

Review treatment plan at every session.

are available (Bryan 2017, n.d.). The CRSP is a straightforward method to decrease an individual's risk for suicidal behavior. See Figures 5–1 and 5–2 for a blank format and a filled-in example. It is important that it be developed collaboratively with the patient and handwritten by the patient himself if possible. At times we use a 4 × 6 index card but as we add more information we sometimes use a whole sheet. A typical plan has the following sections:

1. Personal warning signs
2. Coping strategies
3. Social support
4. Professional crisis support
5. (On the back): Reasons for living

The personal warning signs are signs of an impending suicidal crisis. Coping strategies are uncomplicated actions that can be taken alone to decrease stress and/or serve to distract from the stressful situation. The reasons for living can provide a sense of purpose and meaning in life. All the preceding should be items that personally apply to the patient, not "boilerplate" or generic items. If the patient has trouble thinking of answers for specific items, ask exploratory questions about her motivators and interests in life. The social support portion of the plan can include cellmates, residents of the unit, and family members or friends who will give support during the tough times. Controversial or nonsupportive family might need to be excluded initially and plans made to work out the difficulties, so they become unambivalent sources of support. Professional support in the institution includes correctional officers, chaplain, trusted members of the administration (if accessible), medical, and mental health staff. Correctional systems usually have a local hot line for problems and phone numbers will include contact information for a National Suicide Prevention Lifeline if the person does not feel she can reach anyone else. When the plan is complete, ask the patient what the probability is of her using the plan on a scale of 0–10, and explore low responses.

TABLE 5–8.	Essential features of suicide prevention in corrections facilities

Collaborative approach with administration, corrections, and clinical staff

Specialized administrative staff to ensure adequate mental health care

Training of all staff

Good communications between corrections officers and mental health staff

Mandatory screening of all inmates at intake

Identification of inmates with suicidal ideation

Safe housing

Debriefing after a completed suicide

Treatment of drug and/or alcohol withdrawal

Adequate monitoring of suicidal inmates

Interventions targeted to high risk and suicidal inmates

Adequate staffing

Minimizing bullying and other violence

Improving staff-prisoner relationships

Contacts with community-based services

Restrictive Housing: Suicide Risk and Challenges of Assessment and Treatment

Restrictive housing is a broad term that includes housing that is voluntarily chosen by prisoners for reasons of safety and may also be considered protective custody. *Segregation* or *disciplinary segregation* usually refers to housing that is involuntarily imposed on the prisoner for disciplinary or institutional safety reasons. Often considered to be an equivalent term, the term *solitary confinement* is still widely used to refer to the most highly restricted housing placements. Restrictive housing units have increasingly been viewed as negative and deleterious, and one element of prison reform is the minimization or elimination of solitary confinement, especially for prisoners with mental illness. A position statement by the American Psychiatric Association specifies that:

> Prolonged segregation of adult inmates with serious mental illness, with rare exceptions, should be avoided due to the potential for harm to such inmates. If an inmate with serious mental illness is placed in segregation, out-of-cell structured therapeutic activities (i.e., mental health/psychiatric treatment) in appropriate programming space and adequate unstructured out-of-cell time should be permitted. (American Psychiatric Association 2017)

The Society of Correctional Physicians (SCP) issued a position statement which asserts that restrictive housing of prisoners with SMI violates basic tenets of mental health treatment. The SCP issued recommendations to shift the SMI into a treatment-oriented housing rather than disciplinary, especially when the housing move was a factor in the violation of rules (American College of Correctional Physicians 2013).

Prisoners with mental illness are more likely to be housed in segregation than those without mental illness (Clark 2018). However, all prisoners, even those with no previous mental health services, should be monitored in restrictive housing units. Because of the appearance of the rounds being quick and cursory they are often criticized, but rounds on

Warning signs I am getting suicidal or going to hurt myself   [Side 1]

How can I cope by myself when I start getting into trouble?

Who can I contact?
   Call the National Suicide Prevention Lifeline 1-800-273-8255

Here are my reasons for living   [Side 2]

FIGURE 5–1. Example of a crisis response safety plan (blank format).

Warning signs I am getting suicidal or going to hurt myself [Side 1]

When I'm sleeping less or sleeping poorly

When I stop going to the yard

When I stay in my cell

When I stop eating

When I start to hear voices again

When I think of cutting my arm

When I think I should be dead

When I start to feel guilty about being in prison

When I think abut what my father did to me and I am so mad

When I pick up the razor and start playing with it

How can I cope by myself when I start getting into trouble?

Read a book

Wrap the razor up in a towel and put it away

Do some of my drawings

Read the Bible with the passages I marked and mark some new passages

Go to the yard and exercise or exercise in the cell

Just go to sleep

Do my deep breath

My progressive relaxation that they taught me

My mindfulness exercises

Who can I contact?

My mother 202-×××-××××

My brother 202-×××-××××

Tell my CO now that it is an emergency

Tell the nurse who brings me my medicines

Send in a mental health request

Talk to my cellie

Call the National Suicide Prevention Lifeline 1-800-273-8255

Here are my reasons for living [Side 2]

My family

My children

Suicide is a sin, and I don't want to do that

I like most of the things in life, just not the prison

I can get out in a year

I like watching television

FIGURE 5–2. Example of a crisis response safety plan (filled in).

these units are not meant to administer complete psychiatric assessments. The purpose is to ensure that mental health staff have a presence on the units, screen all prisoners, and improve access to mental health care services (Hughes and Metzner 2015).

Solitary confinement has often been referred to as "the prison within the prison." If the confinement is disciplinary, time out of cell may be limited to an hour a day. Until fairly recently it was common practice for prisoners to spend years in solitary confinement. Hundreds of prisoners were interviewed by Stuart Grassian, a psychiatrist and former faculty member at Harvard Medical School. He found severe mental health issues, including acute suicidal thinking, in a third of the prisoners in solitary. He concluded that solitary confinement may lead to hallucinations, panic attacks, paranoia, poor concentration and memory, poor impulse control, and hypersensitivity to external stimuli. Some prisoners developed debilitating obsessions. In one study of California prisons, nearly half of all suicides from 1999 to 2004 were of prisoners in solitary confinement. A 1995 study found that 63% of suicides took place in solitary or psychiatric seclusion cells (Breslow 2014).

A review of an 11-year period in a disciplinary housing unit of New York State Prison revealed a total of 32 suicides. The median days spent in disciplinary housing before suicide was 63. The recommendation from this review was to increase the observation of prisoners during the first 2 months. The increased scrutiny should include daily screening for suicide risk (Way et al. 2007). A review of medical records in the New York City jail system from January 2010 and January 2013 revealed self-harm to be unquestionably linked with being in solitary confinement. Predictors of self-harm also included length of stay, SMI, and younger age. But change can happen. The jail adopted changes in assigning prisoners with mental illness and who were violating jail rules to more therapeutic settings than solitary confinement (Kaba et al. 2014). Another solution used in New Jersey, after it was noted that single-cell detention had 23 times the suicide rate of the prison system, was to double-cell prisoners placed in detention (Reeves and Tamburello 2014).

Therapy in Restrictive Housing

Therapy in solitary confinement units requires a unified approach and planning for reentry to general population. Everything seems to be limited: time, resources, staffing, and privacy. Too often interactions with prisoners must be conducted through the food port, and if patients are taken to the office, there may be opposition to uncuffing them or at least cuffing them in front. It is difficult to get people out for group psychotherapies. There is a need for daily interaction with prisoners in the restrictive housing and daily suicide risk screenings.

Risk of Suicide on Death Row

There are relatively few people on death row—2553 on October 1, 2020 (Wikipedia 2020b)—so you may never be asked to see one. Such situations do seem ironic, since it seems even more cruel to lessen the suicide risk in a person so he can be killed by the state. Prisoners may find the living conditions on death row to be intolerable and may feel that the only escape from the situation will come with execution (Tartaro 2019).

To give an example from our home state: Scott Dozier was on death row in Nevada and not on suicide watch when he was found dead in his cell on January 5, 2019.

Many times he said he wanted to die rather than live his life in prison and said that suicide watches and segregation were unconstitutional and cruel. His execution was cancelled twice because of legal battles over a drug combination that had never been used for lethal injection. He stated, "Life in prison isn't a life.…This isn't living, man. It's just surviving." "If people say they're going to kill me, get to it." He had been on death row for 11 years at the time of his suicide (Ritter 2019; Romo 2019).

Nonsuicidal Self-Injurious Behavior

Nonsuicidal self-injurious behavior (NSSIB) is not a current DSM-5-TR diagnosis, but DSM-5-TR does include nonsuicidal self-injury as a "condition that may be a focus of clinical attention" and presents nonsuicidal self-injury disorder as a "condition for further study." Self-injurious behaviors are unlike suicidal behaviors and do not *seem* to have the purpose of ending one's life. Although the lethal intent is *apparently* not there, self-injurious behavior can result in death. Self-injurious acts may include cutting, scratching, inserting foreign objects, biting, head-banging, amputation, enucleation, and evisceration. Cutting is the most common. Early detection of persons at risk for self-injury is crucial. The person may use a shared implement to cut, and this will increase the risk of a blood-borne disease (Helfand et al. 2010; International Society for the Study of Self Injury 2018; Young et al. 2006). The approach to NSSIB needs to be multidisciplinary and involves careful and sometimes complex treatment planning. Institutional change may be necessary as NSSIB may be closely related to poor coping with institutional policies (Thomas et al. 2006).

Differences Between NSSIB and Suicidal Behaviors

Opinions of researchers differ as to the ability to distinguish NSSIB and suicidal behaviors, but the current trend is that although they are not the same, they may be mistaken for each other during the assessment and treatment processes. NSSIB differs from a suicide attempt as far as intent, methods, prevalence, lethality, and chronicity. The objective in NSSIB is not to end life but to adjust it. Although both are self-destructive actions, it is important to recognize that NSSIB is a dysfunctional method of coping to control overwhelming emotions and to endure life, whereas an attempt at suicide is a desire to escape and terminate one's life (Butler and Malone 2013). The problem, even if the two behaviors can be distinguished, is that a person who engages in NSSIB may also be or become suicidal, so the tendency to "dismiss" NSSIB as "merely" manipulative can lead to inadequate management.

A very large study of self-harm and suicide from 2004 to 2009 in England and Wales (Hawton et al. 2014) identified 139,195 incidents in 26,510 prisoners. Teenagers of both sexes were included in this study. The study authors found that 5%–6% of male and 20%–24% of female prisoners self-harmed every year, the rate being 10 times higher in females. In the females there was much repetition with a group of 102, accounting for 17,307 incidents. The most common methods were scratching or cutting (65% of 69,634 incidents in males and 51% of 69,548 incidents in females). The next most frequent methods in males were poisoning, overdose, or swallowing objects not intended for ingestion (9%) followed by hanging (7%) and self-strangulation (5%). The second most common method in females was self-strangulation (31%), and other methods included impact injury, wound aggravation, ligature, and biting (less than 5%).

Of course, there is interest in the relationship of self-harm and completed suicide. The same study mentioned above recorded 109 suicides, which amounts to an annual rate of 411 per 100,000 among those 26,510 individuals who had self-harmed. Deaths by suicide consisted of 95 male deaths (rate of 450 per 100,000) and 14 female deaths (rate of 259 per 100,000). In the population of prisoners who did not self-harm, the estimated suicide rates were 79 in males and 98 in females. The authors found that about 50% of the people who died by suicide in prison had a history of self-harm, which increased the odds of suicide in custody between 6 and 11 times (Hawton et al. 2014).

The difficulty in dealing with NSSIB is made clear by a study that reported that 18% of 242 men engaged in self-injurious behavior *while in a California prison psychiatric hospital* (average stay over 100 days). Many of them had been admitted for the same behavior. The major predictive factor for self-harm was not a (former) Axis I disorder but personality disorder and high psychopathy. These persons also had more than eight times the risk of hurting staff members. The authors suggest that the basic defect in harming self or others is a failure of inhibition and that a relapse prevention model could lessen such behaviors (Young et al. 2006).

Assessing NSSIB

During assessment it is important to avoid negative, judgmental conceptions about NSSIB such as that the behavior is "attention seeking" or "manipulative." Although NSSIB is not the same as suicidal behavior, it is important to assess for any suicidal thinking, either concurrently or in tandem with the NSSIB assessment. Decreasing anxiety will result in more honest responses. Details to obtain include asking about the onset, frequency, and methods. You may want to ask, "When was the first time you cut yourself?" or "When was the last time?" rather than vaguely "How often?" Be specific and ask, "How many times a week do you cut?" To determine the methods used you can ask, "What do you typically do or use?" Other areas to assess for are aftercare, reasons, and stages of change. There may be an increased risk for infection and scarring with the lack of wound care. Ask, "After the injury how do you take care of the wounds?" and "Have you ever hurt yourself so badly that you needed stitches?" To establish your treatment plan and provide interventions, ask about the reasons for engaging in NSSIB. You can validate that the NSSIB may be a coping mechanism without condoning the behaviors. You may say, "It sounds like this has helped you. In what way does it help?" Some self-injuring persons may want to discontinue the behaviors but be frustrated as to how to stop. Others see no need to change the behaviors. In such cases, you will want to ask, "Is this something you want to stop?" In summary, the three key questions (as presented by Westers et al. 2016) are:

- Suicidality: "Are you thinking about suicide when you self-injure?"
- Aftercare: "How do you take care of your injuries?"
- Reasons: "In what ways is this helping you?"

A final item to keep in mind is that persons with self-regulation problems leading to self-injury also have problems involving violence with others, this relationship being noted from the onset of both behaviors in adolescence (Richmond-Rakerd et al.

2019). So your treatments to lessen self-injury should also be helpful in reducing interpersonal violence.

Suicide and Mental Illness

A widely held assumption is that most people who attempt suicide (usually about 90% of patients who die by suicide) have a mental illness (Arsenault-Lapierre et al. 2004). We think this is still probably true. Although DSM-5 proposed suicidal behavior disorder as a "Condition for Further Study" (including criteria involving a suicide attempt within 24 months of the diagnosis), and this item was retained in the first printing of DSM-5-TR, it was subsequently dropped. An interesting discussion is found in the volume by Bering (2019), who refers to the concept of "predicament suicide" or the kind of thing that is widely prevalent in prison and occurs to people without pre-existing mental conditions. He gives an example of a sex offender who has been living in an isolated location but has to return to a crowded society. Why, thinks the man, go through the trouble? So does he have a mental illness? How much of suicide is predicament related? There are those we refer to as "narcissistically wounded," who kill themselves soon after arrest or arraignment. A widely discussed case was that of Jeffrey Epstein, the American financier and convicted sex offender who apparently killed himself in 2019 while awaiting trial on new charges. Bering is a psychologist and writer who has chronicled his own experiences with suicidal thinking (Bering 2018), and some of his self-observations may also apply to chronically suicidal people. As to whether everyone feels better that they have been saved, that is kind of a self-fulfilling prophecy, since persistently suicidal people can find fatal methods to kill themselves if their plan recurs.

Suicide and Serious Mental Illness

Word spreads rapidly via "Inmate-dot-com" of an individual suicide or attempt in the building. Personality-disordered patients will take glee in chiding your department for failing to prevent it. Patients with SMI who have suicidal voices become worried of their weaknesses or inability to prevent themselves from ending up the same way, so discuss this with them or explore their worries while at the same time, citing HIPAA, noting that you can't tell them the details of the individual case. If the patient begins to allude to the ease of committing suicide and getting it over with, you should explore the thoughts, although (as in the following example), you should know your patient's history.

Case Vignette

THERAPIST: Are your voices telling you to hurt yourself? If you feel like obeying them, I would like to know about it. If you jump from the tier, you could really hurt yourself or even kill yourself. A few years ago, there was someone who jumped, and he broke his ankle. But the point is, he regretted it and he is glad he is okay now.

PATIENT (*proudly*): Oh, that's nothing. Eight years ago, I jumped off the Hoover Dam, and I also broke my leg.

THERAPIST (*gobsmacked*): Oh, let's talk about that…(*to self:* Was that in his record? Was that a fantasy or is it even possible?)

Programs for Reducing Suicide Risk

In several places we discuss programs that in their original forms and forensic modifications appear to reduce suicide attempts or attempts at self-harm. These include dialectical behavior therapy (Linehan 1993; see also Bohus et al. 2000), various forms of CBT, and therapies in the so-called third wave of CBT such as acceptance and commitment therapy (ACT) (Hayes et al. 2016). A similar-sounding program, ACCT (Assessment, Care in Custody and Teamwork), is used in England and Wales (HM Prison Service 2005). A manualized program combining CBT and DBT, called MACT (manual-assisted cognitive therapy), has been developed (Boyce et al. 2001). (For brief reviews and discussion of other programs and approaches, see Labrecque and Patry 2018.)

Of course, we interview patients who have attempted suicide, after the safety issues have been dealt with, to determine the reasons they made their attempt as well as the current risk going forward. We find that our impressions are consistent with findings of a study based on interviews with 24 prisoners in Oregon state prisons who had attempted suicide (Suto 2007). The conclusion was that multiple factors (we would probably call it a "perfect storm" after the movie of the same name) often converge to cause a particular suicide attempt. From our review, the salient reasons are:

- Depression or worsening depression, especially when associated with hopelessness.
- Threats, either acute or ongoing, from other prisoners that had not been dealt with.
- Issues getting along with officers leading to some so-called manipulative suicide attempts.
- Boredom, especially for time in the cell, and lack of useful activities (see also Harris 2007).

Prisoners had multiple recommendations that they thought would help, including the availability of crisis counseling before they needed an actual suicide watch to prevent them from becoming suicidal. There should be a process by which they can obtain crisis counseling and list it on their CRSP. Keep in mind that—in some individuals—suicidal ideation through suicidal action can develop and occur within minutes to hours seemingly out of nowhere, meaning that crisis services need to be available on weekends and 24 hours a day. A common theme in suicides is that they are not well thought out, and this explains why most people are grateful when they are saved from it. The existentialist philosopher Albert Camus was much fascinated by this and tells us that the supposedly obvious causes of suicide are not actually the most powerful, and it is almost impossible to find out after the fact what the real causes are. Possibly these are some personal sorrow or illness, says Camus, but he wonders if the final triggering event could be some slight from a friend of the suicide victim. If so, says Camus, that is the guilty person (Camus 1942/2018, p. 5)!

Worsening depression probably explains (but still cannot predict) many suicides. However, there are other factors in chronic suicidal thinking that may concern therapists. In fact, even the concepts of being and becoming suicidal are brought into question by a practitioner whom we shall discuss. (But we will add a "grain of salt" to his advice.)

What Do You Say After You Say "Hello"? (Updated)

In an earlier chapter, we characterized therapy as basically a set of decisions about what to say after you say "Hello." To drill down on such choices, we can say that these decisions should always and continuously consider suicide risk. So what you say after you say "Hello" is (tactfully and tastefully and strategically), "Are you—in any way, shape, or form—suicidal?" You need to do your initial assessments and reassessments as required by your institution's policies but include:

- Medical patients newly admitted to the infirmary.
- Your regular patients who happen to be in the infirmary (conduct daily assessments, or "wellness checks").
- Hospital returns, both psychiatric and medical.
- Court returns.
- Returns from visitation if the person appears to be upset.

And you need to put in place a process to make it easier to see prisoners who have received bad news.

One frustrating experience of doing suicide assessments is the receipt of ambiguous answers or refusals to answer. One authority (among many) says to err on the side of caution (Canning and Dvoskin 2018). All it means is maybe spending a little effort but possibly preventing one more suicide. But as we discuss later, you *cannot* put every chronically suicidal patient in the infirmary every time they tell you that they are suicidal. Those patients may need special and often creative monitoring outside the infirmary. You put people in the infirmary when there has been an onset of new suicidal thinking or a worsening of chronic suicidal thinking.

By now the deleterious effects of segregated housing, especially for those with preexisting mental illness, have been extensively documented. In a later chapter, we talk about gang dropouts and note that even these individuals can become suicidal after they choose to move into protected custody. A history of childhood maltreatment does increase suicide risk, but trauma is so prevalent that it cannot be used as a risk factor (Canning and Dvoskin 2018).

Chronically Suicidal Patients

Chronic suicidal thinking is a major problem in corrections. Later in the book, we discuss personality disorders, but here we focus on suicide risk and its mitigation through psychotherapy.

Patients with borderline personality disorder (BPD) are a well-known subset of chronically suicidal patients. While these patients present special problems in the community, there are actually advantages to treating them in prisons. For example, the most common suicidal behavior in the community is an overdose of pills, which can be mitigated in prison by use of directly observed pill administration, use of crushed or liquid medication, and prevention of hoarding. Self-cutting is another form of self-harm but is not usually fatal (by intent) even though it can be accomplished under supervision or control of sharp objects. Observers such as correctional officers or cellmates may also report on changes in behavior or forestall completion of a suicide or self-harm attempt, though such reports are not 100% preventive.

According to Paris (2006), who addressed this condition in the community, chronic suicidality should be managed differently from acute suicidality. Now, we mentioned earlier that we are trying to avoid the use of "suicidality" in place of more precise substitutes, but Paris even questions the use of the term "suicidality" because patients expressing such worries have a low rate of actual suicide and self-harming behaviors are not usually intended to be fatal. He believes that hospitalization should be avoided whenever possible, in lieu of options such as day treatment with experienced treatment teams. He reports on a patient with BPD who noticed that his self-destructive episodes started after he became aware that the mental health system was obliged to respond to his behavior. He says that hospitals reinforce the behaviors that therapists try to extinguish (Paris 2002), and presumably this would be true for prisoners being sent outside the institution to emergency departments or mental health units. His antihospitalization recommendations reinforce the advantages of keeping a patient in the prison environment, with its stepped care ranging from general population to one-to-one observation. Therapy should focus on helping the patient to solve his problems and improve his functioning and supporting his reasons for living (Paris 2006).

Another recommendation (derived from DBT) is that suicide should be discussed *first* in the therapy session because the patient cannot get on to the supposed issues of the day until she deals with the suicide issue and because this turns out to be a form of negative reinforcement for the suicidal ideation itself. In line with this, the clinician should not be overly anxious when hearing about the suicidal ideation (Paris 2002). However, some of the reasons that hospitalization is undesirable or counterproductive are worth noting. The hospital environment provides a social support system that may be missing for a patient with BPD who lives in the community, and self-harm behaviors while there result in more attention and a longer stay. A better alternative to full hospitalization is the day program, since patients with BPD do better in structured programs.

Paris points out that there is always a risk of suicide and a potential for it to occur, but the risk of losing a community lawsuit is low. Yet in the prison setting it is true that suicides can and will be litigated, and this will lead clinicians to be extremely cautious in treating patients with high-risk histories and current suicidal behaviors. The fundamental claim is that the hospitalization doesn't lower the risk anyway so it still should be avoided. However, as part of a treatment process, we have found that hospitalization provides a way to acquire additional data and professional opinions about a person's condition and behavior and, frankly, shows that an attempt was made at the highest level of care to see what could be done for the patients. Sometimes you just learn something new.

Worsening depression is not the cause of chronic suicidal thinking, which according to Paris is substantially due to personality disorder (and in prison populations, a strong contribution of borderline personality disorder). Drawing on data from the general population, he argues that the ratio of attempts to completions is extremely high and that a majority of outpatients who die by suicide do so on the first attempt. Prisons are different, however, and have a tremendous concentration of mental illness and substance abuse.

You will see more data about this in subsequent chapters. Mental illness and substance abuse are both risk factors for suicide, so the ratio of attempts to completions is lower, and the ability to predict suicide, while still evasive, has more grounding in the risk factors. DuRand et al. (1995) found that the rate of completed suicides among prisoners with past attempts (in a Detroit jail) was 100 times that of the general population. There are other risk factors as well. Conviction for manslaughter or murder meant 19 times the risk for suicide compared with other charges. All the suicides were by hanging, and most occurred within 31 days of admission. There are a lot of useful data just from this one small study. So that is the "grain of salt" we mentioned above. The lesson we received in the outpatient world—that "suicide is impossible to predict"—is less valid in prison. Attempts, including so-called parasuicidal behaviors, are much highly correlated with actual suicides *in prison*. Sad to say, given the tremendous baseline rates of serious risk factors (e.g., depression, personality disorder, substance abuse) and attempts, there is still much that needs to done to lower the suicide rate in correctional institutions.

All by Myself

What is it that leads a person who is not suicidal in the morning to become suicidal by noon? Let us turn to our science fiction source with an example. Dr. Conway, a physician in the mammoth hospital of alien patients, hooks himself up to an "educator tape" to learn more about a race of telepathic aliens, one of whom is his sick patient. Pretty soon he starts to feel terribly alone and misses the company of his fellow human beings. He feels unwanted and unloved, and soon he wishes he had never been born (White 2001, pp. 61–62). What has happened? Not being telepathic like his patient, Dr. Conway finds that sinking into his educator tape has cut him off from the normal ways he used to communicate with other people, and the profound isolation makes him suicidal. So imagine the situation in the following vignette.

Case Vignette

PATIENT: I am sorry I tried to kill myself, Doc. I just wasn't myself.
THERAPIST: Then who were you?
PATIENT: You know what I mean. I was beside myself.
THERAPIST: You mean like you were outside yourself looking in, like dissociated?
PATIENT: No, not really, I mean like something had gotten into me.
THERAPIST: Like coronavirus? I guess that could do it.
PATIENT: No, not sick in that way. I was demoralized.
THERAPIST: So was your suicide attempt a moral decision?
PATIENT: C'mon, Doc, you're just making fun of me now. You *know* what I mean!
THERAPIST: Do I?

Does he? The ability to show patients that we do know what they mean is important. It is important to convince patients that we can and do know what it is like to feel their pain and become suicidal in the way that they are.

An initial step in dealing with chronic suicidal thinking in patients with BPD is identification of "acute on chronic" episodes, a term that is probably derived from medical illnesses such as acute on chronic respiratory disease and has an analogy to the diagnostic gradations of schizophrenia such as "chronic with acute exacerbation." In addition to chronic risk factors, added acute factors may include depression and hopelessness. In the community, suicide risk increases after hospitalization (Links and Bergmans 2016), which does suggest that hospitalization per se does not reduce the risk. Links and Bergmans (2016) give the following advice:

- Do not rely on intuition or gut feelings, but use objective evidence such as legal difficulties, affective instability, or worsening of a major depressive episode.
- Work out the early warning signs for the individual patient. This is the approach taken when preparing a CRSP. In prison, these are typically avoiding others, staying in the cell, pacing in the yard, not eating, irritability, having urges to cut, and so forth.
- Help patients to process rather than control emotions using what Links and Bergmans call their own personal "sealing" methods or we would call the coping methods on the CRSP.
- Help the patient to understand the psychological meaning of the chronic suicidal thoughts. Links and Bergmans give an example of a patient who realized that she tried to be a rebellious child to get attention.
- Using a "side-by-side" therapeutic relationship, diminish shame and increase self-agency.
- Using a model derived from the concept of alexithymia, help patients to learn the difference between feeling unsafe and being unsafe. Reinforce that they are likely to be safe when they have chosen a behavior, the behavior is time limited, and they remain in control.
- Using a method from solution-focused therapy, teach them to rate themselves as safe (green), at-risk (yellow), or unsafe (red). As they develop the capacity to observe and rate the emotional distress, their scale becomes more refined (which is conveyed to the therapist).
- Foster a curiosity in their own minds of what is going on, which creates an observing self-distance that they did not have before. Links and Bergmans use the analogy of Dorothy being swept up in the tornado: That is how patients with BPD feel before they develop an awareness of the emotions that drive them.

There are many therapies with varying effectiveness to treating chronic suicidal thinking, typically in persons with BPD. These include mentalization-focused treatment, transference-focused psychotherapy, and DBT. In keeping with our preference for supportive techniques, we mention in particular a set of recommendations based on common factors psychotherapy described by Yager and Feinstein (2017). (As mentioned in Chapter 1, psychotherapies based on common factors are supportive.) We summarize below their recommendations (modified for work in prison), but it's worth reading the original article (which is readily available) with one reservation (noted below). These techniques are offered for use with all chronically suicidal patients, but because of the prominence in prison of BPD, we would expect that these techniques would be used frequently with BPD.

- Learn to "listen with the third ear," a term made famous by psychoanalyst Theodor Reik (1949). That is, don't wait for them to raise an issue; see what is implied and locate those elephants in the room.

- Determine the actual motivations and prior thoughts behind actual suicide attempts, including cultural beliefs (e.g., motives of revenge or self-punishment).
- Identify coping strategies and defenses to suicide (typical strategies of supportive psychotherapy); pay attention to failed defenses leading to suicidal actions; this includes examining the role of trauma.
- Help patients manage emotions better and tolerate psychic pain.
- Examine the effects of taunts or encouragements by patient's peers to self-harm for the enjoyment of the others. (Useful in prison)
- Explore patient's fantasies (sadistic or otherwise) of how others will react to her death and encourage discussion of their unrealistic nature (e.g., visiting their own funeral as Tom Sawyer did) and support that the friends and family will need to get over the patient's death.
- Develop religious (e.g., faith-based) supports or existential issues that oppose suicide.
- Determine the right balance of exploration and support (our preference is the latter). Depressed and suicidal patients tend to deteriorate when they sense that they are not getting support (Yager and Feinstein 2017, p. 215).

Of course, all this is part of a multidisciplinary, multimodal therapy, including the use of a CRSP and involvement (to the extent possible) of outside family and friends.

Clinicians need to manage their countertransference reactions and their own stress, a topic we addressed in the previous chapter.

We do disagree on one issue: the use of what Yager and Feinstein admit might seem to be "irreverent" tough talk such as asking the patient what we are supposed to tell his survivors after he kills himself (Yager and Feinstein 2017, p. 216). These recommendations were intended for ongoing outpatient work, but we think that the intense therapist-patient relationship in the prison environment encourages dangerous acting out in response to such remarks.

Paris emphasizes that chronic suicidality serves a psychological function of relieving dysphoria and communicating distress and is part of the borderline personality structure. His advice (Paris 2014, pp. 161–188):

- It is *not* necessary for the patient to work through childhood trauma.
- The patient needs to find meaningful work and relationships.
- Talk to the healthy part of the patient.
- Ask the patient to reappraise his incidences of emotional reasoning—for example, when he interprets negative remarks as total rejections or when there is a tendency to react with hopelessness.
- Remember that developing a working alliance with a patient with BPD can be difficult. Paris quotes Adler (1979), who says that patients with borderline personality do not even share the concept of "we."

Patients with BPD are known to desensitize themselves to death and engage in a variety of dangerous behaviors such as driving fast in traffic. This leads to one more point: Identify and diffuse any ambivalence to death. This is discussed elsewhere by Paris (2004) under the rubric of "half in love with easeful death," a phrase from John Keats's "Ode to a Nightingale." Here are a few more lines for the context:

My heart aches, and a drowsy numbness pains
My sense, as though of hemlock I had drunk,
Or emptied some dull opiate to the drains
One minute past, and Lethe-wards had sunk:…
Darkling I listen; and, for many a time
I have been half in love with easeful Death,
Call'd him soft names in many a mused rhyme,
To take into the air my quiet breath;
Now more than ever seems it rich to die,
To cease upon the midnight with no pain…

Keats (1795–1821) penned this in 1819 and considered it to be an excursion into his "negative capability," which does seem to be a poetic flirtation with themes of death. A few years later, when he was in great pain, it has been speculated that he was depressed and suicidal and wanted laudanum (an early medicinal form of an opiate) from his doctor, who withheld it. Keats died of tuberculosis, and it is thought that he had already contracted it by 1819 (Smith 2004). The peak of the pandemic was about the year 1800. "By the dawn of the 19th century, tuberculosis—consumption—had killed one in seven of the people that had ever lived" (PBS 2020), including his mother and two of his brothers. Yes, there were pandemics before COVID-19.

In conclusion, Paris urges empathy for patients who are in such psychological pain that they think of suicide as often as daily, sometimes as a way of giving them a sense that they have some control over their lives. These patients experience psychological pain, emptiness, and hopelessness. They are in severe and continuous distress. "The feelings that the chronically suicidal patient is trying to cope with are beyond the experience of most people. Empathizing with these states of mind requires some imagination" (Paris 2014, p. xv).

Women and Suicide in Prison

The situations that affect women are different enough to warrant some differences in advice. We will highlight some of them here and discuss these issues more in Chapter 11. In this respect, there is much useful data and advice in a monograph by Walker and Towl (2016), who point out that there is a problem attempting to lessen suicidal thinking and behavior: If you pay attention to the patients who are clearly at risk (in suicide risk assessments), you will spend a lot of time on false positives, because most of them will not die by suicide. In the United Kingdom, where much of their research was based, there has been a redirection of efforts away from merely identifying at-risk persons and toward positive and proactive strategies (Walker and Towl 2016, p. 81). However, while it is true that clinicians need to address the fact that many suicides occur in persons without prior or "static" risk factors, the at-risk group (even when we use the data from their own book) still needs close scrutiny. Especially for women, the strongest risk factor for suicide is a history of self-injury (Walker and Towl 2016, p. 97, citing Joiner et al. 2005).

Of course, we like to point out the effectiveness of supportive psychotherapy in the therapeutic situations we discuss in this book. An obvious question would therefore be, "What interventions can reduce suicide?" Walker and Towl (2016) discuss two interventions in U.K. prisons. One used a modified DBT program, including individual psychotherapy. It was promising but had no control group. The other study was called WORSHIP II (Women Offenders Repeat Self-Harm Interventions Pilot II) and used an intervention called *psychodynamic-interpersonal therapy*, a reasonable approach that involved discussing the events and interpersonal situations that led to a patient's suicide attempts. Unlike the others, this study had an active control that consisted of meeting with a staff member and performing a positive activity such as playing cards, but not discussing personal business. The actual event of a suicide is still too rare to support a small research study, but a useful proxy is a measurement of suicidal thinking with a scale such as the Beck Scale for Suicidal Ideation. Both groups improved on that scale on thoughts of suicide, self-harm repetition, and self-harm severity. Unfortunately, this randomized controlled trial was a failure: there was no difference between the active controls and the intervention group. What does this mean? It means supportive interventions can lessen suicidal thinking. Just spend the time and it is likely to help your patients! But, okay, there is still more than "happy talk" involved. Individual interventions include:

- Do not keep people waiting in intake—see them within 45 minutes.
- Have a First Day in Custody program.
- Ask about being bullied, as you won't be told unless you tease it out; this includes taxing, extortion, and ostracism (Walker and Towl 2016, p. 89).
- Analyze the situations that led to suicidal behaviors.
- Find ways to increase time outside of the cell.

Other interventions include:

- Interface with officers to reduce the incidents that trigger self-harm.
- Work also with officers, bullies, and victims to create an antibullying ethic and environment to deconstruct bullying situations.

Medication

Medication plays a role in the treatment of most serious disorders and often in the treatment of suicidal behavior. In a previous chapter, when we covered insomnia, we discussed the choice "to medicate or meditate." As we emphasized then, insomnia plays a role in suicidal thinking, and failure to recognize this puts to shame those organizations that decry the use of medications for insomnia yet claim to have proactive suicide prevention policies. So, of course, medication should be considered and patients evaluated for medication for the dual purposes of ameliorating the symptoms of their mental illnesses and lessening suicidal thinking. Certain medications, such as clozapine and lithium, have a strong evidence basis. For example, clozapine was found more effective than olanzapine and is FDA approved for suicide risk reduction in persons with schizophrenia. However, these results were found almost 20 years ago (Meltzer et al. 2003), and no other medication has since received approval. Although the clozapine study involved comparison with olanzapine, the use of olanzapine itself has been suggested to reduce suicidal behavior in other patients. So has quetiapine, but that medication is severely restricted in corrections because of its widespread abuse. The clozapine study took 2 years, so it is not a quick fix for suicidal behavior.

Suicidal ideation that is clearly linked to depression or psychosis should be targeted by possible medication treatment. However, as we noticed when we studied insomnia, it is not just SMI that merits attention. The situational factors that create suicide risks begin with the first few days in jail or the "bad day in court." Increased anxiety is related to suicidal thinking and so forth. The suicide risks caused by these situational factors can also be addressed by temporary medication "fixes" along with coping techniques such as mindfulness, meditation, and guided imagery techniques. To be sure, medicine is not the be-all and end-all in treating suicidal ideation. But whether you are a prescriber or not, be prepared to remind your patient about the possibility of taking some medicine if you think it will help.

Key Points

- Any psychotherapist will become involved at some time in crisis management or grief counseling. The difference this makes to you is that you are not just a crisis worker but a skilled psychotherapist, and your work with patients is ongoing and not limited.

- Many people suffering ordinary grief do not want or need grief counseling. You can follow up with wellness checks, but these differ from grief counseling in that you are there to talk but not about the grief.

- Complicated grief, however, which is extended in time and does not undergo the normal resolution to integrated grief, is more likely to be encountered in corrections.

- Disenfranchised grief is also particularly applicable to prisoners, who have multiple losses of people, jobs, finances, and opportunities that are not normal or socially discussed objects of grief.

- The risk of suicide is always on the minds of therapists, and the points of risk are many.

- Static risk factors for suicide may not be changed but can provide important information to stratify risk and plan interventions.

- Dynamic risk factors can be the object of therapeutic interventions by therapists or via systemic institutional changes.

- It is common practice to use a crisis response safety plan, usually a two-sided card or page that the patient writes himself with the therapist's cooperation. On the front is a list of warning signs, coping methods, and resources to contact. On the back are the patient's reasons to live.

- Chronic suicidal thoughts and behaviors, frequently found in patients with borderline personality disorder, require different management from acutely suicidal behavior. In such cases, hospitalizations may be counterproductive or reinforce suicidal behaviors.

- In women, the greatest predictor of suicide risk is a history of self-harm. Women with those histories need special attention and therapy from the start.

- Individual therapy should be accompanied by systemwide training and policies.

- Medication therapy for suicidal thoughts or behavior should not be forgotten.

References

Adler G: The myth of the alliance with borderline patients. Am J Psychiatry 136(5):642–645, 1979 434239

American College of Correctional Physicians: Position statement on segregation of prisoners with mental illness. July 2013. Available at: http://accpmed.org/restricted_housing_of_mentally.php. Accessed January 11, 2021.

American Psychiatric Association: Position statement on segregation of prisoners with mental illness. December 2017. Available at: http://nrcat.org/storage/documents/apa-statement-on-segregation-of-prisoners-with-mental-illness.pdf. Accessed January 11, 2021.

Arsenault-Lapierre G, Kim C, Turecki G: Psychiatric diagnoses in 3275 suicides: a meta-analysis. BMC Psychiatry 4(37):37, 2004 15527502

Aviram RB, Hellerstein DJ, Gerson J, Stanley B: Adapting supportive psychotherapy for individuals with borderline personality disorder who self-injure or attempt suicide. J Psychiatr Pract 10(3):145–155, 2004 15330220

Bering J: Suicidal: Why We Kill Ourselves. Chicago, IL, University of Chicago Press, 2018

Bering J: Sometimes you won't feel better tomorrow. Slate, February 15, 2019. Available at: https://slate.com/technology/2019/02/mental-illness-suicide-rational-thought-getting-help.html. Accessed November 29, 2020.

Bohus M, Haaf B, Stiglmayr C, et al: Evaluation of inpatient dialectical-behavioral therapy for borderline personality disorder—a prospective study. Behav Res Ther 38(9):875–887, 2000 10957822

Bonanno GA: The Other Side of Sadness: What the New Science of Bereavement Tells Us About Life After Loss. New York, Basic Books, 2010

Boyce P, Oakley-Browne MA, Hatcher S: The problem of deliberate self-harm. Curr Opin Psychiatry 14(2):107–111, 2001

Breslow JM: What does solitary confinement do to your mind? Frontline, April 22, 2014. Available at: www.pbs.org/wgbh/frontline/article/what-does-solitary-confinement-do-to-your-mind. Accessed June 2, 2020.

Bridges to Recovery: What are the signs of complicated grief disorder? 2020. Available at: www.bridgestorecovery.com/complicated-grief/signs-complicated-grief-disorder. Accessed October 25, 2020.

Bryan CJ: The crisis response plan (CRP). 2017. Available at: https://crpforsuicide.com. Accessed September 29, 2020.

Bryan CJ: Crisis response plan (web log post). Military Suicide Research Consortium. n.d. Available at: https://msrc.fsu.edu/blog/msrc-common-data-elements-cde.

Butler AM, Malone K: Attempted suicide v non-suicidal self-injury: behaviour, syndrome or diagnosis? Br J Psychiatry 202(5):324–325, 2013 23637106

Campbell S: Can therapy make your loss worse? Psychology Today, August 2, 2002; last reviewed June 9, 2016

Camus A: The Myth of Sisyphus (1942). Translated by Justin O'Brien. New York, Vintage, 2018

Canning RD, Dvoskin JA: Preventing suicide in detention and correctional facilities in The Oxford Handbook of Prisons and Imprisonment. Edited by Wooldredge J, Smith P. New York, Oxford University Press, 2018, pp 551–578

Carson A, Cowhig MP: Mortality in state and federal prisons, 2001–2016—statistical tables. NCJ 251920. Washington, DC, Bureau of Justice Statistics, February 2020. Available at: www.bjs.gov/content/pub/pdf/msfp0116st.pdf. Accessed October 30, 2020.

Casey P: The course and prognosis of adjustment disorders, in Adjustment Disorder: From Controversy to Clinical Practice. Edited by Casey P. New York, Oxford University Press, 2018, pp 111–122

Center for Complicated Grief: New York, Columbia University, 2020. Available at: https://complicatedgrief.columbia.edu/professionals/complicated-grief-professionals/overview. Accessed August 9, 2020.

Chamberlain M: Be observant: 10 warning signs of suicidal inmates. Lexipol May 2019. Available at: www.lexipol.com/resources/blog/be-observant-10-warnings-signs-of-suicidal-inmates. Accessed October 20, 2020.

Chiles J: Clinical Manual for the Assessment and Treatment of Suicidal Patients, 2nd Edition. Washington, DC, American Psychiatric Association Publishing, 2018

Chiles J: Suicidal behavior and the Three I's. Psychiatr News 54(2):22–23, 2019

Clark K: The effect of mental illness on segregation following institutional misconduct (abstract). Criminal Justice and Behavior 45(9):1362–1382, 2018. Available at: https://journals.sagepub.com/doi/abs/10.1177/0093854818766974?journalCode=cjbb. Accessed January 11, 2021.

Coley RY, Johnson E, Simon GE: Racial/ethnic disparities in the performance of prediction models for death by suicide after mental health visits. JAMA Psychiatry 78(7):726–734, 2021 33909019

Columbia University: Columbia-Suicide Severity Rating Scale (C-SSRS), Version 2.0. February 2013. Available at: https://cssrs.columbia.edu/wp-content/uploads/ScoringandDataAnalysisGuide-for-Clinical-Trials-1.pdf. Accessed July 9, 2020.

Crosby AE, Ortega L, Melanson C: Self-directed Violence Surveillance: Uniform Definitions and Recommended Data Elements, Version 1.0. Atlanta, GA, Centers for Disease Control and Prevention, National Center for Injury Prevention and Control, February 2011. Available at: www.cdc.gov/violenceprevention/pdf/Self-Directed-Violence-a.pdf. Accessed December 20, 2020.

Crumlish J: Suicidality in correctional facilities: challenges in assessing and treating. CAMS Care February 24, 2020. Available at: https://cams-care.com/resources/educational-content/suicidality-in-correctional-facilities-challenges-in-assessing-and-treating. Accessed September 7, 2020.

Daniel AE: Preventing suicide in prison: a collaborative responsibility of administrative, custodial, and clinical staff. J Am Acad Psychiatry Law 34(2):165–175, 2006 16844795

Doka K: Disenfranchised Grief: Recognizing Hidden Sorrow. New York, Lexington Books, 1989

Doka KJ (ed): Disenfranchised Grief: New Directions, Challenges and Strategies for Practice. Champaign, IL, Research Press, 2001

Doka KJ, Tucci AS (eds): When Grief Is Complicated. Washington, DC, Hospice Foundation of America, 2002

Ducasse D, Holden RR, Boyer L, et al: Psychological pain in suicidality: a meta-analysis. J Clin Psychiatry 79(3):44–51, 2018 28872267

DuRand CJ, Burtka GJ, Federman EJ, et al: A quarter century of suicide in a major urban jail: implications for community psychiatry. Am J Psychiatry 152(7):1077–1080, 1995 7793448

Eisma MC, Rosner R, Comtesse H: ICD-11 prolonged grief disorder criteria: turning challenges into opportunities with multiverse analyses. Front Psychiatry 11(752):752, 2020 32848929

Ferszt GG, Leveillee M: Telling the difference between guilt and depression. LPN 5(3):12–13, 2009. Available at: www.nursingcenter.com/wkhlrp/Handlers/articleContent.pdf?key=pdf_01212983-200905000-00003. Accessed March 8, 2022.

Frey LM, Fulginiti A, Sheehan L, et al: What's in a word? Clarifying terminology on suicide-related communication. Death Stud 44(12):808–818, 2020 31088336

Gallagher M: Suicide in prisons and jails: a growing concern. Georgetown Law, O'Neill Institute for National and Global Health Law, November 16, 2018. Available at: https://oneill.law.georgetown.edu/suicide-in-prisons-and-jails-a-growing-concern. Accessed June 6, 2020.

Gold LH: Suicide risk assessment, in The American Psychiatric Association Publishing Textbook of Suicide Risk Assessment and Management, 3rd Edition. Edited by Gold LH, Frierson RL. Washington, DC, American Psychiatric Association Publishing, 2020, pp 3–15

Gold LH, Joshi KG: Suicide risk assessment, in The American Psychiatric Association Publishing Textbook of Forensic Psychiatry. Edited by Gold LH, Frierson RL. Washington, DC, American Psychiatric Association Publishing, 2018, pp 403–420

Harris T: Foreword, in Suicide in Prisons: Prisoners' Lives Matter. Edited by Towl GL, Crighton DA. Hampshire, UK, Waterside Press, 2007

Hawton K, Linsell L, Adeniji T, et al: Self-harm in prisons in England and Wales: an epidemiological study of prevalence, risk factors, clustering, and subsequent suicide. Lancet 383(9923):1147–1154, 2014 24351319

Hayes LM: National Study of Jail Suicide 20 Years Later. Washington, DC, U. S. Department of Justice, National Institute of Corrections, 2010a. Available at: https://s3.amazonaws.com/static.nicic.gov/Library/024308.pdf. Accessed July 5, 2021.

Hayes LM: Toward a better understanding of suicide prevention in correctional facilities, in Handbook of Correctional Mental Health, 2nd Edition. Edited by Scott CL. Washington, DC, American Psychiatric Publishing, 2010b, pp 231–254

Hayes SC, Strosahl KD, Wilson KG: Acceptance and Commitment Therapy: The Process and Practice of Mindful Change, New York, Guilford, 2016

Hedegaard H, Curtin SC, Warner M: Increase in suicide mortality in the United States, 1999–2018. NCHS Data Brief No 362. Hyattsville, MD, U.S. Department of Health and Human Services, Centers for Disease Control and Prevention, National Center for Health Statistics, April 2020. Available at: www.cdc.gov/nchs/data/databriefs/db362-h.pdf. Accessed October 30, 2020.

Helfand SJ, Sampl S, Trestman RL: Managing the disruptive or aggressive inmate, in Handbook of Correctional Mental Health, 2nd Edition. Edited by Scott CL. Washington, DC, American Psychiatric Publishing, 2010, pp 197–230

History.com Editors: Cuban missile crisis. History.com Jan. 4, 2010; updated June 10, 2019. Available at: www.history.com/topics/cold-war/cuban-missile-crisis. Accessed August 15, 2020.

HM Prison Service, Safer Custody Group: The ACCT Approach. Caring for People at Risk in Prison. London, HM Prison Service, 2005

Hughes KV, Metzner JL: Suicide risk management, in Oxford Textbook of Correctional Psychiatry. Edited by Trestman RL, Appelbaum KL, Metzner JL. New York, Oxford University Press, 2015, pp 237–244

Iglewicz A, Shear MK, Reynolds CF 3rd, et al: Complicated grief therapy for clinicians: an evidence-based protocol for mental health practice. Depress Anxiety 37(1):90–98, 2020 31622522

International Society for the Study of Self Injury: What is self injury? International Society for the Study of Self-Injury, May 2018. Available from: https://itriples.org/about-self-injury/what-is-self-injury. Accessed October 10, 2020.

Joiner TE Jr, Conwell Y, Fitzpatrick KK, et al: Four studies on how past and current suicidality relate even when "everything but the kitchen sink" is covaried. J Abnorm Psychol 114(2):291–303, 2005 15869359

Jordan JR: Postvention is prevention—the case for suicide postvention. Death Stud 41(10):614–621, 2017 28557579

Kaba F, Lewis A, Glowa-Kollisch S, et al: Solitary confinement and risk of self-harm among jail inmates. Am J Public Health 104(3):442–447, 2014 24521238

Kanel K: A Guide to Crisis Intervention, 5th Edition. Stanford, CT, Cengage Learning, 2012

Kaster TS, Martin MS, Simpson AIF: Preventing prison suicide with life-trajectory-based screening. J Am Acad Psychiatry Law 45(1):92–98, 2017 28270467

The Kim Foundation: Suicide risk and protective factors. 2020. Available at: www.thekimfoundation.org/suicide-risk-protective-factors. Accessed October 1, 2020.

Knoll JL, Kaufman AR: Suicide in correctional settings: epidemiology, risk assessment and prevention, in Principles and Practice of Forensic Psychiatry, 3rd Edition. Edited by Rosner R, Scott CL. New York, CRC Press, 2017, pp 581–591

Kramer-Howe K: Care for the dying and those who grieve, in Essentials of Psychiatric Mental Health Nursing: A Communication Approach to Evidence-Based Care, 2nd Edition. Edited by Varcarolis EM. New York, Elsevier, 2013, pp 468–487

Labrecque MR, Patry MW: Self-harm/suicidality in corrections, in The Practice of Correctional Psychology. Edited by Ternes M, Magaletta PR, Patry MW. Cham, Switzerland, Springer, 2018, pp 235–257

Linehan M: Cognitive-Behavioral Treatment of Borderline Personality Disorder. New York, Guilford, 1993

Links PS, Bergmans Y: Managing suicidal and other crises, in Integrated Treatment for Personality Disorder. Edited by Livesley EJ, Dimaggio G, Clarkin JF. New York, Guilford, 2016, pp 197–210

Maciejewski PK, Maercker A, Boelen PA, Prigerson HG: "Prolonged grief disorder" and "persistent complex bereavement disorder," but not "complicated grief," are one and the same diagnostic entity: an analysis of data from the Yale Bereavement Study. World Psychiatry 15(3):266–275, 2016 27717273

Maine Department of Health and Human Services: Action Planning for Crisis, Prevention, and Recovery: Crisis Plans. 2021. Available at: www.maine.gov/dhhs/samhs/mentalhealth/rights-legal/crisis-plan/home.html. Accessed February 14, 2021.

Mandracchia JT, Smith PN: The interpersonal theory of suicide applied to male prisoners. Suicide Life Threat Behav 45(3):293–301, 2015 25312533

Meagher T, Chammah M: Why jails have more suicides than prisons: a new report and a growing phenomenon. The Marshall Project, 2015. Available at: www.themarshallproject.org/2015/08/04/why-jails-have-more-suicides-than-prisons. Accessed October 10, 2020.

Meltzer HY, Alphs L, Green AI, et al; International Suicide Prevention Trial Study Group: Clozapine treatment for suicidality in schizophrenia: International Suicide Prevention Trial (InterSePT). Arch Gen Psychiatry 60(1):82–91, 2003 12511175 [Erratum: Arch Gen Psychiatry 60(7):735, 2003]

Mumola CJ, Noonan ME: Deaths in custody: state prison deaths 2001–2007—statistical tables. Washington, DC, Bureau of Justice Statistics, October 28, 2010. Available at: www.bjs.gov/index.cfm?ty=pbdetail&iid=2093. Accessed February 14, 2021.

Myer RA, Lewis JS, James RK: The introduction of a task model for crisis intervention. J Ment Health Couns 35(2):95–107, 2013

National Commission on Correctional Health Care and American Foundation for Suicide Prevention: National response plan for suicide prevention (with link to suicide prevention resource guide). National Commission on Correctional Health Care, October 11, 2019. Available at: https://www.ncchc.org/suicide-prevention-plan. Accessed November 2, 2020.

Novalis PN, Singer V, Peele R: Clinical Manual of Supportive Psychotherapy, 2nd Edition. Washington, DC, American Psychiatric Association Publishing, 2020

Obegi JH: Probable standards of care for suicide risk assessment. J Am Acad Psychiatry Law 45(4):452–459, 2017 29282236

Paris J: Chronic suicidality among patients with borderline personality disorder. Psychiatr Serv 53(6):738–742, 2002 12045312

Paris J: Half in love with easeful death: the meaning of chronic suicidality in borderline personality disorder. Harv Rev Psychiatry 12(1):42–48, 2004 14965853

Paris J: Managing suicidality in patients with borderline personality disorder. Psychiatric Times, July 2, 2006. Available at: www.psychiatrictimes.com/view/managing-suicidality-patients-borderline-personality-disorder. Accessed October 22, 2020.

Paris J: Half in Love with Death: Managing the Chronically Suicidal Patient. New York, Routledge, 2014

PBS: The Forgotten Plague: TB in America: 1895–1954. American Experience. Available at: www.pbs.org/wgbh/americanexperience/features/plague-gallery. Accessed October 22, 2020.

Posner K, Brodsky B, Yershova K, et al: The classification of suicidal behavior, in The Oxford Handbook of Suicide and Self-Injury. Edited by Nock MK. New York, Oxford University Press, 2014, pp 7–22

Pritchard S: Grief vs depression: what you need to know and when to seek help (web log post). Hospice Red River Valley. 2021. Available at: www.hrrv.org/blog/grief-vs-depression-what-you-need-to-know-and-when-to-seek-help. Accessed January 8, 2021.

Ramesh T: Suicide in prison: a new study on risk factors in the prison environment. Penal Reform International, June 13, 2018. Available at: www.penalreform.org/blog/suicide-in-prison-a-new-study-on-risk/#:~:text=Suicide%20in%20prison%3A%20a%20new%20study%20on%20risk,increase%20the%20risk%20of%20self-harm%20and%20suicide%20. Accessed January 9, 2021.

Reeves R, Tamburello A: Single cells, segregated housing, and suicide in the New Jersey Department of Corrections. J Am Acad Psychiatry Law 42(4):484–488, 2014 25492075

Reik T: Listening With the Third Ear. New York, Farrar Strauss, 1949

Richmond-Rakerd LS, Caspi A, Arseneault L, et al: Adolescents who self-harm and commit violent crime: testing early-life predictors of dual harm in a longitudinal cohort study. Am J Psychiatry 176(3):186–195, 2019 30606048

Ritter K: Apparent suicide of Nevada death-row inmate spurs questions. ABC News, January 7, 2019. Available at: https://abcnews.go.com/US/wireStory/apparent-suicide-nevada-death-row-inmate-spurs-questions-60218045. Accessed October 20, 2020.

Romo V: Nevada death row inmate found dead in apparent suicide. NPR, January 7, 2019. Available at: www.npr.org/2019/01/07/683112885/nevada-death-row-inmate-found-dead-in-apparent-suicide. Accessed June 21, 2021.

Roth A: Insane: America's Criminal Treatment of Mental Illness. New York, Basic Books, 2018

Rudd MD: Core competencies, warning signs, and a framework for suicide risk assessment in clinical practice, in The Oxford Handbook of Suicide and Self-Injury. Edited by Nock MK. New York, Oxford University Press, 2014, pp 323–336

Rynearson T: Psychotherapy of bereavement after homicide. J Psychother Pract Res 3(4):341–347, 1994 22700202

Schetky D: Mourning in prison: mission impossible? J Am Acad Psychiatry Law 26(3):383–391, 1998 9785282

Schwartz A: The difference between grief and depression, the DSM-V (web log post). MentalHelp.net 2021. Available at: www.mentalhelp.net/blogs/the-difference-between-grief-and-depression-the-dsm-v. Accessed January 8, 2021.

Shear MK, Skritskaya N, Bloom CG: Treatment of acute and persistent grief, in Textbook of Anxiety, Trauma, and OCD-Related Disorders. 3rd Edition. Edited by Simon NM, Hollander E, Rothbaum BO, et al. Washington, DC, American Psychiatric Association Publishing, 2020, pp 571–583

Shneidman E: The Suicidal Mind. New York, Oxford University Press, 1998

Silverman MM, Berman AL, Sanddal ND, et al: Rebuilding the Tower of Babel: a revised nomenclature for the study of suicide and suicidal behaviors, Part 2: suicide-related ideations, communications, and behaviors. Suicide Life Threat Behav 37(3):264–277, 2007 17579539

Simon NM: Treating complicated grief. JAMA 310(4):416–423, 2013 23917292

Simon RI: Assessing and enhancing protective factors against suicide risk, in Preventing Patient Suicide: Clinical Assessment and Management. Edited by Simon RI. Washington, DC, American Psychiatric Publishing, 2011a, pp 51–58

Simon RI: Suicide risk assessment, in Preventing Patient Suicide: Clinical assessment and Management. Edited by Simon RI. Washington, DC, American Psychiatric Publishing, 2011b, pp. 3–38

Smid GE, Kleber RJ, de la Rie SM, et al: Brief Eclectic Psychotherapy for Traumatic Grief (BEP-TG): toward integrated treatment of symptoms related to traumatic loss. Eur J Psychotraumatol 6(1):27324, 2015 26154434

Smith H: The strange case of Mr. Keats's tuberculosis. Clin Infect Dis 38(7):991–993, 2004 15034831

Stone DM, Simon TR, Fowler KA, et al: Vital signs: trends in state suicide rates—United States, 1999–2016 and circumstances contributing to suicide—27 states, 2015. MMWR Morb Mortal Wkly Rep 67:617–624, 2018. Available at: www.cdc.gov/mmwr/volumes/67/wr/mm6722a1.htm. Accessed July 26, 2020.

Suicide Prevention Resource Center: Step 3: Identify key risk and protective factors. The Kim Foundation. 2022. Available at: www.thekimfoundation.org/suicide-risk-protective-factors. Accessed June 28, 2021.

Suto I: Inmates who attempted suicide in prison: a qualitative study. Doctoral dissertation, Pacific University, July 27, 2007. Available at: https://commons.pacificu.edu/work/sc/27fa646e-1a00-4249-acb6-0bfd8846d151. Accessed October 25, 2020.

Tartaro C: When, where, and how suicides in prisons and jails occur, in Suicide and Self-Harm in Prisons and Jails, 2nd Edition. New York, Lexington Books, 2019, pp 39–60

Therivel J, Kornusky J: Clients and families in grief. Social Work Practice & Skill, 2018. Available at: www.ebscohost.com/assets-sample-content/SWRC-Clients-Families-in-Grief-Skill-Sheet.pdf. Accessed October 15, 2020.

Thomas J, Leaf M, Kazmierczak S, Stone J: Self-injury in correctional settings: "pathology" of prisons or of prisoners? Criminology and Public Policy 5(1):193-202, 2006

Torrey EF, Kennard AD, Eslinger D, et al: More mentally ill persons are in jails and prisons than hospitals: a survey of the states. Treatment Advocacy Center, May 2010. Available at: www.treatmentadvocacycenter.org/storage/documents/final_jails_v_hospitals_study.pdf. Accessed January 9, 2021.

Walker T, Towl G: Preventing Suicide and Self-Injury in Women's Prisons. Hook, Hampshire, UK, Waterside Press, 2016

Walters GD: Changing Lives of Crime and Drugs: Intervening with Substance-Abusing Offenders. New York, Wiley, 1998

Way BB, Sawyer DA, Barboza S, Nash R: Inmate suicide and time spent in special disciplinary housing in New York State prison. Psychiatr Serv 58(4):558–560, 2007 17412861

Western Michigan University Suicide Prevention Program: Protective factors. 2020. Available at: https://wmich.edu/suicideprevention/basics/protective. Accessed January 9, 2021.

Westers NJ, Muehlenkamp JJ, Lau M: SOARS model: risk assessment of nonsuicidal self-injury. Contemp Pediatr 33(7):25–31, 2016

Wetherell JL: Complicated grief therapy as a new treatment approach. Dialogues Clin Neurosci 14(2):159–166, 2012 22754288

White J: Double Contact: A Sector General Novel. New York, Tor Books, 1999

White J: Beginning Operations: A Sector General Omnibus. New York, Tor Books, 2001

Wikipedia: Chinese word for "crisis." Available at: https://en.wikipedia.org/wiki/Chinese_word_for_%22crisis%22. Accessed August 15, 2020a.

Wikipedia: List of death row inmates in the United States, 2020b. Available at https://en.wikipedia.org/wiki/List_of_death_row_inmates_in_the_United_States#:~:text=Federal%20%20%20%20Name%20%20%20,Michigan%2C%20which%20...%20%2010%20more%20rows%20. Accessed January 9, 2021.

Worden JW: Grief Counseling and Grief Therapy: A Handbook for the Mental Health Practitioner, 5th Edition. New York, Springer, 2018

World Health Organization and International Association for Suicide Prevention: Preventing Suicide in Jails and Prisons (HV 6545). Geneva, Switzerland, World Health Organization, 2007. Available at: https://www.who.int/mental_health/prevention/suicide/resource_jails_prisons.pdf. Accessed August 11, 2020.

Yager J: Addressing patients' psychic pain. Am J Psychiatry 172(10):939–943, 2015 26423477

Yager J, Feinstein RE: A common factors approach to psychotherapy with chronically suicidal patients: wrestling with the angel of death. Psychiatry 80(3):207–220, 2017 29087254

Young MH, Justice JV, Erdberg P: Risk of harm: inmates who harm themselves while in prison psychiatric treatment. J Forensic Sci 51(1):156–162, 2006 16423243

Zisook S, Simon N, Reynolds C, et al: Phenomenology of acute and persistent grief, in Textbook of Anxiety, Trauma, and OCD-Related Disorders, 3rd Edition. Edited by Simon NM, Hollander E, Rothbaum BO, et al. Washington, DC, American Psychiatric Association Publishing, 2020, pp 557–570

Zoll LS: Disenfranchised grief: when grief and grievers are unrecognized (supplemental material). The New Social Worker 2021. Available at: https://www.socialworker.com/feature-articles/practice/disenfranchised-grief-when-grief-and-grievers-are-unrecogniz. Accessed January 18, 2021.

6

Trauma

It is a truism that stress is a normal part of life. It includes the mundane, such as getting to work on time, and the extreme, such as observing or experiencing violence, accidents, or natural disasters. Traumatic experiences themselves are nearly universal in human lives. It is estimated that 90% of people will encounter at least one traumatic experience in their lifetimes. Many experience repeated or chronic exposures to trauma, such as persistent emotional abuse, neglect, racism or misogyny in work or social situations, bullying, or frustrations arising from an emotional or physical problem. Stressors such as those involved in committing crimes, being apprehended (or avoiding detection), going through jail, appearing in court, and adapting to prison life likely add to the cumulative effects of lifetime stress.

Bessel Van der Kolk (2015) wrote a comprehensive and popular book on the ways trauma affects people and strategies for treating patients, *The Body Keeps the Score*, which returned to the best seller lists in 2021. In an interview with Ezra Klein (The Ezra Klein Show 2021), van der Kolk discusses the ways in which trauma affects the body, mind, and social well-being of people. To summarize: when you are afraid of the people who take care of you, you become angry and oppositional, and this imprints you irrationally for life.

When you are discussing therapy in instances where there has been trauma, it is important to be aware that in most cases, emotional distress arising from trauma does not indicate a psychiatric diagnosis, but therapy may be indicated to prevent further exacerbation of the distress. Being aware of the possible stress and trauma exposure of the individual in prison over his life span (including before and after incarceration) is essential to understanding the nature of the person's stress reactions and behavior in prison. Continuity of care, including obtaining records from before incarceration and creating linkages to services upon release, should improve outcomes for your patients (Fulks 2014).

In addition to personal harm from one event or chronic exposure to personal abuse, the conditions of the community as a whole can be traumatic to its residents. This is manifest in poor communities, on Native American reservations, and among racial

193

minorities. The conditions in communities, whether characterized by violence, food insecurity, homelessness, lack of health care, the effects of structural racism, and so forth, can be serious stressors on individuals living in these environments. For example, a survey of Black Americans in communities that experienced police killings of unarmed Black people found that these events were associated with an increase in the number of days that survey participants reported poor mental health. Police shootings of armed Black persons were not associated with such reactions (Herd 2021).

Robert T. Carter, a noted researcher of psychology and education, has studied the mental and emotional harm caused by disparities in treatment of individuals who are discriminated against. Carter created a trauma scale that measures the harm of the stressor of racism (Carter and Murchow 2017; Levine 2020). He describes the effects of racial discrimination as emotional trauma. Reactions identified include irritability, anger, rage, low self-esteem, and other markers of chronic stress reactions. Most individuals will recover from these experiences over time, but for some, such experiences can lead to short- or long-term adjustment disorders and other dysfunctions.

Historical trauma is similar in effect. For communities that have been exposed to harsh conditions such as discrimination, poverty, war, or oppression, the cultural reactions may include adjustments such as avoidance of certain places, lack of acculturation into the general society, ongoing mislabeling of behaviors, and feelings of ostracism. Immigrants, for example, face language, social, and employment barriers that can accumulate as a complex trauma. In earlier parts of the twentieth century, Jews were excluded from many locations and activities (such as golf clubs), and in the nineteenth century, the Irish encountered many such limits ("Irish need not apply"). These hurdles, as well as the myriad microaggressions that people encounter, can lead to stress reactions (Hashmi 2017; London 2020). As discussed in Chapter 12, this is true of formerly incarcerated individuals as well. Jäggi et al. (2016) used the National Survey of American Life to review the complex relationship among poverty, racism, and crime, describing the relationship between trauma experienced in high crime and poor communities and interactions with the criminal justice system, including the repeated and cumulative effects of interactions with police, violence, and crime beginning in childhood and persisting through the juvenile system to adult arrests and incarceration. Hypervigilance, fear, and traumatic response are more common in those who report trauma in the past. The more incidents, the stronger the response to each successive event.

Resilience in the face of difficulties is a valuable human trait, the loss of which can lead to physical and psychosocial problems. Trauma-informed care can help provide the skills that traumatized individuals need in learning or relearning the skills and techniques that will help them reestablish that resilience (Southwick et al. 2015). The Substance Abuse and Mental Health Services Administration (SAMHSA) (2014) of the National Institutes of Health describes the three E's of trauma:

1. Events: actual or extreme threat of physical or psychological harm.
2. Experience: the individual's reaction, which is unique to each person and in fact may not be perceived as traumatic by another individual exposed to the same event.
3. Effects: the way(s) in which the event affected the individual. Effects may be immediate or have a delayed onset. These include psychological and physical symp-

toms, the inability to cope with normal day-to-day problems, and the inability to trust, to manage cognitive processes such as memory or attention, to regulate behavior, or to control emotions.

In the general population, the lifetime prevalence of PTSD is 3.6% for men, 9.7% for women, and 6.3% overall. In prison populations, PTSD occurs much more frequently, and the prevalence may be as high as 33% (Javier and Owen 2020). However, PTSD is the most extreme of conditions caused by stressors. In prison, adjustment disorders and acute stress disorders are more prevalent. We discuss these diagnoses in this chapter, along with recommendations for treating patients and taking care of oneself. Prison work for almost all staff is stressful, and for those of us charged with direct care of trauma-stressed patients, the "secondary" trauma may be very damaging.

Trauma-Informed Care

SAMHSA recommends that all individuals seeking mental health services or substance use disorder treatment undergo assessment for trauma in their lives. All people entering a correctional facility should be assessed for stressor-related adjustment disorders as a means to determine the type of treatment and programs that may be necessary (Substance Abuse and Mental Health Services Administration 2014). As discussed in Chapter 3, entering jail or prison can cause a crisis in a person's life. Something similar may occur to people who are being released, as discussed in Chapter 14.

Stressor-Related Disorders

PTSD and other stressor-related disorders may result in many physical and psychological symptoms as follows (based on Milkman et al. 2008):

- Increased arousal such as exaggerated startle response or reaction to noise, insomnia, inability to concentrate, irritability, hypervigilance, and "patrolling" the environment for dangers
- Hyperarousal, when the individual is "primed" to react to his surroundings and any danger that might be present, even when no other people around him notice anything
- Intrusive memories at any time, usually with some event that "triggers" the memories, which may be frightening and impair the functioning of the individual
- Dissociation causing the individual to feel detached from his surroundings and perhaps to "zone out" during an activity or interaction
- Attachment disorders causing the individual to have problems relating to others around him
- Violence, aggression, and uncontrolled rage, where the individual cannot control his behaviors in the face of some stimuli that causes anger or impulsive behavior
- Commonly, major depression comorbid with trauma disorders due to feelings of helplessness, guilt, or low self-esteem resulting from the trauma
- Other psychological problems, including anxiety and eating disorders
- Complex PTSD when individuals are repeatedly exposed to trauma, either emotional or physical abuse, over a long period of time

- Complicated grief—grief over the death of a loved one that becomes pathological and difficult to deal with
- Suicidal thoughts and/or behaviors (see Chapter 5)
- Reexperiencing of the trauma through flashbacks, nightmares, intrusive memories, and reactions to triggers that remind the person of the event
- Emotional numbing such as feelings of dissociation, detachment, apathy, and loss of interest
- Avoidance of reminders, triggers of memories, or reexperiences of the trauma
- Neurobiological changes such as alterations in electroencephalographic activity; changes in brain structures, such as a smaller hippocampus and abnormal activation of the amygdala; and changes in memory and fear responses
- Physical changes such as headaches, digestive problems, immune system changes, breathing problems, dizziness, chest pain, and chronic pain
- Social dysfunction such as interpersonal problems, low self-esteem, substance abuse, employment problems, homelessness, criminal activity, and self-destructive behaviors such as suicide attempts, risky sexual behaviors, and self-injury

In DSM-5 (and DSM-5-TR), trauma and stressor-related disorders form a new class of disorders that include adjustment disorders, acute stress disorder, and PTSD. While stressor-related disorders are often comorbid with other psychiatric diagnoses, the differentiating factor in stressor-related disorders is the presence of a traumatic event or series of events in the person's life. Acute stress disorder and adjustment disorder can be precursors to PTSD. They often resolve more quickly and do not have lingering symptoms but left untreated may develop into PTSD.

The DSM-5-TR criteria for these PTSD and stressor-related disorders are extensive and detailed, and for them we refer you to the source (DSM-5-TR, pp. 301–304, 313–315). However, a quick way to remember the criteria is that there *must* be symptoms from four categories:

- *Intrusive:* includes nightmares and recurring, involuntary, or intrusive memories
- *Avoidant:* persistent avoidance of stimuli associated with the traumatic event
- *Negative:* alterations in cognition or mood
- *Reactive:* changes in arousal or reactivity

The remaining criteria may be roughly summarized as follows:

- Exposure to actual or threatened serious harm or death
- Duration of more than 1 month
- Clinically significant distress or impairment in functioning
- Not the result of use of drugs or alcohol or other medical conditions

Much of the trauma that leads to posttraumatic stress among prisoners is of a prolonged or repeated exposure to violent events or abuse. People who have been incarcerated often experience stressors, sometimes extreme, while entering the institution, serving their sentences, and reentering society. The experiences encountered while incarcerated may trigger memories and trauma-related reactions. Understanding the nature of the symptoms, therefore, will contribute to treating each patient. Most institutions assess the mental health of individuals entering the system and screen for substance use. Assessment should include screening for trauma exposure, since many mental health and other disorders are more effectively treated if the history of trauma exposure is known (Kubiak and Rose 2007).

Haney (2020) describes a "risk factors model" of psychological development that considers a person's surroundings, quality of life, and stressors, creating a life history that increases the likelihood that the individual will develop troubled behaviors and social connections. These include abuse, poverty, and traumatic events that have been shown to cause a person to develop psychological problems and perhaps lead to crime. Given these risk factors in prison populations, there is a need to assess prisoners for a complete history in addition to ascertaining the immediate reason the individual is incarcerated so as to effectively understand the need for trauma care. Haney emphasizes that it is not just one thing or one type of risk, but rather the cumulative effects of experiences and risk factors that compound over time. For example, childhood neglect may seem perfectly normal to a child but will lead to a lack of understanding about how the world works, which in turn may lead to misbehavior and punishment in school. This in turn may cause the child to misbehave further and develop a habit of doing so as the punishments continue. Then, other difficult circumstances, such as family stress, abuse, or homelessness, can add to and inflame the stress. While the individual might not consider this progression to be traumatic in that it is "the way of life," the cumulative problems will affect the person's development and world view and increase the risk of criminal or risky behavior.

The principles of trauma-informed care have been summarized in the acronym of SHARE (safety, hope, autonomy, respect, and empathy) (Levenson and Willis 2019). You should try to avoid retraumatization, create a safe space, and help your patients to learn and practice new skills but to still hold patients accountable for the past. They can learn that their violence can be a response to shame and embarrassment. You should also be aware that the power imbalance inherent in psychotherapy can be a reminder of their helplessness in the face of past traumatic victimization (Bloom 2010; Levenson and Willis 2019; Miller and Najavits 2012).

Stressor-related disorders (including PTSD) are defined by a continuum of symptoms related to a patient's past experiences. They differ from other mental health disorders in that they are precipitated by an event or a series of events that occur in the person's life rather than a change that is "internal" to the individual. One of the defining features of these diagnoses is the element of time: most people confronted with a traumatic experience will react. Some will have an immediate reaction that will resolve itself in a few days or weeks. Others will find their functioning affected for months and years, with symptoms often occurring intermittently. While clear demarcations between different disorders and between normal reactions and more dysfunctional responses are rarely present in assessing psychiatric problems, there is a continuum of criteria and diagnoses that enables the clinician to assess the severity of responses and the need for treatment. Distress and impairment are the deciding factors that lead to a psychiatric diagnosis. The diagnoses of stressor-related disorders, including adjustment disorders, acute stress disorders, and PTSD, rely on clinical judgment concerning the acuity of distress and impairment and duration of symptoms. Patients with subthreshold disorders—circumstances that do not meet the full criteria of PTSD but indicate that there is significant possibility that, left without support, the circumstances of the patient might lead to another diagnosis—should be considered for an appropriate level of follow-up.

Adjustment disorders are short-term reactions to stressors such as traumatic experiences and adverse events in a person's life. Often the symptoms may not meet enough of the DSM-5-TR criteria for acute stress disorder or PTSD but may be indications for follow-up to clarify the diagnosis and provide treatment if necessary (Casey and Strain 2016).

Acute stress disorder is a more complex combination of symptoms occurring within the first month after a traumatic experience. Acute stress disorder is characterized by symptoms of dissociation, depression, intrusive memories, avoidance, hyperarousal, and panic attacks. It is considered an indication that the individual will likely develop PTSD. However, in the experience of the authors, within 2 weeks of entering an institution, adjustment disorders (not acute stress disorders) are the most common new diagnoses among incarcerated populations and are more commonly observed among individuals seeking treatment in the institution.

PTSD is chronic but can be intermittently symptomatic in nature, with symptoms being triggered by memories or such things as loud noises, visual stimuli such as a photo of similar events, or other reminders of the time or site or concurrent events of the traumatic event. PTSD may persist for months or years. Traumatic experiences may be caused by natural disasters such as storms, earthquakes, or the sudden death of a close relative, or human failure such as accidents, malevolence, war, or fire. In addition, DSM-5-TR recognizes trauma caused by repeated abuses, such as sexual assault, abuse, neglect, or maltreatment that occurs over time in childhood or with intimate partners. This includes racism and other forms of bigotry that constitute microaggressions that traumatized individuals may have encountered throughout their lives. Some researchers and clinicians consider these to be in a group of stressor-related disorders that they call *complex PTSD* or *disorders of extreme stress not otherwise specified* (DESNOS). However, others have noted that the majority of these would be diagnosed within PTSD categories in DSM-5 and that the evidence basis for the others was not sufficient to warrant a separate category of disorder (National Center for PTSD 2020). Also, of importance was the belief that the treatments for them would be similar to those for the other forms of PTSD.

Posttraumatic Stress Disorder

PTSD and related disorders can have a broad array of symptoms that overlap with or are comorbid with symptoms of other mental disorders, including depression (Sun 2014) and borderline personality disorder (Lewis and Grenyer 2009). Some researchers even think that borderline personality disorder is actually an adjustment disorder related to complex trauma (Lewis and Grenyer 2009; Kulkarni 2017). The differentiating factor of trauma-related disorders is the presence of an event or events that precipitate these symptoms and that are external to the individual. Indeed, as discussed below, people with existing or underlying mental disorders may be more prone to developing adjustment disorders after such events (Casey and Strain 2016). Diagnosis can be difficult because many individuals with PTSD and other disorders are reluctant to confront the memories of the traumatic events and avoid discussing them with therapists, even going so far as to terminate treatment. Also, since adjustment disorders are often comorbid with other mental disorders and the symptoms are similar, it is possible that apparent diagnoses of major depression, personality disorders, or other problems may in fact be an adjustment disorder or PTSD. Additionally, because many PTSD patients have experienced complex and recurring trauma, ongoing mental health problems may have led to a predisposition to adjustment disorder in the face of new stressors.

Adjustment Disorders

Now, more than ever, it is important to talk about adjustment disorders. Why? For two reasons:

- *They are trauma-related.* After being an orphaned and subsyndromal diagnosis, the disorder was moved to the DSM-5 chapter on trauma- and stressor-related disorders and is thus of interest as reflecting what we know to be the overwhelming presence of trauma in the lives of prisoners.
- *They are common and in the absence of other disorders may be the most frequent new diagnosis in prisoners, even those who have been incarcerated for many months.*

The definition of adjustment disorder is simple and contains five criteria (Box 6–1). Despite the move to a trauma- and stressor-related group of disorders, questions remain concerning the use of this diagnosis, and it is impossible for us to discuss all the issues. For example, there are differences between the criteria in DSM-5-TR and ICD-10.

Box 6–1.   DSM-5-TR Diagnostic Criteria for Adjustment Disorders

A. The development of emotional or behavioral symptoms in response to an identifiable stressor(s) occurring within 3 months of the onset of the stressor(s).
B. These symptoms or behaviors are clinically significant, as evidenced by one or both of the following:
   1. Marked distress that is out of proportion to the severity or intensity of the stressor, taking into account the external context and the cultural factors that might influence symptom severity and presentation.
   2. Significant impairment in social, occupational, or other important areas of functioning.
C. The stress-related disturbance does not meet the criteria for another mental disorder and is not merely an exacerbation of a preexisting mental disorder.
D. The symptoms do not represent normal bereavement and are not better explained by prolonged grief disorder.
E. Once the stressor or its consequences have terminated, the symptoms do not persist for more than an additional 6 months.

Specify whether:
   F43.21 With depressed mood: Low mood, tearfulness, or feelings of hopelessness are predominant.
   F43.22 With anxiety: Nervousness, worry, jitteriness, or separation anxiety is predominant.
   F43.23 With mixed anxiety and depressed mood: A combination of depression and anxiety is predominant.
   F43.24 With disturbance of conduct: Disturbance of conduct is predominant.

F43.25 With mixed disturbance of emotions and conduct: Both emotional symptoms (e.g., depression, anxiety) and a disturbance of conduct are predominant.

F43.20 Unspecified: For maladaptive reactions that are not classifiable as one of the specific subtypes of adjustment disorder.

Specify if:

Acute: This specifier can be used to indicate persistence of symptoms for less than 6 months.

Persistent (chronic): This specifier can be used to indicate persistence of symptoms for 6 months or longer. By definition, symptoms cannot persist for more than 6 months after the termination of the stressor or its consequences. The persistent specifier therefore applies when the duration of the disturbance is longer than 6 months in response to a chronic stressor or to a stressor that has enduring consequences.

How frequently would one expect to diagnose an adjustment disorder in jail or prison? One review (Glancy and Treffers 2015) found just a few studies of prevalence, finding the prevalence to be 11% in a small group of male remand (i.e., presentence) prisoners and a comorbidity of 7.7% in a larger New Jersey sample of prisoners with (what were previously called) Axis I disorders. The review authors cited another study in a Danish remand prison showing rates of 80%–90% (oddly enough, with the lesser rate for those in solitary confinement). Those authors suggested that the availability of treatment for long-term prisoners would presumably lessen the rate (Glancy and Treffers 2015).

Perhaps the best-known fact in corrections is that suicide is a risk for anyone entering jail or prison. Thus, when you're seeing patients with adjustment disorder, a major issue is the risk of suicide or perhaps the additional contribution to the risk of suicide created in a prisoner who develops an adjustment disorder upon entering prison. Of interest, a study comparing suicidal risk in patients with adjustment disorder versus those with major depression found that the former group had less education and lower socioeconomic status and were more likely to be unmarried—a description that may apply to many other prisoners (Polyakova et al. 1998). Half the patients reported being orphaned, coming from unstable families, and having experienced emotional deprivation during childhood. It is significant that 28% of suicide victims in a study of New York prisons had a diagnosis of adjustment disorder (Way et al. 2005). Also noted was that 41% had received a mental health service within 3 days of the suicide. Of course, adjustment disorder has been viewed as a potential transition to major depressive disorder, so consideration should usually be given to change the patient's diagnosis to that of a major depressive disorder once it is clear that symptoms have been present for at least 2 weeks.

In a more recent review article (Frank et al. 2016) and the aforementioned review (Glancy and Treffers 2015), supportive psychotherapy is the first listed of the many individual therapies, which include cognitive-behavioral therapy (CBT), interpersonal therapy, mindfulness-based therapy, and internet-based therapy. A previous Cochrane review did not study supportive psychotherapy but did find some benefit in lessening time in return to work for problem-solving therapy yet no benefit to CBT (Arends et al. 2012, citing Strain et al. 1998). De Leo (1989) compared supportive psychotherapy with an antidepressant, a benzodiazepine, and a nutritional supplement (*S*-adenosylmethionine). All the treatments resulted in improvement, and there were no significant differences among the four interventions. However, the groups receiving supportive psychotherapy or *S*-adenosylmethionine had higher mean scores.

A review of both psychotherapy and psychotropic medications concluded that there is more solid evidence for the use of psychotherapy than for the use of psychotropic medication when treating adjustment disorders (Carta et al. 2009; see also Akiki and Abdallah 2018). Another factor in favor of psychotherapy is that effective medications often include herbal or natural supplements (e.g., kava or the *S*-adenosylmethione in the De Leo study), the antidepressant trazodone (which many correctional prescribers prefer to avoid), and the benzodiazepines (which virtually no one in corrections would use in these cases). Lee et al. (2016) conducted a systematic review of psychotherapy versus pharmacotherapy for PTSD and concluded that trauma-focused psychotherapy is recommended for those suffering with PTSD as a first-line treatment. Certain medications showed effectiveness as a second-line treatment along with stress inoculation psychotherapy. Similarly, Hassanmirzei et al. (2017) found that web-based supportive psychotherapy was effective in adolescents following natural disasters.

Psychotherapy for adjustment disorder, at least in the community, would seem to be a matter of common sense with few surprises. "The goal of treatment in AD is to reduce the impact of the stressor, reduce the symptoms that have resulted, enhance the individual's ability to cope with stressors that cannot be reduced or removed, and establish a support system to maximize adaptation" (Casey 2018, p. 98). In a similar vein, Frank et al. (2016; following Strain et al. 1998) describe the goals of psychotherapy as the following:

- Analyze the patient's stressors and determine how to eliminate or minimize them.
- Illuminate the patient's concerns and conflicts.
- Clarify and interpret the meaning of the stressor for the patient.
- Reframe the meaning of the stressor.
- Identify a means of reducing the stressor.
- Teach or reinforce coping skills.
- Help the patient gain perspective on the stressor, establish relationships, attend support groups, and manage himself and the stressor.

This advice is useful in planning psychotherapy for arriving prisoners, although it is certainly possible for a prisoner to develop an adjustment disorder months later. However, despite the commonsense tone of the recommendations ("If the patient is stressed out, reduce the stressor"), prisons do not always follow the rules of common sense. It is not possible to "eliminate the stressor" as the commonsense admonitions might suggest. However, it is thought possible that an adjustment disorder can be the net result of multiple stressors, so you might be able to eliminate some of them (e.g., unrealistic worries about being abandoned by spouse and children). Using what we have learned about adjustment disorders, we compiled a list of therapy reminders in Table 6–1. Of course, this assumes that a person is being seen after or in conjunction with the full initial mental health assessment.

Although Criterion C for adjustment disorder would seem to preclude the comorbidity of an adjustment disorder with major depressive disorder, in practice it does not seem to preclude simultaneously diagnosing PTSD, anxiety disorder, or personality disorder. Although this does seem to contradict Criterion C, DSM-5-TR goes on to say that "[a]djustment disorders can accompany most mental disorders and any medical condi-

---

TABLE 6–1.   **Therapy reminders when treating patients with adjustment disorders**

Determine what incarceration means for this individual, not your generic assumptions, which may not apply.

Reframe the stressors that cannot be eliminated (e.g., prison does not mean that he is a failed human being, but that he made a mistake and has to plan to use that time for personal growth).

Find positives: a chance to think clearly and "find yourself" in a mostly drug-free environment, room and board for a homeless person, a chance to finish GED, and also ability to engage in psychotherapy.

Mitigate what you can (e.g., fears about abandonment, lack of medical or mental health care for an existing condition, fears of sexual victimization).

Somewhere along the line, determine suicide risk group and whether patient's condition constitutes a crisis warranting crisis monitoring and management (see Chapter 5).

Determine or sketch out the concurrent diagnoses. Although adjustment disorders are not considered difficult to treat, overall risks will be lowered by looking for and attempting to treat comorbid psychiatric disorders, including substance use disorders, PTSD, and personality disorders.

Remember that for adjustment disorder in isolation, psychotherapy, rather than medication, is the preferred treatment at this early stage of the treatment.

Refer for medication for potentially treatable impairments or risks either from the adjustment disorder or from comorbid conditions.

Teach coping skills for anxiety *that they can use that very night*, such as deep breathing, progressive relaxation, guided imagery, and mindfulness.

---

tion. Adjustment disorders can be diagnosed in addition to another mental disorder only if the latter does not explain the particular symptoms that occur in reaction to the stressor. For example,…an individual may have a depressive or bipolar disorder and an adjustment disorder as long as the criteria for both are met" (p. 322).

Note that adjustment disorders do not appear to have a minimum duration, as would be the case with major depressive disorder, which has a two-week minimum. However, in practice, we have learned that diagnosing an adjustment disorder based on a single interview is a ticket to overdiagnosis. How frequently have we encountered that someone seen on the evening of his admission to prison is acutely distraught and nonfunctional but 3 days later returns thoroughly adjusted and worry-free? There are also differential diagnosis issues between adjustment disorder and acute stress disorder. In the short term, we urge you to consider the Z codes for "Incarceration" (Z65.1) and several others for various aspects of psychosocial circumstances (Z65.8 for specified and Z65.9 for unspecified circumstances). However, if there is a history of developing symptoms in another correctional facility (e.g., jail), you might determine that he has a continuing adjustment disorder. Also note that an adjustment disorder, which is normally limited to 6 months' duration, may last longer if the stressor (presumably incarceration) has not been removed, which is typically the case for prisoners.

Here are some choices of diagnoses for patients who have histories of trauma or who develop symptoms as a result of the incarceration itself:

- They may have one or more traumatic events in their personal history. They may have a personal history of trauma (coded Z91.4), but no other condition or code may apply. There are also various codes for histories of childhood or adult physical and sexual abuse.

- They may have an acute stress disorder (which according to DSM-5-TR lasts no more than a month) (F43.0).
- They may develop an adjustment disorder with anxiety and/or depression with or without a disturbance of conduct (F43.23 or F43.24, etc.), and since conduct is frequently a focus of treatment in prison, such a diagnosis is definitely relevant.
- They may have preexisting PTSD or develop the full-blown illness (F43.10 unspecified, F43.11 acute, or F43.12 chronic). Keep in mind, though, that this requires symptoms from four different categories, not just one symptom such as nightmares. There is still some difference of opinion about the supposed differences between an acute stress disorder (F43.0) and acute PTSD (F43.11), but since each of these is time-limited to 30 days, the net effect on treatment is not major.
- They may have a reaction to severe stressors, coded as an "other specified" trauma- and stressor-related disorder (F43.8). They may have a condition referred to as other specified or unspecified stressor-related disorders (F43.8 and F43.9, respectively). These include conditions that do not meet all the criteria for another trauma- and stressor-related disorder. These include:
  - Adjustment-like disorders with delayed onset of symptoms (>3 months after the stressor)
  - Adjustment-like disorders of prolonged duration (>6 months) without prolonged duration of the stressor
  - Pathological grief disorder

We're not expert coders, but we urge the accurate diagnosis of stressor-related disorders rather than "casually" diagnosing PTSD in persons with a history of trauma who have one or two symptoms such as nightmares and depression.

Factors That Make Someone More Likely to Have a Stressor-Related Disorder

In the general population, past trauma is reported by 90%, but the prevalence of diagnosed PTSD is less than 4% in men and 9% in women (Javier and Owen 2020). How do people recover from such experiences in such large numbers, and why is PTSD more prevalent among those who are incarcerated? A key factor may be "resilience," which is the ability to adapt to stressors such as trauma, tragedy, or threats or experiences of life-threatening events (Southwick et al. 2015). In other words, some persons who experience trauma have the ability to bounce back from adversity and do not develop a disorder. Resilience is complex and may be more available to an individual in one circumstance but not another. But why does one person have resilience and not another, and why does the same individual have different responses to trauma at different times? In some cases, biophysical responses, such as those involving the sympathetic nervous system and serotonergic systems, are factors. Developmental factors such as repeated stress, neglect, abuse, or events outside of one's control can prevent the individual from developing appropriate and flexible responses to stressors later in life. In contrast, the ability to control events can give the person skills and attitudes that help develop resilience. The ability to focus on problem-solving, positive attitudes, and engagement with positive social support and involvement are also key factors in resilience. Physical activity may also mitigate the effects of the stress. These issues are explored by the researcher we referenced previously who has found that many people have a natural resilience in the face of trauma and that PTSD is not the automatic outcome of a traumatic experience (Bonnano 2021).

Factors that contribute to the likelihood of PTSD include family background, socioeconomic status, lack of community structure, education, and early childhood development. Reactions to stress as with other aspects of life are conditioned on an individual's physical and mental development. Individuals at most risk for developing PTSD are those:

- Who are directly exposed to the event or were severely injured.
- Whose experience of trauma is of long duration.
- Who believe their lives were in danger.
- Who had a dramatic reaction to the event at the time.
- Who felt helpless during the event.
- Who had experienced earlier traumas, such as childhood abuse.
- Who have experienced mental health problems themselves or in their immediate family.
- Who are without strong social support.
- Who have substance use problems.
- Who experience the sudden death of a loved one (Milkman et al. 2008).
- Who attribute the cause of the trauma to someone else.
- Who feel shame as a result.
- Who are unable to remember positive things (Bryant 2016).

PTSD and other stressor-related disorders have physiological, neurological, and genetic components, the contributions of which are just beginning to be understood. For example, people susceptible to adjustment disorders as well as other psychiatric disorders may have smaller hippocampi and may have family members who have psychiatric disorders. Attachment disorders (Javier and Owen 2020) are hypothesized to arise from severe disruptions in an individual's development of healthy interpersonal relationships and the ability to process difficult circumstances and events as they mature.

The central feature of stressor-related disorders is response to fear that is not resolved and is strongly predicted by negative attitudes and the inability to learn how to eliminate the memories (Bryant 2016). Traumatic experiences are a normal part of human life, and the nervous system and psychological development combine to give people the ability to adapt, but individuals who develop PTSD rather than resolving their reactions suffer from prolonged feelings of fear, vulnerability, loss of control, and depersonalization (Crighton and Towl 2008). Factors that have been shown to increase these feelings include the quality and nature of parental and community support, lesser intelligence, and the amount of family conflict as well as histories of abuse, neglect, or other possibly repeated trauma.

Trauma and Physical Health

Traumatic experiences, particularly chronic exposure to interpersonal violence and abuse, can lead to physical ill-health. For prison populations, where health and access to health services have been limited both before incarceration due to poverty and in prison due to the limits of in-prison services, this effect may be exacerbated. Health problems that have been associated with trauma include cardiovascular, metabolic, endocrine, and respiratory complaints (Schnurr 2014). Some of the problems can be attributed to poor health practices by the patient, such as smoking, diet, and substance abuse. Others may be associated with comorbid psychiatric disorders such as major depression.

Trauma and Substance Abuse

It is estimated that 30% of people with PTSD also have a history of substance use disorder (SUD). When comorbid with PTSD and/or adjustment disorders, although not studied as extensively, the incidence of SUD is likely to be much higher. This comorbidity tends to be more difficult to treat and is associated with more rapid relapses. There is also evidence that PTSD patients suffer greater negative consequences than do those without PTSD (Milkman et al. 2008). Najavits (2002) points out that many substance abuse programs begin with the principle that the substance abuse needs to be treated before other mental health problems are dealt with, when in the experience of mental health professionals, the substance abuse may be a form of self-medicating, and if either the mental health problem or the substance abuse is to be treated successfully, both need to be addressed together. Although the connection has been questioned, substance abuse is sometimes thought to reflect a form of self-medication. Kubiak and Rose (2007) note that the high prevalence of SUD and PTSD in prison populations is a likely indicator of the high comorbidity. In prison, substance use is less common, but in coming to jail and prison, individuals may be dealing with withdrawal both physical and emotional.

Other Comorbid Disorders

Major depression, anger and impulsive behavioral problems, and personality disorders are possible comorbid diagnoses common in trauma-affected individuals. Dass-Brailford (2007) reports that as many as 84% of those diagnosed with PTSD may have another lifetime diagnosis and that the risk for suicidal ideation is significantly higher for this population. Comorbidity is also related to long-term exposure to traumas. It is recommended that co-occurring disorders be treated together rather than consecutively.

Complex Trauma

Complex PTSD, sometimes called disorder of extreme stress not otherwise specified, is a condition caused by prolonged or repeated exposure to traumas and is thought to affect prisoners, women and children who suffer long-term abuse, and captives held and abused by their captor. The symptoms experienced in complex trauma are often more persistent, complicated, and difficult to isolate compared with a single incident of trauma. These include altered affect, impulsivity, altered sense of self, attention difficulties, changes in relationships, physical and medical issues, and difficulty in realistically assessing the meaning of events and thoughts about their situation. Patients have reduced self-esteem and may be vulnerable to self-harm or harming others. Dass-Brailford (2007) relates that such individuals are often diagnosed with depressive, personality, or dissociative disorders and may find that therapy will take longer and encounter more resistance. Since DSM-5-TR does not specify what complex PTSD is, many clinicians consider it an enduring personality change, so we will avoid ascribing a specific code to it.

Trauma and Criminality

Trauma among people who have been involved in the criminal justice system is most often interpersonal (Wolff et al. 2015). For incarcerated males, stressor-related disorders are most often caused by observing or participating in violent acts, such as fights, crime, or combat. They are less likely to have been sexually abused than women but more likely to have participated in violent acts. Potentially traumatic events such as interpersonal violence, sexual assault, and other mistreatment are likely to occur among the incarcerated as well. It is likely that a significant portion of incarcerated women have suffered physical, sexual, or emotional abuse prior to their incarceration and have suffered more incidents of traumatic experiences than women who have not been imprisoned. Indeed, as Milkman et al. (2008) observe, abuse among women may lead to criminality because the abused person may be anxious to escape the abuse. Having experienced substance abuse on the part of family members or others close to them, they may seek substances as a form of escape or self-medication. They often score lower on intelligence tests, have less education, and have less financial security. Childhood victimization may lead to substance abuse, running away, getting involved with prostitution, and selling drugs or robbery for daily support. Living this way is in itself stressful and leads to low self-esteem, anxiety, depression, and possibly aggression and impulsivity. Kubiak and Rose (2007) point to trauma exposure, risky behavior (including illegal activity such as drug-seeking), and violence as risk factors.

Trauma and Incarceration

Among incarcerated people, the prevalence of a history of abuse, violence, and other trauma is as high as three times that of the general population. The incidence of mental health problems, including substance abuse, is also significantly elevated (Wolff et al. 2015). Rates of substance abuse and mental health problems are higher for those who reported previous trauma and abuse than for those who do not report past trauma. Women were more likely to have been under the influence of drugs when they committed the crime for which they were incarcerated, while men were more likely to have been under the influence of alcohol.

Institutions in the justice system are known for violence: robbery and sexual and physical assaults occur more frequently within institutions than in the general population. Wolff et al. (2015) report that the rate of violence in prisons is 1 in 10 for physical abuse and 1 in 5 for robbery, with an overall rate of 1 in 2 for all crimes. Sexual assault frequency in the population studied by Wolff et al. was estimated at more than 3% for women and 1.5% for men. Inappropriate sexual contact was found to be more than 21% for abuse by other prisoners and nearly 8% for abuse by staff. The rates of abuse for those who reported abuse prior to incarceration were higher, as were the rates for those with mental health problems. "[P]rison may be a production site of new traumatic experiences, as well as triggering traumatic memories" (Kubiak and Rose 2007, p. 449).

Trauma and Violence

One of the principal symptoms of stress disorders is the inability to control affect and behavior. Common among these is violence toward others, property, and self. People with PTSD may have an increased expectation of danger, leading to heightened arousal and hypervigilance about their surroundings and a "readiness for aggression" (Grieger et al. 2011, p. 207). A strong relationship exists between stress disorders and anger and aggression; this is especially true among people with military experience. Chronic PTSD and stress disorders resulting from violent traumatic experiences appear to increase aggression over time if left untreated. As we've noted, the proportion of incarcerated people who have reported traumatic experiences and interpersonal violence approaches 50% among women and 30% among men. Violence with intimate partners and even children may be increased. In addition, the risk for suicide and self-harm is increased with people who have experienced trauma, especially those subjected to interpersonal violence (Baranyi et al. 2018).

Treatment

Because trauma is generally externally caused, recovery might be considered as "putting the pieces back together." In her memoir, ER doctor Michele Harper describes the Japanese art of *kintsukuroi*, mending pottery. This is a tradition of repairing broken pottery with the precious metals of gold, silver, or platinum that provides a tribute to what the vessel has undergone in life. As a result, the vessel is made more beautiful. The same applies to people who can mend after being broken in life (Harper 2020, p. xiii). While the availability of gold, silver, or platinum is nil in prisons, the effort to repair injuries due to trauma is, in our opinion, more valuable. The point, as with the pottery, is to provide a new identity for the victim and help her develop life-affirming strengths and attitudes. There are many strategies for this covering much of the variability in causes, effects, and individual reactions to trauma.

As prisons develop more programs to improve the skills and attitudes of incarcerated people with the goal of reducing recidivism and improving the likelihood of success once released, the study of how trauma affects individuals should lead to an understanding of how improving response to trauma can help a person be successful in adapting to life challenges. Trauma-informed care begins with an assessment of the trauma experiences of the individuals in the institution. Ideally, this occurs as the person enters the justice system, since it has implications for the causes of previous criminal behavior. Certainly, upon incarceration the individual should be assessed for mental health problems and for past trauma experiences. Assessment via interviews or questionnaires is needed. The PTSD Checklist is one recommended vehicle for assessing the level of trauma in individuals (Friedman 2015; Wolff et al. 2015).

As we have emphasized, however, PTSD is not the only diagnosis available for persons who have experienced trauma. Most people will have temporary reactions, and others will have symptoms that persist, but not enough of them to be characterized as PTSD. More importantly, not all people with symptoms need intensive treatment, and in fact, learning coping mechanisms may be the only treatment needed. The point is to not overdiagnose PTSD and to not overmedicalize adjustment disorders, but to be sensitive to what individuals may have encountered and the nature of the assistance needed. Johnson and Lubin (2015) describe an approach that may be useful in approaching the treatment of people who have experienced trauma. They identify the constructs of patient and therapist approaches as schemas that explain the emotions and attitudes toward the trauma and the therapy itself:

1. Trauma schemas serve to reduce the emotions of fear and shame associated with trauma.
2. The patient and therapist will both avoid addressing the trauma at least some of the time.
3. The patient will never address the trauma completely, so the work of therapy is ongoing.
4. Trauma often indicates the need for protection from another person.

Treatment Stages

Because of the anxiety and fear associated with the events, treatment is often divided into three stages. First, in order to engage the patient in therapy, it's necessary to establish a safe place to discuss symptoms and teach coping skills. A present-focused program or therapy treatment plan addresses symptoms and behaviors that affect the patient's day-to-day functioning. Once the patient is more comfortable in addressing the trauma directly, then, in the second stage, past experiences may be explored and addressed. The third stage is for the individual to find and establish her own identity, not as a victim, but as a person who can take what has been learned about her experiences and the ways she has coped with it to develop resilience and a new perception of her role in the world (Herman 2015).

Trauma-informed care includes sensitivity to issues that people with stressor-related disorders might face while interacting with all members of a facility and committing to reducing those things that might trigger a traumatic stress reaction. While admittedly difficult within a prison or jail setting, promoting trauma awareness and understanding among the staff can help the new individual entering the facility to get the help needed.

The Substance Abuse and Mental Health Services Administration (2014) has published several guidelines for creating a trauma-informed care approach. The National Center for PTSD, which is part of the U.S. Department of Veterans Affairs, delves into the research about the best practices for trauma-informed care through its PTSD Research Quarterly. In its TIP 57, SAMHSA lays out a detailed programmatic approach to treatment of stress-related disorders. Other programs have successfully approached PTSD treatment, include Seeking Safety (Najavits 2002), Trauma Recovery Improvement Model (Wolff et al. 2015), different forms of exposure therapy, and straightforward psychotherapy (Horowitz 2020).

It is important to note and emphasize that therapy works (Cottraux et al. 2008; Ehlers et al. 2010). For the professional in an institution, access to certain programs may be limited because of budgetary factors, policy, or training. But as discussed in Chapter 1, most approaches to psychotherapy proceed from common factors, with enhancements, techniques, and methods adapted to specific problems or therapeutic styles. Most important is the therapeutic alliance, including the ability of the therapist to listen and respond with the patient to the problems and their realistic solutions.

Therapeutic Alliance

All approaches begin with establishing a therapeutic alliance in order to provide a safe environment in which the patient may feel able to directly address the trauma that was experienced. Establishing that alliance can be challenging, especially in a prison setting where patients are skeptical of institutional services, the environment is punitive, and interpersonal relationships are often strained and may be abusive (Sun 2014).

Because of the history of trauma, in order to succeed in therapy, safety is the key objective in establishing the therapeutic relationship. Patients are resistant to talking about their experiences because bringing up the memories is frightening and uncomfortable. The first task in establishing safety is to educate the patient that symptoms were developed by the person as a way of coping. Traumatic events, especially those of an interpersonal nature, cause damage to them, and damage is also caused by the social structure and participants in a person's surroundings (Herman 2015). In prison environments, many of these relationships are far from what might be considered "normal." Relationships with family are constrained by distance, infrequent contact, and perhaps interpersonal stress due to the incarceration itself. Relationships within prison may be difficult because of the structure of the institution (e.g., roommates are not voluntary; many of the people one interacts with are there in a professional capacity to control the individual's activities, including when to sleep and eat; and trusting peers who are criminals is fraught with risk). In many cases, the therapist is the only person the prisoner can rely on for emotional support. Thus, the therapeutic alliance takes on a deeper importance in dealing with trauma.

Commonalities Across Psychological Treatments

Psychoeducation, emotional regulation, and coping skills are the primary topics of stress-disorder treatment. Common methods for dealing with the memories and understanding their meaning are often based on imaginal exposure to the memories with the objective of reducing their power to negatively affect the patient (Schnyder and Cloitre 2015). Physical exercises and physical health are other dimensions in the programs of treatment. Treatment modalities include supportive psychotherapy, CBT, and psychodynamic therapy. While these treatment approaches are often described as independent of one another, careful reading of the techniques and approaches shows that the approaches, whatever their primary theoretical underpinnings, are intertwined. For example, it is our opinion that much of CBT is in fact psychoeducation and that supportive therapy as a discipline is largely educational. Many CBT programs are manualized, while supportive psychotherapy is more often interactive between the therapist and the patient. However, all approaches need to be sensitive to the reactions of the patient. Although it's unlikely that revisiting memories of trauma will lead to long-term recurrence of PTSD or other stress disorders, such memories are quite upsetting to the patient, and the therapist needs to be sensitive to how to best help the patient when his or her reaction is extreme (Gramigna 2020, citing Peirce et al. 2020). We have observed in reviewing research studies and meta-analyses that comparing different approaches, such as CBT versus supportive therapy, or different programs often depends on the definitions of the alternative approaches. For example, Cottraux et al. (2008) compared CBT with "Rogerian" supportive therapy in a study in France. They established strict criteria for each approach and a structured program for each. But they defined supportive therapy differently than we do in this book (their approach was more Rogerian). For example, their supportive program specifically eliminated education and advice giving to the patients—not our intent at all. Ehlers et al. (2010) looked at meta-analyses of comparisons of CBT with other approaches and concluded that the criteria for including studies and for evaluating their effect can bias the results dramatically.

Psychotherapy (Mostly of the Supportive Type)

Horowitz (2020) stresses that the alliance between patient and therapist can help the patient reduce the acuity of symptoms and reduce feelings of isolation, irritability, and despondency. As therapy progresses, the patient and therapist form a partnership in which the roles of each are defined and refined. The therapist acts as advisor, and the patient helps to regulate the direction of the discussions, with the therapist guiding the conversations toward resolution of anxieties, adjusting any medications, and recommending strategies for improving responses. Given the adjustment problems the patient may be facing, a key objective of therapy is to help the patient develop a sense of control over her memories and emotions.

Horowitz begins with supporting the patient in understanding her problems and, as the therapy progresses, moves to addressing specific symptoms:

- Self-medicating (including substance use disorders)
- Physical symptoms such as weight loss, exhaustion, and sleep disturbance. Troubled dreams and nightmares are among the most common symptoms of adjustment disorders
- Anticipation of things that might recall fears and extreme alarm reactions
- Identity disorders such as feelings of guilt, lack of self-worth, hyperarousal, and disorientation

As the therapy proceeds, strategies for coping with these symptoms should be developed with the patient. They begin with listening to patients and assessing how they are coping, and teaching them to listen to themselves, helping patients reexamine their responses and improve their ability to cope and integrate their responses to the memories.

Trauma-centered psychotherapy should proceed from the concept that trauma is the immediate cause of the need for therapy, according to Johnson and Lubin (2015). Immediacy of addressing the issues facing the patient enables the therapist to treat the problem in a serious manner. Avoiding the "elephant in the room" may increase the avoidant behavior and hence prevent addressing emotionally difficult issues: "Trauma-centered psychotherapies will be dispassionate but clear. They will speak about the trauma and tell the client that together they will revisit the pain in order to get it out and that the client will feel better as a result. The therapist will be optimistic but direct" (Johnson and Lubin 2015, p. 49).

Once the immediacy of the problem is put forth, the therapist should demonstrate engagement in an active manner that appropriately mirrors the trauma and emotions and places the therapist "in the story" so that the patient does not feel alone in dealing with the emotions. While many therapists might approach this stage with neutrality, Johnson and Lubin posit that engaging more closely with the story allows the therapist to establish a therapeutic relationship that allows the patient to better share experiences in more detail. This is accomplished in four ways: 1) through gaze (i.e., looking closely at the patient in an interested and engaged manner), 2) posture (leaning into the conversation), 3) questioning in a way that puts the therapist close to the experience, and 4) responding in an affective manner. All this shows that the therapist is interested in what the patient has to say and conveys that interest (Johnson and Lubin 2015).

The therapist should be prepared for the patient to become emotionally upset; traumatic experiences are overwhelming and terrifying, and recounting them is probably no less so. Allowing such emotionality is often thought by therapists to be a form of retraumatizing, but such emotionality, if carefully monitored, is not induced but rather expected. Intense emotions follow from trauma, and the expression of them in therapy shows that the patient is reacting to the trauma. This helps the therapist understand the nuances of the patient's emotional responses and leads to further information about the trauma (Johnson and Lubin 2015).

Johnson and Lubin then describe four techniques to treating traumatic stress. *Using the narrative* is derived from the initial therapy helps the therapist show how the trauma affects current behaviors through *decoding* words or patient affect that seems to have triggered an emotional response. In so doing, the therapist can point out the differences between how that trigger was present in the past and what is happening in the present, *showing the discrepancy* and enabling the patient to see that current events are not the same as the traumatic ones. The fourth technique, *identifying the perpetrator* of the trauma, allows the responsibility for the trauma to be reallocated to the proper party. While most therapy focuses on the patient as the injured party, at this stage, it's important to identify and ascribe responsibility to the perpetrator, rather than to address the trauma as if it were only the patient's: it's important to rephrase—for example "Your father raped you," not "The rape happened to you." The shame that the patient feels for being the victim can now be properly assigned and the focus turned to anger at the perpetrator.

Crisis Therapy or Psychological First Aid?

Psychological first aid is a process developed by the National Center for PTSD in 2006 to mitigate the effects of trauma. It has been widely used as a substitute for various debriefing programs that have in general been found ineffective or even harmful. If your patient experiences a sexual assault, of course, the procedures of PREA will take precedence. While psychological first aid also seems to lack a strong evidence basis (Bisson and Lewis 2009), it also does not necessarily address or reinforce the elements of trauma but merely determines what help is needed. Immediate formal intervention is not automatically recommended for traumatic events because it could exacerbate negative reactions and the trauma itself. So in cases of trauma outside the realm of PREA, we would recommend following the fundamental principle of psychological first aid that reinforcing traumatic memories can be harmful. Counseling should be focused on safety, emotional support, and facilitation of communication. The therapist should answer any questions from patients, normalize distress by affirming that what they are experiencing is normal, educate them about possible symptoms that may arise, and let them know the resources available should they experience problems as time goes on. Brief follow-up should be attempted at intervals to ensure that the person is adjusting, with therapy as needed (Bryant 2016). Of course, if a genuine crisis is present or develops, the usual tasks of crisis management can be used. Notice the parallel to what we said about grief in the previous chapter—that is, not everyone who has experienced a loss needs grief counseling, and not every traumatic event leads to PTSD.

In order to ameliorate stress reactions, we recommend that all prisoners receive education about situations that engender trauma, such as violence, sexual abuse, verbal harassment, and, lately, infectious diseases. Education, as Friedman (2015) notes, should include:

- Meeting basic needs such as safety and security as well as medical needs.
- Orientation to efforts that are being made to recover from the event or situation. For example, in the case of the COVID-19 pandemic, sharing information about safety measures, testing, and medical contingency plans.
- Techniques for reducing psychological arousal such as relaxation techniques and perhaps medication.
- Professional assistance and identification of social support, such as through individual and group counseling.
- Education about the ways in which people respond to trauma and methods for coping, and providing of accurate information in a supportive manner.

Manualized Programs

SAMHSA cites a number of manualized programs for working with trauma-affected individuals and groups (Substance Abuse and Mental Health Services Administration 2014). In addition, the National Center for PTSD has the PILOTS Database on its website that identifies many of the programs available. There are many excellent teaching and training materials on the internet. For example, we found a treatment manual from one of the regional VA medical centers. Most of it is generic to anyone with PTSD, and only a few pages refer to military history (Lynch et al. 2015).

Some programs focus on patients in the early stages of treatment of their adjustment problems, when they will have a need for present-focused approaches in which they are counseled and educated about trauma and coping strategies through cognitive-behavioral techniques and psychoeducational activities. As they progress, past-centered approaches can help them work through the memories and reactions to them in a more comprehensive way. Among them are Seeking Safety, TREM (Trauma Recovery and Empowerment Model), and integrated therapies such as STAIR (Skills Training in Affective and Interpersonal Regulation) and stress inoculation training (Substance Abuse and Mental Health Services Administration 2014).

Seeking Safety and TREM are two of what are known as *first-stage programs* for treating PTSD in that their purpose is to establish a safe place in therapy for patients to understand their trauma history and develop skills for coping. Second-stage treatments are more past-oriented and deal with lessening the power of the memories of the trauma through techniques such as exposure therapy, which we discuss later. Seeking Safety and TREM integrate treatment for PTSD and substance use disorder, but they have also been adapted for PTSD alone.

Seeking Safety and TREM are based on the principle that helping people recover from trauma who also have a substance use disorder requires one to treat both problems at the same time. Often substance abuse is a form of self-medicating or coping for people with a history of trauma. Najavits (2002), the creator of Seeking Safety, holds that you cannot treat either alone.

Seeking Safety is focused on the interpersonal needs and deficits faced by incarcerated population including impulsiveness, maladjustment, and dysregulation. It differs from TREM in that Seeking Safety concentrates on cognitive-behavioral and psychoeducational techniques for developing coping skills and TREM is more oriented toward cognitive restructuring, psychoeducation, coping skills, and meditation. TREM is based on psychodynamic and experiential techniques with the use of peer support. Originally TREM was designed for women, but a program for men is also available, and that is the version that was used by Wolff et al. (2015). In a randomized controlled study comparing the two programs among incarcerated men, both programs saw modest positive effects, and in a review of other studies, Wolff et al. reported that interventions with these programs can be successful in first-stage treatment. The principal components of Seeking Safety and TREM are presented in Tables 6–2 and 6–3, respectively.

Second-stage programs are used when the patients are able to use coping strategies to control their reactions to stimuli that trigger their stress reactions and begin to deal with specific memories. Psychotherapy and CBT are often successful at this stage. Specific strategies that have been shown to be effective include cognitive processing therapy, a manualized program that combines exposure therapy with cognitive-behavioral techniques to help clients recall the trauma and their feelings and thoughts during the event. This is accomplished by having the patient write a detailed account of the event and reading the narrative aloud, helping the individual to work on understanding her safety, trust, control, and self-esteem issues and fix the ways in which those have been distorted by the stress disorders (Substance Abuse and Mental Health Services Administration 2014).

Exposure therapy helps patients work through the specific memories and reactions of traumatic events in an intensive manner evoking often extreme emotions, but with repetition will decrease in intensity, leading to their being better able to process their reactions. However, it has the potential of retraumatizing patients and should be monitored carefully. It is effective when intrusive thoughts, flashbacks, or anxiety symptoms affect functioning. It is not recommended for people with the complex comorbidity of suicidality.

Eye movement desensitization and reprocessing (EMDR) is widely used for PTSD and has been shown to be effective, but requires training and should be supervised closely. It entails revisiting memories while eye movement is initiated by a moving object. The sessions are highly structured around memories, disturbances, and actions (Casey 2018).

Narrative therapy allows patients to explore the narrative of the traumatic experience in terms defined by them, using the repetition of the story to explore reactions, coping, learning, and context of the events in their life, and especially in the present, to give the experience meaning and enable patients to explore alternatives and explana-

TABLE 6–2.	Key elements of Seeking Safety

Safety

Establishing control

Grounding oneself and detaching from emotional pain

Substance use

Asking for help

Taking care of yourself

Compassion

Red and green flags

Honesty

Recovery thinking

Integrating the split self

Commitment

Creating meaning

Community resources

Setting boundaries in relationships

Discovery

Getting others to support recovery

Coping with triggers

Creating a personal safety reminder (see the Crisis Response Safety Plan—Trauma-Informed version; see Figure 6–1 later in this chapter)

Respecting your time

Healthy relationships

Self-nurturing

Healing from anger

Life choices

Source.   Adapted from Najavits 2002.

tions of their feelings. By owning the story and examining its meaning in their life, patients may better self-manage the suffering and symptoms.

Skills Training in Affective and Interpersonal Regulation (STAIR) is a program of CBT followed by prolonged exposure training (Substance Abuse and Mental Health Services Administration 2014). A strong therapeutic alliance is a key factor in this program, emphasizing development of emotion regulation skills before exposure exercises.

Stress inoculation therapy focuses on managing anxiety and fear in day-to-day activities that may generate stress reactions in persons with interpersonal traumatic experiences and uses skills training and exercises that help with relaxation and control over these reactions.

Nightmares

What can be done about nightmares? Even in James White's alien universe, he wonders if it is possible to face the dangerous "undermind" and "phantasms" that create fear in the dreamer and actually make friends with them (White 1987, p 184). Is this itself a science fantasy or fiction, or a scientific possibility or even a current reality?

TABLE 6–3. **Key elements of TREM (Trauma Recovery and Empowerment Model)**

Part 1: Empowerment	Part 2: What Is Trauma?	Part 3: Social Relationships
Self-awareness	Physical reactions	Family, what is it?
Body image	Physical abuse	Current family relationships
Physical boundaries	Sexual abuse	Judgment and decision-making
Emotional boundaries	Emotional abuse	Communicating what one wants and needs
	Institutional abuse	
Self-esteem	Symptoms	Self-destructive behaviors
Self-care	Addictive or compulsive behavior	Blame, acceptance, and forgiveness
Intimacy and trust	Relationships in abusive circumstances	Control
Sexuality		Relationships
		Healing

Note. TREM was originally developed for women, but it has also been adapted for men.
Source. California Evidence-Based Clearinghouse for Child Welfare (Berley 2016).

In our work with nightmare sufferers, we learned that nightmare disorder is not just a childhood disorder: "Among adults, prevalence of nightmares at least monthly is 6%. Among adults in several countries, prevalence of weekly nightmares is 2%–6%, whereas prevalence of frequent nightmares is 1%–5%" (DSM-5-TR, p. 458). There are detailed criteria for nightmare disorder (Box 6–2), but the important ones are that a person becomes wide awake, remembers the dream, and has significant daytime impairment or dysfunction. When patients report vague unremembered nightmares and cannot point to residual distress or impairment the criteria are not met. Imagery rehearsal therapy (IRT) is the best studied and recommended nonpharmacological therapy for nightmares; we have used a version of this as recommended in Chapter 2 (Krakow 2020; Krakow et al. 1995). It is the only treatment strategy recommended for all patients with nightmare disorder according to the American Academy of Sleep Medicine (Morgenthaler et al. 2018). However, numerous other approaches are available, some which will require additional training (Lewis and Krippner 2016).

Box 6–2. DSM-5-TR Diagnostic Criteria for Nightmare Disorder

F51.5

A. Repeated occurrences of extended, extremely dysphoric, and well-remembered dreams that usually involve efforts to avoid threats to survival, security, or physical integrity and that generally occur during the second half of the major sleep episode.
B. On awakening from the dysphoric dreams, the individual rapidly becomes oriented and alert.
C. The sleep disturbance causes clinically significant distress or impairment in social, occupational, or other important areas of functioning.
D. The nightmare symptoms are not attributable to the physiological effects of a substance (e.g., a drug of abuse, a medication).
E. Coexisting mental disorders and medical conditions do not adequately explain the predominant complaint of dysphoric dreams.

Specify if:
  During sleep onset
Specify if:
  With mental disorder, including substance use disorders
  With medical condition
  With another sleep disorder
  Coding note: The code F51.5 applies to all three specifiers. Code also the relevant associated mental disorder, medical condition, or other sleep disorder immediately after the code for nightmare disorder in order to indicate the association.
Specify if:
  Acute: Duration of period of nightmares is 1 month or less.
  Subacute: Duration of period of nightmares is greater than 1 month but less than 6 months.
  Persistent: Duration of period of nightmares is 6 months or greater.
Specify current severity:
  Severity can be rated by the frequency with which the nightmares occur:
  Mild: Less than one episode per week on average.
  Moderate: One or more episodes per week but less than nightly.
  Severe: Episodes nightly.

IRT is based on behavioral assumptions. We explain nightmare disorder as the body's failed attempt at problem-solving and a learned yet unproductive repetitive behavior, and perhaps Freud would have subsumed it under the category of repetition compulsions. We do discuss the relationship to the whole group of PTSD symptoms when there are other symptoms of PTSD. Therefore, without any deep analysis of the dream content, a new dream script can be learned by rehearsal: "Patients are asked to recall the nightmare, write it down, alter its content to a positive outcome, and rehearse the rescripted dream for 10 to 20 minutes each day" (Callen et al. 2018). Such a scenario could include the one suggested to our science fiction alien in the opening quote, of turning the attacker into a friend.

The American Academy of Sleep Medicine also lists treatments to consider (slightly different) for nightmare disorder both associated and not associated with PTSD and covering both pharmacological and nonpharmacological treatments. In alphabetical order, they are as follows (adapted from Morgenthaler et al. 2018):

- For PTSD-associated nightmares: CBT, CBT for insomnia, EMDR, and exposure, relaxation, and rescripting therapy.
- For nightmare disorder: CBT; exposure, relaxation, and rescripting therapy; hypnosis; lucid dreaming therapy; progressive deep muscle relaxation; self-exposure therapy; sleep dynamic therapy; systematic desensitization; and testimony method

Various medications have varying degrees of effectiveness and you probably should refer anyone with a credible diagnosis of nightmare disorder for a medication evaluation.

If you encounter the disorder frequently enough, set your threshold (e.g., based on the severity specifier) to do so.

If you have many patients with nightmares, we recommend you look at the materials on the Krakow website (Krakow 2020). We have had much success and positive feedback using the workbook in a 12-session nightmare treatment course for women, but we can recall two instances, also working with women, in which a single session of instruction (with written handouts) led to significant improvement. This included the proviso that recall, rescripting, and rehearsal of the rescripted dream did not create significant distress and could be done without the presence of a professional. Of course, the use of imagery rehearsal could be considered part of the behavioral armamentarium of CBT, but we do not mind being eclectic and using what works when it works. Besides, it takes a lot of supportive work, such as encouragement and reassurance, to "nudge" people to try these techniques, which can be daunting when they involve aversive content.

Other Techniques and Approaches

In addition to manualized programs, several therapists have developed individual exercises that can be adapted to a treatment program (Curran 2013; Milkman et al. 2008; Sweeton 2019). Curran (2013) approaches these eclectically using art therapy, physical exercises, yoga, and mindfulness, among others, in her workbook. Sweeton (2019) looks at exercises that address the different areas of the brain that are affected by trauma and has a set of activities for each. Table 6–4 gives examples.

Resilience

One of the most important factors in the ability to avoid PTSD or maintain one's recovery from a traumatic event is to develop resilience as the overarching coping mechanism. If a person matures without role models in dealing with problems, fears, or disappointments, resilience is difficult to come by. Children who are neglected or abused, whose parents and caregivers are having trouble themselves with day-to-day problems or who themselves are without strong support in the community, do not have the opportunity to observe and learn coping skills.

Friedman (2015) identifies four ways in which resilience can be fostered in society, beginning at the societal level with laws and policies that encourage and support readiness in the face of large-scale trauma. In prison settings, one might imagine this to be trauma-informed policies and practices. At the community level, Friedman suggests psychoeducation for the community at large, and at the family level, fostering support among family members. In prison this would suggest that interaction with family on the outside should be facilitated. Inside the prison, group activities and counseling might be of value. Finally, at the personal level, try teaching adaptive strategies to develop skill at handling emotional and physical reactions to stress and identifying sources of social support.

Factors that contribute to resilience include optimism, cognitive flexibility, physical health, coping skills, social support network, and a personal moral compass (Casey and Strain 2016). Supportive psychotherapy can address these issues, for example, by helping patients to address their sense of pessimism while encouraging optimism. Learn-

TABLE 6–4.   **Examples of recommended activities for working with trauma survivors**

Mindfulness

Physical exercises

Meditation

Story telling

Art and music: being both a consumer and a practitioner

Guided imagery

Role-playing

Yoga, qigong, tai chi

Gratitude

Working on recovery with a friend

Journaling

Establishing life goals

Finding a role model/advisor

Giving: finding something you can help make better

Education

Occupational training

Self-praise

Source.   Curran 2013; Milkman et al. 2008; Peterson 2006; Rashid and Seligman 2018; Sweeton 2019.

ing coping strategies is of course the underpinning of all of the programs mentioned in this chapter. Improving physical health may be difficult in prisons, where diet and exercise options are closely regulated and medical care may be limited. In many cases, relying on or developing a social support network for prisoners is also a challenge. Finally, developing a personal moral compass may be challenging in a prison environment, but positive psychology principles and supportive psychotherapy can be helpful (Novalis et al. 2020; Peterson 2006). Faith-based services may also be of value.

Positive resilience role models are important to people attempting to develop their own resilience skills. Incarcerated persons with stressor-related disorders may not have had such models before their involvement in the justice system, and during incarceration the opportunities for such models may also be difficult to come by. In the course of therapy, providing the patient with examples of resilience and strategies for learning should be a key goal.

Talking to Trauma-Affected Patients

All the psychotherapy programs that have been developed for trauma-related therapy have as their base technique ways to talk to patients and questions to explore with them. For incarcerated individuals, establishing mutual trust depends on the therapist both understanding the nature of patients' perceived attitudes and avoiding value judgments about their behaviors that led them to the justice system. We are supportive psychotherapists, but that doesn't mean we condone those behaviors. However, understanding the current problems of patients can lead to productive discussions about how to change.

Therapists need to be active and "genuinely present" so they can overcome the dehumanizing effects of trauma (Sanderson 2013, p. 79). A predictable and consistent setting, preferably without outside distractions, is important, although in a prison setting this may require creativity in finding a location. Respecting the individual's autonomy over what is shared and when to put a halt to the discussion may have to suffice if trust is to be established. In addition to the physical space, needs such as a drink, access to a restroom, and the availability of tissues should be considered because stress and anxiety can elicit physical symptoms.

Attachment issues on the part of the patient include trust, control, fear, intimacy, dependence, and rejection. Helping the patient to establish control by establishing a collaborative approach is effective in dealing with the other issues. Boundary setting and readjusting from time to time lend patients confidence in the trust they have given. Pacing is a central ingredient in therapy, so issues and memories are not brought up before the patient is ready and has the skills needed to process the emotions and reactions safely and effectively (Sanderson 2013).

Perhaps the most important issue is to recognize the feeling of shame and guilt the patient is feeling. It is critical to emphasize that the individual did not cause the events leading to the reaction: for victims, these things were caused by another person. Reactions to triggers and other stimuli are typical coping strategies and not aberrant behavior. And going forward, these reactions can be mitigated and eliminated through therapy and self-care. Topics to explore include:

- How do you see yourself now and what would you like to change?
- What is your attitude toward the people who caused your trauma(s) and what are the ways you can change that attitude to help you cope?
- What are the things you see that were caused by the trauma(s) and how can you change these into a positive reaction?
- What would you want your life to be like here in the facility and once you are released? What are some strategies to achieve that?

Establishing a Plan for the Future

As patients learn how their behaviors and feelings result from trauma reactions and improve their coping strategies through therapy, developing strategies for avoiding unwanted behaviors and reactions to triggers and reminders of the traumas should be the goal of therapy. Such strategies should include exercises to maintain mental stability, coping with triggers, and developing a plan of action to further develop a life plan that is empowering.

Plan of Action

One of the goals of therapy and the path to a successful recovery is for the patient to develop a positive plan for living without the symptoms of adjustment disorders. This includes plans for life within the facility as well as a plan for life afterward. The plan should include strategies for establishing and reestablishing relationships that are supportive and encouraging, for education and training for meaningful work, for establishing and renewing goals for meaningful engagement in the outside world through social activities, and, it is hoped, plans for activities that bring joy outside of work. All

Warning signs I am getting suicidal or going to hurt myself   [Side 1]

When I'm sleeping less or sleeping poorly

When I stop going to the yard

When I stay in my cell

When I stop eating

When I start to hear voices again

When I think of cutting my arm

When I think I should be dead

When I start to feel guilty about being in prison

When I think abut what my father did to me and I am so mad

When I pick up the razor and start playing with it

Warning signs of my PTSD

External triggers   Internal triggers
(things seen or heard or felt)   (thoughts, moods, or behaviors)

CO opens and slams door   *Becoming more irritable, angry, or depressed*

Someone touches me unexpectedly   *Having more upsetting dreams or nightmares*

Someone yells at me or gets in my personal space   *Missing people and feeling lonely*

Seeing people in uniforms   *Feeling different from my usual self*

Someone says or does something to me that   *Feeling unsafe or vulnerable*

   makes me feel unsafe or threatened   *Feeling tense and ready to "go off"*

Watching people argue and hit each other   *A resurgence of my PTSD symptoms*

Hearing a police siren or   *such as memories and flashbacks*

   seeing squad car lights go by   *An increase in my pain*

Hearing a firecracker or real gunfire

Upsetting events on a movie, TV show, or

   news such as an accident

Anniversary of something that happened

Certain prisoners or staff who remind me of an abuser

Other things that are special to me _____

FIGURE 6–1. Crisis response safety plan—trauma informed version (CRSP-T).

How can I cope by myself when I start getting into trouble? [Side 1, continued]
COPING WITH THOUGHTS OF HURTING MYSELF

Read a book

Wrap the razor up in a towel and put it away

Do some of my drawings

Read the Bible with the passages I marked and mark some new passages

Go to the yard and exercise or exercise in the cell

Just go to sleep

Do my deep breathing

My progressive relaxation that they taught me

My mindfulness exercises

TRAUMA: COPING WITH MY PTSD TRIGGERS
Do any of the above and more

Use my coping cards

Repeat my mantra

Who can I contact?

My mother 202-XXX-XXXX

My brother 202-XXX-XXXX

Tell my CO now that it is an emergency

Tell the nurse who brings me my medicines

Send in a mental health request

Talk to my cellie

Call the
National Suicide Prevention Lifeline
1-800-273-8255

My reasons for living [Side 2]

My family

My children

Suicide is a sin, and I don't want to do that

I like most of the things in life, just not the prison

I can get out in a year

I like watching television

My resilience strategies

Do my problem-solving exercises

Do my resilience exercises

FIGURE 6–1. Crisis response safety plan—trauma informed version (CRSP-T). *(continued)*

of these will give patients something to focus on rather than the trauma that previously defined their behavior.

Crisis Response Safety Plan— Trauma-Informed Version

One of the tools therapists use for suicidal patients is a crisis response safety plan (CRSP) (see Chapter 5). However, trauma patients often have warning signs or triggers that cause them to have flashbacks, negative impulses, and other negative reactions (Tull and Susman 2020). A CRSP can also be helpful to them. Therefore, as promised in Chapter 5, we suggest some enhancements to the existing items in Figure 6–1.

Added to the front of the card are warning signs or triggers to the patient's symptoms (such as resurgence of nightmares) and the coping strategies to deal with them. Of course, the front of the card will also include the usual contact information for supportive individuals and services. On the other side, in addition to reasons for living, is a list of reasons that the individual has for developing and encouraging self-resilience. As with the CRSP for suicidal thinking, this should be written by the patient, emphasizing that the helping strategy was self-directed, thereby giving the patient an element of control and self-determination. As patients continue along their recovery, the plan can be updated. The contents of the card might be formatted and filled in similarly to Figure 6–1, customized to the person creating it. In Chapter 14, we suggest further enhancements to the CRSP for prisoners leaving for the community. One important discussion to have with a patient who is about to be released is awareness that a return to the outside world and family and social contacts may mean contact or exposure to places and circumstances associated with his or her trauma history. Strategies for coming into direct contact with these stimuli to avoid triggering should be central to pre-release counseling and are discussed there.

Trauma Self-Care

In treating trauma, when a therapist hears and observes secondhand what has happened to the patient, she can have reactions not dissimilar to a stressor-related disorder. Some caregivers feel they have no right to complain about their own lesser problems or that their unpleasant reactions to treating trauma are a sign of weakness (Lipsky and Burk 2009, p. 44).

Trauma experience as seen by therapists is similar to that of the families of trauma survivors or people who respond repeatedly to trauma, such as first responders and professionals who deal with natural disasters. Acknowledging that working and/or living with trauma survivors is in itself stressful is a first step in self-care. Najavits (2002) recognizes that countertransference can occur throughout treatment and includes self-care for therapists throughout the Seeking Safety program. Lipsky and Burk (2009) identify 16 responses that caregivers should be aware of when being exposed to stories of trauma. These are summarized in Table 6–5. Such responses are normal and nearly universal, although, of course, different people will respond differently to the circumstances about which they are hearing. Strategies for coping with these feelings include:

- *Opening an inquiry:* Understand your feelings and how they developed and learn how treating others affects you given that history.

TABLE 6–5.	Signs of secondary trauma in caregivers

Feeling helpless and hopeless

Sensing that you can never do enough

Being hypervigilant

Experiencing a loss of creativity

Being flummoxed by the complexity of the problems you are trying to solve

Dismissing the severity of the problems

Experiencing fatigue and physical problems

Finding yourself unable to listen or avoiding problems

Dissociating

Feeling persecuted

Feeling guilty

Feeling fear

Getting angry or cynical

Becoming numb to what you are hearing

Becoming dependent on addicting substances or behaviors to alleviate the stress

Having feelings of grandiosity

- *Self-care:* Provide yourself with a sense of personal control; involve yourself in meaningful tasks and be active in their pursuit, develop healthy habits, and make sure your social support is available to you as needed.
- *Patience with the course of treatment:* Remember that treating trauma can take time and be time-consuming and sometimes it can't be speeded up despite frustration.
- *Mindfulness:* Be aware of the present: mindfulness in the face of treating the patient and how you yourself are feeling can ground you in the task. But also be aware of when you need to step back (Lipsky and Burk 2009).
- *Recognizing the role of self-care in advocating for your patients:* "Self-care is essential for the work of social justice. It enables us to advocate for others—amplifying our effectiveness and extending our time" (Vinson and Shim 2021, p. 249).

How Treatment Helps

Trauma-informed care and effective treatment of trauma-related disorders may help prevent relapse and, perhaps, problems in adjusting to society once a prisoner is released. (Kubiak and Rose 2007). It is important not to overmedicalize the diagnosis and treatment of individuals with trauma histories and to give patients the skills they need to recognize that their symptoms are a form of protecting themselves from further harm, and that there are more effective coping strategies that can help them not only to reduce or eliminate the symptoms but also to establish a more productive life.

Key Points

- Trauma plays a central role in the lives of many prisoners, prior to entering prison, upon entering the prison, and in the prison life that follows.

- The effects of trauma include many symptoms that are similar to those of other mental disorders. Care must be given to recognize the source of the issues faced by patients to ensure the proper diagnosis is made. Complicating this, adjustment disorders are often comorbid with other disorders, including substance use, depression, and bipolar disorder.

- An adjustment disorder is now considered a stressor-related disorder and is grouped with PTSD. Adjustment disorders are shorter in duration than PTSD, and treating them may be effective in preventing full PTSD.

- We urge careful attention to diagnostic and coding issues because we believe they do have an effect on the use of therapy for these patients.

- We urge clinicians not to overdiagnose persons with histories of trauma. For example, a person with nightmares does not automatically have PTSD. Overdiagnosing impedes the ability to understand the effect of incarceration on people (especially those with histories of trauma) and the selection and monitoring of their therapy.

- A variety of therapies are effective for persons with PTSD. The goal of treatment is to first ensure that the patient is able to feel safe and then give the patient effective coping skills to enhance resiliency. Supportive psychotherapy techniques remain fundamental, even when another therapeutic technique is used or a manualized program is implemented. As an eclectic or integrative therapist, you can and should incorporate techniques from other "schools" of therapy into your regular practice. Most therapists do this throughout their careers.

- Nightmares are a frequent component of PTSD. They can be treated by a variety of methods, but the one with the greatest evidence basis is imagery rehearsal therapy, which we have used and found effective in working with prisoners.

- Treating persons affected by trauma can lead to a form of secondary trauma in caregivers, and therapists should be aware of their own reactions and take self-care seriously.

References

Akiki TJ, Abdallah CG: Are there effective psychopharmacologic treatments for PTSD? J Clin Psychiatry 80(3):18ac12473, 2018 30695292

Arends I, Bruinvels DJ, Rebergen DS, et al: Interventions to facilitate return to work in adults with adjustment disorders. Cochrane Database Syst Rev December 12;12:CD006389, 2012 23235630

Baranyi G, Cassidy M, Fazel S, et al: Prevalence of posttraumatic stress disorder in prisoners. Epidemiol Rev 40(1):134–145, 2018 29596582

Berley RW: Trauma Recovery and Empowerment Model. San Diego, CA, California Evidence-Based Clearinghouse for Child Welfare, 2016. Available at: www.cebc4cw.org/program/trauma-recovery-and-empowerment-model/detailed. Accessed October 13, 2020.

Bisson JI, Lewis C: Systemic review of psychological first aid. Commissioned by the World Health Organization, 2009. Available at: www.researchgate.net/publication/265069490_Systematic_Review_of_Psychological_First_Aid. Accessed October 25, 2020.

Bloom SL: Organizational stress as a barrier to trauma-informed service delivery, in A Public Health Perspective of Women's Mental Health. Edited by Beker M, Levin B. New York, Springer, 2010, pp 295-311

Bonnano GA: The End of Trauma: How the New Science of Resilience Is Changing How We Think About PTSD. New York, Basic Books, 2021

Bryant RA: Early interventions for trauma, in Handbook of PTSD: Science and Practice, 2nd Edition. Edited by Friedman MJ, Keane TM, Resick PA. New York, Guilford Press, 2016

California Evidence-Based Clearinghouse for Child Welfare: Trauma recovery and empowerment model (TREM), 2016. Available at: https://cebc4cw.org/program.trauma-recovery-and-empowerment-model/detailed. Accessed November 18, 2020.

Callen ED, Kessler TL, Brooks KG, Davis TD: Management of nightmare disorder in adults. U.S. Pharmacist 43(11):21–26, 2018. Available at: www.medscape.com/viewarticle/906093#. Accessed November 28, 2020.

Carta MG, Balestrieri M, Murru A, Hardoy MC: Adjustment disorder: epidemiology, diagnosis and treatment. Clin Pract Epidemiol Ment Health 5:15, 2009 19558652

Carter RT, Murchow C: Construct validity of the Race-Based Traumatic Stress Symptom Scale and tests of measured equivalence. Psychological Trauma: Theory, Research, Practice, and Policy 9(6):688–695, 2017

Casey P: Treatment of adjustment disorders, in Adjustment Disorder: From Controversy to Clinical Practice. Edited by Casey P. New York, Oxford University Press, 2018, pp 97–110

Casey PR, Strain JJ: Trauma- and Stressor-Related Disorders. Arlington, VA, American Psychiatric Association Publishing, 2016

Cottraux J, Note I, Yao SN, et al: Randomized controlled experiment of cognitive behavior therapy with Rogerian supportive therapy in chronic post-traumatic stress disorder: a 2-year follow-up. Psychother Psychosom 77(2)101–110, 2008 18230943

Crighton DA, Towl GJ: Psychology in Prisons, 2nd Edition. Malden, MA, Blackwell Publishing, 2008

Curran LA: 101 Trauma-Informed Interventions: Activities, Exercises, and Assignments to Move the Client and Therapy Forward. Eau Claire, WI, PESI Publishing and Media, 2013

Dass-Brailford P: A Practical Approach to Trauma: Empowering Interventions. Thousand Oaks, CA, Sage, 2007

De Leo D: Treatment of adjustment disorders: a comparative evaluation. Psychol Rep 64(1):51–54, 1989 2648447

Ehlers A, Bisson J, Clark DM, et al: Do all psychological treatments really work the same in posttraumatic stress disorder? Clin Psychol Rev 30(2):269–276, 2010 20051310

The Ezra Klein Show: Transcript: Ezra Klein interviews Bessel van der Kolk. New York Times Opinion, August 24, 2021

Frank JB, Bienenfield D, Benton TD, Talavera F: Adjustment disorder. Medscape, November 1, 2016. Available at: https://emedicine.medscape.com/article/2192631-overview. Accessed September 26, 2020.

Friedman MJ: Posttraumatic and Acute Stress Disorders, 6th Edition. Cham, Switzerland, Springer International Publishing, 2015

Fulks TA: Diagnosing mental illness: what does the DSM-5 mean for corrections? Correctcare 28(3): 2014

Glancy GD, Treffers SR: Adjustment disorders, in Oxford Textbook of Correctional Psychiatry. Edited by Trestman RL, Applebaum KL, Metzner JL. New York, Oxford University Press, 2015, pp 95–98

Gramigna J: PTSD exposure therapy does not cause drug relapse, psychiatric symptoms. Helio News, July 24, 2020. Available at: www.healio.com/news/psychiatry/20200724/ptsd-exposure-therapy-does-not-cause-drug-relapse-psychiatric-symptoms. Accessed September 15, 2020.

Grieger TA, Benedek DM, Ursano RJ: Violence and aggression, in Clinical Manual for Management of PTSD. Edited by Benedek DM, Wynn GH. Arlington, VA, American Psychiatric Publishing, 2011, pp 205–225

Haney C: Criminality in Context: The Psychological Foundations of Criminal Justice Reform. Washington, DC, American Psychological Association, 2020

Haney C: The Psychological Impact of Incarceration: Implications for Post-Prison Adjustment. Washington, DC, U.S. Department of Health & Human Services, Office of the Assistant Secretary for Planning and Evaluation, December 1, 2001. Available at: https://aspe.hhs.gov/reports/psychological-impact-incarceration-implications-post-prison-adjustment. Accessed May 19, 2020.

Harper M: The Beauty in Breaking. New York, Riverside Books. 2020

Hashmi AM: Trauma across cultures: assessment, treatment, and prevention. Psychiatr Ann 47(3):120–121, 2017

Hassanmirzei B, Soltani SK, Haratian Z, et al: Web-based supportive psychotherapy to prevent posttraumatic stress disorder: a cross-sectional study on the Iranian national under-14 girls football team after Nepal earthquake in 2015. Asian Sports Medicine 8(4):e13778, Dec 2017

Herd DA: Pain of police killings ripples outward to traumatize black people and communities across US. Reprinted from The Conversation, Talking Points Memo. May 29, 2021. Available at: https://talkingpointsmemo.com/news/pain-police-killings-tripples-outward-traumatize-black-people-communities-us. Accessed May 30, 2021.

Herman J: Trauma and Recovery. New York, Basic Books, 2015

Horowitz MJ: Treatment of Stress Response Syndromes, 2nd Edition. Washington, DC, American Psychiatric Association Publishing, 2020

Jäggi LJ, Mazuk B, Watkins DC, Jackson JS: The relationship between trauma, arrest, and incarceration history among black Americans: findings from the National Survey of American Life. Soc Ment Health 6(3):187–206, 2016 27795871

Javier RA, Owen EA: Trauma and its vicissitudes in forensic contexts: an introduction, in Assessing Trauma in Forensic Contexts. Edited by Javier RA, Owen EA, Maddox JA. Cham, Switzerland, Springer Nature International, 2020

Johnson JR, Lubin H: Principles and Techniques of Trauma-Centered Psychotherapy. Washington, DC, American Psychiatric Association Publishing, 2015

Krakow B: Turning nightmares into dreams (DVD/digital). 2020. Available at: https://barrykrakowmd.com/product/turning-nightmares-into-dreams. Accessed November 13, 2020.

Krakow B, Kellner R, Pathak D, Lambert L: Imagery rehearsal treatment for chronic nightmares. Behav Res Ther 33(7):837–843, 1995 7677723

Kubiak SP, Rose IM: Trauma and posttraumatic stress disorder in inmates with histories of substance use, in Handbook of Forensic Mental Health With Victims and Offenders: Assessment, Treatment and Research. Edited by Springer DW, Roberts AR. New York, Springer, 2007, pp 445–466

Kulkarni J: Complex PTSD - a better description for borderline personality disorder? Australas Psychiatry 25(4):333–335, 2017 28347146

Lee DJ, Schnitzlein CW, Wolf JP, et al: Psychotherapy versus pharmacotherapy for posttraumatic stress disorder: systemic review and meta-analysis to determine first-line treatments. Depress Anxiety 33(9):792–806, 2016 27126398

Levenson JS, Willis GM: Implementing trauma-informed care in correctional treatment and supervision. J Aggress Maltreat Trauma 28(4):481–501, 2019

Levine J: "Changing the outcomes, not just the symbols." Columbia University Teachers College Newsroom, New York. July 23, 2020. Available at: www.tc.columbia.articles/2020/july/changing-the-outcomes-not-just-the-symbols. Accessed May 30, 2021.

Lewis JE, Krippner SE (eds): Working With Dreams and PTSD Nightmares: 14 Approaches for Psychotherapists and Counselors. Santa Barbara, CA, Praeger, 2016

Lewis KL, Grenyer B: Borderline personality disorder or complex posttraumatic stress disorder? An update on the controversy. 2009. Available at: https://ro.uow.edu.au/hbspapers/3401. Accessed January 18, 2020.

Lipsky LV, Burk C: Trauma Stewardship: An Everyday Guide to Caring for Self While Caring for Others. Oakland, CA, Berrett-Koehler Publishers, 2009

London RT: Can experiencing bigotry and racism lead to PTSD? Clinical Psychiatric News 48(10) October 2020

Lynch J, Mack L, Benesek J, et al: PTSD Recovery Program Treatment Manual, 3rd Edition. Richmond, VA, Hunter Holmes McGuire VAMC, October 2015. Available at: www.mirecc.va.gov/docs/visn6/PTSD_Recovery_Group-Client_Manual_3rd_edition.pdf. Accessed October 25, 2020.

Milkman HB, Wanberg KW, Gagliardi BA: Criminal Conduct and Substance Abuse Treatment for Women in Correctional settings: Female-Focused Strategies for Self-Improvement and Change—Pathways to Responsible Living: Adjunct Providers Guide. Los Angeles, CA, Sage, 2008

Miller NA, Najavits LM: Creating trauma-informed correctional care: a balance of goals and environment. Eur J Psychotraumatol 3:1–8, 2012 22893828

Morgenthaler TI, Auerbach S, Casey KR, et al: Position paper for the treatment of nightmare disorder in adults: an American Academy of Sleep Medicine position paper. J Clin Sleep Med 14(6):1041–1055, 2018 29852917

Najavits LM: Seeking Safety: A Treatment Manual for PTSD and Substance Abuse. New York, Guilford, 2002

National Center for PTSD: Complex PTSD. January 31, 2020. Available at: www.ptsd.va.gov/professional/treat/essentials/complex_ptsd.asp. Accessed March 5, 2022.

Novalis PN, Singer V, Peele R: Clinical Manual of Supportive Psychotherapy, 2nd Edition. Washington, DC, American Psychiatric Association Publishing, 2020

Peirce JM, Schacht RL, Brooner RK: The effects of prolonged exposure on substance use in patients with posttraumatic stress disorder and substance use disorders. J Trauma Stress 33(4):465–476, 2020 32598569

Peterson C: A Primer in Positive Psychology. New York, Oxford University Press, 2006

Polyakova I, Knobler HY, Ambrumova A, Lerner V: Characteristics of suicidal attempts in major depression versus adjustment reactions. J Affect Disord 47(1-3):159–167, 1998 9476756

Rashid T, Seligman M: Positive Psychotherapy Clinician Manual. New York, Oxford University Press, 2018

Sanderson C: Counseling Skills for Working With Trauma: Healing for Child Sexual Abuse, Sexual Violence and Domestic Abuse. Philadelphia, PA, Jessica Kingsley Publishers, 2013

Schnurr PP: A guide to the literature on partial PTSD. PTSD Res Q 25:1, 2014

Schnyder U, Cloitre M (eds): Evidence-Based Treatments for Trauma-Related Psychological Disorders: A Practical Guide for Clinicians. New York, Springer International, 2015

Southwick SM, Pietrzak RH, Tsai J, et al: Resilience: an update. PTSD Res Q 25:4, 2015

Substance Abuse and Mental Health Services Administration: Trauma-Informed Care in Behavioral Health Services. Treatment Improvement Protocol (TIP) Series 57; HHS Publ No (SMA) 13-4801. Rockville, MD, Substance Abuse and Mental Health Services Administration, 2014. Available at: https://store.samhsa.gov/sites/default/files/d7/priv/sma14-4816.pdf. Accessed November 12, 2020.

Strain JJ, Smith GC, Hammer JS, et al: Adjustment disorder: a multisite study of its utilization and interventions in the consultation-liaison psychiatry setting. Gen Hosp Psychiatry 20(3):139–149, 1998 9650031

Sun K: Treating depression and PTSD behind bars: an interaction schemas approach, in Forensic CBT: A Handbook for Clinical Practice. Edited by Tafrate RC, Mitchell D. New York, Wiley, 2014, pp 456–470

Sweeton J: Trauma Treatment Toolbox: 165 Brain-Changing Tips, Tools and Handouts to Move Therapy Forward. Eau Claire, WI, PESI Publishing and Media, 2019

Tull M, Susman D: How to develop a safety plan for PTSD symptoms: Verywell Mind (Dotdash Publishing), April 27, 2020. Available at: www.verywellmind.com/developing-a-safety-plan-for-ptsd-symptoms-2797577. Accessed October 12, 2021.

Van der Kolk B: The Body Keeps the Score: Brain, Mind, and Body in the Healing of Trauma. New York, Penguin, 2015

Vinson SY, Shim RS: Social justice and mental health: a call to action, in Social (In)justice and Mental Health. Edited by Shim RS, Vinson SY. Washington, DC, American Psychiatric Association Publishing, 2021, pp. 239–251

Way BB, Miraglia R, Sawyer DA, et al: Factors related to suicide in New York state prisons. Int J Law Psychiatry 28(3):207–221, 2005 15950281

White J: Code Blue Emergency. New York, Ballantine Books, 1987

Wolff N, Huening J, Shi J, et al: Implementation and effectiveness of integrated trauma and addiction treatment for incarcerated men. J Anxiety Disord 30:66–80, 2015 25617774

7

Substance Use Disorders

There are a moderate number of prisoners who have neither mental health nor substance or alcohol use disorders[1] (20% in state prisons and 28% in federal prisons). There are also a moderate number of "pure" substance abusers (those without co-occurring mental health disorders) in jails and prisons. Slightly less than a quarter (24%) of state prisoners and a fifth (19%) of local jail prisoners had presentations that met the criteria for substance dependence or abuse only (Bronson et al. 2017).

A good indicator of the prevalence of substance users in prison is the percentage of positive drug screens for eight drugs and alcohol at admission. This percentage is 70%–77% at time of arrest; that group includes 36% reporting heavy drug use in the 30 days preceding arrest and 40% at risk for alcohol and drug dependence at the time of arrest (Stephens 2011, p. 237). However, comorbidity is high. An estimated 42% of people in state prisons and 49% in jails were found to have both a mental health problem and substance dependence or abuse. Other surveys report higher numbers. By gender, 54% of female and 41% of male prisoners have both substance use and mental health disorders. Over 70% of persons with a severe mental illness have comorbid substance use disorder (Ternes et al. 2018, reporting data from others). From a different survey, according to Bureau of Justice Statistics data (Bronson et al. 2017), 30%–35% of prisoners (jails and prisons) who do not have mental problems have alcohol use disorder, and among those with mental problems the rates are 44%–54%. Combined alcohol and substance abuse ranges from 53%–56% for those without mental problems to 74%–76% for those with mental health problems. The latter percentage (75%) is typically the one we have heard over the years for comorbidity of mental health and substance abuse problems. A higher percentage of women in prison (47%) and jail (60%) used drugs in the past month compared with men in prison (38%) and jail (54%) (Bronson et al. 2017). As mentioned, the terminology for substance abuse and dependence has been changed into degrees of severity, so older surveys use different terminology.

---

[1]The terms *substance abuse* and *substance dependence* in the older literature were replaced by graded severities of substance use disorders in DSM-5.

Of the persons with substance use disorder, 28% of prisoners and 22% of those in jail were in a drug treatment program at the time of admission (Bronson et al. 2017). Of course, it is not just availability but willingness to participate or a similar concept (e.g., readiness for treatment) that determines who is in a program, but there is a long way to go. What is astounding to us is not our nation's "drug problem," as it is frequently called, but our nation's prisoners' drug problems. (Part and parcel of it is our nation's *drug law problem*.)

In the classic movie *It's a Wonderful Life* (Capra 1946), at the tail end of the 1918 influenza pandemic, Mr. Gower, the Bedford Falls pharmacist, receives the news that his son has died of the disease. He binges, mistakenly puts the wrong compound in a capsule, and would have killed a customer with the poisonous prescription had not a young George Bailey (Jimmy Stewart) intervened.

There are many theories about why people use substances. It is also thought that the reasons people start using substances (e.g., curiosity or peer pressure) may be different from the reasons they continue to use them (e.g., addiction). There are many interventions to prevent, moderate, or mitigate the effects of substance use. Much is also written about how mentally ill persons "self-medicate" their anxiety or depression with substances. This theory plays a role in several of the treatment strategies discussed in this book. However, if that is the explanation for persons with mental illness, what is everybody else—that is, that majority of persons who don't have mental illness—doing? Are they just using substances for fun? Is it fun to be a heroin addict? Is it fun to have binge-eating disorder? Is it enjoyable to have a gambling addiction (the non-substance-related disorder in which the "substance" is thought to be a neurotransmitter, dopamine)? Do people do everything they do for a reason, such as to feel better? Does a pedophile entice children for the fun of it? Do people with deviant behavior need to learn more socially appropriate means of satisfying their needs? (Although you probably think we are leading you into a blind alley here, you will need to think about this when you learn more about the Good Lives Model [which we introduced in Chapter 1] for treating sex offenders.) In a recent review of his lifelong work, which includes his association with the self-medication hypothesis of substance use, Khantzian asks us to consider that addiction can be conceived of as a self-regulation disorder and therapy as a way of addressing disordered self-care, disordered self-esteem, and disordered relationships (Khantzian 2012).

The National Institute on Drug Abuse (2016) identifies 13 principles of drug abuse treatment for criminal justice populations (Table 7–1).

What Works?

What works in correctional settings for substance users? According to the previous "review of reviews" (Ternes et al. 2018), motivational interviewing (MI) is best suited for getting people into treatment and retaining them. However, a review of 59 studies between 1993 and 2010 showed significant immediate effects but not in the long term. Twelve-step approaches were thought to be less effective than other approaches, but later we will discuss a Cochrane Library review that is rather positive for these. Therapeutic communities have a high dropout rate within the first 90 days, especially among women, who tolerate the interpersonal hostility of these programs less well than do men. For opioid dependency, opioid substitution therapy is still the best practice. Of the

TABLE 7–1. **National Institute on Drug Abuse principles of drug abuse treatment for criminal justice populations**

1. **Drug addiction is a brain disease that affects behavior.**
   Drug addiction has well-recognized cognitive, behavioral, and physiological characteristics that contribute to continued use of drugs despite the harmful consequences. Scientists have also found that chronic drug abuse alters the brain's anatomy and chemistry and that these changes can last for months or years after the individual has stopped using drugs. This transformation may help explain why addicted persons are at a high risk of relapse to drug abuse even after long periods of abstinence and why they persist in seeking drugs despite the consequences.

2. **Recovery from drug addiction requires effective treatment, followed by management of the problem over time.**
   Drug addiction is a serious problem that can be treated and managed throughout its course. Effective drug abuse treatment engages participants in a therapeutic process, retains them in treatment for an appropriate length of time, and helps them learn to maintain abstinence. Multiple episodes of treatment may be required. Outcomes for drug-abusing offenders in the community can be improved by monitoring drug use and by encouraging continued participation in treatment.

3. **Treatment must last long enough to produce stable behavioral changes.**
   In treatment, the drug abuser is taught to break old patterns of thinking and behaving and to learn new skills for avoiding drug use and criminal behavior. Individuals with severe drug problems and co-occurring disorders typically need longer treatment (e.g., a minimum of 3 months) and more comprehensive services. Early in treatment, the drug abuser begins a therapeutic process of change. In later stages, he or she addresses other problems related to drug abuse and learns how to manage them as well.

4. **Assessment is the first step in treatment.**
   A history of drug or alcohol use may suggest the need to conduct a comprehensive assessment to determine the nature and extent of an individual's drug problems, establish whether problems exist in other areas that may affect recovery, and enable the formulation of an appropriate treatment plan. Personality disorders and other mental health problems are prevalent in offender populations; therefore, comprehensive assessments should include mental health evaluations with treatment planning for these problems.

5. **Tailoring services to fit the needs of the individual is an important part of effective drug abuse treatment for criminal justice populations.**
   Individuals differ in terms of age, gender, ethnicity and culture, problem severity, recovery stage, and level of supervision needed. Individuals also respond differently to different treatment approaches and treatment providers. In general, drug treatment should address issues of motivation, problem-solving, and skill-building for resisting drug use and criminal behavior. Lessons aimed at supplanting drug use and criminal activities with constructive activities and at understanding the consequences of one's behavior are also important to include. Tailored treatment interventions can facilitate the development of healthy interpersonal relationships and improve the participant's ability to interact with family, peers, and others in the community.

6. **Drug use during treatment should be carefully monitored.**
   Individuals trying to recover from drug addiction may experience a relapse, or return to drug use. Triggers for drug relapse are varied; common ones include mental stress and associations with peers and social situations linked to drug use. An undetected relapse can progress to serious drug abuse, but detected use can present opportunities for therapeutic intervention. Monitoring drug use through urinalysis or other objective methods, as part of treatment or criminal justice supervision, provides a basis for assessing and providing feedback on the participant's treatment progress. It also provides opportunities to intervene to change unconstructive behavior—determining rewards and sanctions to facilitate change, and modifying treatment plans according to progress.

TABLE 7–1.	National Institute on Drug Abuse principles of drug abuse treatment for criminal justice populations *(continued)*

7. **Treatment should target factors that are associated with criminal behavior.**
   "Criminal thinking" is a combination of attitudes and beliefs that support a criminal lifestyle and criminal behavior, such as feeling entitled to have things one's own way, feeling that one's criminal behavior is justified, failing to accept responsibility for one's actions, and consistently failing to anticipate or appreciate the consequences of one's behavior. This pattern of thinking often contributes to drug use and criminal behavior. Treatment that provides specific cognitive skills training to help individuals recognize errors in judgment that lead to drug abuse and criminal behavior may improve outcomes.

8. **Criminal justice supervision should incorporate treatment planning for drug-abusing offenders, and treatment providers should be aware of correctional supervision requirements.**
   The coordination of drug abuse treatment with correctional planning can encourage participation in drug abuse treatment and can help treatment providers incorporate correctional requirements as treatment goals. Treatment providers should collaborate with criminal justice staff to evaluate each individual's treatment plan and ensure that it meets correctional supervision requirements, as well as that person's changing needs, which may include housing and child care; medical, psychiatric, and social support services; and vocational and employment assistance. For offenders with drug abuse problems, planning should incorporate the transition to community-based treatment and links to appropriate postrelease services to improve the success of drug treatment and reentry. Abstinence requirements may necessitate a rapid clinical response, such as more counseling, targeted intervention, or increased medication, to prevent relapse. Ongoing coordination between treatment providers and courts or parole and probation officers is important in addressing the complex needs of these reentering individuals.

9. **Continuity of care is essential for drug abusers reentering the community.**
   Offenders who complete prison-based treatment and continue with treatment in the community have the best outcomes. Continuing drug abuse treatment helps the recently released offender deal with problems that become relevant after release, such as learning to handle situations that could lead to relapse, learning how to live drug-free in the community, and developing a drug-free peer support network. Treatment in prison or jail can begin a process of therapeutic change, resulting in reduced drug use and criminal behavior post-incarceration. Continuing drug treatment in the community is essential to sustaining these gains.

10. **A balance of rewards and sanctions encourages prosocial behavior and treatment participation.**
    When providing correctional supervision of individuals participating in drug abuse treatment, it is important to reinforce positive behavior. Nonmonetary "social reinforcers" such as recognition for progress or sincere effort can be effective, as can graduated sanctions that are consistent, predictable, and clear responses to noncompliant behavior. Generally, less punitive responses are used for early and less serious noncompliance, with increasingly severe sanctions issuing from continued problem behavior. Rewards and sanctions are most likely to have the desired effect when they are perceived as fair and when they swiftly follow the targeted behavior.

TABLE 7–1. **National Institute on Drug Abuse principles of drug abuse treatment for criminal justice populations (continued)**

11. **Offenders with co-occurring drug abuse and mental health problems often require an integrated treatment approach.**
    High rates of mental health problems are found both in offender populations and in those with substance abuse problems. Drug abuse treatment can sometimes address depression, anxiety, and other mental health problems. Personality, cognitive, and other serious mental disorders can be difficult to treat and may disrupt drug treatment. The presence of co-occurring disorders may require an integrated approach that combines drug abuse treatment with psychiatric treatment, including the use of medication. Individuals with either a substance abuse or mental health problem should be assessed for the presence of the other.

12. **Medications are an important part of treatment for many drug-abusing offenders.**
    Medicines such as methadone, buprenorphine, and extended-release naltrexone have been shown to reduce heroin use and should be made available to individuals who could benefit from them. Effective use of medications can also be instrumental in enabling people with co-occurring mental health problems to function successfully in society. Behavioral strategies can increase adherence to medication regimens.

13. **Treatment planning for drug-abusing offenders who are living in or reentering the community should include strategies to prevent and treat serious, chronic medical conditions, such as HIV/AIDS, hepatitis B and C, and tuberculosis.**
    The rates of infectious diseases, such as hepatitis, tuberculosis, and HIV/AIDS, are higher in drug abusers, incarcerated offenders, and offenders under community supervision than in the general population. Infectious diseases affect not just the offender, but also the criminal justice system and the wider community. Consistent with Federal and State laws, drug-involved offenders should be offered testing for infectious diseases and receive counseling on their health status and on ways to modify risk behaviors. Probation and parole officers who monitor offenders with serious medical conditions should link them with appropriate health care services, encourage compliance with medical treatment, and reestablish their eligibility for public health services (e.g., Medicaid, county health departments) before release from prison or jail.

Source. National Institute on Drug Abuse 2016 (public domain).

programs studied there, the ones based on cognitive-behavioral therapy (CBT) do well overall.

Supportive psychotherapy does have a good track record in treating substance abuse, although it usually does not get compared in these studies. For example, it is an effective treatment for cocaine abuse (Crits-Christoph et al. 2008) and was used to treat what was called marijuana dependence (Grenyer et al. 1995).

SAMHSA Treatment Improvement Protocol (TIP) 34 (Substance Abuse and Mental Health Services Administration 2012) is an extensive presentation of brief interventions for substance abuse. This is not to say that only brief psychotherapies should be used; but they do have advantages in many cases, especially in short-stay jail settings. One supposed drawback of brief therapies is that they do not guarantee abstinence, but this is not generally a problem in correctional settings (although some prisoners continue to have access to illegal drugs). Brief therapies can supplement a patient's institutional abstinence by building personal defenses against relapse and improve the chances of success in the community. Institutional abstinence is one of three kinds of exceptions that occur in a substance user's life, the others being deliberate and random. We give examples, derived in large part from the SAMHSA TIPS, on how to capitalize on all three in your therapy in Table 7–2.

TABLE 7–2.   **Capitalizing on the three exceptions to substance use**

Deliberate exceptions are situations in which a client has intentionally maintained a period of sobriety or reduced use for whatever reason. For example, a client who did not use substances for a month in order to pass a drug test for a new job has made a deliberate exception to his typical pattern of daily substance use. If he is reminded that he did do this in the past[,] it will demonstrate that he can repeat the behavior.

Random exceptions are occasions when a client reduces use or abstains because of circumstances that are apparently beyond her control. The client may say, for example, that she was just "feeling good" and did not feel the urge to use at a particular time but cannot point to any intentional behaviors on her part that enabled her to stay sober. This type of exception is more difficult for the therapist to work with, but can also be used to help the client perceive her own efficacy. In such instances the therapist can ask the client to try to predict when such a period of "feeling good" might occur again, which will force her to begin thinking about the behaviors that may have had an effect on creating the random exception.

Forced exceptions include *institutional abstinence* (inability to access the substance due to incarceration or possibly a medical hospitalization) but could also occur at other times, and more examples developed during the COVID-19 pandemic when substance users lost access to their normal supplies of substances (e.g, a client on a cruise ship became quarantined for 2 weeks and ran out of his supply). Ask the client how he feels. Are his urges to use gone? If not, what do they feel like? Unlike times in the community when an urge will lead immediately to drug-seeking behavior, drugs are generally not available in the prison, and to the extent that the urge can be tolerated, it can be talked about. *Frustrated action can be converted into talk.*

Source.   The first two definitions are reprinted from Substance Abuse and Mental Health Services Administration 2012, pp. 89–90.

Supportive-expressive psychotherapy, one of the early models of supportive psychotherapy (Luborsky 1984) (see Chapter 1), is the main therapy described in the TIP 34 section on brief psychodynamic therapies for substance abuse, with additional references about the evidence basis for this type of therapy (Substance Abuse and Mental Health Services Administration 2012). It is also described as one of 10 models of brief psychodynamic psychotherapy for substance abuse. A second model of brief supportive psychotherapy is the one described by Pinsker et al. (1991), whose work was also referenced in Chapter 1.

> The term "supportive" refers to the techniques aimed at directly maintaining the client's level of functioning—that is, "supporting" the client. The term "expressive" refers to techniques that intend to facilitate the client's expression of problems and conflicts and their understanding….Change comes about through three curative factors: a positive helping relationship, gains in self-understanding, and internalization of these gains. (Substance Abuse and Mental Health Services Administration 2013a, p. 138)

Important goals of these supportive therapies are to:

- Develop a good therapeutic alliance.
- Formulate and respond to central relationship patterns (a technique that is also used in the interpersonal psychotherapy of depression).
- Attend to and respond to concerns about separation (therapy termination).
- Make interpretations (what we call "explanations") that are appropriate to the patient's level of awareness.

- Recognize the patient's need to test the therapeutic relationship by developing transference problems.

The techniques (which reflect supportive psychotherapy of all types) are:

- Framing symptoms as problem-solving or coping attempts (a commonality with therapies called "problem-solving").
- Reducing anxiety and boosting self-esteem.
- Providing reassurance, praise, and encouragement.
- Improving adaptive skills and ego functions.
- Respecting adaptive defenses and challenging maladaptive ones.
- Providing clarifications, reflections, and interpretations.
- Providing rationalizations, reframing, and giving advice.
- Using modeling, anticipation, and rehearsal.

SAMHSA TIP 34 (published in 1999 and last revised in 2012) is a broad review of multiple therapies, including cognitive-behavioral, solution-focused, and some others that are fairly rare these days, such as Gestalt therapy, but also existentialist/humanist therapies (such as that of Carl Rogers), which have much to offer and are a kind of predecessor to our own version of supportive psychotherapy. One difference between humanist psychotherapies and modern supportive psychotherapy is that the latter is more educational and directive, but both therapies share common concepts of empathy and the positive therapeutic alliance. It is worth reading, or at least skimming, TIP 34, which is available online, not to transform yourself into an existential or Gestalt therapist, but to assimilate some of the useful techniques or concepts that are literally scattered about the various therapies and add them to your repertory, which is typical of what we have called "eclectic psychotherapy" in the first chapter.

It is true that you should *not* just collect therapeutic techniques from every available psychotherapy that has ever been practiced! Rather, experienced therapists find that a variety of techniques can be added to their own practice effectively. Examples of some applicable techniques include psychoeducation, role-playing, journaling, letter-writing, workbooks, mindfulness, grounding, narrative techniques, and so on. There are many therapists out there using the "empty chair" technique of Gestalt therapy and the "miracle question" of brief solution-focused therapy. Primal screams? Recovered memories of Satanic abuse? No, thank you. You need judgment in looking at the technique and the background in which it is used. Consider that TIP 34 itself presents a wide range of brief psychotherapies, some of which have already had their 15 minutes of fame but that at one time seemed promising. One more example: Existential psychotherapy has been used to address questions of meaning in older prisoners to prevent suicide, and there is a relationship to the existential philosophies. (For example, we mentioned Camus' elucidation of the causes of suicide in Chapter 5.) These therapies suit older patients who are facing "purpose in life" issues.

Humanistic and existential therapies penetrate at a deeper level to issues related to substance use disorders, often serving as a catalyst for seeking alternatives to substances to fill the void the client is experiencing. The counselor's empathy and acceptance, as well as the insight gained by the client, contribute to the client's recovery by providing opportunities for her to make new existential choices, beginning with an informed decision to use or abstain from substances (Substance Abuse and Mental Health Services Administration 2012, p. 106).

Early on, we introduced the concept of psychological defenses and described how they can promote and maintain criminal ways of thinking. Such defenses, as TIP 34 points out, are fundamental in substance users, particularly denial and grandiosity. One of our favorite quotes is from the newly admitted substance user who declares during his assessment that "I don't need drug abuse treatment because I know now that I'll never use drugs again." Particularly with this group of clients, handling defenses can degenerate into an adversarial interaction, laden with accusations; for example, when a therapist admonishes the client by saying, "You are in denial" (Substance Abuse and Mental Health Services Administration 2012). We think that the problem with such declarations of one's future actions is the difficulty people have in their personal *affective forecasting*, or the ability (or inability) to predict one's behavior brought about by one's emotions. This is a much-discussed concept that affects health care decision-making (Ellis et al. 2018), but it does not seem to be well studied in the substance use field. However, we use it as a talking point when starting work with those substance users who declare, "That's the last time. I've had enough." Of course, we also discuss the concepts of social cues and setting in causing relapse, although we probably do not tell them the depressing statistic that "[m]ore than 85% of people with addictions who stop using a drug begin using it again within a year" (National Institute on Drug Abuse 2019).

A more neutral approach is to *ask the patient* to tell you the pros and cons of addressing his 1) mental illness, 2) substance use, and 3) criminality *now* (Stephens 2011). Other therapeutic strategies to avoid adversarial interactions include the following (Substance Abuse and Mental Health Services Administration 2012):

- Working with the client's perceptions of reality rather than arguing
- Asking questions
- Sidestepping rather than confronting defenses
- Demonstrating the denial defense while interacting with the client to show her how it works

There are many common components in substance use counseling with other therapeutic modalities. Two that come to mind are social skills training and assertiveness training. These can be useful for substance users, for persons with mental illness, and even for prisoners who have neither of those problems. These components are best taught through workbooks and homework assignments, but they can certainly be taught in individual sessions, not just in groups. You will need additional resources for these, but examples are given in TIP 34 and include a brief educational workbook for alcohol abusers.

Many therapists feel more comfortable tailoring their interventions to the stages of change that were elucidated almost 40 years ago by Prochaska and DiClemente (1984):

- Precontemplation
- Contemplation
- Preparation
- Action
- Maintenance

This is the approach taken in a separate TIP, No. 35 (Substance Abuse and Mental Health Services Administration 2019). Keep in mind that MI is effective, but no more so than many of the other therapies we have discussed along the way. According to the Recovery Research Institute (2020), a nonprofit institute of Massachusetts General Hospital, "Compared to no intervention, or a non-therapy-based intervention (e.g., assessment only or waitlist control), Motivational Interviewing and Motivational Enhancement Therapy have strong empirical support, though they do not do any better than other kinds of interventions." Our concerns with MI were expressed in Chapter 2, including that it is less directive than supportive psychotherapy because of its stated and underlying belief that people know best what to decide with minimal direction. We also think this is the weakness of nondirective humanistic or Rogerian psychotherapy. However, there is a wealth of information and a lot to be learned about conducting psychotherapy from TIP 35. Here is an example of some supportive and motivational techniques, which, as is often the case, seems like "found money" supplied by the patient.

Case Vignette

Mr. Roberts is a 25-year-old single man who is in his fourth month of prison for a drug deal. When he first came into the prison, he was taking a sedating antidepressant prescribed by his jail psychiatrist. However, he asks the prison psychiatrist to change the medicine to something else "because my girlfriend looked it up and she says it can raise my cholesterol." The psychiatrist agrees but notes that the baseline cholesterol is normal. However, each month Mr. Roberts comes back and asks for more medicine. Finally, he asks to go back on his sedating antidepressant despite the cholesterol risk.

The following week, Mr. Roberts meets with his therapist and complains of having protracted heroin withdrawal symptoms that he describes as periodic vomiting, nausea, and sweating, accompanied by intense craving. He asks the therapist to get him Seroquel (brand name for quetiapine), a well-known antipsychotic/mood stabilizer that is known for its abuse in prisons. The therapist explains that she doesn't prescribe medicine and asks why the patient didn't ask the psychiatrist about it. The patient says "I didn't think he would believe me, so I saved this up for you. Why don't you ask him?" The therapist asks about the connection between the reported withdrawal symptoms and the request for Seroquel. Mr. Roberts says, "I need to feel high again. I have been using heroin since I was 13, and there is no reason why I would want to stop."

The therapist praises Mr. Roberts for his honesty but suggests that he does not need an antipsychotic, and certainly not one for the purpose of being abused. Mr. Roberts is irritated and boasts, "Then I will get some Thorazine [another brand name for a sedating antipsychotic] from somebody else." The therapist says, "I'm sure you could, and that would have a whole bunch of risks and side effects by itself. But what I find strange is that the person telling me this is the same person who stopped his old medicine because he was worried about increasing his cholesterol! Isn't there a kind of disconnect between worrying about your future health at the age of 25 and not caring if you take something which will ruin—hmm, let me think—I can think of four things—your future health, your current life, your sobriety, and your trusting relationship with your girlfriend?"

Mr. Roberts agrees that there is a discrepancy, and the therapist works on finding ways to motivate him to find another way to deal with his protracted withdrawal syndrome. She points out, using what we called the "induced dichotomy of personality" in Chapter 2, that "it seems like a part of you really wants to tell me the truth even though the other part wants to continue to lie to me." Mr. Roberts agrees that there could be a part of him that wants to be truthful and that it opposes the part of him that wants to get high. Mr. Roberts admits that he might be "exaggerating" his withdrawal, but "it really is bad." The therapist develops a plan for anxiety management and has him meet with his group counselor. She agrees to inform the psychiatrist about the anxiety problem and see if there is some nonsedating medicine that Mr. Roberts can take in the morning to manage his anxiety during the day. Finally, she explores Mr. Roberts' relationship with his girlfriend as a motivating factor for staying clean and sober.

But wait, there's more. In this institution, where there is interdisciplinary cooperation, the therapist calls the psychiatrist after the session. The psychiatrist is concerned that one of his patients could be selling Thorazine and calls the nursing staff to pay special attention to the two Thorazine-using patients that night. The nurse catches one of them "cheeking" his medicine. The cell is tossed, and custody finds six pills under the mattress. The psychiatrist calls in the patient and confronts him. The patient is inclined to lie about the hoarded pills and claim that he was "set up" by someone else, thus proving some variety of the adage "I may have schizophrenia but that doesn't mean I can't be antisocial as well." However, the patient eventually confesses that he likes to save a few extra pills so he can go to sleep when he wakes up late at night. The psychiatrist says he sympathizes with the need, but breaking the rules is dangerous and the pills will have to be crushed and floated. The psychiatrist refers the patient back to the therapist for sleep hygiene management so he can learn to relax and go to sleep naturally without pills. Meanwhile, the therapist makes arrangements to get Mr. Roberts into a methadone clinic when he is released.

As the vignette illustrates, it helps to have the various disciplines talk to one another. It also shows how motivational techniques (along with our usual supportive work) are useful in the early stages of precontemplation and contemplation of giving up substances. In the (mostly) forced abstinence environment of prison, however, the therapy that comes to mind immediately is that of relapse prevention. Such therapies were developed by Marlatt and others (Marlatt and Gordon 1985; Parks and Marlatt 1999) and are especially suited to the maintenance phase of addiction treatment. Treatment in prison is designed to help prevent relapse in the high-risk situations that will occur after release, such as when individuals are dealing with negative emotional states, interpersonal conflict, and social pressure. According to Parks and Marlatt (2011), relapse prevention therapy teaches patients to:

- Understand the process of relapse.
- Identify and cope effectively with high-risk situations.
- Cope with urges and craving.
- Minimize the damage from a relapse.
- Stay engaged in treatment after a relapse.
- Create a more balanced lifestyle.

Numerous resources for relapse prevention therapy, including patient workbooks, are available. SAMHSA's Knowledge Application Program (KAP), which produces the SAMHSA TIPs, also produces, without a hint of humor, TAPs, including TAP-19, *Counselor's Manual for Relapse Prevention With Chemically Dependent Criminal Offenders* (Substance Abuse and Mental Health Services Administration 1996). While SAMHSA has labeled this document out-of-date, it is still quite useful, since it includes a complete workbook for patients from which you can pick and choose your handouts even if the entire program has been superseded by newer ones. The comprehensive, modular group program of Wanberg and Milkman (2008) has a module on relapse and recidivism and covers just about everything else including working with criminal thinking and lifestyle development.

There is both art and science to making substance use interventions effective. Interventions are best based on the assessments that measure readiness to change. You also need to be reasonable in what you think you can accomplish. Perhaps Mr. Roberts' therapist lessens his chances of relapse through his therapy in combination with his group work, but keep in mind that the lessons from implementation of the risk-need-responsivity (RNR) model indicate that effective programs require many hours of contact. One of our colleagues, a licensed substance abuse counselor, ran a program in a medium security prison that ran 3 hours a day for 6 months. After working in a community facility, she found it a "breath of fresh air" (except for the spreading coronavirus!) to work with institutionally abstinent clients who could benefit from interventions and not relapse between sessions. There is admittedly an actual disadvantage of working with prisoners—namely, that it can be difficult to know if your interventions are really going to work when they get out. You can only hope that Mr. Roberts will not become a Saturday night heroin overdose victim when he gets out. However, there are assessment instruments that assist counselors in knowing whether interventions have "taken," and it is usually a pleasure to work with abstinent drug users, most of whom feel better, although some do continue to crave for months or even years.[2] Also it is gratifying, through the work that you do in building a supportive relationship and therapeutic alliance, of watching a hostile, resentful, angry, and avoidant patient begin to profit from his therapy and become thankful for the work that you do. (Now, now, don't even imagine that you are really being groomed for some favor!)

Co-occurring Disorders

To avoid confusion or stigmatization, the preferred term for having both substance use and mental disorder is *co-occurring disorders*, or COD.

More than 20 years ago, a foundational article elucidated some principles for combined substance abuse and mental illness treatment. Principles based on that article and addressing incarcerated persons specifically were formulated and included (Drake et al. 1998):

- One program for both conditions.
- Treatment by the same clinicians.
- Clinicians who have appropriate training, including training in assessment and knowledge of psychopathology.
- Treatment that differs from traditional substance abuse treatment because it is tailored for persons with mental illness who have substance abuse.
- Focus on preventing increased anxiety rather than breaking through denial.
- An emphasis on trust, understanding, and learning rather than confrontation, criticism, and expression.
- In some programs: Addressing substance use reduction or harm reduction (controversial even today).

---

[2]The neurobiology of such prolonged states continues to be studied, and we noted with perhaps some amusement that one researcher proposed another Greek word, *hyperkatifeia*, for the state of protracted abstinence and "negative urgency" leading to impulsive actions and relapse exacerbated by stress from the COVID-19 pandemic (Koob et al. 2020).

- A slower pace and longer-term perspective rather than rapid withdrawal (already done if in prison) and short-term treatment.
- Use of stagewise and motivational counseling rather than confrontation or front-loaded treatment
- Increased availability of supportive clinicians rather than just in office hours.
- Availability of 12-step groups.
- Availability of medication (pretty much noncontroversial now).
- A combination of services that includes groups, individual counseling, psychosocial rehabilitation, medication, housing, case management, family psychoeducation.
- Recognition of medical comorbidity (at that time HIV and more recently hepatitis C) in COD patients.

The above principles remain essentially true today, but there is extensive additional guidance available, starting with SAMHSA TIP 42 and related publications (see Substance Abuse and Mental Health Services Administration 2020). What is new in the last 20 years is probably the emphasis of the recovery model, as in the following guiding principles in treating patients with COD (Substance Abuse and Mental Health Services Administration 2020, p. 14):

1. Employ a recovery perspective.
2. Adopt a multiproblem viewpoint.
3. Develop a phased approach to treatment.
4. Address specific real-life problems early in treatment.
5. Plan for the client's cognitive and functional impairments.
6. Use support systems to maintain and extend treatment effectiveness.

SAMHSA urges clinicians to have "empathic detachment" for patients with CODs (Substance Abuse and Mental Health Services Administration 2020, p. 40):

- Acknowledge that the provider and client are working together to make decisions to support the client's best interests.
- Recognize that the provider cannot transform the client into a different person but can only support change that he or she is already making.
- Maintain an empathic connection even if the client does not seem to fit into the provider's expectations, treatment categories, or preferred methods of working.

SAMHSA recognizes that "[a] supportive and empathic counseling style is one of the keys to establishing an effective therapeutic alliance with clients who have CODs" (Substance Abuse and Mental Health Services Administration 2020, p. 151).

SAMHSA promulgates the following guidelines for developing successful therapeutic relationships with patients with COD (Substance Abuse and Mental Health Services Administration 2020, p. 142):

1. Develop and use a therapeutic alliance to engage clients in treatment.
2. Maintain a recovery perspective.
3. Ensure continuity of care.

4. Address common clinical challenges (e.g., countertransference, confidentiality).
5. Monitor psychiatric symptoms (including symptoms of self-harm).
6. Use supportive and empathic counseling; adopt a multiproblem viewpoint.
7. Use culturally responsive methods.
8. Use motivational enhancement.
9. Teach relapse prevention techniques.
10. Use repetition and skill building to address deficits in functioning.

These are fairly straightforward, but we restate them because of the emphasis on supportive methods. For more program details incorporating Drake's work and including a variety of handouts, see the guide by Mueser et al. (2003).

Although it is clear now that mental illness and substance use disorder are "both primary" as far as treatment goes, we did find some interesting distinctions between the ways patients with these disorders present and the approaches needed:

- Chronically mentally ill substance abusers who are using drugs to get high or for what they think are self-medicating reasons need to have the adverse consequences and self-destructive nature of the drug use demonstrated in a nonconfrontational manner.
- Similarly, substance users are relatively unaware of the ways in which substances cause or worsen psychopathology (e.g., cocaine causing paranoia) and need to understand the connection.
- Other substance users may have to develop a degree of trust in order to face their maladaptive and rejecting style of personality (McDuff and Muneses 1998).

Addressing Men's Issues

The majority of packaged or manualized programs for substance use disorders are designed for men or attempt to cover issues in a manner that is not gender-biased. In addition to the many resources from SAMHSA, there is a great amount of material from nongovernment agencies and private sources. This includes a recovery workbook for group or individual work by Daley (2011) that addresses issues of denial and obstacles to relapse and presents a lifestyle improvement program and help in managing emotions, including positive emotions as are found in those relating to the field of positive psychology. These are issues that appear to resonate most strongly in men. There are multiple manuals for women by Stephanie S. Covington and associates (e.g., Covington 2019). However, those authors also have one for men (Covington et al. 2011) that is (we think) strengths based—the approach that is often favored for women but applicable to all. It can be used in groups or one-on-one with a counselor. It does *not* try to motivate men to stop using or give them relapse-prevention strategies. Rather it builds strengths in the four areas those authors believe are the triggers for relapse and of the greatest change in recovery: self, relationships, sexuality, and spirituality. As we'll see in Chapter 12, men have particular issues in recognizing and expressing feelings, and Covington and associates' manual has a chapter that recognizes that communicating feelings may be difficult for men. So it is a good adjunct to substance use treatment programs based on other methods (e.g., MI).

Gender Bias and Stereotyping

SAMHSA has identified several issues that arise in the therapy of men with men and women with men. These are presented in Table 7–3. Therapists can address these in various ways. Male therapists need to recognize that they can go into "competition" mode with a male patient, but that can oscillate into a "homophobic" mode if they experience any attraction. Such attractions can be discussed in supervision, but the male therapist may be reluctant to do so. In their own experience, female therapists may expect to be belittled or demeaned by male patients; their strongest feelings are likely to be fear and unresolved anger (Substance Abuse and Mental Health Services Administration 2013b, p. 35). They may tend to defer to male authority or develop emotional or sexual feelings. (The mirror image of this, deference to a woman's authority and sexualization of the countertransference, is of course a risk when men are therapists for women.)

The Other Comorbidity

We have talked about the co-occurrence of substance use and mental illness in prisoners. However, consider the co-occurrence or comorbidity of substance use disorder and criminal conduct. Both involve behavior. Although there are some people whose behavior is not treatable or whose criminal behavior was a one-and-done, the sheer number of people in prison with both criminal conduct and substance abuse warrants attention. We have written about some of the programs that address criminogenic thinking and criminal lifestyles, and there are some comprehensive programs that simultaneously address both criminality and substance use, such as the one we mentioned above of Wanberg and Milkman (2008). Although the general format of the treatments is for groups, there is much material that can be used in individual work.

Walters (1998) addresses several recommendations to help people change their lifestyles that combine criminality and substance use. In Chapter 4, we recommended his use of a crisis as a catalyst for change. He also has a lifestyle change program for persons with substance use. It is not manualized but a brief and straightforward set of recommendations for interventions and changes, such as the following (Walters 1998):

1. Utilize the "shaman effect" (Walters' emphasis on the therapeutic alliance as a source of prosocial modeling, especially for young offenders).
2. Reduce access to substances through changing the environment.
3. Help substance users to regulate affects, such as depression and anger, which trigger relapses.
4. Through cognitive reframing, help substance users change attitudes toward lapses and relapses.
5. Help substance users to manage their fears and redefine their values. (Walters has assessment instruments for both.)
6. Expand their options, such as in the areas of education and employment.
7. Foster involvement and commitment in a nondrug/noncriminal lifestyle.

Speaking of the first item above, research has shown for years that positive outcome in treatment is associated with longer retention ("more is better") and client-perceived

TABLE 7–3.	Addressing gender bias and stereotyping when working with men

Female counselors

Explore your own gender biases and refrain from stereotyping men.

Be curious and transparent. Make no assumptions about a client's lived experience based on gender.

Don't be afraid to challenge male clients' psychological defenses and behavior in a nonjudgmental, nonshaming way.

Take the client's preference for the gender of his counselor into consideration and match client and counselor when possible.

Raise the issue of gender in the assessment phase and as a therapeutic issue.

Explore your own countertransference issues in clinical supervision.

Male counselors

Explore your own gender biases and refrain from stereotyping men.

Be curious and transparent. Make no assumptions about a client's lived experience based on gender.

Don't be afraid to be supportive and help male clients touch upon emotional content.

Take the client's preference for the gender of the counselor into consideration and match client and counselor when possible.

Raise the issue of gender in the assessment phase and as a therapeutic issue.

Explore your own countertransference issues in clinical supervision.

Source. Substance Abuse and Mental Health Services Administration 2013b, p. 33.

empathy is a variable associated with frequent attendance and favorable outcomes (Fiorentine et al. 2002). Also recall our last mention of the "shaman" in discussing Jerome Frank's paradigm of psychotherapy in Chapter 4. And finally, we will invoke another one of our science fiction analogies comparing psychologists with wizards: Psychologists are said to have the ability to change what was previously an art into an actual science by elucidating laws of human behavior and understanding the otherwise insubstantial structures of the mind. Although they are scientists, these psychologists might appear to others as if they are wizards casting spells using words, observations, and even silence. Thus, it is that these psychologists can remove the internal sicknesses of their patients and attune their patients to external reality (White 1987, pp. 82–83). Now, doesn't this describe what a psychotherapist does? The power and effects of the healing relationship in psychotherapy have been much researched and are known to be a factor in the response of patients to psychotherapy.

Since group work is a mainstay of treatment for those with co-occurring substance use and mental illness, some additional guidelines are needed for individual therapists working with patients who are also in groups (possibly run by the same therapist) (Hendrickson et al. 2004). Like group therapy, individual therapy can:

- Educate the patient about addiction.
- Give specific information about drugs.
- Discuss craving and advocate for abstinence (but see our discussion of harm reduction later in this chapter).
- Stress accountability for individual choices.
- Identify triggers to relapse.

- Strengthen self-esteem.
- Show how patterns of self-destructive behavior may have originated in survival behaviors from childhood.

As in most individual therapy sessions (although cognitive therapists may not wish to talk about childhood history), the purpose is (as noted above) to support self-esteem but also, as appropriate to each issue, point out psychological defenses such as denial that enable continuation of self-destructive drug-using behavior. However, it is important not to allow the group and individual processes to work at cross-purposes. Recommendations, made by Hendrickson et al. (2004, p.131), include:

- Don't allow the individual sessions to compromise the group process (e.g., with a patient who does not speak in group but talks one-on-one).
- It may help to portray the group process as requiring a "higher" level of skill than working with you individually.
- Don't let patients skip the group while continuing to have one-on-one substance use counseling with you.
- Don't split by siding with the patient against the group.
- When you talk about issues in individual therapy, explain how they could be brought up in the group.

It would also be a stretch of terminology, but not a particularly new revelation, that therapeutic interventions often need to address the existing "trimorbidity" or "tri-occurring" disorders of substance use, mental illness, and criminal conduct. One of our authors calls attention to what *we* would call the "fearful synergy" of criminal thinking and substance-user thinking. Being criminal means being suspicious of other people—and, in prison settings, having downright paranoia—and this only worsens the denials and suspiciousness of being a substance user and mentally ill (Stephens 2011, p. 237).

Finally, it is evident that many people writing on the subject think that much of drug use is a victimless crime, even including the selling of smaller quantities of drugs. The possession of marijuana has been decriminalized in many states. In November 2020, Oregon became the first state to decriminalize possession of small quantities of all street drugs ("Oregon Decriminalizes Possession of Street Drugs" 2020). Your opinions on this may affect the way you do drug counseling. It is pointed out that Portugal decriminalized much of drug use in 2001, and the consequences have been fairly benign compared with the predictions (Ingraham 2015).

Case Vignette

Jonathan is a 41-year-old man who was returned to the county jail on a probation violation for a positive drug screen. He has been in and out of prison for nonviolent property offenses partly related to his poor job history and payment for drugs. He is angry with the system and with himself for his relapse. He had obtained his GED in prison and completed 2 years of college. He was raised in group homes and foster care. His three brothers have substance use disorders of stimulants and opioids. Both parents had severe alcohol use disorder. There is no history of suicide attempts. He has had previous diagnoses of ADHD, SUD (stimulants), and intermittent explosive disorder. His first stimulant use was at the age of 15. His last use was at the time of his arrest. He had relapsed after 2 years clean. He reported he was "just dumb and got messed up." He denies depression, anxiety, and mood swings. His projected release date is in 3 months. His plans are to return to working in landscaping with his uncle's business and to live with his girlfriend.

This vignette describes a person who has issues with criminal behavior and a substance use disorder without significant mental illness. Jonathan has some insight into this as well. Jonathan's therapist assured him he was not "dumb" but that he had just made some unwise choices. She addressed the anger issues with him and suggested anger management classes. He became irate with that suggestion and stated, "I have done those classes, and they don't work." The anger management classes were addressed again in the second session, and Jonathan agreed to attend. Later in therapy, he admitted that when he attended the classes the first time he did so "just to look good when I went in front of the Parole Board. I really did not pay too much attention in the classes to be honest."

There is a need for ongoing patient education to manage the long-term treatment of substance abuse. The education materials may be formal and/or informal and include verbal and written materials (Laffan 2013). Over the next several sessions the therapist provided Jonathan with information on the self-help groups available in the community and provided him with handouts and a list of reading materials he could obtain from the jail and county libraries. Jonathan attended several 12-step meetings before he was released to a halfway house and was enrolled into the drug court program. He verbalized a desire to stay away from drugs and to avoid being involved in illegal activity.

Women and Substance Use

For some time it has been known that needs of women who abuse substances are different from those of men. For example, women may get involved with substances to deal with feelings created by early trauma in their lives. As a result, programs for substance abuse need to be different because, as Baletka and Shearer (2005) note:

- Vocational training is more effective with women.
- Women have a high need for family therapy and higher motivation with low resistance to parenting skills training.
- Women have a greater need for treatment of PTSD versus personality disorders in men.
- Confrontational techniques and anger management are more threatening and hence less effective with women than for men. This is because these techniques are less effective in addressing the reasons women become addicted, such as physical and sexual abuse, low self-esteem, and desire to please others.
- Group therapy is of very limited effectiveness for women but is moderately effective for men. (We don't agree entirely with this assertion.)
- Empowerment training is highly effective for women but of limited need for men.

Baletka and Shearer (2005) did a survey of an assessment instrument called FOCI (the Female Offender Critical Interventions Inventory), which can be used to help programs to determine if they are meeting the needs of their clients. The list of topics surveyed is a good indication of what a therapist might want to cover in treatment:

dependency problems, AIDS awareness, lifestyle alternatives to drug abuse and addiction, alcohol dependency and recovery from alcohol and substance use, violence in relationships, childhood physical and sexual abuse, stress and temptation, emotional abuse of the patient and those around her, sexual abuse, self-esteem, available treatment programs, and skills. Society is still more demeaning of women who use drugs or alcohol. Women also have the anger and shame of losing custody of their children as a result of substance use disorder. Turning once more for advice from SAMHSA, there is the usual wealth of material available, including a summary of skills which they think substance use counselors should possess (see Table 7–4).

Substance Use and Suicidality

Substance users have an increased risk of suicide, but the programmatic responses must differ for substance users in the community versus those in prison. For example, research shows that persons with opioid use disorders are at a higher risk of suicide. SAMHSA TIP 50 (Substance Abuse and Mental Health Services Administration 2015) addresses clinician and program administrator responses to the problems but is not specific to correctional environments. The "good news" for those of use in the residential correctional setting is that there are much higher risks of suicide for acutely intoxicated persons and persons with transient substance-induced depression. In addition, there is the lesser availability of suicidal methods for overdose or weapons-related suicide.

One more acronym is introduced: GATE, a four-step process (Gather information, Access supervision, Take responsible action, Extend the action) for addressing suicidal thoughts and behaviors in substance use disorder treatment. Of interest, and perhaps not entirely intuitive, is that persons in substance abuse *treatment* are at higher risk for suicide for a number of hypothesized reasons:

- They enter treatment when their substance use is out of control.
- They enter treatment at the time of a concurrent life crisis. (In the case of our patients, this would be the crisis of the incarceration and the life crises associated with it.)
- They enter treatment at the peak of their depressive symptoms.
- They have concurrent mental health problems (CODs).
- Crises occur during the substance use treatment itself.

By now you should be familiar with the following from previous discussions:

- Static or historical risk factors for suicide such as age, gender, race, or ethnicity
- Dynamic or changeable risk factors specific to the correctional setting, which include legal setback, health problems, changes in marital situation or child custody, rejection from or termination from a treatment program, interpersonal criticism as simple as a problem with a cellmate or correctional officer, and (of obvious importance) a "rupture" in the therapeutic relationship

When assessing suicidality, counselors are advised to maintain an empathic stance and to avoid extremes such as becoming a "suicide interrogator" or the opposite of being afraid to discuss sensitive topics because it upsets the patient (Substance Abuse and Mental Health Services Administration 2015, p. 5).

TABLE 7–4.	Competencies for counseling women with substance use disorders

Goals

To maintain a nonjudgmental, supportive, and respectful manner

To understand the diverse experience of women from different cultural groups, abilities, sexual orientations, and gender identities (e.g., be aware of attitudes toward race, sex, and disability)

To be committed to women's issues

To uphold a sense of hope

To demonstrate unconditional acceptance of and positive regard for the client

Skills

To engage women with empathy, warmth, and sincerity

To develop a treatment alliance with female clients that is mutual and collaborative, individualized, and continually negotiated

To have clear professional boundaries (neither distant nor abandoning) and maintain confidentiality

To remain consistent in caring and availability and possess the ability to set limits in a calm and supportive manner

To conduct assessments that are thorough and trauma-informed

To develop individually focused and outcome-oriented treatment plans

To work with multidisciplinary teams

To perform crisis intervention

To apply trauma coping skills

To tolerate one's own distress in hearing trauma information

To deliver client-led treatment (e.g., help the client learn how to manage her distress without shutting down or becoming overwhelmed—a central focus of treatment)

To maintain and ensure self-care

To support clients' cultural and racial identities and sexual orientations

To ask for and participate in supervision, in part to explore personal biases in ongoing processes, and to be invested in ongoing training

To be a visible advocate for women who use/abuse substances for stigma reduction and for treatment (within treatment teams, the community, and the system)

To be an appropriate role model for women, including on the topic of parenting

To develop professional, respectful, mutually supportive, and collaborative relationships with coworkers

Knowledge

To be culturally informed and knowledgeable

To be trauma-informed, including awareness of the prevalence and impact of trauma on women's lives

To understand the psychological growth and development of women

To recognize the centrality of relationships for women, particularly parenting and social roles and the socialization process

To be knowledgeable about the physiology of women as it relates to substance use and abuse

To understand the etiology of substance abuse in women

To be familiar with the co-occurring disorders that commonly occur in women

To understand the context of abuse and patterns of use for women

TABLE 7–4.	Competencies for counseling women with substance use disorders *(continued)*

Knowledge *(continued)*

To identify the consequences of substance abuse (e.g., legal, general health, infectious diseases, family and relationships, psychological)

To understand the treatment and recovery experience of women

To identify family dynamics (e.g., family of origin, parenting, child development)

To be familiar with a woman's process of recovery

To be knowledgeable about relapse prevention for women; relapse triggers such as family reunification; recovery resources; maintaining a safe place for the client; and loss, grief, and mourning

To understand issues related to sexuality, sexual orientation, and gender identity for women and their relationship to substance abuse

To know confidentiality rules and guidelines

Source. Substance Abuse and Mental Health Services Administration 2013a, pp. 191–192.

Assessment of Substance Use

Despite the expertise required to understand and treat substance use disorders, it is now (but it wasn't always) apparent that substance users are understandable because their behavior follows the same laws of human behavior that other people follow. This was the point of a foundational article a few years ago by Miller (the originator of MI) and Brown (another distinguished researcher) (Miller and Brown 1997). Assessment should, if possible, employ instruments that include the nature and extent of alcohol and drug use as well as the consequences of that use. A popular instrument is the Addiction Severity Index, which was developed in a U.S. Government project and is in the public domain. So is one of our favorites, the Drinker Inventory of Consequences, which was developed as part of the famous MATCH project, which investigated how to match clients to one of three therapies: cognitive-behavioral coping skills, motivational enhancement theory, or 12-step facilitation therapy. The latter was meant to encourage working the "acceptance" steps 1–5 of a 12-step program but did not include AA attendance. The study concluded that matching was not necessary for positive outcomes. The manuals for the entire project, as well as newer materials, are readily available (National Institute on Alcohol Abuse and Alcoholism 2020).

Of course, the therapy that comes to mind when working with the "pure" substance users is motivational interviewing, which is related to the motivational enhancement therapy used in Project Match. Motivational enhancement therapy differs in some particulars such as by using patient feedback sessions. It should be pointed out that MI was developed at a time when substance abuse treatments were highly confrontational.

You should certainly familiarize yourself with MI techniques—and some say that MI is an attitude and not just a set of techniques—but the same could be said of supportive psychotherapy. MI developed as an outgrowth of the patient-centered (but also known as nondirective) psychotherapy of Carl Rogers. The term "patient-centered" seems to have survived, but the appellation of "nondirective" seems to have been forgotten by historians (and many remaining practitioners) of this type of therapy. In retrospect, Rogerian therapy strikes us as a form of "waiting for the patient to change," whereas MI strikes us as "reinforcing the patient's realization that he needs to change." Supportive psychotherapy is more along the lines of "Coming down on one side of the patient's ambivalence to change" or "supporting, encouraging, and directing the change needed by patients." In other words, we think that supportive psychotherapy is further along the spectrum of directive therapies, and we believe it needs to be so to work effectively with prisoners.

However, patients who are prisoners are (except for some alcoholics) rarely substance users "in pure culture." So methods are needed to deal with criminal activity and the psychological defenses that accompany it. MI is good at getting people to stop using drugs, but jail and prison settings are full of people who have already (for the most part) stopped, if temporarily.

Assessment of substance use should also include the relationship of substance use to suicide attempts and criminal behavior (more about this later). The relationship may be none, incidental, strongly connected, and unidirectional or multidirectional. The connection between substance use and crime is of course of great interest, and one foundational article (Goldstein 1985) described it as being of three types:

- Economic-compulsive—the crime is committed to pay for the drugs
- Psychopharmacological—the drugs change behaviors that become criminal
- Systemic—the drug user is a drug distributor

This division is fairly broad, and the actual connections have a lot of exceptions. For example, crack cocaine was used by dealers to impair women's decision-making and entice them into prostitution. Or drugs are often purchased as part of the proceeds of crime. Or drugs are used to get the "courage to offend." Later researchers recommended renaming the third category "lifestyle factors" (Bennett and Holloway 2009). But in any case, your individualized understanding of the relation of these three categories will help you to personalize your psychotherapy interventions.

"I'm Not Like the Others Here"

This is a common lament of persons with alcohol use disorder ranging from mild to severe who are in prison for alcohol-related DUI charges or other alcohol-related behaviors, typically assaults occurring while intoxicated. There is indeed truth in that lament. Most of them (unless there is something else in their history) are not career criminals, and their criminal charges are due to alcohol-related impairments, although (as usual) their decisions to drink are made while relatively sober. By the way, there are many other people in prison who are not like the others—people with singular crimes who are not criminals or substance abusers either, just people who have gone wrong.

Persons with severe alcohol use disorders do have special issues in therapy. One issue that arises both in prison and in outpatient settings is the relationship of individual therapy to the group program. Both can teach:

- Progressive muscle relaxation (We have avoided putting in a specific protocol for this, however, because many of our patients have chronic pain and back problems and may need medical clearance or appropriate warnings.)
- Stress reduction

- Guided imagery
- Self-assertion
- Substance refusal skills
- Systematic desensitization (for social anxiety or specific phobias)
- Problem-solving
- Prosocial modeling with role-playing
- Behavioral self-control

This last item certainly overlaps with the goals of individual psychotherapy for substance users. The individual psychotherapy of substance users assists in teaching emotional management by managing emotions while sober and developing a repertoire of behaviors to avoid relapse when they get out. A crisis response safety plan (see below) can be used to list their triggers for using and their coping behaviors to prevent relapse.

Peer support groups such as Alcoholics Anonymous work in prisons and jails and in the community, and for many prisoners, especially upon release, such programs may be attended more often than the programs of community agencies, as many released prisoners fail to follow up on their outpatient referrals. In addition, it should be mentioned that there are formulations of AA Steps and creeds that are gender-neutral or do not require a spiritual higher power. Consider the 12 Steps of AA and 12 Promises of AA, which are widely reprinted (e.g., Alcoholics Anonymous 2020; Wikipedia 2020). There are other programs, several of which hold groups, although not all (e.g., Rational Recovery) do. The community, and if fortunate the facility, may have in-person groups, and there are online groups for SMART (SMART Recovery 2020) or Women for Sobriety (https://womenforsobriety.org). The latter has a series of acceptance statements that cover similar ground as the AA Promises. For example, Acceptance Statement #9 says, "No longer am I victimized by the past. I am a new woman" (SMART Recovery 2020), and is similar to AA Promise #2, which says, "We will not regret the past nor wish to shut the door on it." For descriptions of these programs and some correlations, see the book by Lewis et al. (2015). The 12-Step facilitation (TSF) therapy manual of Project MATCH may also be of interest but is mostly applicable to alcoholics who are currently drinking.

What is interesting, such as in the 12 Promises (which were an initially unnumbered exposition of the ninth step) but basically in the statements of most peer support groups, is that they frequently correspond to familiar tasks of psychotherapy. To explain this, we turn to an account of integrative psychotherapy for alcohol abuse (Knack 2009). Knack (2009) states that psychotherapy and AA both share the premises of psychotherapy proposed by Jerome Frank that we recounted in Chapter 4, briefly:

- A structured, "trusting, confiding, emotional" relationship that boosts the patient's morale
- A treatment setting with an aura of safety and sanctuary
- A conceptual scheme or explanatory model providing a rationale for treatment and relief
- Therapeutic procedures consistent with the conceptual scheme that relieve the patient's anxiety and encourage new behaviors

Of course, these assumptions would probably also apply to the other peer support groups we have mentioned, as there is no requirement for a spiritual higher power. AA offers all these components of successful psychotherapy even though it does not refer to psychotherapy as one of its methods. It proposes personality change, which is also a goal of long-term psychotherapies. The first four promises offer a new freedom, happiness, serenity, and peace, allowing a way to move forward from the past. The second promise offers the seemingly impossible outcome of neither regretting the past nor forgetting it. The seventh promise is to remove the feeling of uselessness and self-pity, and other promises point to a life of selflessness and giving to others. The eleventh promise talks about developing intuitive social skills, and so forth. The promises might appear grandiose but are a source of inspiration and aspiration to millions of AA members. In keeping with the four premises of Jerome Frank's paradigm, Knack describes psychotherapy as:

1. Establishing, consolidating, and maintaining a sense of self.
2. Establishing a sense of relatedness to others.
3. Improving self-care and ameliorating self-soothing deficits.
4. Building affect tolerance and managing affect and behavior.
5. Moderating the narcissistic grandiosity common in alcoholics.

To comment: AA teaches its members to be "right sized," which means being neither self-deprecating nor self-aggrandizing (Knack 2009, p. 99). And in our own work with patients with personality disorders, we have recognized that inability to self-soothe (without substances) is a feature of their personalities.

The advantage, of course, of working with alcohol and other substance users in prison is that they are usually abstinent. From the standpoint of stages of change, they are in an institutionally sustained maintenance even though their emotional state may be as undeveloped as in the case of the precontemplative person in the vignette we presented earlier. They are then working steps 6–12 of AA, making amends and reaching out to others and (in Step 10) continuing to look open-mindedly at their wrongs. Steps 9 and 12 are action steps to practice their new social skills and actuate their new personalities. Of course, as with Mr. Roberts in the vignette, your patient's heart might not be in the action steps, but the patient may be feeling instead a prolonged withdrawal craving that can last many months. During this time "[t]he therapist's role must remain rather supportive, parental and instructional" (Knack 2009, p. 103). We tell substance abusers that they may find themselves not depressed, but unable to feel any emotions for months after withdrawal because they have deadened their neurotransmitters. But since they are locked up with limited opportunities, what better time is there to get used to life without a substance and to work on their relapse prevention skills?

It is obvious that alcoholics have particular problems with shame and guilt. Potter-Efron (2002) has written a monograph on those emotions alone. He distinguishes shame from guilt as follows, although he admits that other therapists or patients may define them differently:

- *Shame* is something you feel about yourself and involves a lot of bodily sensations.
- *Guilt* is what you feel about what you have done to others and is less bodily than a recognition of culpability.

Potter-Ephron makes a good point that the goal of therapy is to turn an alcoholic's *trait shame or guilt* (the continuous feeling not linked to anything specific) into *state shame or guilt* (in response to the things they do or did).

We differ from Potter-Ephron in emphasizing many of the other emotions that afflict alcoholics and in addressing their denials and rationalizations of behavior—both of those being psychological defenses of the sort we have explained in earlier chapters. Alcoholics use alcohol not only to mask feelings of shame but also to disinhibit themselves in order to neglect the rights of others and injure them. Anger is a dominant emotion, inflamed by the disinhibition of alcohol use. You can, of course, ask patients how they feel. Do they feel ashamed, guilty, neither, or both? Also shame and guilt are linked to the low self-esteem typically found in alcoholics. In accordance with Potter-Ephron's advice, we would like them to feel better about themselves in general but not better about the individual acts they have done that have hurt people, thus melding with Step 10 by admitting their wrongs. We notice an advantage in working with the denials and rationalizations of alcoholics versus the denials and rationalizations of criminals. The former usually offer no excuse for the results of their drinking (e.g., the person they injured or killed with their automobile). The latter usually rationalize away the damage (e.g., "They deserved it" or "It wasn't permanent" or, basically, "My needs were more important than theirs").

Earlier, we noted that many prisoners, like Mr. Roberts, may be somewhat abstinent of necessity but still in the precontemplation state of change. However, useful work can be done both in group and individually to advance them through the stages so they catch up to the maintenance stage that has been forced upon them by incarceration.

A useful adjunct in relapse prevention teaching is to draw a matrix of positive and negative consequences of abstinence and using substances. Larimer et al. (1999) draw one with eight boxes to show the immediately and delayed consequences of using alcohol. Combining the early and late ones, we wrote a sample one for an alcoholic considering using again after he leaves jail or prison (see Table 7–5).

Other lessons for primary alcoholics (presumably who want to deal with eventual release) are:

- Remember that psychoeducation (about damage that can be caused by alcohol and other substances) may be less important than it used to be and can be done more efficiently in a group mode.
- Building upon the understanding of the dominance of denial and rationalization defenses, anticipate that their "drinking mind" will come up with these after they are faced with genuine temptation after relief. Arm them with counterarguments in advance.
- Recognize that relapse can occur over several finite steps that take time. Recognize the earlier steps (such as feeling overwhelmed paying a bill) and how to get help. A good analogy is to view the road to recovery as a highway with warning signs (Larimer et al. 1999).
- Teach "urge surfing," a technique similar to "riding the wave" for people with panic attacks, emphasizing that the urge does pass after a few minutes if one does not give in to it.
- Teach the new lifestyle, especially one that doesn't tangle with alcohol, such as going to a health club, swimming, working out with weights, or going on a wilder-

TABLE 7–5. **A decision-making matrix for an alcoholic returning to the community**

	Consequences	
	Positive	**Negative**
Remain abstinent	Save money Earn respect from friends and family Do better at work Go to school Live up to my promises to God and my family Get my 30-day chip Tell a success story at AA	Miss old friends Can't go to the bar Can't go to games Miss shopping for liquor Feel anxious Get depressed Find it hard to make friends
Drink alcohol	Feel good Feel less anxious in public Go to the old bar Be with drinking friends Go to football games with others Be less inhibited Give a stupid "drunkalog" in the AA meeting	Lose my job Get another DUI Violate parole Go to prison again Be unable to pay rent Get evicted Lose respect of family and friends End of marriage Loss of custody Health problems Die

Source. Modeled after Larimer et al. 1999.

ness hike without alcohol in the backpack; it may be too early to go bowling or to attend football games.

- Teach drink refusal skills.
- Teach or role-play scenarios of what alcoholics returning to the community will face the first few days out such as
  - Driving past the liquor store.
  - Finding the bottle of bourbon they had secreted in the basement.
  - Going to the neighbor's welcome home barbecue and being offered a beer (that's when their drink refusal skills are needed).
- Teach them to avoid the abstinence violation or "What the hell!" effect by which a single drink is so demoralizing that it turns into a binge. Teach them to label a single drink a slip and two drinks a slightly bigger slip, and so forth.
- Counsel them that they may not have to jettison their drinking friends but that they may need to see them in alcohol-prohibited situations.
- Teach healthy obsessions, which could simply include work. "Being a workaholic is better than being an alcoholic." (But protection needs to be made for leaving in the evening, facing their past demon-triggers of going past the bar or liquor store on the way home, using the drink as a reward for a hard day's work, and so forth.)
- Keep in mind that in the community, medications can be helpful in preventing relapse to alcohol and certain other substance uses. A few prisons are beginning to use medications as well.

SAMHSA recommends the use of a safety card consistent with the crisis response safety plan that we have described for suicide (see Chapter 5) and then for trauma-related crisis (Chapter 6) (Substance Abuse and Mental Health Services Administration 2015, p. 9). Since the jail or prison environment is relatively substance-free, the need for this plan may not be apparent until individuals are released. In Chapter 14, the various coping skills and personal professional resources can be added to what we describe as the *response safety plan* for persons being released combining all the issues (suicidality, traumatization, drugs, and criminal recidivism).

- Situations or triggers they expect to face as we have discussed above
- Coping skills—for example, stress reduction, relaxation, guided imagery, chanting mantra or reading the AA Promises, reading the support books and Big Book, fleeing the situation, drug and alcohol refusal skills and verbiage, "urge surfing," and looking up the next available AA meeting to attend
- People to contact, including sponsor, clinics, drug use hot-lines, local support groups, chat rooms, starting some e-mails
- Reasons for sobriety—including the benefits we showed in the matrix in Table 7–5

"The Three (Dangerous) Amigos": Understanding the Relationships and Therapies for Suicidality, Problematic Substance Use, and Criminal Behavior

Looking back on what we have discussed here and in the previous chapters of this book, we would like to highlight some similarities in both understanding and treating three behaviors: suicidal behavior, problematic substance use, and criminal behavior. After all, you are one person, and you have to assess and treat these three behaviors *along with* the conditions of crisis and mental illness that accompany them. We have encapsulated our thoughts about assessing and treating these conditions in Table 7–6. Three messages we would like to impart from that table are that:

- All three behaviors can be viewed as being on a spectrum from one-time, occasional, frequent, to continuous.
- Supportive psychotherapy is a common method to supplement group therapy or packaged programs designed to treat specific conditions.
- However: What you talk about and how you talk about it obviously depend on the goals of your interventions and what behavior you are treating. *Treatment is always individualized.*

TABLE 7–6.   **Suicidality, problematic substance use, and criminal behaviors**

Feature	Suicidal behavior	Problematic substance use*	Criminal behavior
Does it have acute and chronic forms?	Yes Ranges from isolated, occasional, frequent to chronic suicidality (see Chapter 5)	Yes Problematic use ranges from one-time use to mild, moderate, and severe substance use disorder	Yes Crime can be a "crime of opportunity" to adult antisocial behavior to career criminality with criminal lifestyle
Does it have established "packaged" or group programs?	Some Dialectical behavior therapy and some cognitive-behavioral therapy programs target suicidal behaviors	Yes, as in therapies based on relapse prevention, stages of change, and AA and NA	Multiple, such as Reasoning and Rehabilitation, moral reconation therapy, group programs combining substance use and criminality
Does the supportive psychotherapist have a common role?	Yes Establish a therapeutic alliance and expectation of improvement (common factors of all therapies)	Same	Same
Does supportive psychotherapy have specific techniques to offer these problems?	Yes Ensure observation, safety, and stepped care for acute episodes, identifying triggers to events and intervene with causes (e.g., via personal narratives obtained from attempters)	Yes Direct supportive techniques at emotional regulation and improvement of self-esteem issues that lead to use and relapse (e.g., denial is the major defense and shame is the dominant emotion in alcoholics).	Yes Identify criminal thinking and defenses, foster prosocial modeling and thinking
Is the therapy different for acute versus chronic forms?	Yes Identify causes of acute events, have 1) special programs for those with high risk and 2) psychosocial interventions and identification systems to lessen attempts in those with low risk. Depression is the major problem in acute attempts, while personality disorder is the major problem in those with chronic suicidality.	Yes Develop strategies for maintenance based on the causes, such as opportunity and frequency of drug craving	Yes Do not treat noncriminals like criminals, but provide education and community resources to help them to succeed when they leave prison. Not all patients/prisoners are even criminals or have criminal thinking.

*This term (used by some researchers) is meant to encompass a wider range of substance use, even those incidents not qualifying to be a substance *disorder*.

Controversies, Conundrums, and Catastrophes: Ethical Challenges for Psychotherapists Treating Substance Use and Antisocial Behavior

Most of what follows relates to the alcohol user, but some also applies to substance users and persons who have committed crimes.

We get to this point (the second of our discussions on ethics in psychotherapy) as we wrap up our discussion of comorbidities, and in particular the co-occurrence of substance use disorders and criminal behavior. We mentioned twice the program of Wanberg and Milkman (2008). We turn to the preface to their book on that program rather than the program itself. The authors express their concern that Freud's concept of psychopathology was good enough in its day but "failed to address an epidemic psychopathology—sociopathy" (p. xiv). Note that the term "sociopathy" is being used to cover all forms of antisocial behavior, not just the subset of persons often called "sociopaths" or "psychopaths."

They note that we have seen the prisons fill with more than 2 million people, violence dominates the themes in movies and television, a rash of traffic accidents "mostly caused by carelessness and irresponsibility," moral irresponsibility in business, and an "enormous amount of public littering…[and] graffiti" (p. xv).

We take issue with several of their assumptions:

- The conflation of violent crime with lesser offenses such as littering
- The implication that some moral failing or shortsightedness of psychotherapy is responsible for it
- The assumption that the program they offer in their book is going to correct it

We should mention to readers who are unfamiliar with Wanberg and Milkman's program that, according to the authors, their program has been given to more than 75 *thousand* people (and that was back in 2008). We wish to suggest that it is still not going to remake our society unless there is systemic and transformational change in our society as a whole, and in particular the correction of the social injustices we have discussed throughout this book. The causes of crime and violence cannot be addressed by individual or group therapy alone. To amend Julius Caesar's opinion: "The fault, dear Brutus, is not in ourselves, but (to a large part) in our society, that we are products of it." Our fictional protagonist, George Bailey, knew that in 1946 when he financed low-cost housing that had made it possible for residents like Mr. Martini to buy rather than rent their houses and finance their own businesses in Bedford Falls. In December, 74 years later, at the high point of the coronavirus pandemic, Mackenzie Scott, the ex-wife of Amazon owner Jeff Bezos, donated $4.2 billion to 384 organizations to remedy what she called the "long-term systemic inequities that have been deepened by the crisis" (Picchi 2020). Now you might recall that the famous Sector General Hospital at the edge of the galaxy also has 384 levels, and as Harry Bosch (from a different fictional world) told us in the introduction to our book, "There are no coincidences." So perhaps that number is meant to draw our attention to the fact that there are so many needy places in the world that it takes 384 levels to heal them! (And according to the previous article, Ms. Scott started with a list of 6,490 organizations.)

But okay, we already talked about the travesty of mass incarceration in Chapter 1, and how it is not the result of some fin de siècle degeneration of morals. It is in part the result of a massive misunderstanding of the nature of substance use and also the result of systemic racism that created numerous crimes where none existed before.

There is tremendous power and responsibility in conducting psychotherapy of either the group or individual mode. But psychotherapy should not be social control. It is, to invoke the paradigm of Jerome Frank that we used a few pages ago, a form of persuasion and healing (Frank and Frank 1993), and we ourselves have called it a kind of benevolent direction. What it is not is indoctrination or brainwashing. This is particularly important in considering the treatment of substance use disorders. We believe that you have a responsibility to avoid the tendency to *indoctrinate* patients but should rather *inform* them (thus maximizing their autonomy to make treatment decisions, one of the cornerstones of supportive psychotherapy) of the alternatives they have in treatment. We think this is something you *can* do in individual therapy but does not always happen in groups. Group therapy in the criminal justice system is often coercive, and the peer pressures create a kind of "group think" that stifles dissent.

Consider the therapy techniques proposed by Logan and Marlatt in their depiction of harm reduction therapy: "At its core, harm reduction supports any steps in the right direction. Critics may contend that harm reduction somehow enables or excuses poor choices. Although abstinence may be the ultimate goal, and is of course the only way to avoid all negative consequences associated with substance abuse, the harm reduction practitioner seeks to meet with the client where he or she is in regards to motivation and ability to change" (Logan and Marlatt 2010).

Most of Freud's patients came to him because they were bothered by their neuroses, but we do not think he thought psychoanalysis was a form of social control to make these aberrant individuals into paradigms of Victorian virtue. Let the historians decide that, however. Yet we do find it easy to discuss social learning and prosocial modeling when we treat prisoners. What were therapists saying a few years ago when they told their patients that using marijuana reflected a moral failing (unless they had a medical marijuana card)?

Now return to the issue of treating criminality. (Note: In Chapter 10 we address the definitions and treatability of psychopathy.) We have probably already "made our bed" in Chapter 1 by agreeing that as correctional therapists, we ought to do something about it via the various methods of RNR and confronting criminogenic thinking. But we still resist the consideration of psychotherapy as a form of social control or brainwashing. (This will be addressed again when we discuss feminist theories of psychotherapy in Chapter 11.) You probably feel the same way, because if you objected to your role as psychotherapist, you could vote with your feet and skedaddle. But your patients cannot do the same, and therefore you need to take additional cautions when you talk to them. All the ills of today's society like the litter on the street and the graffiti on our bridges—most of which would be absent if we had an authoritarian government like in Singapore or Beijing—are not due to a fault that psychotherapy is too individualistic and lacks a sociocentric focus. The respect for individual autonomy, even in prison, is still important. Wanberg and Milkman's (2008) warnings about social degeneration might have been better directed at George Orwell's fear of what society would have become in 1984 when the Thought Police used psychological therapy (those psychologists do love their rats) to "correct" his protagonist Winston's rebellious tendencies and socially unsanctioned love. (Does that remind you of psychotherapies to "correct" homosexuality?)

Consider the use of medications in prison. Normally, psychoactive medications are taken voluntarily with informed consent. The threshold for involuntary administration of medication is high and involves grave disability, or danger to self or others, as determined by a professional review board as described by the U.S. Supreme Court. That is because the Supreme Court considers it a serious invasion of privacy for a substance to be entered into the body. But there are fewer restrictions for the thoughts that are "injected" into people's minds. And our social ills will not be ameliorated by individual psychotherapy with your littering and graffiti-spraying recalcitrant prisoners.

Now let's return to the issue that occasioned this, the problem of counseling alcoholics. Oh, what a long and storied history we have of that (Locke 1991). Consider U.S. Prohibition, which lasted from 1920 to 1933. Moralistically supported by pillars of society such as John D. Rockefeller, who himself was considered a not-so-moral robber baron, it was grossly violated and yet persisted. The two issues we ask you to consider in your counseling alcoholics are:

- Recommending abstinence as opposed to harm reduction therapy.
- Recommending AA, other 12-step programs, something else, or nothing at all.

We introduced the first subject above with the credible opinion of Logan and Marlatt.

Both abstinence and 12-Step programs have their critics, some of whom object to what they describe as the coercive spiritual foundation of AA and the total abstinence concept that makes anyone who takes a drink feel like a failure. Some also point out something that we have also noted with respect to criminals, that there is a high rate of spontaneous recovery for alcoholics. However, just as we were kind of on the cusp of demoting AA out of this chapter, we discovered that the Cochrane Library had published a meta-analysis of 27 studies, comprising 10,565 people, of the efficacy of AA, TSF programs, and cognitive-behavioral programs. The effect was synergistic: "The evidence suggests that 42% of participants participating in AA would remain completely abstinent one year later, compared to 35% of participants receiving other treatments including CBT. This effect is achieved largely by fostering increased AA participation beyond the end of the TSF program" (Cochrane Library 2020).

The evidence is complex, and one of the well-known vocal critics, Stanton Peele (2020) argues that the study did not address harm reduction. He then goes on to make various counterclaims. And so it goes. But as we can only do our best to sift through the knowledge regarding treatments, we recommend that you take an open attitude toward your patients. A neurological basis for the change that AA creates through socialization and mutual help has also been proposed (Galanter 2014).

As for alcohol: Tell your patients what you believe. If they are curious, let them hear the evidence you follow as you know it, and describe the reported effectiveness of AA and TSF programs, as well as the respected viewpoints of harm reduction. Try to avoid outright moralizing. The United States learned about this during Prohibition.

Alcohol is legal. What is illegal is using it and then putting people's lives at risk. And what is immoral is using it as an excuse to hurt other people (e.g., via intimate partner violence). Make clear those distinctions. If you are opposed to what you consider the spiritual or sexist or coercive "group think" basis of AA, explain your position and give them the opportunity to choose their own path, since the evidence basis is that it does work for many people.

As for other drugs: Recognize that your patients' attitudes toward drugs may vary from precontemplation to maintenance (the paradox of being an institutionally abstinent prisoner), and work with them to decide for their future.

For both alcohol and other drugs: Point out to your patients that the advantage of the maintenance stage is that they are abstinent now, even if they may be uncomfortable with it. Recognize that society's attitudes toward drug use, especially the possession of small quantities of drugs for personal use, is changing, but they have to deal with reality of the laws that govern their current behavior. Recognize that the first thing they do when they get out may be to use a substance, but teach them to avoid the abstinence violation effect, perhaps view it as a slip, and refer to their crisis response safety plan, which they can also call a "crisis response sobriety plan" or something else catchy!

And as for all three: If prisoners want to desist from their alcohol, drug use, or criminality without help, you can still review the stories of people who have come to their substance abuse or criminal "rock bottoms" or "change or die" realizations and worked their way out.

Key Points

- Although there are some prisoners who have no drug or mental health problems, and some have only a substance use problem, there is a high level of co-occurrence.

- The National Institute on Drug Abuse identifies 13 principles of drug abuse treatment for criminal justice populations.

- The Substance Abuse and Mental Health Services Administration (SAMHSA) recommends a number of brief therapies for substance use disorders, including supportive psychotherapy.

- SAMHSA has issued recommendations about differences in treating men and women.

- The lifestyle recommendations of Walters are a sound approach to the "other comorbidity" of criminal behavior and substance use.

- Suicide risk is increased even in abstinent substance users in prison.

- Standardized assessment instruments for substance users should be used.

- In addition to supportive psychotherapy, motivational interviewing, stages of change, and relapse prevention therapies have a role in treating alcohol and substance using prisoners, who usually embody a combination of institutionally enforced abstinence but an early stage of change.

- Suicidality, problematic substance use, and criminal behavior can be viewed as spectrum disorders ranging from acute to chronic, or mild to severe, or one-time to chronic criminality. Supportive psychotherapy should be individualized to the severity and needs of individual patients.

- Alcoholics anonymous (AA) attendance, and the use of psychotherapies that facilitate AA attendance, have been shown to improve abstinence, but we still urge psychotherapists to help their patients make informed decisions about the choice of what program to attend and whether to seek total abstinence or harm reduction.

- While we endorse the use of supportive and directive therapy, we do not view psychotherapy as a form of social control.

- And while we do endorse the use of group and individual psychotherapy to lessen criminal behavior, we propose that no amount of psychotherapy will create the reductions in crime we desire unless there is systemic change in the society we live in.

- A version of a crisis response safety plan, one designed for substance use disorder, may be prepared for patients returning to the community with triggers, coping skills, and resources to maintain sobriety.

References

Alcoholics Anonymous: Alcoholics Anonymous ("Big Book"), 4th Edition. New York, Alcoholics Anonymous World Services, 2001. Available at: www.aa.org/pages/en_US/alcoholics-anonymous. Accessed December 20, 2020.

Baletka DM, Shearer RA: Assessing program needs of females who abuse substances, in Substance Abuse Treatment With Correctional Clients: Practical Implications for Institutional and Community Settings. Edited by Sims B. New York, The Haworth Press, 2005, pp 227–242

Bennett TH, Holloway K: The causal connection between drug misuse and crime. Br J Criminol 49(4):513–531, 2009

Bronson J, Stroop J, Zimmer S, Berofsky M: Drug Use, Dependence, and Abuse Among State Prisoners and Jail Inmates, 2007–2009. BJS Special Report; NCJ 250546. Washington, DC, Bureau of Justice Statistics, June 2017. Available at: www.bjs.gov/index.cfm?ty=pbdetail&iid=5966. Accessed December 26, 2020.

Capra F (dir): It's a Wonderful Life. Republic Films, 1946

Cochrane Library: New Cochrane Review finds Alcoholics Anonymous and 12-Step Facilitation programs help people to recover from alcohol problems. March 11, 2020. Available at: www.cochrane.org/news/new-cochrane-review-finds-alcoholics-anonymous-and-12-step-facilitation-programs-help-people. Accessed December 10, 2020.

Covington SS: Helping Women Recover: A Woman's Journal, 3rd Edition. Special Edition for Use in the Criminal Justice System. San Francisco, CA, Jossey-Bass, 2019

Covington SS, Griffin D, Dauer R: Helping Men Recover: A Man's Workbook—A Program for Treating Addiction. San Francisco, CA, Jossey-Bass, 2011

Crits-Christoph P, Gibbons MB, Gallop R, et al: Supportive-expressive psychodynamic therapy for cocaine dependence: a closer look. Psychoanal Psychol 25(3):483–498, 2008 19960117

Daley DC: Co-occurring Disorders Recovery Workbook: Strategies to Manage Substance Use and Mental Health Disorders. Independence, MO, Herald Publishing House/Independence Press, 2011

Drake RE, Mercer-McFadden C, Mueser KT, et al: Review of mental health substance abuse treatment for patients with dual disorders. Schizophr Bull 24(4):589–608, 1998

Ellis EM, Elwyn G, Nelson WL, Scalia P: Interventions to engage affective forecasting in health-related decision-making: a meta-analysis. Ann Behav Med 52(2):157–174, 2018 29538630

Fiorentine R, Hillhouse MP, Anglin MD: Drug-use careers, in Treatment of Drug Offenders: Policies and Issues. Edited by Leukefeld CG, Tims F, Farabee D. New York, Springer, 2002, pp 273–282

Frank JD, Frank JB: Persuasion and Healing: A Comparative Study of Psychotherapy, 4th Edition. Baltimore, MD, Johns Hopkins University Press, 1993

Galanter M: Alcoholics Anonymous and Twelve-Step Recovery: a model based on social and cognitive neuroscience. Am J Addict 23(3):300–307, 2014 24724889

Goldstein P: The drugs/violence nexus: a tripartite conceptual framework. J Drug Issues 15:493–506, 1985

Grenyer BFS, Luborsky L, Solowij N: Treatment Manual for Supportive-Expressive Dynamic Psychotherapy: Special Adaptation for Treatment of Cannabis (Marijuana) Dependence. Technical Report No 26. Sydney, Australia, National Drug and Alcohol Research Centre, 1995. Available at: https://ndarc.med.unsw.edu.au/sites/default/files/ndarc/resources/T.R%20026.pdf. Accessed October 25, 2020.

Hendrickson EL, Schmal MS, Eckleberry SC: Treating Co-occurring Disorders: A Handbook for Mental Health and Substance Abuse Professionals. New York, The Haworth Press, 2004

Ingraham C: Why hardly anyone dies from a drug overdose in Portugal. Washington Post, June 5, 2015. Available at: www.washingtonpost.com/news/wonk/wp/2015/06/05/why-hardly-anyone-dies-from-a-drug-overdose-in-portugal. Accessed June 20, 2021.

James DJ, Glaze LE: Mental Health Problems of Prison and Jail Inmates. BJS Special Report; NCJ 213600. Washington, DC, Bureau of Justice Statistics, Revised December 14, 2006. Available at: www.bjs.gov/content/pub/pdf/mhppji.pdf. Accessed December 26, 2020.

Khantzian EJ: Reflections on treating addictive disorders: a psychodynamic perspective. Am J Addict 21(3):274–279, 2012 22494231

Knack WA: Psychotherapy and Alcoholics Anonymous: an integrated approach. J Psychother Integration 19(1):86–109, 2009

Koob GF, Powell P, White A: Addiction as a coping response: hyperkatifeia, deaths of despair, and COVID-19. Am J Psychiatry 177(11):1031–1037, 2020 33135468

Laffan S: Alcohol and drug withdrawal, in Essentials of Correctional Nursing. Edited by Schoenly L, Knox CM. New York, Springer, 2013, pp 81–96

Larimer ME, Palmer RS, Marlatt GA: Relapse prevention: an overview of Marlatt's cognitive-behavioral model. Alcohol Res Health 23(2):151–160, 1999 10890810

Lewis JA, Dana RQ, Blevins GA: Substance Abuse Counseling, 5th Edition. Stamford, CT, Cengage Learning, 2015

Locke SJ: Counseling the Alcoholic: a century of elusive success. M.A. thesis, Marquette University, Milwaukee, WI, May 1991. Available at: https://epublications.marquette.edu/theses/1121. Accessed December 20, 2020.

Logan DE, Marlatt GA: Harm reduction therapy: A practice-friendly review of research. J Clin Psychol 66(2):201–214, 2010 20049923

Luborsky L: Principles of Psychoanalytic Psychotherapy: A Manual for Supportive-Expressive (SE) Treatment. New York, Basic Books, 1984

Marlatt GA, Gordon JR (eds): Relapse Prevention: Maintenance Strategies in the Treatment of Addictive Behaviors. New York, Guilford, 1985

McDuff D, Muneses T: Mental health strategy: addiction interventions for the dually diagnosed, in Addiction Intervention: Strategies to Motivate Treatment-Seeking Behavior. Edited by White RW, Wright DG. New York, The Haworth Press, 1998, pp 37–53

Miller WR, Brown SA: Why psychologists should treat alcohol and drug problems. Am Psychol 52(12):1269–1279, 1997 9414605

Mueser KT, Noordsy DL, Drake RE, Fox L: Integrated Treatment for Dual Disorders: A Guide to Effective Practice. New York, Guilford, 2003

National Institute on Alcohol Abuse and Alcoholism: Project MATCH Monograph Series. 2020. Available at: https://pubs.niaaa.nih.gov/publications/ProjectMatch/matchIntro.htm. Accessed December 20, 2020.

National Institute on Drug Abuse: Principles of Drug Abuse Treatment for Criminal Justice
    Populations: A Research-Based Guide. 2016. Available at: www.drugabuse.gov/publications/
    principles-drug-abuse-treatment-criminal-justice-populations-research-based-guide/
    principles. Accessed October 30, 2020.

National Institute on Drug Abuse: Cues gives clues in relapse prevention. Science Highlight,
    April 8, 2019. Available at: www.drugabuse.gov/news-events/science-highlight/cues-
    give-clues-in-relapse-prevention. Accessed August 29, 2021.

Oregon decriminalizes possession of street drugs, becoming first in nation. (The) Oregonian,
    updated November 4, 2020; Posted November 03, 2020. Available at: www.oregon-
    live.com/politics/2020/11/oregon-decriminalizes-possession-of-street-drugs-becoming-
    first-in-nation.html. Accessed November 12, 2020.

Parks GA, Marlatt GA: Relapse Prevention Therapy for Substance-Abusing Offenders: A Cog-
    nitive-Behavioral Approach in What Works: Strategic Solutions: The International Com-
    munity Corrections Association Examines Substance Abuse. Edited by Latessa E. Lanham,
    MD, American Correctional Association, 1999, pp 161–233

Parks GA, Marlatt GA: Relapse prevention therapy: a cognitive-behavioral approach. The Na-
    tional Psychologist, September 1, 2000; last updated May 31, 2011. Available at: https://
    nationalpsychologist.com/2000/09/relapse-prevention-therapy-a-cognitive-behavioral-
    approach/10491.html. Accessed June 23, 2021.

Peele S: So Alcoholics Anonymous is "proven" to work after all? Not so fast. Filter Magazine,
    March 18, 2020. Available at: https://filtermag.org/alcoholics-anonymous-cochrane. Ac-
    cessed December 20, 2020.

Picchi A: Mackenzie Scott, ex-wife of Jeff Bezos, says she gave $4.2 billion to charity. CBS News
    Moneywatch, December 16, 2020. Available at: www.cbsnews.com/news/mackenzie-
    scott-donates-charity-4-2-billion. Accessed December 25, 2020.

Pinsker H, Rosenthal R, McCullough L: Dynamic supportive therapy, in Handbook of Short-
    Term Dynamic Psychotherapy. Edited by Crits-Christoph P, Barber JP. New York, Basic
    Books, 1991, pp 220–247

Potter-Efron R: Shame, Guilt, and Alcoholism: Treatment Issues in Clinical Practice. New York,
    Routledge, 2002

Prochaska JO, DiClemente CC: The Transtheoretical Approach: Crossing the Traditional
    Boundaries of Therapy. Homewood, IL, Dorsey/Dow Jones-Irwin, 1984

Recovery Research Institute: Motivational interviewing and motivational enhancement thera-
    pies. 2020. Available at: www.recoveryanswers.org/resource/motivational-interviewing-
    motivational-enhancement-therapies-mi-met. Accessed November 1, 2020.

SMART Recovery: Introduction to SMART Recovery. 2020. Available at: www.smartrecovery.org/
    intro. Accessed December 19, 2020.

Stephens DJ: Substance abuse and co-occurring disorders among criminal offenders, in Correc-
    tional Mental Health: From Theory to Best Practice. Edited by Fagan TJ, Ax RK. Thousand
    Oaks, CA, Sage, 2011, pp 235–256

Substance Abuse and Mental Health Services Administration: Counselor's Manual for Relapse
    Prevention With Chemically Dependent Criminal Offenders, Technical Assistance Publi-
    cation (TAP) Series 19; DHHS Publ No (SMA) 96-3115. Rockville, MD, Substance Abuse
    and Mental Health Services Administration, 1996. Available at: http://lib.adai.washington.edu/
    clearinghouse/downloads/TAP-19-Counselors-Manual-for-Relapse-Prevention-with-
    Chemically-Dependent-Criminal-Offenders-109.pdf . Accessed November 2, 2020.

Substance Abuse and Mental Health Services Administration: Brief Interventions and Brief
    Therapies for Substance Abuse. Treatment Improvement Protocol (TIP) Series No 34;
    DHHS Publ No (SMA) 12-3952. Rockville, MD, Substance Abuse and Mental Health Ser-
    vices Administration, Center for Substance Abuse Treatment, 1999; latest revision 2012.
    Available at: https://store.samhsa.gov/sites/default/files/d7/priv/sma12-3952.pdf.
    Accessed November 1, 2020.

Substance Abuse and Mental Health Services Administration: Substance Abuse Treatment: Addressing the Specific Needs of Women. Treatment Improvement Protocol (TIP) Series No. 51; DHHS Publ No (SMA) 13-4426. Rockville, MD, Substance Abuse and Mental Health Services Administration, first printed 2009; revised 2013a. Available at: https://store.samhsa.gov/sites/default/files/d7/priv/sma15-4426.pdf. Accessed March 8, 2022.

Substance Abuse and Mental Health Services Administration: Addressing the Specific Behavioral Health Needs of Men. Treatment Improvement Protocol (TIP) Series No. 56; DHHS Publ No (SMA) 13-4736. Rockville, MD, Substance Abuse and Mental Health Services Administration, Center for Substance Abuse Treatment, 2013b. Available at: https://store.samhsa.gov/sites/default/files/d7/priv/sma14-4736.pdf. Accessed March 8, 2022.

Substance Abuse and Mental Health Services Administration: Addressing Suicidal Thoughts and Behaviors in Substance Abuse Treatment. Treatment Improvement Protocol (TIP) Series 50; DHHS Publ No (SMA) 154381. Rockville, MD, Substance Abuse and Mental Health Services Administration, Center for Substance Abuse Treatment, October 2015

Substance Abuse and Mental Health Services Administration: Enhancing Motivation for Change in Substance Use Disorder Treatment. Treatment Improvement Protocol (TIP) Series No. 35; DHHS Publ No 19-02-01-003. Rockville, MD, Substance Abuse and Mental Health Services Administration, 2019. Available at: https://store.samhsa.gov/sites/default/files/d7/priv/tip35_final_508_compliant_-_02252020_0.pdf. Accessed November 1, 2020.

Substance Abuse and Mental Health Services Administration: Substance Use Disorder Treatment for Persons With Co-occurring Disorders. Treatment Improvement Protocol (TIP) Series No. 42; DHHS Publ No PEP20-02-01-004. Rockville, MD, Substance Abuse and Mental Health Services Administration, 2020. Available at: https://store.samhsa.gov/sites/default/files/SAMHSA_Digital_Download/PEP20-02-01-004_Final_508.pdf. Accessed November 1, 2020.

Ternes M, Goodwin S, Hyland K: Substance use disorders in correctional populations, in The Practice of Correctional Psychology. Edited by Ternes M, Magaletta PR, Patry MW. Cham, Switzerland, Springer, 2018, pp 39–67

Walters GD: Changing Lives of Crime and Drugs: Intervening With Substance-Abusing Offenders. New York, Wiley, 1998

Wanberg KW, Milkman HB: Criminal Conduct and Substance Abuse Treatment: Strategies for Self-Improvement and Change, 2nd Edition. The Provider's Guide. Thousand Oaks, CA, Sage, 2008

White J: Code Blue Emergency. New York, Ballantine Books, 1987

Wikipedia: Twelve-step program, 2020. Available at: https://en.wikipedia.org/wiki/Twelve-step_program. Accessed December 20, 2020.

PART III

Key Disorders

8

Serious Mental Illness

Concepts of Care

Introduction to Serious Mental Illness

According to the National Institute of Mental Health (NIMH), *serious mental illness* (SMI) is defined as "a mental, behavioral, or emotional disorder resulting in serious functional impairment, which substantially interferes with or limits one or more major life activities. The burden of mental illnesses is particularly concentrated among those who experience disability due to SMI" (National Institute of Mental Health 2021).

Definitions of SMI in correctional settings vary somewhat but usually include diagnoses of schizophrenia, bipolar disorder, major depressive disorder (moderate to severe levels), and schizoaffective disorder. Some systems consider PTSD to be in the SMI category. Additionally, when other mental illnesses cause significant functional impairment and substantially limit life activities, or when they result in suicidal behavior, they also may count as an SMI. These are based on U.S. federal definitions in legislation and surveys of severity (Mental Illness Policy Org 2020).

In addition to persons with SMI, there are many other individuals and groups of persons with single or multiple disabilities, including those related to hearing, vision, cognitive function, ambulatory status, self-care, and independent living. Three in 10 state and federal prisoners and 4 in 10 local jail prisoners report having at least one disability (Bronson et al. 2015). Depending on applicable statutes, services at various levels will be required for them (Dumond and Dumond 2010). We have already written about supportive psychotherapy for persons with intellectual disabilities (Novalis et al. 2020) and we offer some advice in this area in Chapter 13.

The actual percentages of persons with SMI in correctional settings vary greatly depending on definitions, surveys, and methods. A review of previous surveys (Prins 2014) found a wide discrepancy. For example, estimates of the prevalence of major depression varied from 4% to 30%, but one has to consider that the disorder comes with rated severity, from mild to severe. Schizophrenia and bipolar disorder fell within much smaller ranges: about 2% to 4% for schizophrenia and 4% to 7% for bipolar disorder. The estimates for PTSD ranged from 4% to 21%, but the actual prevalence may be higher (see Chapter 6 for details).

SMI in the world outside prison is thought to be found at a prevalence of 4%–5% (Stanford Justice Advocacy Project 2017), or as the NIMH in 2019 estimated, 5.2% (National Institute of Mental Health 2021). Although you will often see the in-prison percentage of SMI reported as 16% based on Bureau of Justice Statistics data or 15%–30% based on other sources, there are some indications that those rates are low. For example, according to the Stanford Justice Advocacy Project (2017), "Close to a third of California inmates have a documented serious mental illness according to the California Department of Corrections and Rehabilitation." Other surveys come up with similar figures. "Overall, approximately 20% of inmates in jails and 15% of inmates in state prisons are now estimated to have a serious mental illness. Based on the total inmate population, this means approximately 383,000 individuals with severe psychiatric disease were behind bars in the United States in 2014 or nearly 10 times the number of patients remaining in the nation's state hospitals" (Treatment Advocacy Center 2016, p. 10). To achieve this level, "2 million people with mental illness are booked into jails each year. Nearly 15% of men and 30% of women booked into jails have a serious mental health condition" (NAMI 2019).

We will concentrate here on persons with SMI who are incarcerated, not those who have been diverted to other parts of the criminal justice system. Mental health courts, drug courts (since there is much comorbidity), and other diversion programs, or just the court-ordered release of nonviolent prisoners, have helped to keep down the numbers of severely mentally ill prisoners. This is not to say that non-incarcerated persons have fundamentally different therapy needs, but therapy is different for them by virtue of the different environments and availability of family and community involvement. Having introduced the role of advocacy for clinicians in Chapter 1, we mention that there are substantial resources available for addressing the concerns of mentally ill persons as they become involved with the criminal justice system at various times using what is called the *sequential intercept model* (Judges & Psychiatrists Leadership Initiative et al. 2017). While the title might imply that the resources are for persons working outside prison, it is a valuable brief document with resources for addressing criminogenic factors in the lives of those with mental illness. And not irrelevant for those interested in the historical causes of inadequate mental health treatment, there is renewed interest in the place that mental health treatment occupies in infrastructure (Frances 2021).

U.S. jails and prisons now house the majority of mentally ill persons in this country. Despite the reasonable assumption that incarceration is not good for mental health, the research seems to show that prisons in general do not cause severe mental illness, although psychological dysfunction due to the harsh conditions and a virtually total disassociation from life before prison (and after) does create negative and long-lasting change. As Haney (2002) notes, "In general terms, the process of prisonization involves the incorporation of the norms of prison life into one's habits of thinking, feeling, and acting" (p. 3). Prisoners gradually become accustomed to and to some degree internalize the restrictions that prisons impose, beginning with a loss of autonomy and freedom to make many of their own choices, from what to eat, what to wear, and what time to get up to what work to do. "The process of institutionalization renders some people so dependent on external constraints that they gradually lose the capacity to rely on internal organization and self-imposed personal limits to guide their actions and restrain their conduct" (Haney 2002, p. 3). In addition, prison conditions can lead to hypervigilance due to threats or personal risk in an often-violent environment, emotional overcontrol, alienation and psychological and social distancing, and diminished sense of self-worth and personal value. Prison culture makes any outward sign of weakness an opportunity for others to exploit, leading some individuals to the opposite extreme of obtaining a reputation for toughness, with force and domination becoming measures of success. Prison may also be so stressful for some individuals that it leads to stressor-related disorders as discussed in Chapter 5.

The Criminalization of the Mentally Ill

Obviously, there are many incarcerated mentally ill persons, but why? One theory, which has several forms, has been called the "criminalization of the mentally ill." This theory asserts that mentally ill persons are put into criminal justice institutions unfairly, or for behaviors that arise from their mental illness, or (probably the most prominent assumption) that they are arrested for relatively minor offenses. How and why did the theory of the criminalization of the mentally ill become prominent? Several developments contributed. The invention of powerful psychotropic medications contributed to the emptying out of psychiatric hospitals in the 1950s and 1960s. The U.S. Civil Rights movement added a series of legal decisions requiring that persons with mental illness live in the least restrictive environments. The term "deinstitutionalization" was used to explain what had happened to all the persons in mental hospitals. But we are reminded that:

> Whether deinstitutionalization has ever occurred remains a matter of debate. While the number of current public hospital psychiatric beds represents about 3 percent of the 1955 peak, people with serious mental illness are found in many locations providing 24-hour care....Some who live "free" in the community are under the supervision of mental health courts or experience Assertive Community Treatment teams as unduly interfering in their lives or feel intensive case managers run their lives. Counted among those who may be totally unfettered by the mental health system are the shelter residents and the homeless. This has led the critics of deinstitutionalization to instead label it "transinstitutionalization." (Geller 2019, p. 23)

Thus, the mentally ill may never have been deinstitutionalized but may have instead been transinstitutionalized, with prisons taking up much of the transfers. This process did not end in the 1960s; it continued with the 1999 U.S. Supreme Court *Olmstead* decision (*Olmstead v. L.C.*, 527 U.S. 581, 1999), which required state hospitals to develop lists of persons who could be treated in the community (Atlanta Legal Aid Society 2020).

Now we return to the "criminalization of the mentally ill" hypothesis. One credible source concludes that most mentally ill people are in prison not because of their mental illness but because they have committed crimes and that the response of the correctional system should be similar to the way it treats those who are not mentally ill. However—and this is a serious "but"—the evidence also suggests that the prison environment does not meet the goals of reducing their recidivism (Manchak and Morgan 2018, p. 584). Several studies support the notion that recidivism among those who are mentally ill is due to criminogenic issues rather than mental illness (Skeem et al. 2014), and there are even those who call for greater attention to criminogenic factors when evaluating people in emergency departments, contending that it is "misguided" to prioritize their psychiatric needs (Badre and Lehman 2019). As the title of an article by Lamb and Weinberger implies, however, some perspective is needed, because to address mental health needs in the community requires additional systems with 24-hour care (Lamb and Weinberger 2013).

This is not an isolated opinion. Others assert that "the criminalization hypothesis is a limited explanation of the overrepresentation of people with SMI in the criminal justice system because it downplays the social and economic forces that have contributed to justice system involvement in general and minimizes the complex clinical, criminogenic, substance use, and social service needs of people with serious mental illness" (Bonfine et al. 2020, p. 355).

So on the one hand, we are told that mentally ill persons do commit crimes for the same reasons as other persons. On the other hand, we are told that prisons are not a good place for them. But there are major differences of opinion among researchers and advocates, and many still believe that there is a criminalization of the mentally ill as defined above.

Policy-makers and politicians need to consider such issues, while we in our primary role as therapists need to provide the appropriate therapies. Policy-makers need to consider both the needs of the mentally ill and the needs of the society at large. We can do our part as advocates but keep in mind: Most violent crimes are still committed by antisocial persons, and persons with mental illness (not just SMI) can still be antisocial. They can display criminogenic thinking equal to or greater than that of non–mentally ill offenders.

As we have implied, the changeable things (other than heredity)—that is, the life trajectory—that make people into criminals, which in general are the things reflective of social injustice in all societies, transform people into criminals years prior to the things (environmental factors) that give people mental illness (and—this should not be omitted—substance abuse). So you may have to treat all three—mental illness, criminality, and substance abuse. (In Chapter 7 we even dubbed this a "trimorbidity.") This requires you to take your own measure of reality. In certain cases you may say to yourself, "Were it not for mental illness, this person would not be in prison," but this can create a false sympathy because the person you are treating also has criminogenic thinking. Then, you can think that the person is in prison because their SSI payments for their mental illness could not prevent them being homeless and committing crimes to supplement their income. But, as a generality, mentally ill persons are still in prison for the same reason as other persons: they committed crimes.

Through history and screenings, prisoners may be placed in an SMI category mandating a certain level of treatment. Since diagnosis is not merely an activity of psychotherapists, we will not spend any more time on the inclusion criteria but assume that you know which individuals in your institution and your caseload have SMI and how you must document your time and services to them.

There are actually some stabilizing factors in dealing with mentally ill persons in correctional institutions, as recognized by some clinicians (Goomany and Dickinson 2015): You can always find your patients, and they can always find you if they want to. Medication and therapy are available at no charge. Patients who would normally be (or were previously) homeless now have medical care and a clean (and sober) and relatively safe environment, even though they may be subject to harassment and abuse by other prisoners or staff. However, persons with SMI encounter multiple difficulties as well, not just harassment and discrimination but also separation from friends and family, loss of meaningful work, and most of the disadvantages of being incarcerated just like everyone else (Manchak and Morgan 2018).

So when you encounter patients who have antisocial personality disorder (ASPD) comorbid with an SMI, consider that ASPD (which is not per se an SMI) typically develops *first*, so that having a life history of disrespect of others is an expression of criminogenic values prior to developing their mental illness. Combinations of these disorders—ASPD, bipolar disorder, and borderline personality disorder (BPD)—are particularly "toxic" because persons with such diagnoses can be impulsive, break rules, use drugs and alcohol, and/or become violent. For example, research shows that the cohort of antisocial and borderline personality "demonstrated higher trait anger, trait impulsivity, and aggression scores, resulting in an overall higher score on psychopathy" (Sansone and Sansone 2009, p. 18).

The combination of bipolar disorder and BPD also creates management arguments between staff and custody and among members in each group. Misbehavior may be attributed to the bipolar disorder and the patient declared "baseline unstable" and hence not culpable, or attributed to the borderline personality or declared "baseline stable" and suitable for discipline. Differences in recommended treatment will fester among staff members, exemplifying the well-known phenomenon of splitting as staff members become adversaries. Persons with BPD and ASPD also tend to act out or malinger while in therapy.

As with any place that assigns people to programs that provide privileges, there are sometimes issues of misuse of services. Persons with ASPD may talk their way into mental health units and become predators to the other residents. Conversely, persons with symptomatic mental illness may feel they have to appear to be symptom free to get into certain programs such as forestry camp. Because of their behavioral problems, persons with mental illness often end up in disciplinary housing (which is poorly tolerated), with longer sentences because of disciplinary action and, as mentioned above, denial of access to "privilege" programs. So they end up with longer sentences, as well as lack of good time, and are more likely to serve their full sentences.

Psychopathy

Even in the future world of James White, there are sentient predators in every species who cause disruption and suffering that is out of proportion to their actual number (White 1988, p. 146). Although the attribution of "psychopath" has been used in various settings, this is normally used to apply not to persons with SMI (except for those with diagnosed SMI who are also psychopaths), but to a group of persons with a type of disorder, often considered a personality disorder but not delineated as such in DSM-5, who commit crimes out of a constitutional callousness and disregard for the rights of others. Psychopaths lack empathy and do not show remorse. They do not form real relationships with others. They can be deceptive and manipulative and cruel, and their irresponsibility frequently brings them into contact with the criminal justice system (Hare 1993). Psychopaths constitute about 15%–25% of offenders according to Hare's well-known Psychopathy Checklist—Revised, but the percentage of men in prison with ASPD is often considered to be as high as 80% (Hare 1993, pp. 166–167). We will discuss psychopathy more in Chapters 10, 12, and 14.

Another descriptor, "adult antisocial behavior," is applicable to many persons in prison but says nothing else about the other characteristics a person might have. Therefore, as a therapist, you should keep in mind and distinguish these three categories, that is: psychopath, adult with ASPD, and adult with antisocial behavior. Somebody who has committed a crime (or even several crimes) may have done something antisocial but does not necessarily have an antisocial personality or is not necessarily a psychopath.

In the most recent discussion of psychopathy, however, the effect of current thinking about dimensional models of personality is reflected. As we discuss in Chapter 10, DSM-5 recognizes that in the future there will be additional models of personality that are dimensional in nature. The different personality disorders will reflect different proportions of various characteristics that are the defining characteristics of that personality disorder. The same applies to psychopathy. People have varying degrees of the defining characteristics that constitute a psychopathic personality. We have found that to be true in the patients we see in our own practice. Patients who are pathological liars, for example, may have that as a psychopathic trait even if they do not meet the full criteria for psychopathic personality. Keep in mind, of course, that Hare's Psychopathy Checklist is itself a scored item. A person may score high on certain items but not have a score high enough to pass the threshold for psychopathy.

Despite the "cubbyholes" that researchers have established when treating persons with SMI and other diagnoses, questions remain about the other categories of offenders. To many researchers, sex offenders seem to be in a class of their own. There are also many pathways to *violence*. Violent offenders may have different diagnoses, but because of their dangerousness, society has to have a way to deal with them. Violent offenders may have mixed personality disorders, including ASPD, psychosis, narcissistic personality disorder, and/or paranoid personality disorder. In California, there are psychiatric hospitals for end-of-sentence violent offenders or sex offenders. As discussed in Chapter 10, some jurisdictions, such as the United Kingdom, have special legal categories for violent offenders with personality disorders.

"R" Is for Recovery

Perhaps it's just a linguistic accident, but the field of corrections, including the word *corrections* itself, embraces the R's of retribution, rehabilitation, and recidivism. The RNR (Risk-Need-Responsivity) theory promotes the concepts of risk and responsivity. But the most important concept for persons with SMI is recovery. When you think of recovery, you may naturally think of recovery from an accident, recovery from a physical illness, or recovery from an addiction, as in "I am a recovering alcoholic." The Substance Abuse and Mental Health Services Administration (2020) defines it as follows:

> Recovery is a process of change through which people improve their health and wellness, live self-directed lives, and strive to reach their full potential. There are four major dimensions that support recovery:
>
> - Health—overcoming or managing one's disease(s) or symptoms and making informed, healthy choices that support physical and emotional well-being.
> - Home—having a stable and safe place to live.

- Purpose—conducting meaningful daily activities and having the independence, income, and resources to participate in society.
- Community—having relationships and social networks that provide support, friendship, love, and hope.

This concept certainly echoes the goals of supportive psychotherapy. The "R" of rehabilitation encompasses those programs that "rebuild" people who have been broken down by disease or criminal behavior. When they are rebuilt, they are recovered. It can be difficult to implement all the components of recovery programs in a prison. For example, recovery programs typically involve peer support groups. It is difficult to bring outside persons into correctional institutions, so the peers in the support groups may have to be drawn from the prison population. But models of recovery are certainly worth knowing.

Mental Illness and RNR

As we have discussed on several occasions, effective programs in the RNR model require hundreds of hours of therapy—often given in structured group formats. You may find that your role is just to provide "ordinary" psychotherapy with some adjunctive interventions that you think supplement the general approach of the RNR programs in your criminal justice system. So the combination of RNR procedures and mental health treatment is a fortuitous one.

Also relevant, if true, is that according to the RNR theory of recidivism, treating mental illness per se does not reduce recidivism. This is because, as we anticipated in Chapter 1, the onset of criminal activity is years earlier than that of most mental illnesses such as schizophrenia or bipolar disorder. But by the time somebody has become mentally ill, he has usually been a criminal for years. We did just say "if true." It is probably true in most instances of mental illness, but some researchers identify a small group of persons with SMI for whom the criminal actions are a direct result of treatable psychosis.

An example of a structured program is Changing Lives and Changing Outcomes, which is presented in an accessible manual with a considerable amount of supplemental online material (Morgan et al. 2018). After the preliminaries, its second module is "Mental Illness and Criminalness," and CJ-PMI is their acronym for "Criminal justice involved persons with mental illness." They state that CJ-PMI persons are responsible for managing their illness, avoiding criminal behavior, and meeting their life goals. The Changing Lives and Changing Outcomes program holds them responsible for prosocial and productive behavior, despite the fact that they may have grown up in unfavorable environments (Morgan et al. 2018, p. 5). Even for us (and you know that we generally hold persons with SMI responsible for most of their behaviors), this seems to be a tall order.

Supportive Psychotherapy and Education for Persons With SMI

As a therapist, you are also an educator about behavioral health. Education about one's condition has increasingly been recognized as an important factor in medical compliance and cure. We print out relevant information about a patient's condition from the internet, and there is a rack of handouts in our waiting area. We bookmark our favorite reliable sites and have some preprinted materials available. We urge you to pre-screen anything that you recommend and be prepared to discuss, agree, or disagree with it. Patients can selectively use statements from other sources to augment resistance to the therapy, or they may discover unorthodox or dangerous treatments and insist that these be undertaken instead of standard treatments.

Most prisoners do not have access to the internet, but their friends and families do. There is a considerable amount of antimedication, antipsychiatry, and antitherapy material online, and your patients may have questions about sites with that material and the validity of their information. They will also have a lot of information from chat boards and prisoner advocates (and often anticorrections) websites. Hopefully, they will not be more knowledgeable than you are about their illness. But you should also familiarize yourself about the usual mental and emotional conditions that prisoners experience, such as admissions depression and prerelease jitters.

Your major therapeutic questions will concern the extent to which specific types of information should be provided to a prisoner at a specific time. You may be concerned that education about the illness will not be understood or will generate stigma or irresponsibility. The stigma of mental illness in prison is major. Moreover, the consequences of ascribing an SMI diagnosis should be considered since it may involve change of housing and programs. Education requires considerable time and repetition and is often best presented in standardized group programs. Educational materials, although subject to their own misinterpretation, carry independent authority. Most therapists can recount an experience in which their patients disagreed with them about some facet of their illness until they found corroboration in the popular press. Materials distributed by the clinic often add to the institutional transference and provide the patient with an emotional link to the clinic. They also help to dispel confusion over verbal statements of the therapist, since patients may misinterpret educational statements because of transferential reasons. For example, you say, "I think your illness can be effectively treated," and the patient may think that you're trying to be kind. On the outside, they or their families may find social media tools effective, although the evidence is still building for that (Torous and Keshavan 2016) as well as applications (Firth and Torous 2015; Linardon 2019; Nott 2013).

Mental Illness and Segregation— Like Oil and Water?

In Chapter 5, we said that segregated or more generally restrictive housing is often thought of as a "prison within a prison." Here we want to talk about *involuntary* segregation, not the voluntary isolation that some mentally ill persons prefer. The deleterious effects of involuntary segregated housing on mentally ill persons are well known. Yet mentally ill persons are also human beings who are, for the most part, responsible for their behavior. How can you sanction such persons for institutional violations once they're already being punished by being in prison? What are the alternatives to disciplinary segregation? Should it be forbidden to segregate a mentally ill patient even for a week? A day? An hour? We, too, have encountered mentally ill patients who declare, "You can't punish me because I am mentally ill!" Has the pendulum of accommodation swung too far? What about non–mentally ill persons who threaten suicide to avoid discipline?

Now that we have your attention, we'll admit that we don't have all the answers. De facto, each institution has developed its own answers, which themselves are in a constant state of evolution. However, therapists, in general, need to "render unto custody what is custody's and to mental health what is mental health's." You will provide input into custody decisions and vice versa. Then custody does what it has to do, and you do what you have to do. When the process breaks down (e.g., the prisoner sent to segregation threatens suicide), the patient is sent from one treatment location (segregated housing) to another (the infirmary). More creative solutions, such as providing suicide watches without moving patients between systems, are constantly being developed out of necessity. Doing supportive work, however, you'll find it difficult to sit back and do nothing much of the time if you feel that segregation is causing undue hardship on a truly mentally ill patient (not an antisocial one who is threatening suicide). This is an undeniable source of job stress. It has frequently happened to us, and no doubt it has frequently happened to you. Our advice is:

- Try not to take it too personally (unless you have proof that it is, i.e., that they don't like you as opposed to mental health people in general).
- Avoid spouting generalizations in return, such as "You officers are heartless!" This does tend to make things worse.
- Keep your skills sharp and choose your battles sparingly and wisely (i.e., those cases you want to challenge up the chain to the warden [or the central office]).
- With your patients, use firm, fair, and predictable metrics for determining who is "baseline" stable and can be sent to segregation and whose punishment should be mitigated. Explain your criteria and the resulting decisions against the background of treating them as responsible human beings.

Restrictive housing, both voluntary and involuntary, raises many more questions, examples of which are given below, but these certainly apply to all types and levels of mental health services:

- How to provide psychotherapy services safely, and if possible not at cell side.
- How to provide as many hours as possible of out-of-cell services with the staff available.
- How to investigate the underlying reasons why mentally ill persons ask for voluntary segregation (e.g., poor socialization, fear of victimization, gang politics) and, if possible, return them to general population.
- How to incentivize mentally ill patients to improve behavior and thus return to general population.

There is specialized programming for services in segregation, such as the Stepping Up, Stepping Out program (Batastini et al. 2019). There are also many other sources for information on services in segregation (e.g., Chaiken and Shull 2007). Chaiken herself describes that her first experience with a prisoner who was "eating" his TV was "overwhelming and disheartening" (Chaiken and Shull 2007, p. 18-8).

Here are some suggestions for trying to engage at cell side with patients, whom perhaps you might be meeting for the first time, to draw them out, avoid a cell extraction, or begin some sort of useful psychotherapy:

- Introduce yourself and ask them to verify their name or number (getting them to pay attention to a simple task).
- Make it clear that you are part of a mental health treatment team.
- If you work for a specialized medical subcontractor, it sometimes helps to emphasize that you are not a state or federal employee, but rather part of the medical services company and that "it's our job to give you medical treatment, not lock you up."
- Try some noncontroversial and calming questions.
- See if they can tell you why they will not leave the cell. Is the reason something you can help them with?
- Use verbal deescalation strategies, but don't endanger yourself.
- Try to state alternatives to cell extraction ("It'll be easier if you can come with me and the officers to the infirmary").
- If you're able to do so: Talk and conduct some kind of a rudimentary therapy that does not escalate them.
- Repeat your request that they see mental health, because this may eventually convince them (Chaiken and Shull 2007, p. 18-6).

Schizophrenia and Psychotic Illnesses

Schizophrenia is the most common form of psychotic illness, but there are many other factors that can cause a person to become psychotic, if only briefly. While we frequently refer to schizophrenia in this section, the interventions are valid for many psychotic illnesses.

Of the many times we have discussed issues regarding the history of social injustice in the United States, this is one that applies to the use of one specific diagnosis: schizophrenia. The most salient evidence of the socially unjust use of this diagnosis is the historical overdiagnosis of schizophrenia, especially paranoid schizophrenia, in Blacks, and a continued overdiagnosis of schizophrenia and paranoid schizophrenia and underdiagnosis of mood disorders in Black men (Bolden et al. 2021). Bolden et al. (2021) recount the disturbing history of the use of schizophrenia as a diagnosis for disobedient wives in the 1950s and for protesting Blacks during the civil rights movement of the 1960s. Of course, paranoid schizophrenia has gone away in the DSM, and Bolden et al. think it had its origin in the "protest psychosis." We should keep in mind that at one time schizophrenia was thought to be the result of "schizophrenogenic" parenting and so forth. To put it mildly, or to make a gross understatement, perhaps, diagnostic validity and reliability in mental health are still major issues and are still subject to issues regarding bias and injustice regarding many social groupings. But as for schizophrenia, we urge you to be aware of potential bias in your own diagnoses.

Using the recovery model, the National Institute of Mental Health produced an evidence-based Illness Management and Recovery Kit. The program can be given individually or in a group. There is a strong emphasis on understanding the disease and its treatment with medication. Although you may not be able to offer it, there is also provision for family involvement. There are a number of documents and media items, but the major document is about 350 pages and includes the curriculum and handouts for patients (Substance Abuse and Mental Health Services Administration 2009).

There is not a lot of evidence about the use of genuine (vs. control condition) supportive psychotherapy for schizophrenia. A Cochrane Collaborative Study concluded that "[w]hen we compared supportive therapy to cognitive behavioural therapy…, we again found no significant differences in primary outcomes" (Buckley et al. 2015). Equivalent, perhaps, but their definition of supportive psychotherapy was of a very minimal intervention far less than the psychotherapy we perform. In addition, "[M]any researchers believe that aspects of ST [supportive therapy], such as the therapeutic alliance, the provision of support and advice, and efforts to minimize stress, may be beneficial in their own right…and incorporating lessons learned from ST may strengthen the effect of cognitive behavioral therapy…on schizophrenia" (Penn et al. 2004). This is because in the past few decades, there has been accumulating evidence for the effectiveness of cognitive-behavioral therapy for this syndrome (Opoka and Lincoln 2017; Smits and van der Gaag 2010). However, there is also a major study that found cognitive therapy to be ineffective for schizophrenia (Lynch et al. 2010; University of Hertfordshire 2009). In favor of training in supportive therapy for psychosis, we quote some cognitive researchers: "What is startlingly evident is that a supportive and consistent relationship seems to be of great value to many people with psychosis and can help reduce positive symptomatology" (Lewis et al. 2002, citing Sensky et al. 2000). Further, "A supportive relationship may have a different mechanism of action than CBT" (Dudley et al. 2009, citing Milne et al. 2006). Finally, in a study comparing supportive psychotherapy and treatment as usual in first-episode psychosis, the intervention group was found to be superior (Rosenbaum et al. 2012).

Because what we have characterized above as the destructive effects of prison life, supportive psychotherapy has the "right stuff" for mitigating the stress of the prison environment, preventing decompensation and relapse, and, in due time, facilitating recovery. It accomplishes this by addressing the symptoms of SMI and also improving coping skills, encouraging a healthy lifestyle, providing a long-term perspective (e.g., for depressed patients), and providing (what we hope you will be) a reliable and concerned professional who stays in their lives for the duration.

Treatment of persons with schizophrenia in prison must begin with assessment of their history (both legal, including the presentence investigation, and medical), intelligence, general abilities, and dangerousness using instruments validated for the SMI population. We discussed treatment plans in Chapter 4, but briefly, the reduction of hallucinations or delusions typically finds a place there, hopefully with behavioral measurements or simple behavioral observations such as "Patient will say he is not hallucinating during the day" or "Patient will not appear to be under the influence of delusions," or "Patient will go to 80% of his visits with the therapist and prescriber." It helps to put in something that is relatively unconflicted, such as getting out in the day room, going to the yard daily, and following a "Diet for Health" or similar plan. For more functional patients, there will be goals of staying on their job, meeting family at least once a month, taking their GED class, and so forth.

Here are some things you should do; many of these are discussed in more detail later.

- Address depression in persons recently diagnosed with schizophrenia because the suicide rate is high among these individuals and the rate is even higher the first year after diagnosis. Combined with arrival in jail or prison, which has a high suicide risk, you have "double trouble."
- Assess for comorbid diagnoses, strengths and deficits (e.g., intellectual, learning disability), and violence risk using validated instruments.
- Refer for medication management. You may not be a prescribing provider, but you need to convey your position on this to your patient. You'll also find yourself discussing medication frequently just because you're not the prescriber.
- Even if you're not a prescriber, assess for nonadherence to medication recommendations or for side effects that your patient is not aware of. For example, your patient may admit that he is cheeking his medicine because "it's too strong." Or he may show tremors or hypersalivation of which he is unaware.
- Assess the relationship of criminality to illness to determine how it will help to address criminogenic factors in your patient's life experience.
- Assess, teach, and maximize the patient's current mechanisms for coping with psychosis.
- Teach metacognition (discussed later).
- Teach your patient skills. There are various specialized or manualized modalities of treatment, including skills training (social, occupational, problem solving, and independent living).
- Provide integrated treatment for co-occurring SMI and substance use disorder (Spaulding et al. 2017; see also Chapter 7).
- Teach the cognitive therapy skills and use the handouts provided by Kingdon and Turkington (2004).
- Treat persons with SMI as responsible human beings when they need to be held accountable for their actions.
- Work with the patient to develop a crisis response safety plan to prevent personal crisis, suicide, or reactions to trauma in the prison setting and after release.
- Encourage your institution to have specialized mental health units based on successful models such as the clubhouse model or a therapeutic community for persons with co-occurring mental illness and substance use disorders.
- Provide as many out-of-cell or dayroom activities as you can (although not all residents will want to participate).

Keep in mind that a patient's symptoms will vary depending on the course of illness (influenced by stressors in the patient's life such as arrest, trial, and incarceration) and response to treatments. You'll have a specific agenda as you prepare the patient for release from prison. For more, see Chapter 14.

Important characteristics of supportive psychotherapy in schizophrenia for prisoners include:

1. Understanding the value of a good therapeutic relationship.
2. Using specific emphases in technique during therapeutic sessions.
3. Improving social relationships within and outside the prison.
4. Encouraging education, work, or simply yard time outside of the cell.
5. Promoting identification with the therapist.

TABLE 8–1.   **Value of relating to patients who have schizophrenia in jail or prison**

You may be the only objective person they relate to in the jail or prison.

You are in a position to mediate or even arbitrate issues that arise with custody.

You will probably be asked to determine instances in which they may or may not be subject to discipline.

You can be a sounding board for actions they are thinking of doing.

You are a model for their development of their interpersonal and social skills.

You can improve their reality testing.

You can provide an objective critique of their family relationships.

You are an agent to improve their self-esteem.

You can also become an agent of constructive criticism in areas of criminal behavior.

You can teach them to model your calmness in crisis.

You may have to intervene as a caring person to help them to get better and prevent them from being abused.

The Therapeutic Relationship

Advantages of a good therapeutic relationship are listed in Table 8–1. Patients with good therapeutic alliances show greater acceptance of treatment, better medication adherence, less total medication use, and better long-term outcome on measures of psychopathology, cognitive function and social functioning, and work performance (Frank and Gunderson 1990). By talking about what they do every day, such as their interactions with correctional officers (COs) and other prisoners, you can try to modify their delusional perceptions and social skills deficits. Social functioning is rarely improved by medication alone, yet it is "one of the strongest predictors of current functioning and long-term outcome in schizophrenia" (Penn et al. 2004, p.101).

Many patients with severe mental illness may struggle with their words but are adept at reading your expressions and gestures. Don't betray your words by your expressions! There will also be transference issues. For example, a patient may experience the therapist as overly controlling and react negatively to direction (Meaden and Van Marle 2008). One expert warns us that "[s]ome patients may believe they are putting their lives at risk by talking to the therapist" (Garrett 2019, p. 116). You may want to reassure them that they can talk to you safely, that you will do your best, and that you will make their experience as safe as it can be for a prison. Furthermore, if they are being abused or harassed, you do want to hear about it.

In Chapter 3, we imagined what it would be like to inherit a patient who trashes or, conversely idolizes her previous therapist, leaving you to inherit a residue of resentment and distrust or facing an impossible ideal against which you will undoubtedly fail. Patients with SMI, either before prison or perhaps in prison before they meet you, have probably had more negative experiences than positive. They may have been held down to receive involuntary injections of psychotropic medicine. They may have horror stories of how they were abused in psychiatric hospitals. Ask them open-ended questions about what happened to them in the past. Ask them what "was the best thing" about their previous therapist and what could have been improved. Ask them (but do not require them) to write you a brief history of their doctors and treatments, and try to obtain their previous records.

Patients with schizophrenia also have a large area of function that we call the "non-conflicted sphere." Think of their beliefs as gardens. One of those gardens is full of evil delusional plants that try to devour them and create fear. Other gardens are just as normal as anyone else's. When you diligently ask them to change subjects or direct the conversation to new subjects, you may want to move the conversation to the non-conflicted sphere. There will also be entire periods of life both prior to a first psychotic break and during periods of wellness or illness remission. Recalling the good times rather than swimming in the delusions can improve insight into the value of accepting therapy and being well.

Frequency and Duration of Sessions

As in our earlier recommendations regarding flexibility, and within the guidelines required for SMI in your institution, you should be prepared to "dose" your psychotherapy and divide it between the various members of the treatment team. While patients with personality disorders may demand their time, patients with SMI may best be seen for the time and frequency they need, following concepts of triage.

Repetition

Repetition is often required for a lesson to sink in or be generalized. For example, you may spend some time telling a patient not to yell loudly at his cellmate, and then discover the next day that he is yelling at his neighbor because "that's a different person and you didn't tell me not to yell at him."

Hope: Did You See That Rubber Tree Plant?

In Chapter 4, we did wonder if "hope" is a strategy. But especially for this group of patients, expressing hope and support can be as important as working your therapeutic magic on delusions. "High Hopes" is a song about an ant who decides he can move a rubber tree plant. While the attitude of cognitive therapists might be described as conveying the belief that "We can talk you out of your delusions," the approach of supportive therapy is to say, "We'll get you feeling better," "I'm here to support you," "I don't want those voices to hurt you," or "It must be terrible when your voices get loud? What can we do about that?"

Hallucinations and Delusions

Dealing With Hallucinations

Hallucinations and delusions are prominent features in schizophrenia. We will discuss each in turn. Therapeutic ways of responding to hallucinations are given in Table 8–2. Some patients do not want to get rid of their hallucinations. Hallucinations can be pleasant or grandiose or provide comfort in the isolation and loneliness of the illness. If these patients don't want their hallucinations to go away entirely, they may agree that they don't want to be bothered all the time by them, or not during the day when they are working. You can give them a sense of control by saying, "You can be the judge of how much you want to lower your hallucinations." Tell them that they should not allow themselves to be insulted by their hallucinations and the hallucinations

TABLE 8–2.	Therapeutic responses to hallucinations

Don't demonize; empathize.

Normalize the experience (many people hear voices at some time in their lives).

Don't feel you have to agree with the patient's assumptions about the reality basis for the hallucinations (e.g., they come from God or the Devil).

Examine the circumstances of the hallucinations when it is helpful to do so. (Are they a reaction to being alone or are they a reaction to feeling abandoned?)

Interpret the occurrence (e.g., trauma, disappointment, as a reaction to a blow to self-esteem).

Determine the distraction, damage, discomfort, delusions, or danger posed by the hallucinations; if none, do they need treatment? What does the patient think?

Find out what the patient's current coping mechanisms are (see Table 8–5), and try to improve their existing coping mechanisms and add new ones.

In therapy, deemphasize the hallucinations and focus on positive matters.

Write out "coping cards" with specific strategies of thinking or doing to counteract them.

Use cognitive therapy arguments such as "I'm a good person. I don't need to believe what the voices say" (e.g., see Wright et al. 2014 and Grummisch and Wright 2021).

---

should not be "allowed" to keep them up all night. You can raise questions about dangerous voices. "What makes you sure that God is telling you to cut yourself? Why would God do that? Doesn't God want people to do good things?"

In many instances, hallucinations can be normalized. You can say, "I sometimes hear my name called at night when there is nobody there. That's a normal experience, but you seem to have more of that than most other people." You can point out that many people report having had hallucinations at one point in their lives, or that hallucinations occur in persons with trauma histories, for example, the voices of their past abusers. Hallucinations can occur in psychotic depression, brief reactive psychoses, and psychoses due to substance use both acute and chronically. Because of our own experience in settings with high rates of malingering, we do not overreact to a complaint of hallucinations, especially an isolated complaint without the usual co-occurrence of delusions: If a person comes in with an isolated complaint of hallucinations but no delusions, is it an emergency to treat them? Explore this and ask for details.

Some researchers, especially in the European community, have taken the attitude that hallucinations are a lot more normal than abnormal, and that the problems of "voice-hearers" often arise because of the way society reacts to them (see discussions in Morin 2014). Some working on the content of hallucinations try to direct scrutiny on negative or insulting voices that seem to be the interrogations of other figures who rejected the patient. Specific methods include rescripting imagery (Ison et al. 2014), by which the subjects lessen their distress from the voices. There is also benefit to be found in having people interact with their voices (Shaikh-Lesko 2014, summarizing the work of Marius Romme). Some of these patients have schizophrenia, and some do not. Another resource is a manualized therapy for auditory hallucinations (Jenner 2016).

The degree of distress and disability generated by hallucinations varies greatly. When you are inquiring about hallucinations, it's important to determine the patient's feelings, both individual and in general, in response to the hallucinations. If the hallucinations are pleasant, it's less important to focus on them and more important to turn your attention to disabling psychopathology. We tell patients that we have a particular concern about hallucinations that are hurtful, unpleasant, or command them to do dangerous things. We might say, "Tell me more about that experience, because I have not had that myself and I don't hear that voice" or "I realize that this is an important experience, but maybe there's another way to make sense of it."

It can be helpful to investigate the hallucinations further as part of a process that may weaken them or their influence (which is the most dangerous aspect of having a hallucination). For example, forms are available to describe their psychotic thoughts and consider alternative explanations for their occurrence at this time in their lives (Wright et al. 2014). You can also try to establish the circumstances under which the hallucinations started or tend to recur. The classical psychoanalyst Silvano Arieti contended that an examination of hallucinations will show them to be a reaction to some perceived assault on the patient's self-esteem, and that establishing this will eventually result in the disappearance of this symptom (Arieti 1974). This would be overly optimistic in our opinion, but taking an interest in the origin of the hallucination helps you to form an alliance with your patient. For example, investigation may show that the hallucinations started at a time of loneliness or of interpersonal disappointment, leading to decreased self-esteem. Rather than "argue" about the reality of the hallucination, you can then discuss the disappointment and the effect it had on the patient's self-esteem and self-image. However, we admit that you can only do so much before you run out of time or argument.

Command hallucinations.   Command auditory hallucinations are always a source of concern. Guidelines for treating these have evolved as our understanding has evolved. Treating command hallucinations in a prison is not the same as treating them in a community. In the community, if you met a patient with command hallucinations to kill himself, you would think about hospitalizing him or sending him to a crisis unit. But if you have such a person on your caseload in prison, it may be neither desirable nor necessary to react in that manner. In fact, the rate of compliance with command hallucinations is quite low. Command hallucinations are more likely to be obeyed based on perceived benevolence, perceived omnipotence or power, or connection to other delusions. Command hallucinations alone may not create greater risk for dangerous behavior (Hellerstein et al. 1987). Thus, a command hallucination in isolation is not likely to be followed unless it is connected to delusions (Braham et al. 2004). Other factors affecting the likelihood that a command hallucination will be obeyed are the patient's sense of control over the hallucinations (more control means less likely to obey) (Sarti and Cournos 1990) and the ability to identify the voices (which makes it more likely to obey) (Junginger 1990).

Coping with voices.   Patients who are bothered by their voices use a variety of coping strategies. In the community they may have had access to smoking (including marijuana), using alcohol or street drugs, talking at length to family, exercising or playing sports, playing games on computer or cell phone, using cell-phone apps that absorb time and even ones for mental problems, listening to music, or watching TV at length or all night. In prison, the options are limited, but you can try to be creative, encourage use of headphones, suggest they read books and pray and use their Bible if it helps, do written games like Sudoku, talk to their cellmates if they can, ignore the hallucinations if they are able to, hum over the hallucinations, or talk back to them, engage with them, or tell them to go away. Meditation and yoga can help. Somewhat effective

TABLE 8–3.	Suggested ways of coping with hallucinations in prison

Hum or talk out loud (but not so much as to be disturbing or disruptive to others).

Listen to headphones—whether talk or music, whatever works.

Meditate and/or practice mindfulness.

Use a mantra.

Phone someone.

Pray.

Do paper puzzles, sudoku, crosswords, mandalas, and so forth.

Use diary or journal to distract yourself.

Use TV or game time.

Nap or sleep (but first try active methods).

Talk to cellmates.

Phone friends or family.

Take a shower.

Go out to the dayroom and socialize.

Exercise or practice your yoga in cell or unit.

Go to the yard.

Talk back to or tell hallucinations to stop (not so as to disturb others).

Normalize the hallucinations.

Use cognitive methods to weaken them (list evidence for and against).

Remind yourself that voices don't know much and you don't have to obey them.

Use metacognitive methods (e.g., to act against them).

Source. Cohen and Berk 1985; Northern Ohio Universities Colleges of Medicine and Pharmacy 2020. Coping approaches selected, adapted, and modified for prisons.

but disheartening is the desire (and actual practice) in prisons of sleeping away the time. Of course, this is done by many prisoners regardless of mental health status. But as for persons with SMI, exercise your judgment about whether there is a better way to go. True, some psychiatric medications are sedating, and it is important to determine if your patient wants to sleep as much as he does or wants to sleep less. A variety of coping mechanisms are listed in Table 8–3.

Dealing With Delusions

Most persons with schizophrenia have delusions, often associated with hallucinations. Delusions can be bizarre, nonbizarre, mood-congruent, or mood-incongruent. Purely delusional disorders (i.e., in which there are no hallucinations and only delusions) are much less common. In the past, many purely delusional persons were diagnosed as having delusional disorder or paranoid schizophrenia, but the latter category was eliminated in DSM-5. (It still appears in ICD-10.) This view is consistent with a Cochrane report that concluded that there is a paucity of high-quality randomized trials on delusional disorder. Those authors found only one relevant study comparing supportive psychotherapy with CBT but concluded that there is insufficient evidence to make evidence-based recommendations for treatments of any type for people with delusional disorder (Skelton et al. 2015). However, even if you encounter somebody with a purely delusional disorder, you can certainly work with him as you would with a psychotic disorder.

It can be difficult to understand the reasoning of delusional patients. It is good advice that "[w]hen therapists do not understand what the patient has said, they should not pretend to understand but rather should say that they are attempting to understand, but are not yet certain what the patient is trying to say" (Garrett 2019, p. 120). However, as Garrett (2019) remarks, most delusional systems follow a pattern of a persecuting agency or voices like the CIA and a compensatory set of grandiose beliefs that the patient has special talents and is being prevented from reaching his potential by the persecutors. Delusions have a limited number of plots with a few stereotypical characters. Or maybe (to use a symphonic example) Vivaldi concertos. Once you've heard one, you hear the similarities in all the others.

Insight varies. Many delusional patients recognize that they have a problem and are eager to get help. However, you will invariably encounter patients who are adamantly delusional and who, at the start of treatment, spring the well-known "lose-lose" trap question on you. The usual trap question is: "Do you believe me or not?" Or "So are you just like the others, thinking I am crazy?" Any normal answer—yes, no, maybe—creates a lose-lose situation. If you say you don't believe them or say that they are mentally ill, they will dismiss the whole therapy ("What's the point of talking to you? This is a waste of time.") and walk off in a huff. This may be a preventive action to keep them from engaging in therapy. If you say that you believe them, they'll assume you are patronizing them, because most delusional patients do have a little bit of what the psychoanalysts call "observing ego" that knows, deep inside, that "there be delusions." Even a "maybe" answer stirs suspicion because (since they are paranoid) they assume you are playing games with them.

The best response to the "trap" question is, "Whoa, wait a minute!" Let's explain. You tell them, "Wait a minute. I just met you. I barely know you and you are asking me if I believe you or not? I hardly know what you believe, or who is doing what to you or what bothers you. I am here to help you to feel better and relieve your suffering. And to do that I don't necessarily have to believe what you believe. People can believe different things and still be on speaking terms. Even Republicans and Democrats. Well, maybe that is a bad example, but do we have to root for the same baseball teams to talk to each other? So can you start by telling me what's making you suffer?" In a similar vein, you can tell them that you're keeping an open mind, need more information, and want to understand them better or that you recognize that their statement might strike some people as unusual but you want to hear more (Robinson 2007).

We have had reason to normalize some symptoms such as hallucinations, and we do so to an extent with paranoia and delusions, but *in general* we emphasize that it is not therapeutic to agree in total with the content of a patient's delusions. Such false agreement can increase your patient's anxiety, further confuse his reality-testing skills, and reinforce the psychotic content. However, you can to an extent normalize delusions in a prison, because a prison is a paranoid place even for previously normal people. We introduce the notion of "prison paranoia" early in treatment when we wish to build rapport in the therapy. Here is talk that we give, at least in part, to some paranoid prisoners at a certain point in their treatment:

Mr. Jones, think about this place. Prison can be frightening and overwhelming, and it is hard to know who your friends are or even if you can ever call anybody your friend. It is pretty certain that you have some enemies and that some of them may really want to steal your stuff or attack you. There are loudspeakers with prison staff often yelling commands like "Jones, come downstairs immediately" or "Rack up for count." They listen to and record your phone calls. The prison staff have life-and-death control over you. The courts, the prison, and the Department of Corrections have files on you, and you also have a mental health file, and each of these groups makes various allegations about your behavior. So it is pretty much normal and common to have paranoid thoughts in prison, and these thoughts may take the form of fears about what seem to be all-powerful law enforcement agencies who seem to run the entire country.

Delusional thinking can run a gamut from the beginning of ideas of reference to a long-term fixed delusional system, as the following two vignettes illustrate.

Case Vignette 1: Mr. Victor

Mr. Victor tells his therapist that he thinks that others are talking about him outside the cell. Instead of immediately challenging his "perception," the therapist points out that no one has said anything to his face and moreover no one has physically hurt him—thus helping him feel safer—and that Mr. Victor has the power to ignore them, a power that would illustrate his strength and self-control. Meanwhile, the therapist continues to explore the reality of the delusion. The therapist asks how it is that Mr. Victor knows what he thinks he knows. The therapist does not agree with the delusion but simply explores its origins, makes the patient aware of potentially dangerous consequences (e.g., assaulting the officer), and lessens Mr. Victor's fear and perception of threat so that he is less likely to take dangerous action.

Case Vignette 2: Ms. Lee

Ms. Lee is a 59-year-old woman well known in the mental health community but recently placed in jail because she took a swipe at somebody and nearly blinded her. On this particular occasion, the court could not forgive the assault or divert her to a mental hospital. But Ms. Lee has an issue with her food. She thinks her food is being poisoned by "the Korean gangs" (she is originally from South Korea). As a treatment-refusing homeless mentally ill person, she has been getting by (using her SSI money) purchasing food that is securely packaged to avoid contamination, but now in the jail the food is scooped out from steam tables onto trays. She refuses to eat. The same with water, which she insists must be bottled. After losing 10 lbs. down to 92 (her height is 5' 2"), her appearance concerns the staff. The therapist talks about the safety of the jail food, to no avail. Negotiations ensue. The prison relents and gets her bottled water and commissary food, which is packaged. She eats oatmeal for the most part but remains hydrated and begins to gain weight. Very gently, the therapist attempts to "chip away" at the gang delusion by asking questions that at least appear to be fairly objective. How did these gangs follow her here from Korea? Why is she so important to them that they try to poison her food? Isn't the jail able to prevent them from getting into the facility and its food? She briefly takes medicine (which she has taken in the past) but decides it is also contaminated. However, for a time the food delusion abates, and she begins to take the regular tray. At that stage, the therapist "reminisces" with her about how she used to be afraid of eating the food, and they discuss what has changed. Ms. Lee says that she thinks the gangs are on vacation. These therapeutic "debates" continue throughout her stay. Although she is often oppositional, she obviously enjoys seeing the therapist and seems genuinely happy to see her.

As we see in these vignettes, major issues concern the distortions of reality that take the form of simple ideas of reference to persistent and relatively fixed delusions, including the common one of food being poisoned. Delusions are typically persecutory and can be bizarre (e.g., microchips in a tooth) or "down home" paranoia. In the community they may be delusions about family; in the prison delusions can be about the officers or other prisoners and can include medical staff. Paranoid patients frequently misinterpret visual appearances in the manner of delusional perceptions as well as motives. For example, Ms. Lee sometimes saw a crease in the packaged food and refused to eat it because she decided it had been opened and poisoned. If you find this difficult to believe, consider how people can invent reasons for their behavior under the influence of a posthypnotic suggestion. We have seen that criminals have a distorted perception of reality, including their assessments of themselves and other people. But ideas of reference and delusions take that concept further into the area of impaired perception of reality that is psychosis.

Garrett (2019, p. 117) calls an inquiry an "inference chain" in which you ask, "What would it mean to you if we find evidence that does not support your current belief?" Although he likes to ask this question soon after meeting the patient, we use this kind of question later (see below) in what we call the "double awareness stage."

With people who are actively and fixedly delusional, it helps to normalize a little bit, agree a little bit, but agree to disagree and to chip away at the delusional material with indirect methods, often in conjunction with generally recommending adherence to their medication. Yes, there can be times when you appear to "split" the treatment team by "siding with" your patient when he decides to stop his medication. But this has to be done judiciously for alliance building and not just for being oppositional. Example of a comment we have made: "Of course, I support your right to stop your medicine, but can you tell me why, or can you stop it in steps?"

Speaking of chipping away, cognitive therapy programs take a highly structured approach using the usual table of "evidence for" "evidence against" as they mutually investigate the predecessors, triggers, and meaning of hallucinations and other psychotic thought content. Some of the techniques involve multiple questions about the origin of delusions in perceptions, as in "What was it about the way the CO looked at you that made you conclude that he was thinking of killing you?" Once the patient answers, the therapist drills down on the supposed evidence and questions why that "look in the eyes" really proves that the CO is murderous. For example, "How closely can you see his eyes from 12 feet away? What was the CO doing at the time? Are you sure he was really looking at you?" Delusions are attacked with detailed questioning about why the FBI would target the patient, or how the patients knows what is in the file. Or more personally, "Why is that voice criticizing your looks? Do you have concerns about your looks?"

We have recommended to not completely accept a patient's delusional beliefs. Some people can hold fixed delusions for a lifetime, and some can function tolerably well despite their delusions. There is a timing issue about questioning a delusion, such as when you can mildly challenge them with "I wonder if there is another way to explain that." We find it useful to stage a patient's delusions to determine the type of therapeutic interventions. A delusional patient goes through three phases (Sacks et al. 1974):

1. A fully delusional phase, in which the delusions are very difficult to weaken and anything thought to be a challenge of their delusions can result in hostility. (And since we like to talk about fictional detectives, we would be remiss not to mention that the most famous one of all, Sherlock Holmes, warns us in "A Case of Identity" [1891], citing the medieval Persian poet Hafiz, that it is as dangerous to snatch a delusion from someone as it is to grab a tiger cub.)
2. A double-awareness phase, in which the delusions coexist with more accurate reality testing; the patient may question the delusions, may simultaneously accept and reject them, or may conceal or try to suppress them; some therapists have called this stage "double bookkeeping."
3. A nondelusional phase, in which no delusions or only residuals or memories of the delusion exist.

If the patient has no doubt whatsoever of the reality of the delusion, confrontation should be only mild questioning. If the patient displays any doubt about the reality of the delusions, you can begin to more aggressively and frequently confront the delusions (Rudden et al. 1982). This can be done by reinforcing the "observing ego" of the patient by questioning the reality of the delusion more forcefully and by investigating the circumstances around the formation of delusion. You can normalize delusions by relating them to common beliefs or human nature. For example, if a patient thinks he is entitled to millions of dollars from Workers' Compensation, you might say, "I know that many people have gotten Workers' Comp settlements, but the paperwork is complicated and it is certainly possible to be uncertain if you have won your case or not, especially if you have a natural wish to win your case."

Your patient has probably had many experiences in which he has been lied to and victimized even by persons he considered his friends. You can give your version of the "prison paranoia" talk we related above. And, you go on, "paranoid" exactly describes the belief that there is an FBI sniper trying to get a bead on him when he is in the prison yard. But, you are not aware of anyone who has been shot by the FBI in the prison yard. Sure, shots might be fired if there is a general disturbance, but not by the FBI! You can validate any true themes or elements of reality in the delusion. For example, you may agree that the patient's supervisor is watching him, while questioning whether the supervisor actually works for the CIA. As in: "If he really worked for the CIA, wouldn't he have a better job than in this prison?"

Even firmly held delusions can be explained in a symbolic manner that does not challenge the patient and yet prepares him for the double awareness stage. For example: "The way you've been treated in life, it's no surprise to me that you think the CIA is trying to hurt you."

Recovery from an acute psychotic decompensation takes many forms, on a continuum ranging from denial of or amnesia for the psychotic episode (i.e., "sealing over"), through some awareness of the psychotic symptoms, to partial insight into why certain symptoms may have occurred, and, at times, a fuller understanding and integration of the entire episode (McGlashan et al. 1975). Sometimes a patient factually remembers the episode, such as being sent to the outside prison psychiatric unit, but discounts the significance or danger of the incident, while focusing on the discomfort or

TABLE 8–4. **Therapeutic responses to delusions**

As with hallucinations, normalize delusions to some extent while not totally buying into the patient's delusional system (e.g., relating the delusions to "prison paranoia").

Look for "genetic" sources in personal history of deprivation, abuse, or trauma.

When the patient is ready, express mild questioning or skepticism when appropriate.

If the patient has any doubts whatsoever, begin to confront the delusion and to explore its formation.

If the patient becomes nondelusional, further explore the process of delusional formation and possibly interpret the content.

Offer consensual validation for elements of reality in the delusion.

Interpret the delusion as "poetic truth."

the way he was mistreated. Early in therapy, you may not be able to address total denials, but as your therapeutic alliance develops, you should start to make mild comments that can help your patient integrate the experience.

When the patient is relatively nondelusional, you can build defenses against the recurrence of delusions. Discuss the warning signs (premonitory symptoms) that the patient is getting delusional again and what to do about it. For example, "I'm having a tough time this month, so it's natural to think that the COs are turning against me, but I don't really have any proof of that."

Therapeutic ways of responding to delusional material are summarized in Table 8–4.

Our reviews of long-term therapy of psychotic patients have convinced us that the therapeutic relationship with patients helps them to let go of their delusions. Their delusions have created a meaningful (if negative or grandiose) relationship to the world. Once patients have a positive relationship with another human being, one that has raised their self-esteem and does not require their grandiose compensations, they need their delusions less.

Ideas of Reference

Ideas of reference, such as those experienced by Mr. Victor above, are common in prison and can be normalized with the "prison paranoia" talk we described. Ideas of reference can be chronic but in a relatively nonpsychotic person can be an early warning sign for psychosis. Sometimes we think they are secondary to the development of the anxiety or confusion prisoners develop. In their minds, the "bad feelings" they are experiencing must have a cause, which they assume is because the officers and other prisoners are talking about them in mean ways or actually plotting against them.

Like full-blown persecutory delusions, ideas of reference probably serve a psychological defensive function of projection (of anger toward others) often with a compensatory grandiosity. As negative as the ideas of reference are, if people are talking about him, the prisoner must be important. You cannot address the defensive mechanism directly, but you can suggest that low self-esteem is stirring up the ideas of reference. For example, "Have you been feeling a little depressed lately? Maybe that's why you think these people are talking about you!" Like other psychotic symptoms, ideas of reference can be referred for treatment with medication. Often, we explain the reason

TABLE 8–5. **Levels of therapeutic response to ideas of reference**

Patient's level of awareness	Therapeutic response
A. Strongly held ideas of reference (not safe to challenge cognitively; rapport with therapist uncertain)	Without challenging these ideas, ask the patient to spell out who is saying what about him, when this is happening, and why he thinks it is happening now. Address the fears and concerns the patient is feeling as a result of such thoughts, without agreeing with the content.
B. Moderately held ideas of reference (some rapport with therapist)	Normalize the patient's experience and acknowledge how his beliefs make him feel without agreeing to the validity of his conclusions.
C. Weakening ("dissolving") ideas of reference (subject to discussion)	Discuss and suggest other possible explanations for the experience or observations. Ask for details of why the patient believes what he believes (e.g., the inference chain from a delusional perception to a delusion).
D. Some self-observation occurring (and patient begins to express)	Encourage the patient's ability to observe himself (gently encourage doubts of the delusions).
E. Developing social awareness	Encourage the patient's realization that others will not agree and that it serves the patient poorly if he talks about the ideas of reference (to persons other than the therapist).
F. Double-awareness (i.e., patient has a sense of reality coexisting with the ideas of reference)	When the patient has reached the double-awareness stage, strongly encourage doubts as to the validity of the ideas when it is appropriate to do so. Develop alternative explanations of their beliefs.
G. Predominantly realistic thinking (sometimes with residue of ideas of reference)	At this stage, help the patient to understand the situations in which these ideas develop. Be as current and concrete as possible (say, "When you feel threatened you sometimes think you hear the other prisoners talking about you, but maybe they are not actually saying those things" but not "You are projecting your hatred of others onto them").

for medication as, not because the symptom is psychotic but because it causes distress that can be relieved by medicine.

A supportive psychotherapy approach to ideas of reference, including levels of therapeutic response, is given in Table 8–5. Over time, the therapist hopes to reach the stage at which the patient is predominantly able to think realistically (i.e., Level G), but may often have to be satisfied with the patient being able to have a double awareness (i.e., Level F). With many patients, development of social awareness (i.e., Level E) is all that can be achieved, yet this does still allow them to get on with most of the functions of a normal life.

Psychodynamic therapists attempt to help patients to find meaning in their delusions such as discovering that they are figuratively true while not literally true. We agree that sometimes it is appropriate to provide personally acceptable explanations that help patients understand how they have developed delusions. This can certainly include the explanation that abuse in their family of origin may be partly responsible for their current delusions. Since many persons with schizophrenia have problems such as hypertension or diabetes (and there is an issue of whether some psychotropic medications increase that risk), we also compare having schizophrenia with having an illness like hypertension. We explain that we take patients' "mental status" the way the nurse takes their blood pressure and that if there is a problem we recommend medication just as their provider does for their high blood pressure. Without the relevant medicine, a person is at risk for a stroke or paranoia. A disease model helps to separate the patient from guilt for the mental illness and underscores the need for appropriate treatment. It should not, however, be used as an excuse for dependency, inactivity, and failure. To the patient who says, "I am mentally ill so I can't help myself," you must say, "You have a mental illness, but you must still try to act responsibly and get help to control it." Some advocates suggest using "biological" explanations that are reasonable but probably don't express the full neurobiology. For example, a basically true biological explanation is that "it's typical for hallucinations to get worse at bedtime." Not exactly a lie, but a little inexact, is one that Torrey (1986) suggests to the patient who claims his food is poisoned: that it is common for people with schizophrenia to taste things differently and think they are being poisoned. Perhaps this could have been helpful to Ms. Lee.

However, a complete psychodynamic program probably goes beyond what you would want to do or have time to do. In addition, we don't believe that most delusions have the historical explanations that psychodynamic therapists seek. Delusional thinking is a result of neurobiological deficits in information processing but does not always reflect trauma and real-life losses. Schizophrenia is not a result of poor parenting (the debunked "schizophrenogenic mother" of psychoanalytic theory) or abandonment in childhood. It's true that many patients with PTSD hear voices, but it's obvious that trauma does not cause schizophrenia, or else the prevalence of schizophrenia would be a lot higher than 1%.

If we cannot lessen delusions, we focus on their effects, not their content. We ask the patients if their delusions:

- Are disabling.
- Make them dangerous.
- Make them suffer.
- Create conflicts, and even crimes, and put them in prison.
- Result in costs to them and their families.
- Isolate them from cellmates, staff, friends, and family.
- Impair their ability to work (as with the hallucinations).
- Interfere with their educational classes.
- Make them distrust you and the other mental health staff.
- Make them fearful of going to the medical clinic.
- Result in disciplinary actions.

When these things happen, we discuss them in an open-minded manner if the delusion, whether true or not, is a "troublemaker" in their lives.

TABLE 8–6.	Social skills worth teaching to patients who lack them

Making eye contact with officers and other prisoners (Patient can practice with therapist; does not imply this has to be paranoid or intense; patient may start by looking over once in a while.)

Learning other nonverbal ways to communicate

Reading someone's nonverbal cues (but we suggest that many patients do this well but neglect the cognitive content of messages instead)

Active listening (nodding, saying "Uh-huh")

Using the telephone

Signing up for sick call or requesting an appointment with mental health, medical, or dental

Applying and interviewing for a job within the prison and in the community

Making social conversation with cellmates, neighbors, or others in the unit

Learning self-assertiveness if they feel wronged (to be adjusted for paranoid patients who file grievances daily)

Learning to make pleasant conversation (perhaps even what we called "happy talk")

Developing skills during nonworking time (including filling time of boredom with drawing, puzzles, journaling, conversing, exercising, and doing homework from therapy sessions; avoiding "sleeping away the time")

Solving problems

Combating negative thinking (includes using methods of cognitive-behavioral therapy)

Questioning delusions (includes using methods of cognitive-behavioral therapy)

Source.   Suggested by Bellack et al. (1989); Granholm et al. (2016); Liberman et al. (1985), as modified by us for prison use.

Social Skills Training

Many prisoners, such as those with poor education or chronic mental illness, have impaired cognition and judgment and lack basic social skills. Social skills training, a modular, highly structured program of interpersonal skills training, has received extensive implementation and validation (Liberman 1988; Liberman et al. 1985). Many programs have been around for many years and have reproducible handouts (e.g., Bellack et al. 2004; Granholm et al. 2016). Programs include role playing, videotaped feedback, and the practice of skills in group and community settings. They can also learn what is called self-efficacy training, an important program of self-management based on the work of Albert Bandura (see Fluent 2013). Social skills training has received reemphasis as an implementation of approaches to several of the criminogenic risk factors. These include antisocial peer associations, family/marital tension, and unproductive or unstructured leisure time (Batastini et al. 2018).

With or without a group program, you can help to provide many of the items in formal social skills training, as shown in Table 8–6. Social skills should be addressed as needed in the therapy (such as when a deficit is revealed) or through specific training scenarios rather than as abstract lectures. Not every seriously mentally ill person can learn every skill, but keep trying.

Criminality and Schizophrenia

Individuals with schizophrenia may have issues with criminality, and one source reports that "the association of severe mental illness with criminality, and especially violent criminality, was almost entirely due to schizophrenia" (Hodgins and Klein 2019, p. 251). Since the age at onset for antisocial behaviors usually precedes the age at onset of schizophrenia or bipolar disorder, persons with schizophrenia, like those with other SMI, have often committed crimes before the onset of their psychotic symptoms. However, there is a group in which the onset of criminality coincides with the onset of symptoms. In addition, according to Hodgins and Klein, there is a third group of "callous" individuals who may have brain damage from chronic illness and are particularly dangerous.

Persons with schizophrenia who commit a crime during a psychotic episode may have genuine remorse, even if it is attenuated by their negative symptoms. (In contrast, a psychopath does not have remorse.) A person with schizophrenia may have had an impairment of appreciation of the wrongness of their act at the time of their act. This is comparable to the criteria for a finding of "not guilty by reason of insanity" (NGRI) in many U.S. jurisdictions. However, the actual number of mentally ill persons found to be NGRI is relatively few, and the majority of mentally ill persons who are convicted of a crime are sent to a regular prison.

When you're treating persons with schizophrenia, the question arises whether, how, or if ever you should discuss their crime(s). According to the RNR model, the issues of criminogenic factors can be addressed in the same way as with other criminals. In fact, their negative symptoms may include a lack of appreciation of the seriousness of their past actions. This may actually make it easier to initiate a discussion of their criminal actions. If your institution uses a packaged treatment program for offenders with mental illness, you may choose to incorporate elements of that program into your therapy sessions. However, timing is important when to ask:

- Do you think that you were mentally ill at the time of your crime?
- How do you think that happened? (e.g., Had you stopped taking your medicine? Had you stopped going to your clinic or lost contact with your case manager?)
- What did you believe? (e.g., Did you believe that the victim was trying to kill you?)
- If you begin to have beliefs like this in the future, in the prison or in the community, what would be a better plan of action?

Medical Complaints

You will frequently hear medical complaints. We'll say more about this in Chapter 12. However, the following is advice mostly for patients with schizophrenia: While these may be a deliberate diversion from the mental health business you want to address, you should keep in mind that patients may not appreciate the significance of medical symptoms, and even if they do, they may lack the social skills to get their medical complaints addressed. For example, your patient may remark incidentally that she can't write because her arm is completely numb each morning. She may not notice that tremor and significant weight gain are side effects of her medications. When you hear a medical complaint, you can:

- Address it quickly if it is important to do so. Do a referral or empower your patient to make a medical request. In the next session, check that she actually made the request.
- Look up who she saw and what has been done and, if necessary, jog her memory about it. "You saw Dr. Smith yesterday. Did you tell her that you had a sore throat?"
- See if the discussion does engage her in treatment with you in areas other than the mental illness.
- Tell her why you're doing this: "You know I'm not the medical doctor, but let's take care of this so we can talk about your mental and emotional problems."
- Refer medication side effect complaints to her prescribing provider.
- Help her with lifestyle modifications to stabilize or lose weight to counteract weight gain from psychotropic medications. Psychoeducation or cognitive-behavioral interventions will help prevent weight gain that is common with antipsychotic medications (Alvarez-Jiménez et al. 2006; Evans et al. 2005).

It is also important to address comorbid illnesses and substance use disorders. Fifty percent of patients with schizophrenia have another medical diagnosis (Mitchell and Malone 2006). These patients have higher rates of cardiovascular disease, hepatitis C, cerebrovascular disease, and (even when controlling for their high rate of smoking) lung disease (De Hert et al. 2011). They also have a history of poor oral care that impairs their other life activities. Make sure they are getting their medical and dental care. Prison, of course, being relatively drug- and alcohol-free, is a good time to talk about the benefits and "clear mind" of abstinence. We will discuss depression in schizophrenia below. In many cases, discussing depression with your patient may allow you to move the conversation onto a nondelusional topic. However, if delusional thoughts are the source of the depression, then you will need to address the delusional thinking as you would usually do.

Co-occurring Substance Use

Fifty percent or more of patients with schizophrenia have significant drug or alcohol abuse (Winklbaur et al. 2006). This is a common problem in all persons with SMI, and we discussed the integrated (rather than parallel or sequential) treatment of substance use disorders in persons with mental illness in Chapter 7. In the stress-vulnerability model of the illness, it's thought that persons with schizophrenia are highly sensitive to low doses of substances and that the use of substances results in an earlier onset of schizophrenia. It's unclear if this is really an instance of self-medication, since in the case of persons with schizophrenia it may be that substance use ameliorates certain natural reward-seeking, learning, and processing deficits yet the substances worsen their actual symptoms (Pratt et al. 2020).

Family Contacts

Families being what they are—highly variable—many therapists are secretly if not openly gleeful about the relative lack of family contacts when working in prison. Since you work for the prison system, you should be prepared for much opposition or even outright hostility when hearing from families. Families are often opposed to medication, and we frequently hear from patients that they have stopped medications upon the advice of family members. It's true that many patients believe that their hallucinations have a historical meaning and are not necessarily to be eradicated. For example, we looked at the reviews on Amazon.com of Marcus Romme's book (Romme et al. 2013) and similar ones on hearing voices and found a great of number of positive reviews praising this "new attitude" toward hallucinations that they need to be understood as reactions to past trauma. As mentioned above, we doubt that schizophrenia is caused by trauma even if it can be worsened or modified by it. Moreover, the general tenor of the reviews was hostile to psychiatry and the medical model of treatment. The writers of the reviews almost uniformly trashed the concept of schizophrenia being a brain disease and demonized the bedside manner of prescribers in general.

So, given the context "out there," it helps to remember that families usually have formed an image of you through social media and the "lens" of the patient and you may be:

- Blamed for locking them up in the "hole" (segregation).
- Accused of overmedicating them or overemphasizing the importance of medicine (even if you are not the prescriber) (e.g., "You told them they will have to take medication *forever*!").
- Blamed for alienating them from family members (e.g., "You said he would never be able to have a normal relationship with me [his wife]!").
- Shamed for not "going to bat for them" in writing prerelease reports (which is one of many reasons to separate treatment and forensic functions if possible).
- Criticized on the basis of antimedical as well as anticorrections social media and internet sources, although there are certainly many competent sources that you can recommend to your patient's family (e.g., Smith 2018).

Guidelines for working with families of prisoners with SMI are listed in Table 8–7.

Outside Activities

There are not a lot of outside activities for prisoners, but there are still the yard, socialization activities, education, group therapies, and work. When needed, talk to your patient's supervisor as well as get the input you require from the patient's COs and any other providers.

Stigma

Although some prisoners may malinger having mental illness for personal gain, in general having SMI is stigmatizing in general prison populations. In particular, we have heard that from gang members with genuine mental illness, who emphasized that there was no way they were going to present for treatment until they got involuntarily moved into the mental health track. Many people with SMI know not to talk openly about their symptoms, but sometimes they just can't help it and need to share or offload their worries about their symptoms onto their peers (if they are not yet in a mental health unit). We tell them that other people just don't have the experiences

TABLE 8–7.	Working with the family in the prison environment

Determine the family's attitude toward you (the therapist).

Ask them to help you gather information (past records or names of hospitals).

Gain the family as allies so they can reinforce your supportive relationship to the patient.

Serve as a buffer to overemotional family members as needed.

Help educate the family about the disease.

Encourage them to warn you if the patient is beginning to decompensate.

Note. Mostly indirectly by asking your patient to get the information from his family.

they have and that others might make fun of them or even mistreat them if they talk openly about their voices or delusions.

Metacognitive Approaches

People with schizophrenia have deficits in "thinking about thinking," or in *metacognition*, a lack that contributes to their poor quality of life and their recovery (Lysaker and Dimaggio 2014; Pesek 2009). Metacognitive therapy that specifically targets delusional beliefs improves insight and reduces the severity of delusions and positive symptoms (Balzan et al. 2019). It should be mentioned that patients in the Balzan et al. (2019) study (52 out of 54 completed it) continued to take their antipsychotic medication. Metacognitive treatment approaches that have supportive qualities include:

1. Metacognition reflection and insight therapy (Vohs et al. 2018).
2. Group-based metacognition-oriented social skills training (Inchausti et al. 2017a, 2017b).
3. Metacognition using a focus on narratives (Schweitzer et al. 2017).
4. Metacognition as a way of helping adolescents seeking treatment (Scheyer et al. 2014).
5. Mentalization-based psychodynamic psychotherapy (Brent 2009).

Metacognitive (as well as cognitive) approaches are being used to treat the negative symptoms of schizophrenia (e.g., amotivation, alogia, blunted affect, apathy).

Depression in Schizophrenia

Depression in a patient with schizophrenia is a challenge, especially when a patient is recovering from an acute psychotic episode. Published surveys of depressive symptoms in schizophrenia show a wide range. One site reports that the majority (70%) of persons with schizophrenia will experience a depressive episode in their lives and that 25% are depressed at any given time (Living with Schizophrenia 2016). Opinion is divided over whether such episodes of depression represent new episodes of depression, the revelation of already existing depression previously masked by florid psychotic symptoms, a basic aspect of schizophrenia per se, or a reflection of the stigma of the mental illness itself (Mulholland and Cooper 2000; Taylor 1992).

In some patients, the course of the depressive symptoms is not the same as that for the psychotic symptoms. Strictly speaking, the term "postpsychotic depression" might best apply to the symptoms in this group, but these symptoms are actually defined and called "post-schizophrenia depression" in ICD-10. The greatest concern is for new-onset schizophrenia that is beginning to resolve after treatment, for which it is known that there is a high suicide rate. The lifetime suicide rate has been estimated at 5.6%, but the rate doubles during the first 5 years of illness, and the percentage of attempt-ers prior to hospitalizations was 23%; a suicide attempt was listed as a reason for hos-pitalization in 15% (Ventriglio et al. 2016). Depressive symptoms can also herald the relapse into psychosis (Pratt et al. 2020).

It's obvious that you have to pay attention to any episode of depression. Ask about well-known somatic symptoms such as feeling tired and lacking energy. Also ob-serve: Patients who had been relatively verbal may now become very quiet and less likely to participate in conversational give-and-take. Check collateral data: Are they socializing in the day room and going to the yard? Are they missing their medication sessions? If you think they are depressed, help them to understand the experience as related to their recovery process. At times, especially when fatigue is prominent, it helps to point out that such feelings are common with many medical situations, the most recent example being recovery from COVID-19, but tiredness and slowing down are also side effects of most antipsychotic medications.

Common themes are grieving and mourning, ambivalence toward the psychotic episode, and real-life setbacks that could cause depressive symptoms in anyone. Con-sider the discussions of grief and disenfranchised grief and of suicide in Chapter 5, including the recognition that some patients have already attempted suicide in a dan-gerous or spectacular manner. Sometimes patients may seem more demoralized by their depression than by their floridly psychotic symptoms. One possible comment about the issues leading to depression, serving both to reassure and to promote the therapeutic process, might be: "What previously made you psychotic is now making you depressed. This may be painful, but it's a step forward in the process of your re-covery."

Finally, try to reduce any added risk from vacation or therapist absence. Explain extended absences and the backup plan you have put in place. Staff turnover (including that day when you leave the facility) can create added risk.

A repertoire of therapeutic responses to depression in schizophrenia is provided in Table 8–8.

Other Co-occurring Mental Illnesses

As if having schizophrenia, with or without a substance use disorder, were not enough of a challenge, there is a high co-occurrence of PTSD, panic disorder, anxiety disor-ders, and social anxiety disorder with schizophrenia. The lifetime prevalence of PTSD with schizophrenia ranges from 14% to 53%. In persons with schizophrenia, panic attacks occur in 25%, and panic disorder is found in 15%. Anxiety symptoms occur in 65%, and an actual diagnosis of anxiety is found in 38% (Pratt et al. 2020, reporting the findings of various others). Although we don't have an exact number for social anxiety disorder, they surmise that the percentage in persons with schizophrenia is higher than that in the community, where social anxiety has been reported in 25% of outpatients and 9% of inpatients. So the need to assess for and treat these illnesses is obvious.

TABLE 8–8.	Addressing depression in schizophrenia in prison

Investigate and document the patient's history of depression.

Determine whether this is the first time the patient has become depressed.

If it's not the first time, find out about the course of his previous depression. How long did it last, and what helped it to end (medication, psychotherapy, or did it just spontaneously remit)?

Relate the depression to the stage of illness. When was this person first told he had schizophrenia?

Determine what the patient was told about the illness and what they believe about it.

Review his understanding of the illness and correct misconceptions and provide hope and reassurance that life will get better for him.

Address history of suicide attempts and suicidal thinking. Describe and update in every face-to-face meeting.

In every session, look for signs of and ask about symptoms of depression.

Use a depression rating scale, either one completed by clinicians or one filled out by patients (if you or he is good at filling out such things).

Respond empathically to the patient's depressive feelings and then do something immediately useful about it. For example, "Let's see if we can figure out what is causing this…did you get some news from your family or your attorney?"

Address bereavement reactions for all relevant losses, including losses due to the illness (e.g., help patient to process loss reactions from psychotic episodes).

Address interpersonal (prison, family) conflicts that lead to depression.

Give reassuring explanations. For example, "Now that you are over the psychosis, it is natural to feel a little bit down."

The End Is Insight

Prior to this section, we used the word "insight" on several occasions to refer to a commonly used concept that encompasses many possible aspects of this illness. As mentioned earlier, there are interventions using metacognition that also improve insight into psychosis. There are several scales, including self-report versions, for assessing insight in psychosis that can be used to augment your general impression of what you need to do to measure and report your patient's insight. An example is the VAGUS Insight into Psychosis Scale (Centre for Addiction and Mental Health 2014). This scale contains several simple and typical questions about your patients' illness and three open-ended questions about whether they believe they have a mental illness, whether they have experienced any negative consequences as a result of their symptoms, and whether they think they need treatment. Another article reviews the advantages and disadvantages of seven other scales or subscales, several of them self-rated (Casher and Bess 2012).

Medications

If you're a prescriber, you're already trained in the multiple issues involved, but if you're not, you may find yourself in disagreement with the prescriber if you think your patient is overmedicated or undermedicated. You do not have to stay in *agreement* with the prescriber, but you should try to stay in *touch* with him or her. You may also see various side effects such as tremors, hypersalivation, or a general restlessness called *akathisia* that can sometimes be caused by antipsychotics. Patients may even complain of a subjective restlessness that makes them extremely uncomfortable even though they do not show signs of physical restlessness. In addition to noticing side effects, you will still see the patient after medications have been changed, raised, lowered, or stopped. The meaning to your patient of changes in medication can provide you with essential information and is a fundamental issue in psychotherapy.

You're also in the position to notice premonitory symptoms of decompensation. As our examples suggest, these could include ideas of reference in a currently nonpsychotic patient. They could represent a mood change, which is certainly true in patients with schizoaffective disorder but also in patients with schizophrenia given the frequent co-occurrence of depression discussed earlier. However, many patients have their own warning signs, such as sudden onset of insomnia, worry, irritability, or social withdrawal.

Because of many patients' ambivalence about taking medication, and in particular their opposition to increases in medicine (most patients are happy to take less!), you may not want to argue with them about it or seem to be on the side of the prescriber. True, the prescriber should go through the risks and benefits of the medicine. But if you do feel obliged to refer the patient to the prescriber, a principle that is an "oldie but goodie" is to personalize the benefits for the patient (Diamond 1983). If the patient complains that she can't read her Bible at night, tell her that more medicine might help her to disregard her hallucinations and concentrate, or watch TV without thinking the announcer is talking about her. In other words, emphasize positive, personal benefits that are individualized for your patient's needs. We recognize that mental health works as a team and a psychotherapist is not the "prescriber's assistant," but everyone ought to work as team members.

Guidelines for nonprescribers in discussing medication are given in Table 8–9.

Challenges in Supportive Work With Seriously Mentally Ill Patients

The very success of supportive psychotherapy in enhancing the lives of patients with schizophrenia carries with it the risk of overinvestment in a particular patient to the point where you are not willing to let them go. There will be times when the proper treatment is a move to the infirmary or outside hospitalization, no matter how much you want to get your patient "over" his current psychotic exacerbation. Or you may find yourself spending excessive time with one particular patient even though there are others who seem to need you more.

Then, there is the downside of the work. Working with patients who have schizophrenia can be very difficult, and in particular with prisoners. Although prison systems give such patients a stable, if depleted and dangerous, environment, where medications and basic health care are available, it also deprives them of many of the benefits of mental health programming in the outside world, such as peer groups, family contact, meaningful jobs, and social development. The poor outcome for some patients can be disappointing, and it may even lead you to blame "the system" rather than the inherent course of the disease for the bad results. Or to blame yourself for not being a good-enough therapist. It is, indeed, often a tough disease for either patient or

TABLE 8–9.	Nonprescriber approaches to talking about medications

Determine within your treatment team the role you will play in discussing medications:

  None (refer all questions to the prescriber)

  Partial (answer some of patient's questions, e.g., does medication seem to be helping?)

  Major (discuss medication effects frequently)

Depending on your attitude above:

  Refer to prescriber or monitor as you see fit or feel comfortable:

    Benefits of medication.

    Personal benefits such as better sleep, less anxiety, or relief from torment of voices.

  Be concrete.

  Monitor adherence (casually and unobtrusively or indirectly: "You know, I've noticed that some of the guys are still cheeking their medicines so they can take them later in the night…").

Ask patient to describe his personal attitude toward medication (opposed, accepts, totally rejects).

Ask patient (using an item on an insight scale if you prefer) to describe her belief about the effectiveness of psychotropic medications.

Pay attention to symptoms of relapse (prodromal symptoms) and discuss or refer to prescriber.

Pay attention to changes of mood, not just psychosis, and treat with therapy and/or refer for antidepressants or mood stabilizers.

therapist to live with, and psychotherapy per se is frequently not the sole treatment, but medications are not 100% effective either. This can lead you to develop unrealistic expectations for your patient, if you assume they have learned the lessons you tried to "teach" them, and if so, you can expect to suffer inevitable disappointment when your teaching fails. You may also suffer from undue pessimism that makes you lose interest in your work as you assume your patients will make zero progress. You can begin to mirror the paranoia and depression of your patients and develop professional burnout as discussed in Chapter 4.

On the other hand, it can be very satisfying to work with such patients in prison, or even to make small steps in therapy with them. Because of the nature of the disease, however, you must be prepared for both the ups and downs of the illness. The challenges of supportive psychotherapy in schizophrenia and some suggestions for addressing them are listed Table 8–10.

For long-term patients, you may be interested in psychodynamic psychotherapy. Psychodynamic therapists and psychoanalysts saw psychotic patients all the time prior to the introduction of the antipsychotic medications. However, we have expressed our concerns about using explanations of the illness (or what they will call "interpretations") that we think are simply untrue. Others have warned that so-called insight-oriented psychotherapy can be too intrusive and lead to decompensation and regression (Drake and Sederer 1986), and even the classical psychodynamic therapists often wondered if their patients could drive their therapists into psychosis (Searles 1966). Quoted above on several occasions, Garrett (2019) details his work and success with using an overlapping combination of cognitive-behavioral therapy for psychosis and psychodynamic interpretation. But if you go that route, make sure you are qualified, and we also recommend that you have supervision.

TABLE 8–10.   **Challenges of using supportive therapy for schizophrenia in prison and strategies for dealing with them**

Challenge	Response
For the patient	**For the therapist**
Dangers of inappropriate intensive psychotherapy	Get to know your patient and employ explanations, but don't use psychodynamic interpretations unless you have the time, training, and supervision for this mode of therapy.
Increased depression; risk of suicide	Build in safety by seeking feedback from the patient about these issues and be able to offer extra support when needed.
Premature termination	Maintain appropriate distance; avoid overstimulation and intrusion into patient's life before such issues can be handled.
Countertransference problems	
Mirroring the patient's discouragement, depression, and hopelessness of a long prison term	You may find yourself losing the ability to "think normally" if you spend hours doing psychotherapy with illogical and delusional patients; to compensate, you should seek a mixed caseload that includes nonpsychotic patients.
Overinvolvement (e.g., via sympathy rather than empathy) and subsequent depression	Learn or relearn professional detachment and share feelings with supervisors or mental health group; if too intense, may have to "trade patients" (which creates separation issues with certain patients).
Unrealistic expectations	Understand the course of prognosis of the illness; in particular, become knowledgeable about negative symptoms and cognitive deficits in schizophrenia, and understand the problems caused by co-occurrence of criminal behavior.
Overly pessimistic expectations	Consider that pessimism may be a way of protecting yourself from doubts about your own competency; however, *pessimism can become self-fulfilling.*
Therapist burnout	Avoid staking your reputation on curing any one patient, and balance the challenges of your prison work with some enjoyable nonprofessional activities; refer to another provider if it is necessary for good care.

Key Points

- Connecting with persons who have schizophrenia or other psychotic conditions is one of the greatest challenges in psychotherapy.

- It is important to establish empathy, rapport, and a good relationship early in treatment.

- Severe mental illness or SMI, generally refers to diagnoses of schizophrenia, bipolar disorder, severe major depression, and sometimes other diagnoses.

- There has been a lot of talk about deinstitutionalization of the mentally ill from mental hospitals into the community., What mostly happened, however, is a movement of mentally ill persons into other institutions, including correctional systems, a process called *transintitutionalization*.

- Despite the impression that mental illness per se has been criminalized, the data say that mentally ill persons do commit crimes. However, there are better alternatives than putting them in prison.

- There is some association of violence with mental illness, but for the most part violent crimes are due to other factors and not a mentally ill state, and conversely a mentally ill state is not usually associated with violence (with some exceptions such as manic persons and severely delusional persons).

- Schizophrenia requires special attention. It is important to know the natural course of the illness and how patients deal with the various stages of illness, such as dealing with prodromal symptoms and recovering from a psychotic episode.

- Hallucinations as well as delusions can be "normalized" as a way of helping patients accept their experiences even if the therapist does not share the same "reality."

- You should time your interventions with the stages of the patient's illness (e.g., when the patient is in a "double-awareness" phase of the illness and is amenable to challenges of his delusions, or when the manic patient is in remission).

- Metacognitive therapy is a relatively new form of therapy that addresses deficits in "thinking about thinking."

- You should pay attention to your countertransference when treating patients who express serious symptoms.

- Despite your relative isolation in prison, you must be prepared to deal with family interactions that are often negative.

- Persons with schizophrenia can also have depression and other problems, including substance use disorder.

- Because of a high suicide rate, both lifetime and early in the illness, when the rate is even higher, suicidality must be addressed.

- You need to have a subtext of assessing for suicidality in all patients every time you see them, especially as it relates to depression (including depression in schizophrenia). Although a patient can become suicidal for the first time, knowing the history of suicide attempts can make it easier to design therapeutic interventions.

References

Alvarez-Jiménez M, González-Blanch C, Vázquez-Barquero JL, et al: Attenuation of antipsychotic-induced weight gain with early behavioral intervention in drug-naive first-episode psychosis patients: a randomized controlled trial. J Clin Psychiatry 67(8):1253–1260, 2006 16965204

Atlanta Legal Aid Society: Olmstead Rights: Olmstead v. LC: history and current status. 2020. Available at: www.olmsteadrights.org/about-olmstead. Accessed June 4, 2020.

Arieti S: Interpretation of Schizophrenia, 2nd Edition. New York, Basic Books, 1974

Badre N, Lehman D: Criminals in the psychiatric ED. Clinical Psychiatry News 47(9):7, September 2019

Balzan RP, Mattiske JK, Delfabbro P, et al: Individualized metacognitive training (MCT+) reduces delusional symptoms in psychosis: a randomized clinical trial. Schizophr Bull 45(1):27–36, 2019 30376124

Batastini A, Morgan RD, Kroner DG, Mills JF: Mental Health Treating Program for Inmates in Restrictive Housing: Stepping Up, Stepping Out. New York, Taylor & Francis, 2019

Batastini AB, Hill JB, Repke A, et al: Approaching correctional treatment from a programmatic standpoint: Risk-Need-Responsivity and beyond, in The Practice of Correctional Psychology. Edited by Ternes M, Magaletta P, Patry M. New York, Springer, 2018, pp 283–303

Bellack AS, Morrison RL, Mueser KT: Social problem solving in schizophrenia. Schizophr Bull 15(1):101–116, 1989 2655067

Bellack AS, Mueser KT, Gingerich S, Agresta J: Social Skills Training for Schizophrenia: A Step-by-Step Guide, 2nd Edition. New York, Guilford, 2004

Bolden KA, Choo How P, Rao S, Anglin DM: Social injustice and schizophrenia, in Social Injustice and Mental Health. Edited by Shim RS, Vinson SY. Washington, DC, American Psychiatric Association Publishing, 2021, pp 157–170

Bonfine N, Wilson AB, Munetz MR: Meeting the needs of justice-involved people with serious mental illness within community behavioral health systems. Psychiatr Serv 71(4):355–363, 2020, 31795858

Braham LG, Trower P, Birchwood M: Acting on command hallucinations and dangerous behavior: a critique of the major findings in the last decade. Clin Psychol Rev 24(5):513–528, 2004, 15325743

Brent B: Mentalization-based psychodynamic psychotherapy for psychosis. J Clin Psychol 65(8):803–814, 2009 19572277

Bronson J, Maruschak LM, Berzofsky M: Disabilities Among Prison and Jail Inmates 2011–2012. NCJ 249151. Washington, DC, Bureau of Justice Statistics, December 2015. Available at: www.bjs.gov/content/pub/pdf/dpji1112.pdf. Accessed June 27, 2020.

Buckley LA, Maayan N, Soares-Weiser K, Adams CE: Supportive therapy for schizophrenia. Cochrane Database Syst Rev April 14; 2015(4):CD004716, 2015 25871462

Casher MI, Bess JD: Determination and documentation of insight in psychiatric inpatients. Psychiatric Times 29(4):1–6, April 2, 2012. Available at: www.psychiatrictimes.com/view/determination-and-documentation-insight-psychiatric-inpatients. Accessed June 18, 2020.

Centre for Addiction and Mental Health: VAGUS Insight into Psychosis Scale. Toronto, Ontario, Canada, Centre for Addiction and Mental Health, 2014. Available at: www.vagusonline.com/#:~:text=The%20VAGUS%20was%20designed%20to%20assess%20clinical%20insight,psychotic%20features%2C%20such%20as%20bipolar%20disorder%20or%20depressio. Accessed September 6, 2020.

Chaiken S, Shull J: Mental health treatment of inmates in segregation housing, in Correctional Psychiatry: Practice Guidelines and Strategies. Edited by Thienhaus OJ, Piasecki M. Kingston, NJ, Civic Research Institute, 2007, pp 18-1–18-19

Cohen CI, Berk LA: Personal coping styles of schizophrenic outpatients. Hosp Community Psychiatry 36(4):407–410, 1985 3997104

De Hert M, Correll CU, Bobes J, et al: Physical illness in patients with severe mental disorders. I. Prevalence, impact of medications and disparities in health care. World Psychiatry 10(1):52–77, 2011 21379357

Diamond RJ: Enhancing medication use in schizophrenic patients. J Clin Psychiatry 44(6, Pt 2):7–14, 1983 6133855

Drake RE, Sederer LI: The adverse effects of intensive treatment of chronic schizophrenia. Compr Psychiatry 27(4):313–326, 1986 2873959

Dudley R, Brabban A, Turkington D: Cognitive behavioural therapy for psychosis, in Psychotherapeutic Approaches to Schizophrenic Psychosis. Edited by Alanan YO, De Chávez M, Silver A-L, Martindale B. New York, Taylor & Francis, 2009, pp 267–287

Dumond RW, Dumond DA: Mentally disabled inmates—concerns for correctional managers, in Managing Special Populations in Jails and Prisons, Vol II. Edited by Stojkovic S. Kingston, NJ, Civic Research Institute, 2010, pp 5-1–5-45

Evans S, Newton R, Higgins S: Nutritional intervention to prevent weight gain in patients commenced on olanzapine: a randomized controlled trial. Aust N Z J Psychiatry 39(6):479–486, 2005 15943650

Firth J, Torous J: Smartphone apps for schizophrenia: a systematic review. JMIR Mhealth Uhealth 3(4):e102, 2015, 26546039

Fluent TE: How best to engage patients in their psychiatric care. Curr Psychiatr 12(9):22–36, 2013

Frances A: Ignoring mental health infrastructure will be a costly mistake. Stat. July 9, 2021. Available at: www.statnews.com/2021/07/09/ignoring-mental-health-infrastructure-costly-mistake. Accessed July 11, 2021.

Frank AF, Gunderson JG: The role of the therapeutic alliance in the treatment of schizophrenia. Relationship to course and outcome. Arch Gen Psychiatry 47(3):228–236, 1990 1968329

Garrett M: Psychotherapy for Psychosis: Integrating Cognitive-Behavioral and Psychodynamic Treatment. New York, Guilford, 2019

Geller J: The rise and demise of America's psychiatric hospitals: a tale of dollars trumping sense, Part 2. Psychiatric News 64(6):11, 23, March 15, 2019

Goomany A, Dickinson T: The influence of prison climate on the mental health of adult prisoners: a literature review. J Psychiatr Ment Health Nurs 22(6):413–422, 2015 26122924

Granholm EL, McQuaid JR, Holden JL: Cognitive-Behavioral Social Skills Training for Schizophrenia: A Practical Treatment Guide. New York, Guilford, 2016

Grummisch J, Wright N: Treating psychosis. 2021. Available at: www.treatingpsychosis.com. Accessed February 17, 2021.

Haney C: The psychological impact of incarceration: implications for post-prison adjustment, in From Prison to Home: The Effect of Incarceration and Reentry on Children, Families, and Communities. U.S. Department of Health and Human Services, Office of the Assistant Secretary for Planning and Evaluation, January 2002. Available at: https://aspe.hhs.gov/reports/prison-home-effect-incarceration-reentry-children-families-communities. Accessed June 25, 2020.

Hare R: Psychopathy and crime: a review, in Clinical Approaches to the Mentally Disordered Offender. Edited by Howells K, Hollin CR. New York, Wiley, 1993, pp 165–178

Hellerstein D, Frosch W, Koenigsberg HW: The clinical significance of command hallucinations. Am J Psychiatry 144(2):219–221, 1987 3812793

Hodgins S, Klein S: Severe mental illness: crime, antisocial and aggressive behavior, in The Wiley International Handbook of Correctional Psychology. Edited by Polaschek DLL, Day A, Hollin CR. Hoboken, NJ, Wiley, 2019, pp 251–264

Inchausti F, García-Poveda N, Ballesteros-Prados A, et al: The effects of metacognition-oriented social skills training on psychosocial outcomes in schizophrenia-spectrum disorders: a randomized controlled trial. Schizophr Bull 44(6):1235–1244, 2017a 29267940

Inchausti F, Garcia-Poveda NV, Prado-Abril J, et al: Metacognition-oriented social skills training (MOSST): theoretical framework, working methodology and treatment descriptions for patients with schizophrenia. Psychologists Papers 38(1):204–215, 2017b

Ison R, Medoro L, Keen N, Kuipers E: The use of rescripting imagery for people with psychosis who hear voices. Behav Cogn Psychother 42(2):129–142, 2014 23920004

Jenner JA: Hallucination-Focused Integrative Therapy: A Specific Treatment That Hits Auditory Verbal Hallucinations. London, Routledge, 2016

Judges & Psychiatrists Leadership Initiative, APA Foundation, Council of State Governments Justice Center: Supporting People With Serious Mental Illness and Reducing Their Risk of Contact With the Criminal Justice System: A Primer for Psychiatrists. New York, Council of State Governments, September 2017. Available at: https://csgjusticecenter.org/publications/supporting-people-with-serious-mental-illnesses-and-reducing-their-risk-of-contact-with-the-criminal-justice-system/#:~:text=With%20input%20from%20leading%20clinical%20and%20forensic%20psychiatrists%2C,serious%20mental%20illnesses%20and%20a%20criminal%20justice%20history. Accessed July 11, 2021.

Junginger J: Predicting compliance with command hallucinations. Am J Psychiatry 147(2):245–247, 1990 2301669

Kingdon DG, Turkington D: Cognitive Therapy of Schizophrenia. New York, Guilford, 2004

Lamb HR, Weinberger LE: Some perspectives on criminalization. J Am Acad Psychiatry Law 41(2):287–293, 2013 23771942

Lewis S, Tarrier N, Haddock G, et al: Randomised controlled trial of cognitive-behavioural therapy in early schizophrenia: acute-phase outcomes. Br J Psychiatry Suppl 43:s91–s97, 2002 12271807

Liberman RP (ed): Psychiatric Rehabilitation of Chronic Mental Patients. Washington, DC, American Psychiatric Press, 1988

Liberman RP, Massel HK, Mosk MD, et al: Social skills training for chronic mental patients. Hosp Community Psychiatry 36(4):396–403, 1985 3997101

Linardon J: Can smartphone apps improve your mental health? Break Binge Eating. Oct.16, 2019. Available at: https://breakbingeeating.com/mental-health-apps/#Do_mental_health_apps_work. Accessed July 11, 2021.

Living with Schizophrenia: Depression and schizophrenia. 2016. Available at: https://living-withschizophreniauk.org/information-sheets/depression-and-schizophrenia/#:~:text=In%20fact%20some%20experts%20maintain%20that%20the%20majority,15%25%20of%20people%20in%20the%20general%20population.%203. Accessed November 20, 2020.

Lynch D, Laws KR, McKenna PJ: Cognitive behavioural therapy for major psychiatric disorder: does it really work? A meta-analytical review of well-controlled trials. Psychol Med 40(1):9–24, 2010 19476688

Lysaker PH, Dimaggio G: Metacognitive capacities for reflection in schizophrenia: implications for developing treatments. Schizophr Bull 40(3):487–491, 2014 24636965

Manchak SM, Morgan RD: Offenders with mental illness in prison, in The Oxford Handbook of Prisons and Imprisonment. Edited by Wooldredge J, Smith P. New York, Oxford University Press, 2018, pp 579–600

McGlashan TH, Levy ST, Carpenter WT Jr: Integration and sealing over: clinically distinct recovery styles from schizophrenia. Arch Gen Psychiatry 32(10):1269–1272, 1975 1180660

Meaden A, Van Marle S: When the going gets tougher: the importance of long-term supportive psychotherapy in psychosis. Adv Psychiatr Treat 14:42–49, 2008

Mental Illness Policy Org: What is "serious mental illness" and what is not? 2020. Available at: https://mentalillnesspolicy.org/serious-mental-illness-not. Accessed June 4, 2020.

Milne D, Wharton S, James I, Turkington D: Befriending versus CBT for schizophrenia: a convergent and divergent fidelity check. Behav Cogn Psychother 34(1):25–31, 2006

Mitchell AJ, Malone D: Physical health and schizophrenia. Curr Opin Psychiatry 19(4):432–437, 2006 16721177

Morin R: Learning to live with the voices in your head. The Atlantic, November 5, 2014. Available at: www.theatlantic.com/health/archive/2014/11/learning-to-live-with-the-voices-in-your-head/382096. Accessed February 5, 2021.

Morgan RD, Kroner DG, Mills Jeremy F: Changing Lives and Changing Outcomes: A Treatment Manual for Justice Involved Persons With Mental Illness. New York, Routledge, 2018

Mulholland C, Cooper S: The symptom of depression in schizophrenia and its management. Adv Psychiatr Treat 6(3):169–177, 2000

NAMI (National Alliance on Mental Illness): Responding to Crises. 2019. Available at: www.nami.org/Learn-More/Public-Policy/Jailing-People-with-Mental-Illness. Accessed November 10, 2019.

National Institute of Mental Health: Mental illness. 2021. Available at: www.nimh.nih.gov/health/statistics/mental-illness. Accessed February 17, 2021.

Northern Ohio Universities Colleges of Medicine and Pharmacy: Best Practices in Schizophrenia Treatment (BeST) Center List of 60 Coping Strategies for Hallucinations, Available at: https://southbayprojectresourcedotorg.files.wordpress.com/2015/09/list-of-60-coping-strategies-for-hallucinations.pdf. Accessed June 26, 2020.

Nott L: iPhone app helps schizophrenics block voices. Mental Health, August 7, 2013. Available at: www.elementsbehavioralhealth.com/mental-health/iphone-app-helps-schizophrenics-block-voices. Accessed January 31, 2020.

Novalis PN, Singer V, Peele R: Clinical Manual of Supportive Psychotherapy, 2nd Edition. Washington, DC, American Psychiatric Association Publishing, 2020

Opoka SM, Lincoln TM: The effect of cognitive behavioral interventions on depression and anxiety symptoms in patients with schizophrenia spectrum disorders: a systematic review. Psychiatr Clin North Am 40(4):641–659, 2017 29080591

Penn DL, Mueser KT, Tarrier N, et al: Supportive therapy for schizophrenia: possible mechanisms and implications for adjunctive psychosocial treatments. Schizophr Bull 30(1):101–112, 2004 15176765

Pesek MB: Therapy and quality of life of patients with psychosis. Psychiatr Danub 21(Suppl 1):146–148, 2009 19789502

Pratt S, Bennett M, Brunette MF: Co-occurring disorders and conditions, in The American Psychiatric Association Publishing Textbook of Schizophrenia, 2nd Edition. Edited by Lieberman JA, Stroup TS, Perkins DO, Dixon LB. Washington, DC, American Psychiatric Association Publishing, 2020, pp 205–249

Prins SJ: Prevalence of mental illnesses in US State prisons: a systematic review. Psychiatr Serv 65(7):862–872, 2014, 24686574

Robinson DJ: My favorite tips for exploring difficult topics such as delusions or substance abuse. Psychiatr Clin North Am 30(2):239–244, 2007 17643840

Romme M, Escher S, Dillon J, et al: Living With Voices: 50 Stories of Recovery. Herefordshire, UK, PCCS Books, 2013

Rosenbaum B, Harder S, Knudsen P, et al: Supportive psychodynamic psychotherapy versus treatment as usual for first-episode psychosis: two-year outcome. Psychiatry 75(4):331–341, 2012 23244011

Rudden M, Gilmore M, Frances A: Delusions: when to confront the facts of life. Am J Psychiatry 139(7):929–932, 1982 6979944

Sacks MH, Carpenter WT Jr, Strauss JS: Recovery from delusions: three phases documented by patient's interpretation of research procedures. Arch Gen Psychiatry 30(1):117–120, 1974 4808730

Sansone RA, Sansone LA: Borderline personality and criminality. Psychiatry (Edgmont) 6(10):16–20, 2009 20011575

Sarti P, Cournos F: Medication and psychotherapy in the treatment of chronic schizophrenia. Psychiatr Clin North Am 13(2):215–228, 1990 1972273

Scheyer R, Reznik N, Apter A, et al: Metacognition in non-psychotic help-seeking adolescents: associations with prodromal symptoms, distress and psychosocial deterioration. Isr J Psychiatry Relat Sci 51(1):34–43, 2014 24858633

Schweitzer RD, Greben M, Bargenquast R: Long-term outcomes of metacognitive narrative psychotherapy for people diagnosed with schizophrenia. Psychol Psychother 90(4):668–685, 2017 28544223

Searles H: Collected Papers on Schizophrenia and Related Subjects. Madison, CT, International Universities Press, 1966

Sensky T, Turkington D, Kingdon D, et al: A randomized controlled trial of cognitive-behavioral therapy for persistent symptoms in schizophrenia resistant to medication. Arch Gen Psychiatry 57(2):165–172, 2000 10665619

Shaikh-Lesko R: Imagining voices: a look at an alternative approach to treating auditory hallucinations. Stanford Medicine Scope, November 13, 2014

Skeem JL, Winter E, Kennealy PJ, et al: Offenders with mental illness have criminogenic needs, too: toward recidivism reduction. Law and Human Behavior 38(3):212-224, 2014 24377913

Skelton M, Khokhar WA, Thacker SP: Treatments for delusional disorder. Cochrane Database Syst Rev (5):CD009785, 2015 DOI: 10.1002/14651858.CD009785.pub2 25997589

Smith B: Helpful hints about schizophrenia for family members and others. PsychCentral, October 8, 2018. Available at: https://psychcentral.com/lib/helpful-hints-about-schizophrenia-for-family-members-and-others. Accessed January 31, 2019.

Smits CT, van der Gaag M: Cognitieve gedragstherapie bij schizofrenie [Cognitive behavioural therapy for schizophrenia] (in Dutch). Tijdschr Psychiatr 52(2):99–109, 2010 20146181

Spaulding WD, Silverstein SM, Menditto AA: The Schizophrenia Spectrum, 2nd Edition. Boston, MA, Hogrefe Publishing, 2017

Stanford Justice Advocacy Project: The Prevalence and Severity of Mental Illness Among California Prisons on the Rise. Stanford, CA, Stanford Justice Advocacy Project, 2017. Available at: https://www-cdn.law.stanford.edu/wp-content/uploads/2017/05/Stanford-Report-FINAL.pdf. Accessed June 5, 2020.

Substance Abuse and Mental Health Services Administration: Illness Management and Recovery: Practitioner Guides and Handouts. DHHS Publ No. SMA-09-4462. Rockville, MD, Center for Mental Health Services, Substance Abuse and Mental Health Services Administration, U.S. Department of Health and Human Services, 2009

Substance Abuse and Mental Health Services Administration: Recovery and recovery support. Updated April 23, 2020. Available at: www.samhsa.gov/find-help/recovery. Accessed November 28, 2020.

Taylor MA: Are schizophrenia and affective disorder related? A selective literature review. Am J Psychiatry 149(1):22–32, 1992 1728181

Torrey EF: Management of chronic schizophrenic outpatients. Psychiatr Clin North Am 9(1):143–151, 1986 2870477

Torous J, Keshavan M: The role of social media in schizophrenia: evaluating risks, benefits, and potential. Curr Opin Psychiatry 29(3):190–195, 2016 26967314

Treatment Advocacy Center: Serious mental illness prevalence in jails and prison. September 2016. Available at: www.treatmentadvocacycenter.org/evidence-and-research/learn-more-about/3695. Accessed June 4, 2011.

University of Hertfordshire: Cognitive therapy is of no value in schizophrenia, analysis of studies suggests. ScienceDaily, June 26, 2009. Available at: www.sciencedaily.com/releases/2009/06/090625074512.htm. Accessed July 20, 2020.

Ventriglio A, Gentile A, Bonfitto I, et al: Suicide in the early stage of schizophrenia. Front Psychiatry 7:116, 2016 27445872

Vohs JL, Leonhardt BL, James AV, et al: Metacognitive reflection and insight therapy for early psychosis: a preliminary study of a novel integrative psychotherapy. Schizophr Res 195:428–433, 2018 29108671

White J: Federation World. New York, Ballantine Books, 1988

Winklbaur B, Ebner N, Sachs G, et al: Substance abuse in patients with schizophrenia. Dialogues Clin Neurosci 8(1):37–43, 2006 16640112

Wright NP, Turkington D, Kelly OP, et al: Treating Psychosis: A Clinician's Guide to Integrating Acceptance & Commitment Therapy, Compassion-Focused Therapy and Mindfulness Approaches Within the Cognitive Behavior Therapy Tradition. Oakland, CA, New Harbinger Publications, 2014

9

Mood Disorders

The mood disorders we discuss here mostly fall in the serious mental illness (SMI) group, especially bipolar disorder. In the case of depression, however, it is common to assign a severity to episodes of an illness or the course of illness. Therefore, mildly depressed individuals may not be in the SMI category, although most moderately depressed and all severely depressed individuals will probably be included.

A recent study by Zimmerman (2019) on the ubiquitous Patient Health Questionnaire–9 (PHQ-9) has had a significant effect on the assignment of a severity measurement. The author showed that the PHQ-9 underdiagnoses mild depression and overdiagnoses severe depression. The author says that the PHQ-9 can still be used to measure progress in therapy but emphasizes that the clinical interview should not be used as the basis for the severity measurement. We think this is especially important in corrections, where being placed in an SMI category can have major implications for treatment.

As for the evidence basis for supportive psychotherapy: There is no recent Cochrane review of psychological therapies for adult depression. Ijaz and colleagues (2018), in their Cochrane review of psychological therapies for treatment-resistant depression, did not examine supportive psychotherapy, but they did find that the psychotherapies studied were equally effective. Supportive therapy came to clinicians' attention when it showed effectiveness even as a minimalist placebo–clinical management treatment condition in the National Institute of Mental Health Treatment of Depression Collaborative Research Program study (Elkin et al. 1989). More recent evidence is readily available (Jacobs and Reupert 2014). Various forms of short-term psychodynamic psychotherapy (STPP), which includes both supportive and expressive elements, were evaluated in a meta-analysis and found to be effective in the treatment of depression (Driessen et al. 2010), and the supportive and expressive modes of STPP were found to be equally effective. For adolescents, there is also a positive study of STPP (Dil et al. 2016) and other positive studies for specific subcategories of depressed persons. Note that we do believe that depression, especially if severe or psychotic, requires consideration of somatic treatments as well as psychotherapy. We remind you of a study showing that cognitive therapy is ineffective in schizophrenia, because that study also showed that it was of minimal effectiveness in depression (Lynch et al. 2010;

University of Hertfordshire 2009). Despite its widespread use, and certainly its use in programs to prevent recidivism, there are disadvantages of cognitive therapy. For example, it is not effective with many unmotivated, illogical patients and has decreased effectiveness in depressed patients with social dysfunction (Sotsky et al. 1991).

There are many similarities between supportive psychotherapy and interpersonal psychotherapy (IPT). IPT employs elucidation of psychic conflicts only when necessary, preferentially using education, antidemoralization measures, social manipulations, and problem-solving techniques. Therapists are specifically trained to be supportive but not overly active or directive (Klerman et al. 1984; Rousanville et al. 1984). In a major meta-analysis that compared several psychotherapies, including cognitive-behavioral therapy (CBT), nondirective supportive treatment, and interpersonal psychotherapy, IPT was found to be somewhat more efficacious, but the nondirective therapy they used would naturally be less efficacious than the directive therapies we advocate here (Cuijpers et al. 2008). Therefore, it did not surprise us (since it was several years in the making) that there was finally a large study of IPT for depressed prisoners (Johnson et al. 2019). A cost-effective group IPT treatment (provided by trained master's-level nonspecialists) improved time to remission of major depression as measured by Quick Inventory of Depression scores. But you need to pay attention to the other measures in the study. The treatment did not improve time to recovery. The study also investigated, specifically because of their importance, many important variables in prison life, namely:

- Suicidal ideation assessed directly
- Aggression and victimization
- Correctional programs started and completed
- Discipline and incident reports
- Time spent in punishment/isolation
- Perceived social support
- Reported loneliness
- Other prison services

That is a long list, and *none of the items on that list were improved by the treatment*. So this study is an impetus to learn more about IPT, but we would not say that it affected all the variables that are important for psychotherapy in prison. In fact, the above is a good list of the items you should consider when you do supportive psychotherapy for depression in prison. However, the positive findings in the study have increased our interest in the components of interpersonal therapy that make it especially suitable for persons undergoing role transitions as in the transition into prison. Thus, "IPT identifies a current interpersonal crisis in one of four areas (an interpersonal dispute, a change in life circumstances, grief, or social isolation) as the proximal trigger for the current depressive episode and addresses it by helping the individual to improve communication, change relationship expectations, or adapt to changes within the context of building or better utilizing a social support network" (Johnson et al. 2019, p. 393).

It is likely that psychotherapy is synergistic to medication and may improve a different set of symptoms than does pharmacotherapy. In addition to IPT, therapies that embrace some supportive measures include social learning (Lewinsohn et al. 1980), social skills (Hersen et al. 1984), self-control and reward programs (Rehm 1984), behavioral activation (Tull 2020), and, as we have emphasized in Chapter 1, positive psychology (Seligman 2002; see also the references in Chapter 1). An instructive early version of supportive therapy for depression was developed by Hollon (1962), who described a short-term psychotherapy that utilized a "maximum activity program" with a log of daily activities, attention to food, and a detailed recollection of the patient's life history that was used to enhance the patient's reality testing. The express aim was to create gratifying work that would displace the patient's attention from his or her depression. Modern versions of these techniques can be recognized in cognitive therapy, in logs for behavioral activation (Schuldt 2019), and in several of the supportive techniques mentioned later.

Well-Being Therapy

We would like to highlight one particular therapy that developed independently on a parallel track to positive psychology and is now in the positive psychology sphere. It is called *well-being therapy* (WBT), and we introduce it because of its simplicity, accessibility, and adjunctive applicability to any other therapy. WBT has been elaborated over some years by Giovanni Fava (Fava 2016), who reports that it had two sources (Jahoda 1958; Ryff 1989). Jahoda named six criteria for mental health that were further explored by Ryff: autonomy, environmental mastery, positive interpersonal relationships, person growth, purpose in life, and self-acceptance. Ryff developed psychological well-being scales to measure these characteristics. WBT seeks to develop these areas of a patient's life. Backdating his own therapy, as we did supportive psychotherapy, to the Ancient Greeks, Fava finds affinity with another Ancient Greek concept, *euthymia*, which meant "good soul" (we use modern derivatives such as *dysthymia* to mean "unhappy mood") (Fava and Guidi 2020). The other concept we invoked in Chapter 1 was *eudaemonia*, or "good spirit." Unlike the interventions of positive psychology that address fairly well or normal (nonpatient) populations, WBT was developed by Fava as an add-on therapy for persons who did not respond to cognitive therapy. In fact, and not coincidentally, the foreword to Fava's book was written by Jesse Wright, whom you may recall is an international expert on cognitive therapy cited in Chapter 3. Wright and his daughter, Laura McCray, wrote a self-help book incorporating WBT methods that includes reproducible handouts (Wright and McCray 2011).

Fava's impetus for developing WBT was his realization that cognitive therapy trained its users to recognize negative aspects of their lives and minimize them. WBT looks instead at the positive qualities of a patient's life and seeks to maximize them. A basic eight-session program is presented in Fava's handbook (Fava 2016). In each session the patient presents his 2-week diary in which he records four items: the situation, well-being (rated 1 to 100), interfering thoughts and behaviors, and (in later sessions) an observational comment. Even the eight-session plan can be adjusted to need, and in fact when we use WBT techniques we often draw a grid with the four categories above and ask for positive experiences in the next session. WBT has been used mostly for depression, anxiety, and cyclothymic disorder.

Supportive Psychotherapy for Mood Disorders

Supportive psychotherapy approaches to several disorders with affective components are summarized in Table 9–1. As the table indicates, there are several diagnoses in the mood area that we have already discussed in various chapters of this book. We have learned that prisoners can suffer may kinds of mood disorders, ranging from the ones they bring with them to the facility and the ones they develop after arrival. Table 9–2 presents more strategies for the treatment of depressive disorders in prison.

Supportive psychotherapy also has an important role in treating depressed patients with other psychiatric problems or those who deny or somatize their illness, and in working with medically ill patients. We have also mentioned the potential need for adjunctive medication, but in addition the most available somatic treatment for mildly to moderately depressed prisoners (if medically clear for such) is now thought to be exercise. "While there has been some controversy, the most recent systematic reviews suggest large effects of supervised, moderate intensity aerobic exercise to decrease depressive symptoms, compared to no treatment, and a moderate effect in comparison to TAU [treatment as usual]" (Cowen 2020, p. 809, citing Kvam et al. 2016).

In prison, depressed patients present in many ways. They may be self-referred, directed from the intake assessment, or sent by medical providers who find them anxious in their offices, or by correctional staff. If self-referred, they may be anxiously seeking relief and pinning all their hopes on you; or perhaps they just want a referral for sedatives and don't care one whit about talk therapy. Patients who don't want to be seen may parade their irritability and defensiveness.

Supportive interventions are good for patients who passively express helplessness and do not volunteer information. They may not need a lot of time, and (except as provided in your department rules of service) can often be helped with very brief interventions. Mood-congruent psychotic features (e.g., delusions of worthlessness or persecution) are generally not worth challenging directly at first but can be worked with in the ways we previously described for psychotic patients (see Chapter 8).

On previous occasions we have talked about dealing with patients who appear for therapy but have medical complaints. When you are treating depression, it should be remembered that *somatic complaints* are fundamental to the DSM-5-TR definition of depression and that somatic complaints should be taken seriously and addressed as were the medical complaints we described for patients with schizophrenia. However, with a patient who is also depressed, somatic complaints should be clarified (since they are a fundamental part of the illness in these patients), and discussion of the complaints can be useful as a displacement from more painful psychological issues.

Primary Techniques and Emphases in the Treatment of Depression

Giving Reassurance

A starting point for many patients, cooperative or not, is the giving of appropriate hope and reassurance. Regardless of whether patients are living in a prison or at home, they can be told that there is light at the end of the tunnel and that their depression will probably be of finite duration. We are talking not about giving reassurances about prison terms or outside problems, but simply about emphasizing that they have an illness and that it can be treated and that they will likely recover. Initially this reassurance may be rejected but they will remember it when the recovery process begins. To bypass the conscious rejection of reassurance, some therapists have effectively used

TABLE 9–1. Supportive psychotherapy approaches to disorders with affective components

Disorder	Major defense mechanisms	Immediate source of disturbance	Effect on self-esteem	Supportive approach to treatment
Grief	Normal defenses typical for the individual (at times exaggerated); denial	Extrinsic	Traditionally said to be intact	Environmental supports, providing time perspective for self-healing and development of new social relationships (see Chapter 5)
Depression or adjustment disorder with depressed mood	Introjection of ambivalently regarded love object; regression or fixation at oral stage of development	Sometimes extrinsic (i.e., exogenous depression or adjustment disorder), but usually involving endogenous biological and genetic factors, especially if patient has bipolar disorder	Acutely decreased	Improvement of self-esteem; improvement of cognitive and interpersonal processes to prevent depressive reactions to life events; displacement of aggression into reinforcing activities, often as adjunct to biological treatments (see Chapter 6)
Persistent depressive disorder	Defective defenses and coping capacity in a stable self	Mostly intrinsic (i.e., life history and genetic factors)	Chronically low	Restructuring dysfunctional defenses and counteracting chronically learned helplessness with improved coping strategies
Borderline personality disorder	Splitting and other primitive defenses in an inadequately matured self	Mostly intrinsic (i.e., poor parenting, early trauma, some genetic association to mood disorders)	Defectively and unrealistically regulated; dependent on external supports	Limit setting; controlled provision of a gratifying primary object relationship; confrontations of dysfunctional behavior; improvement of skills in controlling impulsive behavior (see Chapter 10)
Mania	Denial and grandiosity, possibly as defenses against underlying depression and low self-esteem	Intrinsic (i.e., strong genetic factors)	Increased, but may oscillate dramatically in mixed states	In acute manic state, limit setting and protection from destructive acts; as manic state subsides, compliance issues, defense mechanisms, and personality dysfunction can be addressed

---

TABLE 9–2.   **Treating the depressed patient in prison**

Know your patient's history and risk factors for suicide (what suicide attempts did your patient have in the past?).

Reiterate your ongoing advice about suicide prevention ("Tell your therapist or another medical worker or the corrections officer when you are feeling like you may harm yourself").

Despite the potential for malingering, at the start, take the patient's distress at face value.

Educate about the biological aspects of illness (i.e., "It's a chemical imbalance").

Provide educational materials or journals.

Instill hope that the depression will get better rather than last "forever," as many patients feel it will ("There is light at the end of tunnel").

Divide and conquer (address multiple "subcomplaints" separately).

Deal with bereavement not only about death but also about losses from the transition to prison.

Discuss medication issues, efficacy, and side effects (as you see fit and are qualified if you are not the prescriber; you may actually be more credible because you are not the prescriber).

Counter feelings of self-blame and responsibility for the depression.

Counsel patient not to make major decisions while depressed.

Prevent blaming and "bridge burning" with family and other prisoners (e.g., accusing them of putting them in prison, displacing anger by "telling off" other prisoners).

Cautiously and judiciously improve social support from family, other prisoners, and staff (ask patient who they think can help and discuss when and how to ask others for help).

Tell patient not to be so hard on themselves (counter temporary reductions in self-esteem associated with the depression).

While enhancing self-esteem, temporarily put on hold your anticriminogenic talk and agendas ("Now is not a good time to deal with those issues, but we will get to them later").

---

metaphorical reassurance (Barker 1985). Of course, these days there are a lot of analogies and metaphors related to the COVID-19 pandemic, and here is an example of the kind of talk we give:

> Depression can be a serious problem, maybe even a mental equivalent of COVID-19. When someone gets the virus, they may not be able to do the ordinary things of life, and sometimes they can't even breathe for themselves and require a ventilator, but with proper treatment they can recover their full function. So don't worry about your limitations now. When your depression improves, you will have your energy back again to do the things you used to do.

This analogy can be used as their rationale for delaying precipitous decisions as well as warding off suicidal actions. Also well known are the memory complaints found in depression, which are usually a reason to delay a formal workup: "Sure, we can test your memory (and we can do a quick test), but depressed people often forget things, and it would probably be better to wait until you are less depressed." A good resource to discuss, by Scaccia (2019), can be found online. We must note, however, that memory and somatic complaints have proliferated in the aftermath of the COVID-19 pandemic and have become associated with prolonged symptoms, often called "long COVID," and as of our writing are being investigated in specialized neurological clinics.

Reassurances should not be far from the patient's own beliefs and feelings and may need to be softened with statements like, "You might find this hard to believe, but...[give the reassurance here]." Reassurance should not be automatic; rather, it should be based on an assessment of compatibility with the patient's sentence, level of function, and future prospects. But do note that giving reassurance can be hurtful if is patronizing or clearly false. We do like the positive psychology interventions, but they should be based on what is possible for the prisoner in his or her life and not something unrealistic.

Facilitating Medication

Much has been written on medication for depression. If you're a prescriber as well as a psychotherapist, by all means follow your protocols. We'll limit this to a discussion of what to do when medication is offered by a prescriber other than yourself. You'll have to decide the position you want to take on medication: Are you in favor of your patient taking it? Should she be told to tolerate minor or even major side effects in the hope of achieving remission? Did the prescriber address any guilt and fears of addiction or dependency at having to take medication? What attitude did the prescriber convey about the effectiveness of medications? Did he say that antidepressants are always or usually or sometimes effective, or did he waffle on that point? By the way, we do encourage positive expectations and even anticipate a placebo effect when taking medication. Also consider that concerns about medication may be a displacement of concerns about the patient's relationship with you—the therapist. Scorn or derision about the medication may reflect negativity about therapy as well. Ask your patient to clarify.

Addressing Guilt

Many prisoners have guilt about being in prison or the things they did that got them there, including injury to victims in the family or strangers. But keep in mind that they can feel guilty simply about being depressed or taking medication. When they are depressed, you may need to boost their self-esteem and dispel self-accusatory modes of thought, even though usual therapy sessions may target criminal thinking styles and defensive rationalizations for behavior. You don't have to be a hypocrite about this duality; just tell your patient that "now is not the time for morbid thought—that's your depression talking." Silences (used somewhat in psychodynamic psychotherapies) should be avoided in supportive psychotherapy with depressed patients, and if you find a silence that seems to connote guilt, you should discuss it. The patient who does not feel like conversing may feel additional guilt in not holding up her side of the conversation. Hopelessness and failure are common themes in depression. Interestingly, the strongest outcome measure of the Johnson et al. (2019) study mentioned earlier was on the Beck Hopelessness Scale.

Address metacognition—the same type of measure discussed in the previous chapter about schizophrenia. The patient's "depression about depression" needs to be addressed, and the patient needs to be counseled to disconnect the pessimistic meanings attached to depressed feelings. Depression frequently involves a masochistic component, and, without attempt to explain a masochistic defense, it is supportive and consistent to tell depressed patients that "Now is not the time to take it out on yourself."

Managing Dependency

You can allow some dependence with depressed patients, but you must also set limits to it. Some patients evoke a strong countertransference irritation because of their obsessive ruminations or clinging behaviors. Others stir up a profound sadness and an inclination to offer more support than is realistic. As in offering reassurance, there is no absolute rule about the degree of dependency to allow. It depends on the patient's need.

Addressing Loss

There are many losses in entering prison, and Johnson et al. (2019) mention that more than a quarter of prisoners have lost a family member. We do have a modicum of healthy skepticism about death reports (e.g., grandmother who has died five times), but we also recognize that most of them are true. Depressed prisoners often talk about their losses. The loss may remind them of the many other losses experienced in the transition to prison, such as the continued erosion of future plans. These grief reactions, which we discussed as disenfranchised grief in Chapter 5, may be reactions to the separation from family and friends, or the isolation and the separation from the rest of the prisoner's life. The losses eat away at their self-esteem and self-concepts. Knowing your clientele, however, you may not agree with your patients' attributions of responsibility for the loss. Their "lousy bitch" wife or "a-hole" husband might not be the whole source of their problems, but you may just let them ventilate at first. Over the years it has been recognized that bereavement and depression are similar, and it has been clarified in the mental health research community that chronic bereavement can become major depressive disorder or coexist with it. However, since grief for multiple reasons (not just a death but including loss of finances and life opportunities) is so pervasive in prison, we recommend trying to distinguish the treatment of grief and depression. We discussed many distinctions in Chapter 5, but one last reminder is:

> In distinguishing grief from major depressive episode (MDE), it is useful to consider that in grief the predominant affect is feelings of emptiness and loss, while in MDE it is persistent depressed mood and the inability to anticipate happiness or pleasure. The dysphoria in grief is likely to decrease in intensity over days to weeks and occurs in waves, the so-called pangs of grief. These waves tend to be associated with thoughts or reminders of the deceased. The depressed mood of MDE is more persistent and is not tied to specific thoughts or preoccupations. (Black and Andreasen 2021, p. 151 footnote)

We don't exhort patients to get better on their own or work themselves out of it. Experienced therapists find that these exhortations, which might be empowering in other circumstances, create greater guilt and hopelessness in depressed patients who do not believe that they can single-handedly beat the illness, and they are usually right about that. It may be helpful to discuss medical models of depression. For example, according to the stress-diathesis theory of depression, stress creates an excess of the "stress hormone" cortisol and, as a consequence, damages the neurons in the brain. If we think the patient needs medications, we may add that antidepressants help to restore the chemical imbalance created by the cortisol overload and may even help to regrow brain cells. However, there is some commentary that states that chemical imbalance theories, while reducing guilt, can have stigmatizing effects on the way mentally ill persons are perceived (Rathje 2018).

Divide and Conquer

One obstacle in treating depression is the way a patient drops comments about being depressed and seemingly has nothing more to say. "I just feel depressed. It's hopeless."

We find it helpful to divide up the complaints and then spring back with counters for each of their "sub-complaints." For example, "I have no energy" is countered with "Your energy will come back…what else bothers you?" "I sleep all day." "You're not going to die from too much sleep, but why don't you get up an hour earlier tomorrow and see what you can do? What else bothers you?" "I haven't talked to my family." "I'll bet they miss you. Call them when you get back to your unit. What else bothers you?" In this case, we are using encouragement and principles of behavioral activation (for treatment manuals, see Society of Clinical Psychology 2020).

Noticing Improvement

A characteristic of depressed patients is that their behavior often improves before they themselves realize it. Observer ratings of their depressions improve sooner and are leading indicators of response to therapy. Here it does help to point out that the patient is spending more time in productive activities and is smiling more in the session. We are aware, however, that there were warnings from the FDA about suicidal ideation in young patients starting on antidepressants (presumably because the antidepressant gave them the energy they lack to carry out a suicidal plan) and that there is thought to be an increased risk of suicidal behavior during the recovery phase of depression.

Education and Coordination

Educating your patients about the course of the illness and preventing the family from sabotaging treatment are important objectives. If the family tells them not to take medicine, inquire further. Better yet, explore what their family knows about their depression and to whom they have talked. Considering what we said above about blaming family for losses, explore the patient's description of family interactions and try to determine if the patient is ventilating appropriately to receptive family members or is rather "burning bridges" to family members he blames for his depression. Unlike sharing of psychotic thoughts, sharing depressed feelings with other prisoners can be helpful—but within appropriate limits. They should be told to report suicidal thoughts, but not exclusively to close friends. We say: "I don't want to hear from your cellie that you are suicidal; if you are suicidal, I want to hear it from you."

The Depressed Patient in Remission

Patients with severe major depression, even in remission, will probably end up taking medication and participating in therapy indefinitely, so we don't usually worry about losing them to follow-up. An exception would be a patient with a supposedly resolved adjustment disorder with depression, but who really has a major depressive disorder or develops one. All remitted or recovered patients should have a few wellness checks and be primed (e.g., "Don't be ashamed if you need to come back!") to seek additional treatment if symptoms recur. There is much work in trying to see if there is a prodrome to major depression. Fava (the same person who invented WBT) and Kellner found anxiety and irritability prior to onset of major depression (Fava and Kellner 1991), and a more recent study found irritability, anxiety, sleep problems, and fatigability (Pede et al. 2017). Since so many prisoners have had COVID-19 and since fatigue is a common and lasting symptom post-infection, it may be difficult for a while to track or distinguish both prodromes of depression and residual depression during the COVID-19 era.

Issues in long-term therapy will include use of maintenance medications and the memory of the depression itself and its demoralizing effect on self-esteem, and may include damage to family relationships due to allegations the patient made during his depression. It is during remission, or in the maintenance phase, that much effective work can be done. While current opinion favors the view that combined medication and psychotherapeutic treatments are often beneficial, your opinion may differ from that of a prescriber. You also have to decide what to say when a patient announces, after a month on medications, that he has stopped "because I am all better and I don't want to be a mental case." In such cases, talk to the prescriber or discuss the questions with the treatment team: "How important do we think it is for this patient to stay on his medicine? If he stops, how frequently should we follow up?"

Other Types of Depression

The resolution of major depression, while leaving fears of recurrence, may result in relatively normal functioning. Often, however, there are residual symptoms, personality problems, or cognitive dysfunction that may predispose the patient to future depression. After building your history, you may decide that your patient has what used to be called dysthymic disorder and is now called *persistent depressive disorder* (Nübel et al. 2020). This is a DSM-5-TR category with the more severe variety showing early onset, a history of attempted suicide, the patient's self-classification as persistent depression, and treatment resistance. In prison, the combination of personality disorder, chronic stress, and/or medical disorders can result in persistent depression. Patients with depression secondary to medical illness may feel depressed because their capacities and strengths fail to live up to usual cultural expectations. They will benefit from realistic support of self-esteem and a necessary decrease in expectations.

Prisoners with persistent depressive disorder often have a history of loss, trauma, or deprivation. There are also certain prisoners, often persons arrested for the first time, with depressive reactions called "narcissistic wounding." These are patients (who may also have narcissistic personality disorder) who react depressively because their grandiose beliefs (e.g., of invulnerability) have been thwarted. Persistent depressive disorder can also develop insidiously and progress to major depression, thus turning into the infamous "double depression."

Many depressed patients in prison are chronically unhappy, hopeless, and nihilistic, making it a challenge to pull them even a little bit out of their "Slough of Despond." However, we were pleased when one of them came in one day and said, "I always like to see you because you are upbeat and optimistic and I feel better when I leave." Perhaps that was flattery, but the verbal statements and nonverbal aspects of the relationship with an encouraging therapist are likely to be helpful to some chronically unhappy and demoralized prisoners.

Bipolar Disorder

Although bipolar disorder is much less common than unipolar depression, there has been much attention to the development of evidence-based treatments for its various phases.

Both supportive and cognitive-behavioral therapies were found to be equally effective in the treatment of bipolar disorder (Pedersen 2012, reporting findings from Meyer and Hautzinger 2012). A recent review states that there is consistent evidence supporting the use of group psychoeducation (often with care management), family-focused therapy, and interpersonal and social rhythm therapy (IPSRT); however the evidence they reviewed was too mixed to support CBT (Vieta et al. 2020, p. 763). Care management and psychoeducation are of course techniques of supportive psychotherapy, so in the light of current evidence, we feel quite comfortable in treating bipolar patients with supportive psychotherapy. A vital component of all therapies with bipolar patients is establishing and maintaining a therapeutic alliance with patients at all stages of the illness.

Mentioned above, of course, is family-focused therapy, which, while not impossible to carry out, will be of lesser impact in a prison setting. The remaining item on the list is therefore IPSRT (Frank 2007), and it is obvious the management of daily rhythms is going to prove highly interesting and feasible in the carefully controlled prison environment. Despite the uncertainty of the evidence basis for CBT, as the authors above (Vieta et al. 2020) were concerned, as well as the concerns we have raised about it in earlier chapters, we do use CBT, and we have incorporated CBT techniques (e.g., from Basco and Rush 2007) into our presentation. A fundamental tenet of IPSRT is that vulnerable individuals can change moods because of changes in their biological and social rhythms, such as sleep, activity, and light exposure (the signals to the body known as *Zeitgebers*, or "time-givers"). However, a limitation of both IPSRT and cognitive-behavioral therapy is the difficulty of treating acutely manic patients, and it is suggested that IPSRT should be initiated when the patient is either acutely depressed or beginning to recover from a manic or mixed episode (Frank 2007). Therefore, it remains important to discuss supportive techniques that begin at a time when the patient is acutely manic and may then segue into an established or time-limited brief therapy for stabilization. And there is obviously an advantage to the highly scheduled prison routine in encouraging bipolar patients to maintain their daily sleep schedules. We frequently point out to them that a single lost night of sleep can precipitate a manic episode in susceptible persons.

Bipolar illness has a complex relationship to the criminal justice system (Fovet et al. 2015). Consistent with our discussion that persons with SMI have similar criminality to those without mental illness, Fovet's "review of the reviews" notes that bipolar patients generally commit no more crimes when manic, depressed, psychotic, or not psychotic. However, bipolar persons are overrepresented in prisons, and their behavior can lead to the following problems:

- Conflict with prison staff
- Overly familiar or exhibitionist behaviors
- Disciplinary action
- Actual extension of prison terms

The following vignette illustrates how supportive therapy was helpful to a patient who became manic for a period of time but remained in the facility.

Case Vignette

Mr. Jackson is a 55-year-old man who was in prison for several years for some nonviolent drug charges. He had a history of bipolar disorder, but he appeared well on admission. He promised that his attorney would get them some papers from his previous care, but these never arrived. He was very pleasant and agreeable and required only minimal mental health services in general population. After several months he complained of depression and was referred to a prescriber, who gave him an antidepressant. A few months later, Mr. Jackson's behavior underwent a major change. He began to complain of harassment on his unit and made a PREA (Prison Rape Elimination Act) complaint against another prisoner. The complaint was not validated. He started to demand to see the therapist every day and demanded that the alleged perpetrator be moved to another unit. He began to make allegations that a second prisoner was harassing him. He lived on the downstairs tier of his unit, but he would go upstairs and bang on the door of Mr. Low, the alleged harasser. Then he began complaining that he was suicidal.

The mental health team "suddenly" recognized that Mr. Jackson had become manic, possibly as a result of the antidepressant he was taking, and he was sent back to the prescriber for medication adjustments. Over several weeks, Mr. Jackson received a mood stabilizer and both a first- and a second-generation antipsychotic. He was never dangerous enough to be hospitalized, but he had several stays in the infirmary for suicidal threats. He was moved to the mental health unit. He started demanding that various harassers be removed from "his" unit because they did not belong there. The therapist saw him once or twice a week in addition to brief daily wellness checks.

It took 4 months for Mr. Jackson to return to his normal, easygoing self. During that time the therapist worked with him supportively to redirect him when he exhibited disruptive behaviors or had suicidal thoughts. For example, one day, during the COVID-19 crisis, Mr. Jackson declared that he was going to fire his attorney, who was trying to get him released on humanitarian grounds because of Mr. Jackson's age and his medical problems. The therapist asked Mr. Jackson to consider that this would be a bad time to fire his attorney, because he might lose a once-in-a-lifetime opportunity to get released from prison. The therapist had to consider that he did not personally know if the attorney was doing a good or bad job, but that the reasons for poor performance given by Mr. Jackson seemed to be reflective of Mr. Jackson's irritability and impaired judgment from his manic state. Based on what we have said earlier about giving advice, the therapist framed the advice with the usual qualifications but also educated Mr. Jackson that his manic state could be affecting his opinion of the attorney. Mr. Jackson agreed to call his attorney and meet with her, and they worked out their differences, although other circumstances ultimately prevented his release. The therapist salvaged Mr. Jackson's relationships with the other prisoners and staff. The therapist also worked with the precursors to suicidal thinking and forestalled several trips to the infirmary.

Mr. Jackson was probably in a mixed manic state, which may have accounted for the difficulty of treatment and the length of time it took for him to return to normal. As we have suggested, mixed manic states can have a current of suicidal thinking.

In the outside world, an acutely manic patient is usually hospitalized and may be stepped down through a day program or returned to a residential facility. While prison hospitals and infirmaries are still available, medication, simple confinement, and limit-setting may be all that is possible for a manic patient, and supportive psychotherapy can assist the treatment of acute mania and the continued treatment of bipolar illness. In fact, as Rakofsky and Dunlop (2014, p. 43) report, the only forms of psychotherapy that are indicated during acute mania are supportive psychotherapy and psychoeducation. Other psychotherapy trials have not shown short-term efficacy in treating acute mania, and it is difficult to conduct such trials by enrolling acutely manic patients.

Manic patients lack sound judgment yet may have a kind of mental acuity that leads them to pick up on many items that you might miss. Their maneuvers are well known and include:

1. Holding you to promises of a minor nature such as promising to see them at 2 P.M. and chewing you out if you are 10 minutes late.
2. Stretching any promises you make. If you say you will see them at 5 P.M. and they can get to you, they start pacing around your office at 4 P.M. If you say you might release them from the infirmary in "a few days," they demand to be released the following morning.
3. Toying with your feelings—telling you that you are good or bad depending on whether you do things for them.
4. Blaming others for their issues (as do many prisoners).
5. Demanding things you can't supply like air freshener or bottled water.
6. Demanding that you get their medical ailments treated immediately (as if you didn't get enough of this from your euthymic patients).
7. Alienating family members (which is often the outcome of mania, as well as an interpersonal maneuver by the patient).

It is important to set limits both inside and outside the therapy. Proper limit setting in prison requires an authoritarian approach, so don't feel guilty about it. Premature accommodations or privileges, perhaps offered to buttress a shaky therapeutic alliance, will usually lead to rule violations or even assaults followed by discipline that reflects the manic patient's ideas of reference that the correction officers (COs) are scheming against him.

It can be difficult and dangerous to see manic patients in the office. Most of the time, it seems to us that a therapist errs on the side of accessibility or buys into the "macho" orientation of the prison and tells himself that "I can handle this guy alone." This belief is usually self-serving and ends up in a "Code Black" (all officers respond to staff member assault). Once this has happened to you a few times, you will know better and ask for manic patients to be seen in the infirmary. Sometimes, officers may "spring" a manic patient on you by bringing him into your office since you are available or were foolish enough to be the only mental health person working late. Think about the behavioral safety of the patient before allowing the CO to plunk him into a chair.

Assuming you decide to see the manic patient in your office, you can still change your mind. Verbal abuse might be reasonably okay, but as you assess the potential for escalation, call for assistance. You usually need to keep your cool, but acutely manic patients can read your emotions, and firmness and determination are the emotions they should be reading. "I see you are upset, but I'm concerned that you are losing control. Let's get you moved to a safer place and then we can talk." Manic patients are at high risk for violence and assault. If someone is sitting back in his chair and talking loudly, that is one thing. Sitting up, getting louder and closer to you—don't think about this very long but call for assistance.

Despite the stresses, it can be gratifying to work with manic or hypomanic patients and prevent them from destroying their placements and interpersonal relationships with both prisoners and officers, given the limited choices in prison. Each therapeutic tactic should be seen as a reality-enhancing countermove to the manic person's reality-denying defenses.

Acutely manic patients exhibit both thought and mood abnormalities. In some cases, they are totally irrational and cannot be argued out of their grandiosity. However, it is often possible to select some aspects of manic behaviors that are defensive (as opposed to biologically fueled) and interpret them to the patient. Briefly put, being manic or hypomanic is often pleasant and reinforcing. Such enjoyment can reinforce denial and interfere with the patient's adherence to medication and overall treatment goals. These issues must be addressed whenever it becomes a stumbling block to treatment. There is nothing wrong with acknowledging that you know that it is pleasant to be manic but should add that being manic comes with its downside, and you are there to help them mitigate the damage.

An agenda for treating the acutely manic patient is shown in Table 9–3. By putting such an agenda in operation, you increase the chances that your respectful but restraining approach early in treatment will be remembered by the patient later when you do ongoing therapy.

The Bipolar Patient in Remission

Previously manic persons with a normal mood may be as typical as anyone else and benefit from various forms of psychotherapies in addition to maintenance medications. However, they are especially suited for supportive psychotherapy, because bipolar illness has a complex psycho-physiological basis and it is often difficult to use therapies whose core concepts are solely psychological or social. Education about the illness is one of the first items on the agenda. A useful start is the National Institutes of Health brochure "Bipolar Disorder" (National Institute of Mental Health 2018a).

A goal of therapy is to prevent mood disturbances, and specifically to arm the patient against the recurrence of mania or depression. By "arming," we mean giving them "weapons" to fight the recurrence of mood episodes. Knowledge about the disease is probably a weapon of sorts, but there are more active things they can do on a daily basis to make them feel they have some control of the illness. Using IPSRT, for example, when the patient is well enough to implement the techniques helps the patient learn to stabilize her social rhythms, starting with sleep and then moving to behavioral patterns. All of these techniques involve the use of mood monitoring charts or applications. Therefore, in therapy for well patients, we begin with an introduction of social rhythms and provide a mood monitoring chart. Many such charts are available from the relevant treatment manuals and internet sites. One that we recommend (best if you have a color printer) is the National Institute of Mental Health Mood Chart (National Institute of Mental Health 2018b). The existence of the fixed prison routine is in general helpful to having a fixed regimen and regular sleeping hours, although the lack of darkness and frequent awakenings for counts are counterproductive.

Since manic states have a prodrome (with both common features of the illness and features that may be specific to a given individual), it helps to compile a list of warning signs for a possible manic mood escalation. It is recommended that these be things that can be easily recognized or even measured (e.g., hours of sleep), recognized even when there is a small change (e.g., going from 8 to 7 hours of sleep), and monitored on a daily basis (Reinares et al. 2020, p. 68). If the patient has a crisis response safety plan, these data can be kept there. These include:

- Fewer hours of sleep.
- Finding themselves more talkative than usual.

TABLE 9–3.	Treating the manic patient in prison

Be firm, caring, and supportively restraining and explain to the patient that you are doing just that.

Send the patient to the infirmary or hospital if necessary and explain why.

Limit the damage the patient does to his relationships within and outside of prison.

Do not buy into the manic person's point of view (e.g., jump up and accuse the corrections officer of harassing him because the patient says so).

Support the use of medications unless you have serious reservations about what and how much is being used (if so, discuss with prescriber).

Develop a consistent therapeutic and staff approach that counteracts the manic patient's tactics, utilizing the patient's own beliefs about self.

Use many frequent and short interventions when they are effective.

Ask the patient for immediate feedback to determine whether he heard you (e.g., "I promise not to go up on the second tier and bang on Mr. Low's door") to see if your interventions are remembered and accepted.

Set limits within therapy.

  Avoid fruitless interactions so as to reinforce fruitful ones.

  Don't continue talking when you realize it is ineffective in that particular session.

  Don't be a hero by continuing sessions when there is risk of violence.

Set protective limits outside of therapy (including interactions with staff and other prisoners).

Assist family members if they get involved in the patient's treatment.

- Having racing thoughts or new grandiose ideas, which you should personalize to their own historical pattern (e.g., feeling they are "too good for this place" or "much smarter than these jerks").
- Distractibility, irritability, restlessness, or agitation.
- Tendency to pick fights with cellmates, members of therapy groups, officers, and others.
- Increased sexuality.
- Getting psychotic again (if this typically happens) (e.g., hearing the voices again).

Co-occurring Illnesses and Personality Issues

Patients with bipolar illness may have other major mental illnesses, so it must be routine to diagnose all of them. There is frequent substance use disorder that is worth addressing in an abstinent environment. One finding worth mentioning here is that about half of bipolar patients report a history of impairing panic symptomatology (Frank et al. 2002, cited in Frank 2007, p. 59).

The classic study of MacVane et al. (1978) showed no significant differences between a group of 35 lithium-stabilized manic patients and a like number of psychiatrically healthy control subjects. However, we do believe (as do most therapists) that many previously manic patients have interepisodic personality traits, usually narcissistic in nature, that may be seen as reasonable adjustments to their illness. Frank (2007) notes that it is difficult to diagnose personality disorders in persons who have had manic episodes. They may appear borderline, antisocial, narcissistic, or dramatic (Frank 2007, p. 61), but it may not be known whether they really have one disorder or two separate disorders.

The postmanic agenda focuses on protective measures for recurrence of mania (or depression). Patients with bipolar illness are usually interested in understanding their disease and its pharmacological maintenance. Their fear of relapse and of the destructive loss it brings needs to be discussed. Because elevation of mood is associated with nonadherence to treatment plans, the patient needs to learn to associate elevation of mood with that loss and turn to the therapist or prescriber for protection. Listen for talk that they are beginning to doubt the importance of their medicine or having side effects and thinking the medicine is not worth taking. When manic, patients have poorer insight (than when depressed or euthymic) into the effectiveness of treatment or the personal and social consequences of their manic behavior (da Silva et al. 2015). You can work best with bipolar patients to improve their insight when they are either depressed or euthymic. We are all aware of the phenomenon by which these patients' insight evaporates like dew on a hot morning when they start to become manic.

Although many classic psychodynamic approaches interpreted mania as a defense against depression or the expression of a wish to return to an omnipotent childhood state, there are a substantial number of therapeutic issues deriving from the disease itself.

Issues covered in IPSRT (Suppes and Dennehy 2005, p. 67) include:

- Grief over loss (including loss of their healthy self).
- Interpersonal conflicts.
- Role transitions.
- Improving interpersonal skills.

Related issues (Kahn 1990) are:

- Interruption (by the illness) of developmental tasks, such as forming extrafamilial relationships and career progression.
- Discrimination of normal from abnormal moods and the tendency to fear strong emotions.
- Demoralization from fears of recurrence.
- Guilt at destructive efforts.
- Concern about genetic transmission.
- Losses due to the treatment itself (e.g., symbolic loss of self-esteem and the use of treatment as an excuse for unrelated failures).

You can provide education, guidance, and reassurance in most of these areas, mixing these with psychoeducation efforts regarding:

- The complex interrelationship of their bipolar disorder to criminal behaviors and substance use disorders. Consider including the latter in relapse prevention treatment while in prison described in the book by Atkins (2014), an excellent resource that pairs treatment plans for specific mood disorders with substance use.

- The relationship of their relapses to nonadherence to prescribed therapies.
- The (commonly) destructive effect of their manic behaviors on their finances and family relationships.

Manic states, like depressive states, have prodromes. However, the prodromal symptoms of depression, as we discussed above, do not seem very specific or useful. The situation is different in mania. Irritability and lack of sleep are very evident and telling. We instruct all bipolar patients to inform us if there is a change in the number of hours they sleep.

In the prison setting, it is also useful to instruct patients to record their thoughts and emotions, especially "unhelpful" ones to discuss in therapy. One clinician calls the record an "Emotions Library Card" (Reiser et al. 2017, p. 55), which could be a nice addition to their crisis response safety plan.

You should of course notice changes in mood that might signify relapse but resist the urge to instantly clamp down or overreact to their daily excitements and depressions of normal life (e.g., locking them down because of their behavioral excesses). In this regard, we know that the therapist who works in a prison setting is often approached by other medical or correctional personnel with warnings that the patient is getting out of control. Experience does not always allow one to discriminate between false and genuine alarms. Usually you need to call in the patient and determine this yourself.

Key Points

- With mood disorders, just as with psychotic disorders, it is important to establish empathy, rapport, and a good relationship early in treatment.

- Well-being therapy is a therapy within the positive psychology sphere that is simple and easy to add on to other therapeutic methods.

- When patients are depressed, it is important to give reassurance and hope ("There is light at the end of the tunnel") and address dependency, guilt, and loss.

- Depressed patients may need a suspension of the therapeutic interventions involving criminogenic issues while hope and support are given to get them well.

- With both depressed and manic patients, you have to do "damage control" because of their tendency to strike out (verbally and physically) against others, including family, and to "burn their bridges" and damage relationships that they will need later.

- For all disorders, it is important to address co-occurring mental illnesses, including personality issues and substance use disorders.

- Bipolar disorder, especially the manic phase, requires judicious limit-setting. You cannot hospitalize everyone all the time, so you have to manage behavior in the institution and salvage the patient's relationship with others in the institution and family outside.

- Manic patients have a repertory of behaviors that can be countered therapeutically.

- Educational interventions will help manic patients when they are between acute episodes. Education about illness is a general strategy for all persons when they are in a state amenable to such interventions.

- For most patients with serious mental illness, it is important to be aware of somatic complaints.

- As discussed in Chapter 5, you need to have a subtext of assessing for suicidal thinking in all patients every time you see them, but especially as it relates to depression (including depression in schizophrenia) and in mixed manic states. Knowing the history of suicide attempts can make it easier to design therapeutic interventions.

References

Atkins C: Co-Occurring Disorders: Integrated Assessment and Treatment of Substance Use and Mental Disorders. Eau Claire, WI, PESI Publishing and Media, 2014

Barker P: Using Metaphors in Psychotherapy. New York, Brunner/Mazel, 1985

Basco MR, Rush AJ: Cognitive-Behavioral Therapy for Bipolar Disorder, 2nd Edition. New York, Guilford, 2007

Black DW, Andreasen NC: Introductory Textbook of Psychiatry, 7th Edition. Washington, DC, American Psychiatric Association Publishing, 2021

Cowen PJ: Management and treatment of depressive disorders, in New Oxford Textbook of Psychiatry, 3rd Edition. Edited by Geddes JR, Andreasen NC, Goodwin GM. New York, Oxford University Press, 2020, pp. 807–816

Cuijpers P, van Straten A, Andersson G, van Oppen P: Psychotherapy for depression in adults: a meta-analysis of comparative outcome studies. J Consult Clin Psychol 76(6):909–922, 2008 19045960

da Silva RdeA, Mograbi DC, Camelo EV, et al: Insight in bipolar disorder: a comparison between mania, depression and euthymia using the Insight Scale for Affective Disorders. Trends Psychiatry Psychother 37(3):152–156, 2015 26630406

Dil L, Dekker J, Van R, et al: A short-term psychodynamic supportive psychotherapy for adolescents with depressive disorders: a new approach. J Infant Child Adolesc Psychother 15(2):84–94, 2016

Driessen E, Cuijpers P, de Maat SC, et al: The efficacy of short-term psychodynamic psychotherapy for depression: a meta-analysis. Clin Psychol Rev 30(1):25–36, 2010 19766369

Elkin I, Shea MT, Watkins JT, et al: National Institute of Mental Health Treatment of Depression Collaborative Research Program. General effectiveness of treatments. Arch Gen Psychiatry 46(11):971–982, discussion 983, 1989 2684085

Fava GA: Well-Being Therapy: Treatment Manual and Clinical Applications. New York, S Karger, 2016

Fava GA, Guidi J: The pursuit of euthymia. World Psychiatry 19(1), January 10, 2020

Fava GA, Kellner R: Prodromal symptoms in affective disorders. Am J Psychiatry 148(7):823–830, 1991 2053620

Fovet T, Geoffroy PA, Vaiva G, et al: Individuals with bipolar disorder and their relationship with the criminal justice system: a critical review. Psychiatr Serv 66(4):348–353, 2015 25555137

Frank E: Treating Bipolar Disorder: A Clinician's Guide to Interpersonal and Social Rhythm Therapy. New York, Guilford, 2007

Frank E, Cyranowski JM, Rucci P, et al: Clinical significance of lifetime panic spectrum symptoms in the treatment of patients with bipolar I disorder. Arch Gen Psychiatry 59(10):905–911, 2002 12365877

Hersen M, Bellack AS, Himmelhoch JM, et al: Effects of social skills training, amitriptyline, and psychotherapy in unipolar depressed women. Behav Ther 15:21–40, 1984

Hollon TH: A rationale for supportive psychotherapy of depressed patients. Am J Psychother 16:655–664, 1962 13961369

Ijaz S, Davies P, Williams CJ, et al: Psychological therapies for treatment-resistant depression in adults. Cochrane Database Syst Rev 5(5):CD010558, 2018 29761488

Jacobs N, Reupert A: The Effectiveness of Supportive Counselling, Based on Rogerian Principles: A Systematic Review of Recent International and Australian Research. Melbourne, Psychotherapy & Counselling Federation of Australia, May 2014. Available at: www.pacfa.org.au-wp-content-uploads-2012-10-PACFA-SupportiveCounselling-literature-review-2014-Final.pdf. Accessed September 5, 2020.

Jahoda M: Current Concepts of Positive Mental Health. New York, Basic Books, 1958

Johnson JE, Stout RL, Miller TR, et al: Randomized cost-effectiveness trial of group interpersonal psychotherapy (IPT) for prisoners with major depression. J Consult Clin Psychol 87(4):392–406, April 2019

Kahn D: The psychotherapy of mania. Psychiatr Clin North Am 13(2):229–240, 1990 2191279

Klerman GL, Weissman MM, Rousanville BJ, et al: Interpersonal Psychotherapy of Depression. New York, Basic Books, 1984

Kvam S, Kleppe CL, Nordhus IH, Hovland A: Exercise as a treatment for depression: a meta-analysis. J Affect Disord 202:67–86, 2016 27253219

Lewinsohn PM, Sullivan JM, Grosscup SJ: Changing reinforcing events: an approach to the treatment of depression. Psychotherapy (Chic) 17:322–334, 1980

Lynch D, Laws KR, McKenna PJ: Cognitive behavioural therapy for major psychiatric disorder: does it really work? A meta-analytical review of well-controlled trials. Psychol Med 40(1):9–24, 2010 19476688

MacVane JR, Lange JD, Brown WA, Zayat M: Psychological functioning of bipolar manic-depressives in remission. Arch Gen Psychiatry 35(11):1351–1354, 1978 708196

Meyer TD, Hautzinger M: Cognitive behaviour therapy and supportive therapy for bipolar disorders: relapse rates for treatment period and 2-year follow-up. Psychol Med 42(7):1429–1439, 2012 22099722

National Institute of Mental Health: Bipolar disorder (brochure). Revised 2018a. Available at: https://www.nimh.nih.gov/sites/default/files/documents/health/publications/bipolar-disorder/19-mh-8088.pdf. Accessed March 8, 2022.

National Institute of Mental Health: Mood Charting. 2018b. Available at: www.cqaimh.org/pdf/tool_edu_moodchart.pdf. Accessed March 16, 2018.

Nübel J, Guhn A, Müllender S, et al: Persistent depressive disorder across the adult lifespan: results from clinical and population-based surveys in Germany. BMC Psychiatry 20(1):58, 2020 32041560

Pede VB, Jaiswal SV, Sawant VA: Study of prodromal and residual symptoms of depression. Ind Psychiatry J 26(2):121–127, 2017 30089957

Pedersen T: CBT, supportive psychotherapy equally effective for bipolar. July 9, 2012. Available at: https://icmha.ca/cbt-supportive-therapy-equally-effective-for-bipolar. Accessed March 8, 2022.

Rakofsky JJ, Dunlop BW: Treating bipolar mania in the outpatient setting: risk vs reward. Curr Psychiatry 13(11):38–46, 2014

Rathje S: Don't say that depression is caused by a chemical imbalance: the most popular way of talking about mental illness may be misguided ("Words Matter" blog). Psychology Today, August 9, 2018 Available at: www.psychologytoday.com/us/blog/words-matter/201808/dont-say-depression-is-caused-chemical-imbalance. Accessed December 6, 2020.

Rehm LP: Self-management therapy for depression. Adv Behav Res Ther 6(2):83–98, 1984

Reinares M, Martínez-Arán A, Vieta E: Psychotherapy for Bipolar Disorders: An Integrative Approach. New York, Cambridge University Press, 2020

Reiser RP, Thompson LW, Johnson SL, Suppes T: Bipolar Disorder, 2nd Edition. Ashland, OH, Hogrefe Publishing, 2017

Rousanville BJ, Chevron ES, Weissman MM: Specification of techniques in interpersonal psychotherapy, in Psychotherapy Research: Where Are We and Where Should We Go? (Proceedings of the 73rd Annual Meeting of the American Psychopathological Association, New York City, March 3–5, 1983). Edited by Williams JBW, Spitzer RL. New York, Guilford, 1984, pp 160–172

Ryff CD: Happiness is everything, or is it? Explorations on the meaning of psychological well-being. J Pers Soc Psychol 6:1069–1081, 1989

Scaccia A: Can depression cause memory loss? 2016; medically reviewed Legg TJ; updated September 13, 2019. Available at: www.healthline.com/health/depression/depression-and-memory-loss. Accessed January 31, 2019.

Schuldt W: Behavioral activation. Therapist Aid (website). 2019. Available at: www.therapistaid.com/therapy-worksheet/behavioral-activation. Accessed January 3, 2019.

Seligman MEP: Authentic Happiness: Using the New Positive Psychology to Realize Your Potential for Lasting Fulfilment. New York, The Free Press, 2002

Society of Clinical Psychology: Treatment: Behavioral Activation for Depression. 2020. Available at: www.div12.org/treatment/behavioral-activation-for-depression/#treatment-manuals. Accessed June 28, 2020.

Sotsky SM, Glass DR, Shea MT, et al: Patient predictors of response to psychotherapy and pharmacotherapy: findings in the NIMH Treatment of Depression Collaborative Research Program. Am J Psychiatry 148(8):997–1008, 1991 1853989

Suppes T, Dennehy EB: Bipolar Disorder: The Latest Assessment and Treatment Strategies. Kansas City, MO, Compact Clinicals, 2005

Tull M: 8 tips for using behavioral activation for treating depression. Medically reviewed by Block DB, August 4, 2020. Available at: www.verywellmind.com/increasing-the-effectiveness-of-behavioral-activation-2797597. Accessed January 31, 2019.

University of Hertfordshire: Cognitive therapy is of no value in schizophrenia, analysis of studies suggests. ScienceDaily, June 26, 2009. Available at: www.sciencedaily.com/releases/2009/06/090625074512.htm. Accessed January 31, 2019.

Vieta EV, Pacchiarotti I, Miklowitz D: Management and treatment of bipolar disorder, in New Oxford Textbook of Psychiatry, 3rd Edition. Edited by Geddes JR, Andreasen NC, Goodwin GM. New York, Oxford University Press, 2020, pp 757–766

Wright JH, McCray LW: Breaking Free From Depression: Pathways to Wellness. New York, Guilford, 2011

Zimmerman M: Using the 9-item Patient Health Questionnaire to screen for and monitor depression. JAMA 322(21):2125–2126, 2019 31626276

10

(They've Got) Personality (Disorder)

A Challenge in Corrections

Prelude

Everybody has a personality, but some people have a personality *disorder*, or several of them. Or maybe "A Little Bit of This, a Little Bit of That." More about this and that later.

But make a correction: Our college history professor really *had no personality at all*; her lectures were utterly boring, and she even put you to sleep with her monotonous tones when you tried to strike up a conversation with her at the faculty-student mixer. On the other hand, our English professor was so utterly negative and dismissive of things that we called him a sourpuss, which should be a kind of personality disorder, shouldn't it? And it was strange that as an English professor he could hardly write a capital "A," even when followed by a minus sign, but he frequently wrote capital "Bs" and "Cs."

Everybody has a personality (except for our college history professor). Personality is the combination of behavior, emotion, and thought patterns that describe a person. People with personality *disorders* can be the most difficult and complex to treat both in the outside world and in prison because of their maladaptive means of coping and behaviors.

Our interest in certain people with personality disorders is not merely theoretical; it is due to the fact that they *cause trouble*: They commit crimes, sometimes violent, which get them into prison, and act out and incur discipline. Estimates vary greatly, but it is stated that in the United States the prevalence of antisocial personality disorder in the male prison population is between 50% and 80% and that the prevalence of all personality disorders there could be as high as 90% (Bell and Evershed 2004).

The word "personality" comes from the Latin *persona*. In the ancient world, a *persona* was a mask worn by an actor. Hippocrates, in 370 B.C., proposed that personalities and behaviors were the consequences of an imbalance of four temperaments associ-

327

ated with four essential bodily fluids (humors): yellow bile from the liver, black bile from the kidneys, red blood from the heart, and white phlegm from the lungs. Centuries later, the Greek physician and philosopher Galen expanded the theory and proposed that there were four temperaments: the choleric person is bad-tempered, mean, and easily angered; the melancholic person is sad, reserved, sensitive, and emotional; the sanguine person is outgoing, joyful, and optimistic; and the phlegmatic person is meek and reserved and kind of laid-back and lazy (Kagan 2005; see also Clark and Watson 2008). Our English professor probably had something like a choleric temperament.

A personality disorder (PD) is an ongoing, relatively stable or rigid pattern of behavior that deviates from the expectations of the person's culture. Onset is generally in adolescence or early adulthood and leads to distress or impairment. PDs may be partly genetic or a result of abuse, neglect (e.g., poor parenting), social inequities, poverty, and so forth, and these issues need to be addressed in primary prevention. Often, PDs will co-occur with other disorders—usually substance use, PTSD, major depression, generalized anxiety disorder, or bipolar disorder.

The current method of assessing and classifying personality disorders is moving from a categorical model of three clusters to a dimensional model. However, for now, the definitions of PDs in Section II of DSM-5 (and DSM-5-TR) are unchanged from those in DSM-IV. Section III of DSM-5-TR provides an alternative dimensional model of PDs with different criteria for diagnosis.

Thinking ahead to dimensional models, we will avoid talking about the standard categorical clusters (e.g., Clusters A, B, and C) and will discuss the PDs individually. It is important to note that only 6 of the 10 disorders are presented in the alternative model. Left out are dependent, schizoid, paranoid, and histrionic personality disorders. We'll only cover the four personality disorders that are the most prevalent in corrections: borderline personality disorder (BPD), antisocial personality disorder (ASPD), narcissistic personality disorder (NPD), and paranoid personality disorder (PPD) (Virdi and Trestman 2015). PPD is one of the four PDs not covered under the alternative model, but we will discuss it because paranoia is often reported in prison surveys, and whether or not the researchers are identifying PPD or just paranoia, it helps to understand this disorder. There is also suspiciousness in individuals with ASPD and in psychopaths. Of the four PDs, individuals with BPD and ASPD are most likely to carry out two or more acts of violence (Abracen et al. 2014). Three of the PDs—avoidant, dependent, and obsessive-compulsive—do not have a strong association with criminality or violence, and in fact the relationship is most likely an inverse one (Howard and Howells 2010). Histrionic personality disorder is not in the dimensional model, but we do think it has some connection to crime and aggression in prison. In this chapter, for each of these four disorders, we discuss defining features, prevalence in correctional settings, challenges in treatment, and supportive psychotherapy recommendations.

The categorical model defines a PD by the presence or absence of characteristics. The dimensional model differs in using a classification based on the occurrence of traits and the degree to which the symptoms hinder the patient's behaviors and functioning. It is based on the principle that PDs consist of a compound interaction of factors over time (DSM-5-TR). That is, rather than asking "present or absent?," it asks "how much?" The dimensional model has greater specificity and contributes a basic standard for continued research to broaden our knowledge of personality disorders.

The alternative model for PDs was included in DSM-5 "to address numerous shortcomings of the approach in Section II to personality disorders. For example, in the approach in Section II, symptoms meeting criteria for a specific personality disorder frequently also meet criteria for other personality disorders, and other specified or unspecified personality disorder is often the correct (but mostly uninformative) diagnosis, in the sense that individuals do not tend to present with patterns of symptoms that correspond with one and only one personality disorder" (DSM-5-TR, p. 881).

Both models call for significant impairment and inflexibility. In the dimensional system, there must be a) impaired function and b) pathological personality traits. The level of functioning is divided into four elements: 1) identity, 2) self-direction, 3) empathy, and 4) intimacy. Each element is rated on a five-point scale from zero to extreme. The personality traits are organized into five broad domains: Negative affectivity, Detachment, Antagonism, Disinhibition, and Psychoticism.

The DSM-5 dimensional model is not identical to the well-known Five-Factor Model of personality, but in its current state has been called a maladaptive variant of the Five-Factor Model. To clarify, it was not meant to claim that the *model* was maladaptive (whatever that might mean!) but that the DSM-5 model measures maladaptive traits and maladaptation of the individual rather than the degree of adaptation and positive traits in the Five-Factor Model (Widiger and McCabe 2020).

Are Personality Disorders Really Treatable?

To speak of treating a person with PD implies that the person can change, at least somewhat, or that the effects of his behavior can be mitigated. (One way to mitigate the effects is to incarcerate a person, but one would hope to do better than that.) Fortunately, despite the common belief, even among clinicians, that PDs are very stable, they actually do change over time, either spontaneously or because of therapy. Moreover, many people with PDs are eminently treatable, as evidenced by the results of the many treatment programs (including those that involve supportive psychotherapy) that target patients' motivations and behaviors that lead to violence and crime. For example, one review of 14 outcome studies (including one of supportive psychotherapy) concluded that "25.8% of personality disorder patients recovered per year of therapy, a rate sevenfold larger than that in a published model of the natural history of borderline personality disorder" (Perry et al. 1999, p. 1312).

However, if you have an interest in treating someone with a rather "pure" paranoid or histrionic or obsessive-compulsive personality, it will benefit you to look at the articles and books that are specific to these PDs. The ascendence of the dimensional model of personality disorders will probably lead to a deemphasis on treating "pure" versions of those disorders, especially the four that were dropped from the dimensional model. For information on supportive psychotherapy with the other PDs, see our manual (Novalis et al. 2020) and the book by Winston et al. (2020).

Because of the still-prevalent clinical pessimism about treating PDs, especially ASPD and BPD, we do want to make you aware of some concerns that relate PDs to social injustice. For example, if persons with criminal histories tend to be diagnosed as having antisocial personalities, there can be an inherent bias in diagnosing socially disadvantaged persons, including Black prisoners, as having antisocial personalities. *Labeling* these individuals with a supposedly "untreatable" condition isolates and stigmatizes them, leading to a self-fulfilling prophecy for future misconduct despite the treatability of persons with criminal histories. There is a tendency for persons of color to be diagnosed as behaviorally disordered rather than psychiatrically disordered (Freedman and Woods 2021, citing Mizock and Harkins 2011), and the criminalization of Black youth results in an overdiagnosis of ASPD. Freedman and Woods urge much caution when diagnosing PD and recommend treating co-occurring psychiatric disorders without diagnosing PD. Of course, the transition to the alternative model will decrease emphasis on "pure" PDs and (we hope) improve the diagnostic accuracy of any final diagnosis while recognizing antisocial behavior that does not meet the criteria for ASPD. As we have said before, adult antisocial behavior is not synonymous with ASPD. This assertion is well supported by epidemiological data that shows a community prevalence of 4.3% for ASPD and 20.3% for a non-DSM-defined adult antisocial behavioral syndrome without conduct disorder before 15 years of age (Goldstein et al. 2017).

Supportive psychotherapy is used in various forms for PDs. One recent study used what was called "supportive psychoanalytic therapy." Its methods consist of developing the therapeutic alliance, monitoring for emergency situations that threaten the treatment such as suicidal behavior, improving the patient's ability to tolerate unpleasant affects, and developing the patient's sense of identity. Like supportive psychotherapy, this modification of psychoanalytic therapy does not interpret unconscious aspects of the transference (Carsky 2013, p. 443). The psychoanalytic part is minimal, but it does include techniques we have recommended, such as modifying patients' psychological defenses. And despite the impression that certain treatments, such as dialectical behavior therapy (DBT), are supposed to be superior to other forms of psychotherapy in the treatment of conditions such as BPD, such superiority is not found in head-to-head studies such as the study by McMain et al. (2009), which compared DBT with a symptom-targeted medication management and psychodynamically informed therapy based on the guidelines of the American Psychiatric Association called Good Psychiatric Management (GPM). The outcome of the two treatments was not significantly different. We will say more about GPM below. Other studies were referenced in Chapter 1.

In corrections, progress can be slow in treating PDs. As one of the advocacy groups points out, "Although people with personality disorders may appear 'normal'—just obnoxious or difficult—these mental disorders are very real and drive those who have them to behave the way they do" (Human Rights Watch 2003, p. 33). Indeed, these patients may be exasperating to treat, but you must remember that these disorders are real and propel them to behave in the manner they do. Impediments to treatment of persons with PD are listed in Table 10–1.

One expert, W. John Livesley, argues that the successful outcome of psychotherapy for personality disorders is due to the common factors that are shared by most psychotherapies despite the claims that may be found for the success of specific interventions. Therefore, treatment should emphasize those nonspecific elements rather than the specific ones (as described by Howard and Duggan [2010], p. 318). Since we have presented supportive psychotherapy as using the common elements of all psychotherapies, that statement is pretty much an endorsement of supportive psychotherapy. We couldn't have said it better ourselves.

TABLE 10–1.	Barriers to therapy for patients with personality disorder

Shortage of medical, mental health, and corrections staff

High turnover of staff

Staff burnout

Time needed for team meetings

Interruptions

Difficulty accessing paper charts and reports

Difficulty ensuring confidentiality

Prisoners' struggle to adapt to institutional lifestyles

Patients' unfamiliarity with or distrust of treatment by mental health professionals

Overcrowding

Noise

Segregated housing

Prevalence of substance use disorder

Environment of security, not treatment

Lack of anonymity when seeking treatment leading to refusing and resisting treatment

Limited resources

Fears of being the target of a violent outburst

With a focus on bolstering self-esteem and adaptive skills while establishing and preserving a strong therapeutic relationship, supportive psychotherapy is especially applicable in the treatment of most PDs (Winston et al. 2020) and is a starting point for merging other treatment strategies. The goals include placing limits on destructive and disruptive behaviors, preserving the necessary conditions for treatment and protecting the therapeutic alliance. Therapeutic interventions consist of contracting, limit-setting, advice, inspiration, and concern (Caligor and Clarkin 2010). Interventions should be based on knowledge of your patient's history, utilizing established measures to assess the risk of violence and addressing agitation as soon as it is recognized (Ritter and Platt 2016). Interactions with these prisoners require good communication skills and an awareness of when you are being manipulated and getting involved in a power struggle. Staff may be criticized and called incompetent or insensitive. A simple response such as "Maybe I am" without any other comment might be a good way to handle such an encounter (Ritter and Platt 2016).

We now discuss in detail the four personality disorders we mentioned earlier.

Antisocial Personality Disorder

Defining Features of ASPD

DSM-5-TR describes the essential feature of ASPD as "a pervasive pattern of disregard for, and violation of, the rights of others that begins in childhood or early adolescence and continues into adulthood" (p. 748). Other terms have been used, such as *psychopathy*, *sociopathy*, or *dissocial personality disorder*. We shall distinguish psychopathy from ASPD later in the chapter. The criteria for ASPD in the categorical models and alternative models are available in DSM-5-TR.

When a patient has a substance use disorder (SUD), you should carefully consider all aspects of his history before making a diagnosis of ASPD. It is not at all unusual for individuals with SUD to be charged with criminal offenses because of the means used to obtain the illicit substances (Avery and Barnhill 2018). The aggressive behaviors of the person with ASPD should be also distinguished from those of the person with psychosis. The former will have an unmistakable objective for his actions—intimidation, revenge, or some tangible result; the motives of the psychotic patient are more obscure (Baskin 2008).

Because of the lack of a social conscience, individuals with ASPD have a higher rate of violence and acting out aggressively when faced with frustration, anxiety, or helplessness. Their strong need for dominance may surface if they experience others as threatening. Lack of impulse control will lead to legal problems. The comorbidity of SUD will substantially increase the risk of harm to others (Craissati et al. 2015).

Prevalence of ASPD in Corrections

Trestman (2000) describes ASPD as "endemic to correctional settings." The prevalence of ASPD exceeds 70% in substance use disorder clinics, prisons, and other forensic settings (DSM-5-TR; Zeier et al. 2012). However, it is important to recognize that not every individual with a diagnosis of ASPD breaks the law and not every incarcerated person has ASPD (National Institute for Health and Clinical Excellence 2009).

It is generally believed that ASPD is found more frequently in men than in women. A study of Connecticut jails found ASPD present in 27% of women compared with 40% of men (Trestman et al. 2007). However—and this may be an outlier—a study of prisoners newly admitted to the Iowa Department of Corrections came up with a figure of 27% for women and 37% for men, but the difference was not statistically significant, and the authors concluded, "The fact that so many women met criteria for ASPD is a strong indicator that the disorder needs to be included in the differential diagnosis in prison settings, particularly when the presenting complaints involve irresponsibility, aggression, or deceitfulness" (Black et al. 2010, p. 116). Or to reference Michael Connelly's fictional detective Harry Bosch again, when Bosch self-reflectively laments that men are devious, his female partner, Ballard, corrects him and says that everybody's devious (Connelly 2019, p. 293).

Challenges of Working With ASPD Inmates

Challenges of working with prisoners with ASPD include the potential for violence and aggression. Prisoners with ASPD have problems coping with authority and living in the structured environment of a jail or prison (Trestman 2000). Struggles over dominance lead to conflict (Baskin 2008). Your reactions to the person and your awareness of countertransference are crucial. With power differences, countertransference occurs and at times is problematic (Zwirn and Owens 2011). Overall, challenges of working with persons who have ASPD come from traits like deceitfulness, manipulativeness, hostility, and impulsivity. Because of the overlap of ASPD traits with psychopathy, we will have more to say about this later.

Supportive Psychotherapy Techniques and Tips for ASPD

Supportive psychotherapy can improve impulse control and coping strategies (Baskin 2008). However, some ASPD patients may not take the therapy seriously and, perhaps, view it as a means of secondary gain. According to Virdi and Trestman (2015), it is essential to apply the basics of psychotherapy when working with ASPD patients by maintaining a respectful attitude, being direct, and following through with any commitments. You should monitor your own emotional reactions. You may find yourself becoming too passive or even resentful. You should be cautious of becoming overly invested while remaining positive, transparent, and respectful. Try to prevent or reduce the effects of manipulative behaviors, and arrange for the limits placed on the prisoner to be carried out by all staff members. It is important to specify clear boundaries and consequences (Cihlar 2014).

We have already said that it is important to distinguish adult antisocial behavior from antisocial personality disorder and from psychopathy. One of the leading researcher therapists in the field, Michael Stone, has also given us an 11-point gradation of antisociality that seems fairly straightforward but serves as a reminder that some patients with antisociality are more treatable than others (Stone 2000, p. 97). The points summarized and rephrased are:

1. ASPD traits but less than full ASPD or part of another PD.
2. Some antisocial traits with explosive and irritable personality traits.
3. Malignant narcissism.
4. ASPD with property crimes only.
5. Nonviolent sexual offenses (e.g., voyeurism).
6. ASPD with violent felonies.
7. Nonviolent psychopathic behavior (e.g., as with con artist).
8. Violent psychopathic behavior.
9. Psychopathic behavior with sadistic control.
10. Psychopathic behavior with violent sadism and murder but no prolonged torture.
11. Psychopathic behavior with prolonged torture followed by murder.

We will talk more about psychopaths below, but we urge you to think twice before imagining how effective you will be with ASPD patients who are far along on the spectrum.

Borderline Personality Disorder

Defining Features of BPD

The dominant features of BPD are impairments in functioning, difficulties with emotional control, poor impulse control, a distortion of self-image, risk-taking, an unstable mood, and rocky interpersonal relationships. Violence toward a partner or significant other is common as a reaction to an impending rejection or abandonment. Poor long-term judgment and impulsive and reckless acts such as prostitution and substance use due to impaired regulation of emotions are frequent. Attention-seeking behaviors such as fire-setting or other rule breaking acts are prevalent (Craissati et al. 2015).

Prevalence of BPD in Corrections

The prevalence of BPD in correctional settings is quite high but seldom reviewed in the forensic or correctional literature (Conn et al. 2010). BPD in the correctional setting is considerably greater than in the general community and psychiatric clinic settings (Trestman et al. 2007). Prevalence is reported to be between 12.9% and 26.8% for men and between 20% and 54% for women (Black et al. 2007; Tye and Mullen 2006). The prevalence reported in a survey of English maximum security units and prisons, which included much comorbidity, was 69%, making it the most common PD (Coid 1998).

Challenges of Working With BPD in Prison

Patients often present as angry, entitled, and demanding. Splitting of staff is a common occurrence. These individuals may be seductive or create strong countertransference reactions. They may vacillate between mushy thankfulness and abuse. You may find you are spending an excessive amount of time and resources with them.

Patients with BPD create multiple barriers to care due to the impulsive and emotionally labile presentation, self-mutilation, aggressiveness, and suicidal acts (Trestman 2000). Correctional staff often respond with irritation, frustration, and anger, and you may feel threatened by them, drained by them, or avoidant of them (Craissati et al. 2015). Persons with BPD in prison repeatedly find themselves in or create what they feel are catastrophic or crisis situations. Crisis management techniques are useful.

Supportive Psychotherapy Techniques and Tips for BPD

Psychotherapy is fundamental in the treatment for BPD (American Psychiatric Association 2001). A review of psychotherapy treatments for patients with BPD revealed that supportive psychotherapy was associated with improvements in facets of impulsivity (Clarkin et al. 2007). It has also been found effective in reducing self-injurious and suicidal behaviors (Aviram et al. 2004). Even in a complex article by experts discussing such things as transference interpretations in the treatment of borderline personality, a comment was made about the major importance of the nonspecific factors, which we have called the "common factors theory of psychotherapy effectiveness," which is embodied in supportive psychotherapy:

> We know that a good enough therapeutic alliance is a key ingredient in outcome. Although variously defined, the core concept involves the patient's perception that he or she is being helped and is pursuing goals held in common with the therapist [citing Gabbard et al. 1994]. Norcross [citing Norcross 2000] noted from his analysis of numerous approaches to psychotherapy that technique accounts for only 12%–15% of outcomes across all different kinds of therapies. (Gabbard and Horowitz 2009, p. 519)

TABLE 10–2.   **Tips for therapy with the patient with BPD**

Immediately deal with staff splitting.

Keep in mind that these patients are in emotional pain.

Focus on current, not past choices.

Do your limit-setting and boundary management.

Be aware of the potential for aggression and self-harm.

Use nonjudgmental verbiage.

Expect the emotional roller coaster.

Instill hope.

Use a calm voice.

Show empathy and compassion.

Focus on thoughts, not feelings.

Remember that these individuals may be impulsive.

Do not set too many goals.

Recognize the need for a team approach.

Be sensitive to fears of abandonment.

Consider other diagnoses (including other personality disorders).

Provide clear communication with patient and staff.

Provide psychoeducation.

Tips for therapy are shown in Table 10–2. Supportive psychotherapy keeps the focus on the present, not the past, to minimize regression and identity diffusion. Often, patients present with guilt and regret related to the charges that brought them into the legal system. They may say "I should have…," "I didn't do…," or "I did…" And often, "I am so stupid to have…" You can of course acknowledge the patient's feelings. Then you may want to assure her that everyone has made choices and decisions that may not be wise, but that does not make her "stupid." Then work with the person to focus on the present and to set very short-term goals. Have the patient picture herself driving down the road and her eyes never leaving the rearview mirror. Such a rear-looking attitude would obviously be dangerous, wouldn't it? Inform her that she cannot forget the events, but she can change how she sees them and learn from the mistakes. Setting too many goals or goals that are too far in the future can be overwhelming.

Allowing the patient to set goals in collaboration with the therapist helps those who often feel controlled and manipulated by others (Hellerstein et al. 2004). It is essential to be cognizant that most people with BPD have a history of childhood trauma, including sexual, physical, and emotional abuse. This understanding enables the therapist to have some empathy right from the beginning (Battaglia 2020). Empathy is an effective tool of therapy. A therapist can show empathy with the patient's distress at incarceration and concern and understanding for any physical, emotional, and sexual trauma the patient has suffered. Patients also should receive education about BPD and alternative ways to relieve anger, stress, and depression and alternatives to self-injury (e.g., journaling, exercising, seeking someone to speak with).

Validation of feelings is important and conveys the message that the therapist cares. With anger, patients occasionally only get angrier when the feeling is identified. For example, the patient may accuse you: "What would you know about being locked up?

You get to go to your nice house every night." To this an appropriate response would be "Yes, I can leave every night, but I do still care about your feelings and your well-being." Allowing patients to discuss stressful relationships facilitates learning the circumstances leading to their behaviors and inappropriate responses to stressors (Gunderson and Links 2014; Hong 2019).

Patients' remarks, either of praise or of belittlement, may be out of proportion. Try not to react strongly to these remarks. Splitting of staff can occur if you do not recognize it quickly and resolve the issue before it is a problem. Often, the behaviors create animosity with custody staff. Despite your countertransference feelings, keep in mind that prisoners with BPD are not *always* intentionally engaging in manipulative behaviors but are dealing with painful emotions. You need to assist the patient with effective coping skills.

The ultimate goal for the patient with BPD is for her to achieve the ability to manage emotions and have an understanding of her feelings, improve interactions with others, and stop self-destructive behaviors. The feelings of emptiness that many with BPD experience can be addressed by clarification, psychoeducation, and naming feelings. Impulsive behavior should be focused on by increasing choices and reviewing issues when the patient is no longer upset. The difficulties with intense anger can be addressed by offering methods of control. For example, rather than asking the patient with BPD why she did something, you can make a comment that allows the patient to choose to respond or not. Questioning why may be threatening for the patient with a fragile sense of self. There should be no drawn-out periods of silence, as that might arouse paranoia or regression. Supportive psychotherapy is conversational with the therapist guiding the exchange toward mutually agreed-upon goals (Hellerstein et al. 2004). Goals should be realistic and attainable, and you should use easily understandable concepts. You should be aware of manipulative behaviors and set clear and consistent boundaries.

With all prisoners, but especially those with BPD, it is important to assess for suicidal and self-mutilating behaviors, especially during times of stress (Cihlar 2014). Nonsuicidal self-injurious behaviors are common, but an individual who has experienced trauma could be further traumatized when placed in an environment such as being secluded on a suicide watch. Therefore, it is important to teach interventions that help patients to calm themselves to prevent escalation, as well as developing a crisis response safety plan. Continuing to assess for signs and symptoms of depression is crucial. Determination of dangerous behaviors requires collaboration with correctional staff.

Good Psychiatric Management for BPD

BPD was not an official disorder until publication of DSM-III in 1980. The term "borderline" had been used in the 1930s to describe patients who psychiatrists thought were inclined to slide into "borderline schizophrenia" (Salters-Pedneault 2020). As a young psychiatrist, John Gunderson, M.D., was fascinated with these patients. In 1975, he coauthored an article that provided a name and diagnosis for the "borderline schizophrenic" and "borderline neurotic": borderline personality disorder. Gunderson is now known as the "Grandfather of the BPD Diagnosis" (McLean Hospital 2019).

Gunderson developed a supportive and psychoeducational program, called Good Psychiatric Management, which is manualized for a variety of practitioners (Gunderson 2014; see also Choi-Kain and Gunderson 2019). GPM is nonspecialized and avoids being a therapeutic school of its own, and practitioners who have done all they can do with GPM are urged to refer patients to more specialized therapies such as DBT. GPM incorporates case management alongside supportive psychotherapy and uses both psychodynamic and cognitive-behavioral methods. The basics of GPM are practical and intended to be easy to put into action. GPM is easy to learn and emphasizes psychoeducation and the need to focus on social adaptation. The distinctive features of GPM are a focus on the patient's life outside therapy, psychoeducation, goal-setting, and multimodality. There is no specific length or intensity of the therapy, and an effort is made to connect emotions and behaviors to interpersonal stressors. In addition, GPM integrates approaches and interventions from other evidence-based psychotherapies (Gunderson 2014; Gunderson et al. 2018). Suicidal behavior, of course, can be a fundamental issue in treating persons with BPD, as we discussed in Chapter 5. Finally, we mention that Gunderson thought that the evidence shows that BPD and bipolar disorder are separate conditions that would only be found to coexist coincidentally (Gunderson et al. 2014).

Narcissistic Personality Disorder

Defining Features of NPD

DSM-5-TR describes the essential features of NPD as grandiose self-esteem, attention-seeking behaviors, a sense of entitlement, and a need for admiration. The proposed diagnostic features under the dimensional model under criterion A are a moderate or greater impairment in personality function, manifested by characteristic difficulties in two or more of the following four areas: identity, self-direction, empathy, or intimacy. Under Criterion B, the features are grandiosity and attention seeking. However, there are researchers who believe in the heterogeneity of the disorder, and a recognition that only some variants of the disorder predispose to criminality.

Patients with NPD may be vulnerable to extreme reactions when their self-image is damaged or threatened. They may respond with intense feelings of hurt or anger to even the least bit of rejection or criticism (Skodol et al. 2014). Their defensive responses may be intended to punish the person who threatens or damages them (Logan 2008). Comorbidity with mood, anxiety, and SUD are common (Caligor and Clarkin 2010; Eaton et al. 2017). The most common comorbidity is major depressive disorder.

Prevalence of NPD in Corrections

As with BPD, the reported prevalence of NPD in the correctional setting varies considerably. According to Ambardar (2018), the prevalence rate in the forensic population is 6%. Between 50% and 75% of those diagnosed with NPD are male (American Psychiatric Association 2013). Coid (1998), in his study, found a prevalence of 48%.

Challenges of Working With NPD in Prison

Prisoners with NPD may believe they are superior, cannot recognize that they have faults, and are not open to feedback. A notable challenge is addressing the trait of grandiosity—one that leads them to create problematic situations for themselves in the restrictive environment of corrections because they believe they are better than the other prisoners, and this can lead to violence (Trestman 2000). Their behavior and overblown ego can aggravate corrections staff and fellow prisoners. Often, they believe that the only answer to problems is an act of violence, and the violence may be directed toward corrections staff (Coid 2002). It is a challenge to limit the NPD patient's destructive behavior toward others and himself (Caligor et al. 2015).

Supportive Psychotherapy Techniques and Tips for NPD

Unlike therapy for ASPD, most therapists do not recommend group therapy for patients with NPD (Logan 2008). The supportive techniques noted in the early chapters of this text are beneficial because they engender feelings in the patient that he is approved of. When working with the problems of entitlement, specialness, and arrogance, you should not use direct confrontation. You should expect to be provoked by insulting remarks. Do all you can to resist the temptation of a power struggle. If your patient does in fact have a good education, sophisticated tastes, and is well read, then simply acknowledge it in a neutral way. Should the patient verbalize false declarations, you may need to ignore them. Be aware of the power imbalance in the therapeutic relationship and the NPD patient's need to feel superior. Measures you can take to lessen this include encouraging collaborative decision-making, offering choices, avoiding the use of jargon, and underplaying the hierarchy (Craissati et al. 2015). We're reminded of an adage that we found in a science fiction classic, which nicely expresses how you might feel about cultivating the relationship with a smug and superior narcissist: "It is written, If you need something from a dog, call him 'Sir'" (Laumer 2001, p. 556). (Apologies to dog lovers for even quoting this, but you get the point.)

It may not be effective to initially challenge these prisoners' grandiosity because their self-esteem is unstable and they may drop out of the therapy if they find it painful. You want to promote self-awareness and an understanding of the impact relationships have on the self. Do not initially attempt to improve their sense of empathy. Promoting awareness of the vulnerable self should not be rushed. In the *later stages* of therapy, the negative impact that one's behavior has on others needs to be addressed (Dimaggio 2012).

Although GPM, mentioned previously, was developed as a treatment for BPD, it has also been implemented for narcissistic personality disorder. This approach involves seven elements, including psychoeducation (see Table 10–3).

Paranoid Personality Disorder

Defining Features of PPD

People with a PPD present with feelings of mistrust and suspiciousness and tend to hold grudges against others. Often, they are very guarded and distant in their relationships and avoid closeness. They may be hypervigilant and prone to over-reacting to innocuous situations. They interpret the actions and intentions of others as a threat (Craissati et al. 2015). Childhood trauma is prevalent (Lee 2017). Individuals with a

TABLE 10–3.	Good psychiatric management (GPM) for narcissistic personality disorder

Elements of management

Diagnostic disclosure—essential first step

Psychoeducation—genetics, course, vulnerability

Case management—focus on life outside the treatment

Progress—determines duration and intensity of treatment

Treatment—psychodynamic (motives, feelings) and behavioral (contingency accountability)

Multimodality—"It takes a village"

Managing safety (suicidality)—collaborative, but patients are in charge of their own safety

Elaboration of psychoeducational techniques

Heritability: "It is not your fault"

Prevalence: "You are not alone"

Vulnerability: "Be proactive, anticipate difficulties"

Physiological basis: "The difficulties are real, not made up"

Naturalistic course: "Improvements happen over time"

Available treatments: "Treatments can help"

Source.   Weinberg et al. 2019, pp. 263–265.

history of physical, sexual, and emotional abuse may have one or more symptoms of PPD (Tyrka et al. 2009). There is no alternative model for PPD at this time.

Prevalence of PPD in Corrections

PPD is common but not well studied. The prevalence of PPD in the Coid (1998) study was 47%, but as we have noted, this was with an assumed comorbidity with other PDs that included BPD (69%), ASPD (55%), and NPD (48%)—numbers higher than reported in other surveys.

Challenges of Working With PPD in Prison

Prisoners with PPD are difficult to treat. About 70% do not stay in treatment, and the likelihood of them forming a therapeutic relationship is low (Berichon et al. 2019). Treatment plans should encourage cooperation and minimize anxiety and suspiciousness (Cihlar 2014).

Supportive Psychotherapy Techniques and Tips for PPD

According to Skodol et al. (2014), supportive individual psychotherapy may be the best treatment. You should avoid being too "nice" or "friendly," because this could raise the level of mistrust and suspiciousness and you need to provide clear and simple instructions (Cihlar 2014). Provide symptom-centered care addressing anxiety, delusions, and agitation and help the patient to develop positive coping mechanisms (Berichon et al. 2019).

Violent Offenders

Violent offenders are those who have committed violent crimes outside of prison and may be (and often are) at risk for violent behaviors within prison. But what is the relationship between PD and violent crime? While there is a considerable overlap between psychopathy, ASPD, other PDs, and violent crime, the causal elements are still much debated beyond the known co-occurrence. Some major researchers have "found little credible evidence to support a simple unidirectional causal relationship between PD and risk of violence. We are left with a relationship whose nature is unclear and which may be less robust than commonly assumed (although few would doubt that some sort of relationship exists, the epidemiology suggests as much)" (Howard and Howells 2010, p.197, discussing Duggan and Howard 2009). But prisons are full of people who have been violent and some others who will become violent in the future. Many of them have a personality disorder, but of different kinds. Traditional research usually distinguishes planned violence from unplanned violence. For example, from the preceding sections, we think that people with ASPD are more likely to engage in premeditated violence and those with BPD and NPD are more likely to engage in impulsive violence. Everything needs to be kept in perspective, however. Major mental disorders, those that used to be called "Axis I" pathology, still contribute to violence through mediators such as delusions and poor impulse control. Depression plays a role in murder, not just suicide and self-harm. Psychopathy plays a role in violence but barely overlaps with schizophrenia. And we feel obliged to consider the opinion that "[t]he real public health issue concerning mental health disorder and violence is alcohol abuse. Much of the violent crime in the United States occurs under the influence of alcohol" (Beck and Wencel 1998, p. 21).

What about treatment? So far, we have approached the treatment of violence and criminality from the aspect of personality disorders. But violence can also be approached as a thing-in-itself, that is, as a behavior needing improving rather than a personality worth fixing.

There is increasing recognition of the role of self-regulation, or the lack thereof, in the causation of violent behavior. Self-regulation of emotions is a developmental process that starts at birth from a baby's first cry and continues daily until that child is an adult facing a challenging, threatening, or painful situation. Good parents' ability and availability to soothe a crying child, which may happen hundreds or thousands of times over years, leads to a young person who can soothe and regulate his or her own emotions (Groves Gillespie and Seibel 2006; Shonkoff and Phillips 2000). Failure to do so may result in a person who erupts in violence against self or others or suffers "breakdowns" such as immobile depression. Healthy relationships with one's parents are the building block of one's healthy development. There is a relationship of childhood trauma to adult problems in prison (Moore et al. 2020; Shonkoff and Phillips 2000; Wolff and Shi 2012). Both early and late traumatic experiences are associated with development of many psychological problems, including those that may lead to violence. They also tend to live in violence-prone environments that are not conducive to self-regulation. Improvement in self-regulation also plays a role in programs such as the Good Lives Model.

Most researchers believe that the reduction of violence in the world starts with good parenting in homes and the creation of nonviolent communities and, thus, nonviolent cultures. Is it too late to do anything by the time people are put in prison? The measurement we are talking here is recidivism. No, it's not too late, and current research shows that the question "What works?" is answered affirmatively for a number of programs—in general, programs embracing the risk-need-responsivity (RNR) principles. A recent review (Olver and Stockdale 2018) does a thorough job of naming what works, what might work, and what doesn't. Two types of programs work: comprehensive multi-intervention programs such as the Violence Reduction Program (Wong and Gordon 2013) and high-risk specialized treatment units (Polaschek and Kilgour 2013), and focused intervention/single-need programs such as Reasoning and Rehabilitation (Ross and Fabiano 1985), moral reconation therapy (Little and Robinson 1989), Thinking for a Change (Bush and Taymans 1997), and Cognitive Self-Change (Bush and Brian 1993), various anger management programs, behavioral modification programs such as social skills and assertiveness training, relapse prevention, substance abuse treatment, and, last but not least, medication treatments. Of lesser proven effectiveness are some well-known programs such as DBT, aggression replacement therapy (Glick and Gibbs 2020), therapeutic communities, and trauma-focused approaches such as the Seeking Safety program of Miller and Najavits (2012). Of no value are nondirective therapies, and toss into this bucket, prison itself, that is, criminal sanctions applied in isolation.

Although the preferred modality of most of these programs is the group, we have found it useful to "pick and choose" group material for individual therapy. An example of a program based on aggression replacement training can be found in the book edited by Hornsveld et al. (2019). About half the book is a discussion of research and assessment, while the rest is a packaged program with modules and forms for treatment. In Table 10–4 we give an example of a scenario inspired by one from the program for prosocial thinking. It exemplifies a theory of crime that we have not discussed before: Routine Activities (Cohen and Felson 1979). Criminal acts are said to involve a motivated offender (or two of them), an attractive target (or two of them), and the absence of what is called "guardianship." Patients can explore and debate the motivations and behavior of Anton and Jeremy in robbing the young woman and her mother. Excuses and rationalizations (or what Walters calls "mollifications") will be given that the woman is a sitting duck and deserves to be robbed, or that she is well dressed and can easily afford the loss, or that she and her mother are gamblers who throw away their money anyway, and that casinos in general don't have a moral right to keep any of their money because their business is basically dishonest. The therapist points out that Anton and Jeremy make a bad decision together because they're in a hurry and don't think of the risks (e.g., the presence of a security camera) or the consequences (arrest for aggravated assault and robbery charges). The therapist also discusses the effect of antisocial thinking in the pair of men and how Anton originates the criminal idea and Jeremy doesn't even think twice and agrees.

Isolated violent acts can have many explanations and may not be repeatable, such as when a person attacks or kills an abusive spouse. Perhaps Anton and Jeremy are not normally violent robbers but the situation kind of "got away from them." Nevertheless, such persons are violent offenders, even if the risk of further violence is low. Such persons need therapy for their role as violent offenders, not because they are victims, but because they may suffer trauma or remorse from their commission of the offense. Thus, Anton may be remorseful that the elderly women broke her hip—or he

---

TABLE 10–4.   Example of scenario to develop prosocial thinking

Anton and Jeremy like to hang out at the local hotel and casino, but they are getting low in funds so they start walking to their car in the outdoor lot. They notice that the casino security guard has just rounded through the lot, but he is nowhere to be seen now. A woman is assisting her obviously disabled elderly mother to their car, as she obviously holds on to her mother's arm and they walk slowly. Anton takes one look at Jeremy and says: "Two pocketbooks, easy pickings, what do you think? They're not going to fight back—she'll be too worried about her mother." Jeremy agrees: "Sure, let's go quick, before the guard comes back. I'll grab the woman and you grab her mother."

They come up behind the women and grab the pocketbooks, but the women kind of hold on so Anton and Jeremy push them hard to the ground, pick up the pocketbooks, and run. The young woman screams, "Help! We've been robbed!" The elderly woman seems alive but moves slowly as if she has broken something. The guys escape in their car. They get a few hundred dollars in cash and use the credit cards. Three days later, a team of police officers shows up at Jeremy's apartment and arrests him, since he was identified on the casino security cameras from his previous mug shots. Jeremy implicates Anton and says, "It was his idea." Anton and Jeremy are convicted of aggravated assault with serious bodily injury and an elderly enhancement. They are going to be away from that casino for a long time.

Discussion questions:

1. What do you think was Anton's reasoning when he suggested they rob the women?

2. Do you think the women deserved to be robbed since they were playing in a casino (actually, they were just coming out of the hotel)?

3. If the couple had been a young man and his father, would the guys have considered robbing them? If not, why not?

4. What does it mean to pick on women or people who can be overwhelmed and possibly injured or even killed by force? Is it the women's fault for fighting back and resisting injury? If the elderly woman had broken her neck (and maybe she did since the scenario is not clear) when Anton pushed her, would that be Anton's fault or the woman's fault for being weak and frail?

5. Do you think Anton should have ratted out Jeremy?

6. If either Anton or Jeremy had been alone at the time, would either one of them have even thought of robbing anyone? Does having two robbers just make it physically easier or mentally easier for the guys to agree to commit the crime together?

7. Are the guys just stupid, not considering that the parking lot has cameras as well as physical security? Did they forget that fact in the rush to commit the crime? Did they really think about the possible consequences at all when they decided to "go for it"?

Source.   Scenario not the same as, but inspired by, a scenario in Hornsveld et al. 2019, p. 254.

could blame her for resisting him! Not every violent person has a mental illness diagnosis, either, and our brief scenario makes no such assumption. However, there is a recognition that some repetitively violent persons have PDs that may contribute to some of their violent behaviors.

Somewhat fancifully, but with an eye on the treatment programs that have been and are being developed, we present an announcement of a treatment program for violent offenders with ASPD in Figure 10–1. We wish we could get these individuals into therapy by posting a flyer like that on the prison wall or a community bulletin board. However, you can benefit from the observations of Glicken and Sechrest (2003), who studied and wrote about a group of 400 men (we have not quoted these exactly but summarized them incorporating our own experiences):

- Violent people are often embarrassed to self-disclose and view psychotherapy as feminizing and emasculating—an issue relevant to our discussion of what has been called "toxic masculinity" in prison in Chapter 12.
- Violent people may need to save face, so chart a more indirect route to get them to talk. For example, let them talk about other things, and sooner or later the important content will come up incidentally and you can seize on it.
- Violent people do not form therapeutic relationships easily, although they may think they have one with you.
- Consistent with their difficulties in handling emotions properly, violent people release much anger and rage in therapy. Your job is to help them to delay and verbalize before becoming rageful.
- Violent people do not like to admit they are in pain, including emotional pain, so you have to be gentle and persistent in getting them to admit it.
- In therapy with opposite-sex therapists, violent people can be manipulative, but they may also work hard to please, and this can be put to work to make gains in therapy.
- Violent persons are often disorderly and benefit from structure; praise them for their accomplishments and build on their strengths.
- Glicken and Sechrest (2003) advise therapists to avoid diagnostic labels. "The diagnostic category may be true but it certainly will not help the client to know it" (p. 261). This is worth considering, and we understand the basis of this in the defensiveness of the violent group that he worked with. However, we do not think it is always possible to avoid diagnostic labels such as when patients ask about them or get copies of their chart. So we would say: Don't spontaneously bring up the diagnosis, but be prepared to hear about it from the patient and defend it.
- Violent people may have a terrible track record in intimate relationships, but they still have the need and desire to have them. You can try to help them with that, and their failures in intimate relationships may actually have caused regret that can be used to develop positive nonviolent relationships.
- Finally, it may be appropriate to give up if you can't get it to work. Glicken and Sechrest think that 30% of their group (domestic violence perpetrators) cannot benefit from individual talk therapy.

Attachment Theory

Many violent persons who have committed crimes have severe and dangerous PDs, and PDs in this context have been recognized as a distinct category in the United Kingdom, but to a lesser extent in the United States. The United Kingdom has developed an Offender Personality Disorder (OPD) strategy based on a psychoanalytic model of attachment theory and a method to prevent recidivism called the "desistance model." Attachment theory was developed by John Bowlby in the 1940s from his observations of infants and refined by him throughout his life. His collaboration with Mary Ainsworth was significant in the evolution of his theories (Bretherton 1992). Attachment theory also plays a role in at least two theories of criminology, Sampson and Laub's Age-Graded Life-Course Theory (Sampson and Laub 1993) and Gottfredson and Hirschi's theory developed in *A General Theory of Crime* (Gottfredson

Attention all criminals! Yes, this means YOU!

Do you routinely neglect the rights of other people?

Do you always hurt the ones who love you
(because you can't love anybody but yourself)?

Do you have a rocky rap sheet the length of the Atlantic Coast?

Do you fell isolated, lonely, even depressed because
your behavior is a turn-off to other people?

If so, you might have ASPD, an embarrassing but treatable disorder!

Yes, ASPD is treatable,
and there are even noncarceral options that are government-funded.

These treatments, like those monoclonal antibodies ("Mabs"),
will immunize you against your violence: they are called Psychoblab!

If interested, apply to your case manager (if incarcerated) or
to your local mental health clinic (if unincarcerated).

After a few years, you'll be thankful you did
(and so will those who persist in
loving you despite the way you treat them)!

FIGURE 10–1.   A fanciful announcement.

Note.   While the above is fanciful and sarcastic, a program to attract persons with ASPD needs to achieve their buy-in ("What's in it for me?") such as by offering to ameliorate feelings of loneliness or depression that come from their criminal lifestyle. If it is possible that the program will improve their personal relationships to significant others, so much the better. Long-term commitment is needed, and drop-out rates are quite high. It also takes considerable therapist skill and certain personal characteristics to treat persons with ASPD. Of course, the patients are not going to pay for it, and options to continue in community corrections beyond prison are vital to achieving success and lessening recidivism.

and Hirschi 1990). We thought we would research the latter, and we were reminded that "[s]earching online produces over 177,000 scholarly articles and 57 books associated with A General Theory of Crime" (Cook 2016, p. 338). Is that what happens when someone proposes a *general* theory instead of a *specific* theory? Suffice it to say that Gottfredson and Hirschi's "general theory" has been extremely influential.

Attachment theory is helpful in classifying different types of failed attachments and their relationship to future criminal behaviors, including stalking and violent crimes such as spouse battering (Meloy 2003). The relevance of early attachments reminds us of issues we have discussed in assigning the primacy of parental neglect, abuse, and trauma in the lives of many prisoners. For our previously mentioned fictional psychologist/detective Alex Delaware, cruel and often hypocritical nurturing was called "Bad Love" (Kellerman 1994), which was not exactly invented by its author since it was, among others, a 1990 Eric Clapton song. The possibility (raised in the book) that "bad love" could create a psychopath was developed, and it seems unlikely that anyone would doubt that. The nature of love, good and bad, has been written about in fiction and has been the subject of philosophical inquiries (McMurtry 1992). Surprisingly, however, we have not found "bad love" used as a technical term in the mental health literature. Research on the nature/nurture question continues, with recent developments including investigation of the relationship of callous-unemotional traits in childhood and the heritability of psychopathy (according to one source being 50%; Junewicz and Billick 2021). A reasonable position is that there is an interaction between genetic characteristics such as impulsivity and adverse early childhood experiences, particularly when caregivers do not provide a safe and supportive environment for the child, leading to traumatic experiences or disrupted attachments (Campbell and Craissati 2018, p. 14). It is hypothesized that these deficits in early life lead to problems in adulthood, including:

- High levels of anxiety and arousal.
- Difficulty in "mentalizing" (understanding what others are thinking or feeling).
- Great sensitivity to shame and humiliation, which can spark violence and a need to control others and get respect.
- Poor self-identity.
- A feeling of powerlessness and lack of purpose and meaning in their lives.

This is not a list just for ASPD. For example, difficulty in mentalizing is considered to be a fundamental deficit in the personalities of those with BPD. A detailed manual for practitioners is available online (Craissati et al. 2015).

The use of attachment theory, while psychoanalytically based, is thought to be an independent therapeutic method but informs the way case formulations are made. It is also an alternative to cognitive-behavioral methods, which, as we have mentioned, work solely on the surface with behavior and do not investigate a person's psychological past. Since therapy based on attachment theory attempts to remember, replay, and repair a patient's previous deficient attachments, it relies heavily on a supportive relationship with the therapist, so it is eminently compatible with supportive psychotherapy and worth learning about so as to understand how to interview, assess, and treat personality disordered patients. "An attachment framework does not give us a set of exercises or a workbook in the way that cognitive behaviourism can, but it offers us a way of understanding our offenders, re-activating their sense of being understood, and nurturing their understanding of themselves and others" (Ansbro 2008). Detailed histories and relationships to therapeutic practice can be found in articles by Ansbro (2008) and Holmes (2015). "The most significant aspect of the treatment of the antisocial personality is this individual's difficulty with attachment and bonding" (Harris 1995, p. 94).

We have not given up talking of therapy for people with ASPD, but we are going to move on to another topic for a while—psychopathy.

And Speaking of Which—Here Come the Psychopaths

(hopefully not into your house, but into your prison)

> *"I've come to believe that there are people among us that simply aren't human." (Patterson 2019, p. 9)*

Hey, what is this? The opener for a book about a secret alien invasion? No, these "in-humans" (if that is what you believe they are) have been with us since the beginning of civilization. They are the ones we call "psychopaths."

Psychopathy is a topic that occupies and fascinates both laypersons and professionals—and is found in many books, movies, and plays—for psychopaths can be quite charming, enough to charm us out of our money and our lives. Back in 1599, Shakespeare's Octavius tells us that "some that smile have in their hearts, I fear, millions of mischiefs" (*Julius Caesar*, Act 4, Scene 1). And Hamlet muses that "[o]ne may smile, and smile, and be a villain" (*Hamlet*, Act 1, Scene 5). It does appear that no matter how much we talk about psychopaths, new questions come up that prolong the debate of whether they are "bad" or "mad" or "badly raised" or "bad seeds" or something in some proportion. The terminology can be confusing because several terms are often used interchangeably. Psychopathy is a smaller category than ASPD. Most persons with ASPD are not psychopaths. Also, the terms "sociopath" and "psychopath" are used loosely in the movies, novels, and television programs. The first usage of "psychopath" was around 1900 and changed to "sociopath" in the 1930s with emphasis placed on the damage the individuals inflicted on society. The first DSM in 1952 considered antisocial personality as a "sociopathic personality disturbance." DSM-III revised the definition of personality disorders with the addition of *traits*, which was an improvement, but because of the brevity of the descriptions, usually only a sentence or two, the diagnoses had poor validity (Coolidge and Segal 1998). Today, researchers have returned to the terminology of "psychopath." There are various assessment instruments, the major one being the clinician-rated Psychopathy Checklist—Revised (PCL-R) of R.D. Hare (see Hare 2020 for latest versions). Other assessments, such as the Psychopathic Personality Inventory (a self-report inventory), are often discussed in the media (Hirstein 2013).

Psychopaths are often considered untreatable because of their lack of empathy and shallow feelings, need for high levels of stimulation, and lack of moral sense. As noted, DSM-5 recognizes psychopathic traits as related to ASPD. Most researchers consider psychopathy to be a personality disorder closely related to ASPD. So consider:

- It would follow that many people share some characteristics of antisocial persons and some psychopaths, just not to the degree of severity of multiplicity of features found in persons diagnosed with ASPD or those considered to be psychopaths. (In fact, there was an attempt to popularize the concept of what were called "almost" disorders in a series of books by Harvard University clinicians [Schouten and Silver 2012].)

- Many researchers believe that psychopaths are a heterogeneous group, with some of them being treatable and others being very difficult to treat, depending on their particular traits.
- A corollary is that it should be possible to have some empathy and a therapeutic alliance (albeit limited) with some psychopathic patients.

Dr. Marla Patterson spent 24 years with the Federal Bureau of Prisons (BOP) until she retired in 2014, most of it as chief of psychology at USP Marion, one of the two highest security prisons in BOP (the other being the well-known ADX Florence). She supervised a staff of 18, but she states that in her 2019 book she writes only about prisoners she knew personally (Patterson 2019). She says that the people we call psychopaths do not have and are unaffected by normal human motivations and emotions. An example is a person who kills his children and stashes the bodies under his bed until the neighbors become aware of the stench. Is this sickness or evil? She says it's difficult to believe that these psychopaths are not mentally ill or intellectually disadvantaged. Rather they lack empathy and normal human attachments. They cannot be healed or rehabilitated, and they are particularly dangerous because they are able to hide their depravity (Patterson 2019).

British mystery writer Ruth Rendell's renowned Inspector Wexford references a philosophical position when discussing a suspect. It is said that Sara is intellectually brilliant but lacks normal human feelings and this makes her a psychopathic *solipsist* (Rendell 1985, p. 320). But what is this reference to solipsism, and why apply it to a psychopath? *Solipsism* (related to the word *solo*) is a theoretical philosophical position that the speaker or holder of that position can never know if *anyone else* exists. It is one of those "argue me out of this" positions in the philosophical theory of knowledge leading us to explain how it is that, inside our heads, we really know that there is a world with other people out there. There is relevance here to understanding human thought, such as helping an autistic child to relate to other people. To call a psychopath a solipsist implies that the psychopath really does not believe that there is anyone else but him or her in the world. But keep in mind that it is a literary allusion. Rendell's point is that Sara believes she is the only one who *matters*. She lives for "number one," and there is no "number two." The name of the mystery we alluded to, by the way, is *An Unkindness of Ravens*, using the traditional term for a group of ravens (no kidding), just as you can have a *pride* of lions, a *parade* of elephants, or a *clowder* of cats (did you know this?). But if you can have an unkindness of ravens, what would you call a group of solipsists? An impossibility? (Since there can only be one solipsist?) And a group of psychopaths? That might depend on your politics.

We have been talking about one end of the spectrum of beliefs, that psychopaths are unaffectable and untreatable. We even compared them to aliens. Consider the alien race in the original *Star Trek* episode "Menagerie" (Internet Movie Database 2021), the Talosians. Those Talosians were a formerly advanced race of beings with large hat sizes who developed the ability to project illusions upon and deceive anybody at a distance. Captain Kirk and Commander Spock end up in a conflict with them, but they are unable to know if they are winning or not. If you fire your phaser at a Talosian, you don't know if you have hit him (or her, or it, or them), because he can deceive you into thinking you have missed him or that he is somewhere else. So aren't they just like psychopaths, charming you into thinking you have some influence on them, while all the while laughing at you and disregarding your influences and not giving a darn? You don't even know if you have gotten through to them with those phaser-like strikes of your psychotherapy! What do you really know about your Talosian/psychopathic patients? If they have such a consummate ability to deceive, how can you know if they have really decided to be prosocial? Can't they just be fooling you all the time? Do you want to make them better or will that make them better psychopaths when they get out?

Now, we should mention that "ordinary" (i.e., nonpsychopathic) patients have an incredible capacity to deceive their therapists, as shown by numerous studies and books on the subject. For example, a study by Blanchard and Farber (2015) reported that 93% of psychotherapy patients admit that they have lied at least once to their therapist. The lies cover a variety of topics, including their impression of whether the therapy is effective or whether they are feeling suicidal.

So we should not be surprised that nobody does it better than a psychopath.

We have said that we believe that many psychopaths are treatable. Proponents of the Good Lives Model, discussed further in Chapter 13, are even more sanguine (as in one of the four personality types!) about treating psychopaths. Using the factor analysis of Hare's PCL-R, Wong (2013) divides the checklist into the F1 personality and F2 antisocial factors (a division that is used by most researchers). The personality factors are the glibness and charming characteristic by which psychopaths deceive their audiences and in particular disrupt and defeat their psychotherapists through manipulations and boundary violations. The antisocial factors are the ones that describe these individuals' criminality, unstable behavior, and hurts to others. Psychopaths, if properly engaged in psychotherapy with a fostered therapeutic alliance, can be affected by RNR programs, but the therapist has to work hard to defeat their deceptions—like facing those Talosians. (FYI: Many psychopaths, although they do not have huge brains like the Talosians, seem to have deficits in various areas of their brains.)

Wong proposes a two-component method of therapy similar to that of Livesley (2013), who points out some of the deficiencies of treatments like DBT and proposes that personality disorder treatment requires a general nonspecific factor and a specific or technical factor. The generic factor involves supportive engagement to bolster a therapeutic alliance that counteracts the patient's treatment-interfering behaviors (Wong 2013, pp. 6-6–6-7). We think that the optimal use of supportive psychotherapy would be in establishing a therapeutic alliance working on the items in Factor 1 of the PCL, which is responsible for patients' lack of motivation to change (Wong 2018). In general, psychodynamic psychotherapy does not work, but there is also a role for cognitive therapy and social skills training. You may also find that motivational interviewing techniques may help to engage the psychopathic patient in treatment. Deal with resistance (even though the latest version of motivational interviewing avoids that term—but we don't). This helps to focus the therapy on the treatment plan and avert the patient's "meaningless challenges and provocations" (Wong 2018, p. 633). Although there is a role for group therapies, psychopaths can defeat even skilled group therapists with their disruptive behaviors, so it takes a high level of skill and therapeutic expertise to work with them (Wong 2013). Use a team approach with frequent consultations between the team members to discuss progress and avoid splitting, manipulation, and burnout. Countertransference problems can include feelings of despair and exhaustion, a wish to retaliate, or overprotective relationships with boundary violations. There are several advantages, at least, to working with psychopaths in prison, including the ability to observe their out-of-session behaviors, control such behaviors, and take a team approach with frequent consultations with your colleagues.

Wong's optimism is shared by other researchers. For example, Polaschek and Daly (2018) reviewed older research that supports the existence of primary and secondary psychopaths. The former are the stable ones, with shallow emotions and insensitivity to others. The latter are like neurotics and have anxiety and mood disorders and disturbances of emotions such as irritability, reactive aggression, and impulsivity (p. 9, citing multiple historical sources). Those authors believe that secondary psychopaths are treatable and that the primary ones are not. This makes a lot of sense. It is also consistent with the findings (based partly on self-reports of persons considered psychopathic) in Martens (2014). Martens points out that hidden suffering, loneliness, and lack of self-esteem are risk factors for the violent behaviors of psychopaths. He believes that psychopaths do become depressed and disheartened as they age and fail to achieve the usual closeness that others achieve in relationships. We would suspect that Martens' treatable psychopaths are those of the secondary group described by Polaschek and Daly and that they should be fairly easy to identify if they present to you for psychotherapy, either voluntarily or as a result of suicide attempts. Again, and in the opinion of some researchers: Some people are just more psychopathic than others. There is a big overlap between antisocial personality (which you work with all the time) and psychopathy. It's just that psychopaths have "more of the bad stuff" than ordinary folks.

The second component of the therapeutic programs targets the second factor of the Hare checklist, which is responsible for criminal behavior. These programs are consistent with RNR methods, usually with skills training and CBT groups to address empathy, frustration tolerance, and impulse control. Sometimes patients need to attend different groups during the same time periods. Your treatment team should agree on your general approach using Wong's two-component therapy, or you might want to delve into Livesley's Integrated Modular Treatment (Livesley et al. 2018). You are also not limited to Hare's PCL approach, since there are others, such as a triarchic model of psychopathy involving disinhibition, meanness, and boldness (Patrick and Brislin 2018).

To avoid wasting time, experts recommend assessing for motivation when bringing persons with psychopathy into treatment (Hemphill and Hart 2002, pp. 209–213).

Preconditions

- The prisoner is interested in changing, acknowledges personal problems, and freely participates in treatment. He must experience marked emotional distress, guilt, or shame regarding his problems.
- He must have some capacity for self-reflection.
- He does believe that his problems are psychologically based and can be helped by psychotherapy (either group or individual as available).
- He establishes a positive relationship with a therapist and is willing to accept help. He has to have the ability to trust and have confidence in psychotherapy.
- He strives for autonomy and independence. This is compatible with one of the major goals of supportive psychotherapy and works well with persons who have "burned the bridges" of support from their families.

- The therapy should have clear and realistic treatment goals that are doable within the frame of the therapy you can offer and that the patient will accept.
- The patient is willing to exert effort to maintain treatment changes. This is a real problem, given that many individuals with psychopathy drop out of treatment within a year.

Motivational deficits can be shored up by turning some of the supposed deficits of psychopathy into strengths. Such "deficits" include their status orientation, strong desire for and tolerance of novelty, good interpersonal skills, and desire to be in control. The power of these can be harnessed if you do the following (summarized, paraphrased, and elaborated from Hemphill and Hart 2002):

- Build the therapeutic alliance with them—but slowly and carefully. As we have found, psychopaths like to be in control, and they would like to control *you*. Also, Hemphill and Hart (2002) recommend that you warn them in advance that you may compare the statements they make in therapy with factual material from their records and collateral sources.
- Use a formal assessment of motivation for treatment up-front. There is a lot of interest now in what is called "treatment readiness," and there are group therapies to improve motivation for treatment. An unmotivated person with psychopathy is likely to drop out of treatment or if completing treatment, to fail to apply the learning in the treatment.
- Highlight criminal lifestyle as low status. Psychopathic offenders can build on their strengths and train for prosocial jobs that are exciting and benefit from their interpersonal skills. Play up the status of those jobs and downplay the status of the criminal lifestyle.
- Help psychopathic prisoners to understand what a psychological explanation is. Do not expect them to understand sophisticated psychological explanations. Use a few simple examples of cause and effect.
- Get them to understand their personal contribution to their problems—an objective that is, of course, central to undermining the criminal lifestyles. Playing on their "strength" of a need to control things, you can help them overcome their impulsive tendencies when they get into criminally tempting situations.
- Emphasize self-sufficiency. Unlike many other prisoners, psychopaths have the skills to live prosocially and independently. What they lack is motivation and direction. They can be motivated by building a realization of the problems they have caused with family, friends, and the criminal justice system.
- Limit your therapeutic efforts (according to Hemphill and Hart [2002]) to managing antisocial behaviors rather than changing the more enduring personality characteristics of your patient. We do disagree on this point because we are more sanguine (there is that optimistic personality type again) about the possibility of permanent personality change or amelioration from supportive psychotherapy.
- Teach your patients strategies to change their behaviors. Since psychopaths are impulsive and have information-processing deficits, the simple act of *pausing* before acting improves prosocial actions. In conjunction, they need to learn to plan ahead and map out their activities in advance.

- Focus on cognitive strengths rather than affective deficits. Hemphill and Hart (2002) relate this in part to the work done by Wong and Hare, suggesting that programs to improve self-esteem, empathy, and conscience (i.e., affective deficits) do not work. Although we have cited and generally agree with the approaches in Wong's programs, we think there is more positive evidence that you can do something with the affective deficits.
- Develop strategies to maintain behavioral change. There has to be community supervision and follow-up to maintain their prosocial skills and motivation.
- Continuously modify your strategy based on the content of the therapy. Obviously, space has not permitted us to teach you how to use all the components of Livesley's Integrated Modular Treatment, The Good Lives Model, Wong's two-component method, or for that matter the Suzuki method (of learning the violin). But we suspect that they all begin by *listening*! (We also discussed the concept of *active listening* in Chapter 3.)

In determining the treatability of psychopathic patients, we also suggest you "don't try to treat a sadist." Sadistic personality disorder was a proposed category in older editions of DSM to describe persons with cruel, demeaning, and aggressive behavior toward others (not just for sexual arousal). It's not in DSM-5. A recent survey of psychiatrically hospitalized adolescents, for example, found sadistic personality in 14% (Myers et al. 2006). Despite the need to understand such a possible disorder, it was, according to Stone (a previously mentioned author), excluded from recent editions for what some think were political reasons—that including it as a disorder could result in exculpatory mental illness claims for criminals who had it. Stone concludes:

> Has the time not come for the psychiatric profession to make it abundantly clear to the legal community that sadistic personalities, while lamentably they surely exist, are for all intents and purposes untreatable (especially when the person in question has already embarked upon a career of sadistically violating other people) and not to be viewed as an illness justifying exculpation or reduction of sentence? (Stone 1998, p. 49)

We hope that more can be learned about sadistic people. Since we have emphasized the dimensionality of personality disorder, we therefore mention a recent review of multiple studies showing that *boredom* itself increases sadistic fantasies or actual sadistic behavior in several community populations, including military and parents. However, it does not appear that boredom makes everybody sadistic. No. "Only those persons who showed an inclination toward sadism in their personality actually do show sadistic behavior when bored. For most people, boredom does not lead to sadistic behavior" (Ocklenburg 2020, p. 3). Boredom has been widely studied as a factor in juvenile street crimes and on a continuum of other crimes up to and including violence on forensic units. Clearly as the "other side of excitement," boredom is provocative to an antisocial person or psychopath, both in prison and in the community. So please give them something to do.

General recommendations for treating these severe personality disorders (including psychopathy) are presented in Table 10–5. We cannot say everything in a single table, and in fact we highly recommend the other work of Stone, who not only discusses how to treat individual personality disorders but enumerates the behaviors involved

TABLE 10–5.   **Recommendations to treat severe personality disorders and psychopathy (a nonfanciful, basic, supportive approach)**

Determine or *create* your institution's policy for selecting and treating.

Coordinate with and supplement existing group programs.

Address modifications of criminal lifestyle (see Table 10–6).

Research and explore more about the approaches we suggest or the ones you like (read articles and books; interface with your department, with state providers, and with local and national organizations).

Use assessment instruments.

Assess and select your patients for degrees of ASPD, psychopathy, and sadism in particular, but also the other dangerous traits, including narcissistic, paranoid, and borderline.

Determine treatable comorbidities starting of course with substance use disorder, ADHD, and mood disorders; consider a "divide and conquer" strategy.

Avoid boredom (see text); keep patients busy in prison and when they get out.

Prepare yourself for manipulations, allegations of incompetence, and missed or late sessions.

Interface with family (directly or through patient) and emphasize role in community.

Reassess or rethink your treatment plan

  Automatically and periodically.

  If treatment stalls.

  If there is a "rupture" in the treatment process.

Use assessment scales for prosocial attitudes and other measures to monitor progress.

and indicates which are more treatable (i.e., worth addressing in therapy) and which are not. For example, some traits that (if intense) create problems for therapy even in the absence of a diagnosed personality disorder are abrasiveness, bigotry, bullying, greed, jealousy, laziness, quarrelsomeness, rudeness, sanctimoniousness, sensating-seeking, spitefulness, being unforgiving, untrustworthiness, vengefulness, and viciousness (Stone 2006, p. 195). Stone and Brucato (2019) have also provided a detailed elaboration of the degrees of psychopathology that clearly implies lesser treatability as they progress.

In addition to looking at programmatic materials based on our previous discussion, recall the recommendations regarding treatment of criminal lifestyle, based on the work of Walters. In a book drawing together different approaches to treating ASPD, Walters (2006) described his own approach. We summarize components of this approach in Table 10–6. In a later work, Walters (2017) recommends that therapists encourage a kind of existential lifestyle crisis but frame it positively by creating the hope and anticipation of change. To help patients work through this, he recommends that they develop a change plan on a card, listing involvements, commitments, and identifications matched by past problems, present substitutes, and future goals. Keeping in mind what we called crisis response safety plans, we even suggest you can add "Future goals" to the "Reasons for Living" section. Examples of such "Goals=Reasons for Living" might be "Get my G.E.D," "Appeal my case," "Get married," "Have children," or "Get a marketing job."

TABLE 10–6.	A program to modify a criminal lifestyle

Not a school of therapy, but:

  Congenial to existential and humanistic therapies, which emphasize freedom, responsibility, and meaning

  Compatible with most other therapies

Emphasis on four areas:

  Responsibility

  Confidence

  Meaning

  Community

Discuss negative consequences of current criminal lifestyle.

Discuss positive consequences of prosocial lifestyle and new identity.

Use assessment scales, not just to make a diagnosis but to determine areas that need change.

Identify strengths (e.g., intelligence, perceptions, and positive reinforcements for identities):

  "You would be a great salesman"

  "You could be a great mechanic"

Develop social skills for anger management, education, and rehabilitation.

Source. Based on Walters 2006.

Intimate Partner Violence

> The man that lays his hand upon a woman,
> Save in the way of kindness, is a wretch
> Whom 'twere gross flattery to name a coward.
>   John Tobin, *The Honeymoon*, Act 2, Scene 1 (1805)

John Tobin (1770–1804) was an English playwright (and a contemporary of John Keats) who wrote many plays and finally became famous in the last year of his life with *The Honeymoon*. Oh. FYI, he died of tuberculosis. Fortunately, he did live as long as he did, since if he had died at the age of 25 like Keats, we would never have heard of him. But if you are wondering why we are mentioning tuberculosis when we have just lived through a pandemic, it is because there are a lot of pandemics out there. "Tuberculosis is a global pandemic killing someone approximately every 22 seconds—about 1.4 million in 2019.…The TB alliance stands in solidarity with the global fight against COVID-19. We hope the world will emerge from this crisis with renewed commitment to aggressively anticipate and address global health threats and pandemics" (TB Alliance 2020).

"Intimate partner violence" has been used to replace "domestic violence" and does not require that the parties have a sexual relationship. However, we do frequently see people in prison who were charged with domestic violence against a mother-in-law or a brother or some other nonintimate partner.

To give another one of our literary examples, Ruth Rendell's detective Wexford is accused of being soft on abuse of women. The accuser says that as a man and like all men he would think nothing of giving his wife "a little tap" but the same thing if done to a man would be an assault and lead to a prison term (Rendell 1999, p. 243). There are obviously parties on each side of intimate partner violence, but that does not mean that each party is equally responsible, and Wexford's accuser does at least seem to show it was not all that long ago that there was an inherent bias against female victims. Hopefully, it is gone now. In any case we will just write briefly about men who abuse their wives. The usual advice is to "get thee to group therapy." One group program for men is based on the Duluth model for a DAIP (Domestic Abuse Intervention Program), which takes as an assumption the tenets of second-wave feminism (see Chapter 11) that abuse is fueled by beliefs that men should dominate women (see Wolfe 2020 for the accounts given here). However, lately there have been questions about the effectiveness of such programs. While many men seem ashamed and apologetic when they begin these programs, they are readily seen to engage in total denial of the actions that led to their placement, and where they cannot deny outright, they minimize or claim an accident or admit only to the actions that led to arrest. They blame the victim as much as possible and claim to be victims themselves of violence perpetrated by their wives, thus trying to confuse and muddy the waters as to who is the perpetrator. The groups have a male and female facilitator, but the men show hostility to the female. A common method of instruction is a Power and Control Wheel that illustrates abusive tactics such as put-downs and making the woman feel bad about herself. Many of the men have substance and alcohol problems that they also blame for their actions.

Called into question are both the change of philosophy approach of the DAIP (Jackson et al. 2003) and a hybrid using CBT methods to change what the men believe (Arias et al. 2013). An evaluation of two DAIP programs showed that one didn't work and the other was fairly modest in effect. A newer program, developed by Amie Zarling, is called ACTV ("Active" or Achieving Change Through Values-Based Behavior) and addresses multiple causes, including the use of violence to fend off unpleasant emotions, by helping men to tolerate these emotions but not act on them and to choose actions that reflect more positive values. The rationale behind this program makes sense, but we also found conflicting studies about its effectiveness (Gondolf et al. 2019). The ACTV program creates a "non-judgmental and collaborating environment" and "works with offenders to identify what they value in life—often their children–and use their own experience as a guide to making better choices and building a healthier relationship with their partner" (Iowa State University 2017). We would certainly like to see more studies about this program since the use of positive goals and values is similar to the Good Lives Model and is compatible with supportive psychotherapy methods. If you do use individual therapy, we think it should be structured using similar approaches of identifying (in a supportive manner as suggested in the description of ACTV) the emotions that lead to violence and exploring and developing skills to prevent the actual violence while substituting safe behaviors. This includes not only men who have abused women, but both men and women who abuse same-sex so-called "friends" (usually intimate partners) in prison. It is hoped that abusers can change, but to ask a question similar to the one we asked earlier, Inspector Wexford wonders if the abuser can be shocked into changing. He even muses, using our previous notion, whether a leopard can change its spots (Rendell 1999, p. 250)!

When the abusers think of the "other" side, they usually claim that the victim was responsible in some way at least in provoking, if not engaging in, some of the violence. However, there is usually an asymmetry in intimate partner violence situations, with the victim's "contribution" viewed not as being that of a perpetrator or instigator but as tolerating the violence. When we began to work with abused women (and some men, also), we often withheld expressing the obvious question of "Why did you put up with it?" There are many answers for that, certainly many more than the financial dependency and staying together for the sake of the children. Rendell introduces us to Inspector Wexford's daughter, who is knowledgeable of the subject from her work in a women's shelter. Yet Wexford finds himself heartbroken one day to discover that Sylvia's new boyfriend hits her. He asks her how she allows it. She says it's different when a person who seems genuinely good strikes her. Wexford sarcastically replies that "strikes" is certainly the right word but (and here he fails in his understanding) that she has only herself to blame for tolerating it (Rendell 2002, pp. 217–218). Wexford's enlightenment may extend to the condemnation of the domestic violence, but not to an understanding of why it is difficult for victims to extricate themselves from it.

Anger Management

Persons in criminal justice settings have a need for anger management programs. For example, SAMHSA produced a program for anger management for substance users or those with mental health problems (Reilly and Shopshire 2019; Reilly et al. 2019). To give you a sense for its general tone, we excerpted the introduction to the first lesson in Table 10–7. This program *can* be used on an individual basis. One of many non–governmentally produced management programs in prison is Cage Your Rage, from the American Correctional Association, with the published guide now in its second edition (Cullen 2013) and with a leader's manual. It's simple and it needs to be. It educates about the causes of anger and the cycle of anger and recovery from anger episodes. Also consider the program by Tafrate and Kassinove (2019), the former known for his CBT program for prisoners. If the anger is related to intimate partner abuse, recall the two issues we mentioned earlier: 1) attitudes toward women, including toxic masculinity, and 2) the individual vulnerabilities that lead to violence against a partner as a "solution" to low self-esteem and feelings of powerlessness and frustration.

Women also have anger and violence issues. A comprehensive program, one of many developed by Stephanie Covington (2014), covers these. Patients learn to record the triggers to their anger, and in the case of women, there is an emphasis on the relationship of their anger to past trauma and victimization. They learn techniques to control anger, including means of dissipating it by analyzing it and relating it to "old" anger and common "stop and think" methods. Central to this approach, and probably all anger management programs, is an anger log. We provide our own version in Table 10–8. Review historical anger situations and *every* angry situation in prison. Challenge these patients to discuss what the other person (prisoner or officer) did and what they did to provoke or defuse the confrontation. Identify the triggers to violence leading to arrest or disciplinary sanctions. Practice signposting (i.e., the recognition of escalating anger). Learn to justify avoidance of physical violence and seeking interventions from staff. Behaviors resulting in discipline are now being studied as "offense analogue be-

---

TABLE 10–7.   **Myths about anger in Substance Abuse and Mental Health Services Administration Anger Management Workbook**

Myth #1: The Way You Express Anger Cannot Be Changed

One misconception or myth about anger is that the way people express anger is inherited and cannot be changed. Although many of our anger responses are inherited, our behavior is learned, and it is possible to learn more appropriate ways of expressing anger. You can also change the way your nervous system reacts after you get angry. You can learn to calm down more quickly with practice.

Myth #2: Anger Automatically Leads to Aggression

A related myth involves the misconception that the only effective way to express anger is through aggression. There are other more constructive and assertive ways, however, to express anger. You can do this by learning assertiveness skills, changing negative and hostile thoughts or "self-talk," challenging irrational beliefs, and employing a variety of behavioral strategies.

Myth #3: You Must Be Aggressive to Get What You Want

Many people confuse assertiveness with aggression. But the goal of aggression is to dominate, intimidate, harm, or injure another person—to win at any cost—and you can be angry in a way that is respectful of other people and does not blame or threaten them.

Myth #4: Venting Anger Is Always Desirable

For many years people thought that the aggressive expression of anger, such as screaming or beating on pillows, was healthy and therapeutic. However, recent research shows that this is not true and that venting anger in an aggressive manner reinforces aggressive behavior.

Source.   Summarized and abbreviated from Reilly et al. 2019.

havior" (Gordon and Wong 2011). Some studies even "show anger management to be more effective than more intensive multimodal corrections programs" (Polaschek 2019, p. 503).

The Rest of the Story

We said earlier that everybody is "A Little Bit of This, and a Little Bit of That," or, in the case of some patients, "A Lot of This, and a Lot of That." Consistent with the trend of thinking of dimensions in personality disorder, it is thus important to consider the co-occurrence of multiple mental disorders. One recent study, for example, found that prisoners with major depression and BPD, compared with prisoners without BPD, were more likely to perpetuate and be victimized by psychological aggression. "Prisoners with comorbid BPD and ASPD were no more likely than prisoners with ASPD to report disciplinary incidents/infractions but were significantly more likely than those with ASPD only to report perpetrating and being victimized by psychological aggression" (Moore et al. 2018). Our take on this: the borderline, and not the antisocial, component of the personality disorder is the source of much of the pathology in prison behavior.

Another disorder that co-occurs is substance use disorder. Also there is attention-deficit/hyperactivity disorder (ADHD), which itself overlaps with substance use disorders and conduct disorder. Like many disorders, ADHD is highly overrepresented in prison populations, and its presence should be addressed in treatment plans since ADHD affects the ability to learn and perform sustained tasks. ADHD creates issues

TABLE 10–8. An anger log

DAY AND TIME	Describe the incident. Could it have been avoided or managed differently?	How bad (mild, moderate, or severe)? How many minutes did it last?	What were the consequences (injury, discipline, loss of friendship)?
Monday			
Tuesday			
Wednesday			
Thursday			
Friday			
Saturday			
Sunday			

for prescribers because many of the medications used to treat it are controlled substances. Most institutions avoid using such medications and there is a resultant tendency to underdiagnose the disorder. However, there are nonaddicting treatments as well as methods for self-management of the disorder (e.g., Safren et al. 2005). Many institutions do not have ongoing groups for prisoners with ADHD, so it may fall to you to provide patients with workbooks and associated psychoeducation. And another reason for considering both diagnosis and treatment of ADHD is that because of structural racism, ADHD is thought to be underdiagnosed in the Black population, which as we know is overrepresented in prison (Moody 2016).

ADHD, of course, is a disorder that begins in childhood, and there are several other childhood disorders that may need to be recognized in adulthood. These include oppositional defiant disorder, episodic dyscontrol disorder, and intermittent explosive disorder. But also, problems with or disorders of *attachment* have specifically been recognized as contributing to future criminal behavior. They may play the same pervasive role that we now know trauma does in individual life trajectories.

So in treating those multifaceted individuals who are our patients, we must be aware that in addition to just being individual people with a trail of personal and family history, they have mixes of various personality disorders and multiple other "named" disorders, including the high prevalence of ADHD, and each disorder may come, in varying degrees, with its own contribution to functional impairment and ability to learn. We have a section on intellectual disability in Chapter 13. This too is a problem that comes in various degrees along with simply poor educational ability, learning disabilities, or just lack of opportunity or school dropout.

Quarantine Zone

JILL: How about a movie tonight? I think I can get us "Love in the Time of Cholera" on Netflix.

JACK: How romantic! I heard that Gabriel García Márquez was using a pun on the word "Cholera" to refer to the meaning of "Choleric" for the passionate love of Florentino for Fermina.

JILL: You mean "Choleric," like one of the four humors of Hippocrates?

JACK: Exactly. I'm glad you remember our chapter on personality disorders.

JILL: Of course. I'm not phlegmatic like that other personality disorder.

JACK: Then are you sanguine or hopeful that I will see that movie with you?

JILL: Absolutely.

JACK: Forget it. This might make you melancholic, but the movie only rated 25% on Rotten Tomatoes. A bomb, unless you like Shakira.

JILL: I see. Well, at least you do use Google sometimes. What about the mini-series "Love in the Time of Corona?" Too bad they didn't renew it.

JACK: I'm game for that. I hear it's about couples dealing with life during the pandemic…

JILL: Okay, I'll get it from Hulu.

JACK: …and having affairs and cheating on each other?

JILL: On second thought, I'll just read a book. Any suggestions?

JACK: What about Albert Camus' *The Plague*? We already quoted him in the chapter about suicide.

JILL: No, too depressing, like all of his existential absurdity stuff.

JACK: Then try Boccaccio's *Decameron*—another one of those "get together during the plague" books!

JILL: It was Boccaccio who called Dante's *Comedy* "Divine" and gave it the name we know it as today, so you have to give him credit for that, but I am not up to reading 100 stories.

JACK: Then I would recommend you read *A Plague of Prisons: The Epidemiology of Mass Incarceration in America* by Ernest Drucker.

JILL: Did that just come out? Some sort of pun on the coronavirus pandemic like the TV series?

JACK: No, actually, it was last updated in 2013, and it's not just a cute title. It starts by discussing cholera and AIDS and explains how mass incarceration follows the same principles as an infectious epidemic. It describes how imprisonment creates chronic disability and incapacitation just as coronavirus can do, and how a public health model can be applied to "treat" mass imprisonment.

JILL: Really prophetic. I guess I will curl up with that, if that's the sort of book one can curl up with.

Key Points

- A personality disorder (PD) is an ongoing dysfunctional or maladaptive pattern of behavior that deviates greatly from the expectations of a person's culture.

- Contrary to many long-standing assumptions, PDs can often be treated.

- DSM-5 (and DSM-5-TR) retains its long-standing categorical diagnoses of PDs but introduces an alternative model of PDs as well.

- The four most common PDs in corrections are borderline personality disorder (BPD), antisocial personality disorder (ASPD), narcissistic personality disorder (NPD), and paranoid personality disorder (PPD).

- Supportive psychotherapy is applicable in the treatment of most personality disorders. It can be a basic approach that leads into or incorporates the methods used in more specialized treatments such as dialectical behavior therapy.

- Before making a diagnosis of ASPD, the therapist should consider that the history of criminal activity may be related to substance use disorder.

- Aggressive acts of the ASPD prisoner differ from those of prisoners with psychosis and have a focus of intimidation or revenge.

- BPD in corrections is high, and challenges of working with BPD prisoners are numerous.

- Supportive psychotherapy with the BPD patient will keep the focus on the present.

- The greatest obstacle with the NPD prisoner is addressing the trait of grandiosity.

- Do not use direct confrontation with the NPD patient.

- A major goal with the PPD prisoner is to overcome mistrust.

- Awareness and flexibility help overcome the challenges of treating patients with a PD.

- There are many programs with proven effectiveness in treating violent persons.

- Psychopaths and sex offenders are problematic but create a great deal of interest. Many psychopaths are treatable, but certainly not all.

- Psychotherapy for offenders with PDs is described using Livesley's common factors approach, which is exemplified by supportive techniques.

- We concur with Stone's opinion that the least treatable group consists of those with sadistic personality disorder, a category not found in DSM-5.

- There is growing interest in a program called ACTV ("Active": Achieving Change Through Values-Based Behavior), which uses methods similar to those of supportive psychotherapy to treat intimate partner violence.

- Early attachment relationships and attachment theory have increasingly been recognized as playing a role in criminal behavior.

- We recommend that you review anger-producing situations that your patient experiences. The simplest type of "add-on" or "add-in" program for your ongoing psychotherapy for violence would be anger management.

References

Abracen J, Langton CM, Looman J, et al: Mental health diagnoses and recidivism in paroled offenders. Int J Offender Ther Comp Criminol 58(7):765–779, 2014 23640808

Ambardar S: What is the prevalence of narcissistic personality disorder (NPD) in the US? Medscape. Updated May 16, 2018. Available at: www.medscape.com/answers/1519417-101779/what-is-the-prevalence-of-narcissistic-personality-disorder-npd-in-the-us. Accessed July 15, 2020.

American Psychiatric Association: Practice Guideline for the Treatment of Patients With Borderline Personality Disorder. 2001. (Guideline Watch March 2005 also available). Available at: https://psychiatryonline.org/pb/assets/raw/sitewide/practice_guidelines/guidelines/bpd.pdf. Accessed September 27, 2020.

American Psychiatric Association: Diagnostic and Statistical Manual of Mental Disorders, 5th Edition. Arlington, VA, American Psychiatric Association, 2013

Ansbro M: Using attachment theory with offenders. Probat J 55(3):231–244, 2008

Arias E, Arce R, Vilarino M: Batterer intervention programmes: a meta-analytic review of effectiveness. Interv Psicosoc 22:153–160, 2013

Avery JD, Barnhill JW: Personality disorders, in Co-occurring Mental Illness and Substance Use Disorders: A Guide to Diagnosis and Treatment. Edited by Avery JD, Barnhill JW. Washington, DC, American Psychiatric Association Publishing, 2018, pp 83–92

Aviram RB, Hellerstein DJ, Gerson J, Stanley B: Adapting supportive psychotherapy for individuals with borderline personality who self-injure or attempt suicide. J Psychiatr Pract 10(3):145–155, 2004 15330220

Baskin JH: Corrections psychiatry: antisocial personality disorder. A difficult personality disorder and other challenges to treatment (blog). Psychology Today, October 4, 2008. Available at: www.psychologytoday.com/us/blog/cell-block/201810/corrections-psychiatry-antisocial-personality-disorder. Accessed September 27, 2020.

Battaglia J: Doing Supportive Psychotherapy. Washington, DC, American Psychiatric Association Publishing, 2020

Beck JC, Wencel H: Violent crime and Axis I pathology, in Psychopathology and Violent Crime. Edited by Skodol AE. Washington, DC, American Psychiatric Press, 1998, pp 1–27

Bell R, Evershed S: The management of difficult clients, in Applying Psychology to Forensic Practice. Edited by Needs A, Towl G. Malden, MA, BPS Blackwell, 2004, pp 82–96

Berichon M, Birgy TR, Konrath CM, Abraham SP: Challenges of treatment and living with the stigma related to paranoid personality disorder. Int J Soc Res Methodol 12:51–64, 2019

Black DW, Gunter T, Allen J, et al: Borderline personality disorder in male and female offenders newly committed to prison. Compr Psychiatry 48(5):400–405, 2007 17707246

Black DW, Gunter T, Loveless P, et al: Antisocial personality disorder in incarcerated offenders: psychiatric comorbidity and quality of life. Ann Clin Psychiatry 22(2):113–120, 2010 20445838

Blanchard M, Farber B: Lying in psychotherapy: why and what clients don't tell their therapist about therapy and their relationship. Counselling Psychology Quarterly 29(1)90–112, 2016 Available at: https://www.researchgate.net/publication/282197507_Lying_in_psychotherapy_Why_and_what_clients_don't_tell_their_therapist_about_therapy-_and_their_relationship. Accessed March 9, 2022.

Bretherton I: The origins of attachment theory: John Bowlby and Mary Ainsworth. Dev Psychol 28(5):759–775, 1992

Bush J, Brian B: Options: A Cognitive Change Program. Longmont, CO, National Institute of Corrections, 1993

Bush J, Taymans J: Thinking for a Change. Washington, DC, U.S. Department of Justice, National Institute of Corrections, Integrated Cognitive Behavioral Change Program, 1997

Caligor E, Clarkin JF: An object relations model of personality and personality pathology, in Psychodynamic Psychotherapy for Personality Disorders: A Clinical Handbook. Edited by Clarkin JF, Fonagy P, Gabbard GO. Washington, DC, American Psychiatric Publishing, 2010, pp 3–35

Caligor E, Levy KN, Yeomans FE: Narcissistic personality disorder: diagnostic and clinical challenges. Am J Psychiatry 172(5):415–422, 2015 25930131

Campbell C, Craissati J (eds): Managing Personality Disordered Offenders: A Pathways Approach. New York, Oxford University Press, 2018

Carsky M: Supportive psychoanalytic therapy for personality disorders. Psychotherapy 50(3):443–448, 2013

Choi-Kain LW, Gunderson JG (eds): Applications of Good Psychiatric Management for Border-
    line Personality Disorder, Washington, DC, American Psychiatric Association Publishing,
    2019
Cihlar CA: Personality disorders, in Varcarolis' Foundations of Psychiatric-Mental Health
    Nursing: A Clinical Approach, 7th Edition. Edited by Halter MJ. New York, WB Saunders
    2014, pp 457–498
Clark LA, Watson D: Theory and research, in Handbook of Personality, 3rd Edition. Edited by
    John OP, Robins RW, Pervin LA. New York, Guilford, 2008, pp 265–286
Clarkin JF, Levy KN, Lenzenweger MF, Kernberg OF: Evaluating three treatments for border-
    line personality disorder: a multiwave study. Am J Psychiatry 164(6):922–928, 2007
    17541052
Cohen LE, Felson M: Social change and crime rate trends: a routine activity approach. Am So-
    ciol Rev 44(4):588–608, 1979
Coid JW: Axis II disorders and motivation for serious criminal behavior, in Psychopathology
    and Violent Crime. Edited by Skodol AE. Washington, DC, American Psychiatric Press,
    1998, pp 53–97
Coid JW: Personality disorders in prisoners and their motivation for dangerous and disruptive
    behaviour. Crim Behav Ment Health 12(3):209–226, 2002 12830313
Conn C, Warden R, Stuewig J, et al: Borderline personality disorder among jail inmates: how
    common and how distinct. Correct Compend 35(4):6–13, 2010 27065512
Connelly M: The Night Fire. New York, Grand Central Publishing, 2019
Cook KJ: Has criminology awakened from its "androcentric slumber?." Fem Criminol
    11(4):334–353, 2016
Coolidge FL, Segal DL: Evolution of personality disorder diagnosis in the Diagnostic and Sta-
    tistical Manual of Mental Disorders. Clin Psychol Rev 18(5):585–599, 1998 9740979
Covington SS: Beyond Anger and Violence: A Program for Women. Hoboken, NJ, Wiley, 2014
Craissati J, Joseph N, Skett S (eds): Working With Offenders With Personality Disorder: A Prac-
    titioner's Guide, 2nd Edition. NHS England, National Offender Management Service, Sep-
    tember 2015. Available at: www.england.nhs.uk/commissioning/wp-content/uploads/
    sites/12/2015/10/work-offndrs-persnlty-disorder-oct15.pdf. Accessed September 16,
    2020.
Cullen M: Cage Your Rage: An Inmate's Guide to Anger Control, 2nd Edition. Alexandria, VA,
    American Correctional Association, 2013
Dimaggio G: Psychotherapy tips: working with persons with narcissistic personality disorder.
    Psychiatric Times, August 28, 2012. Available at: www.psychiatrictimes.com/view/
    psychotherapy-tips-working-persons-narcissistic-personality-disorder. Accessed October
    4, 2020.
Drucker E: A Plague of Prisons: The Epidemiology of Mass Incarceration. New York, The New
    Press, 2013
Duggan C, Howard RC: The "functional link" between personality disorder and violence: a
    critical appraisal, in Personality, Personality Disorder and Risk of Violence. Edited by
    McMurran M, Howard H. Chichester, West Sussex, UK, Wiley, 2009, pp 19–37
Eaton NR, Rodriguez-Seijas C, Krueger RF, et al: Narcissistic personality disorder and the
    structure of common mental disorders (Abstract). J Pers Disord 31(4):449–461, 2017
    27617650
Freedman D, Woods GW: Social injustice and personality disorders, in Social Injustice and
    Mental Health. Edited by Shim RS, Vinson SY. Washington, DC, American Psychiatric As-
    sociation Publishing, 2021, pp 171–188
Gabbard GO, Horowitz MJ: Insight, transference interpretation, and therapeutic change in the
    dynamic psychotherapy of borderline personality disorder. Am J Psychiatry 166(5):517–
    521, 2009 19411377
Gabbard GO, Horwitz L, Allen JG, et al: Transference interpretation in the psychotherapy of
    borderline patients: a high-risk, high-gain phenomenon. Harv Rev Psychiatry 2(2):59–69,
    1994 9384884

Glick B, Gibbs JC: Aggression Replacement Training: A Comprehensive Intervention for Aggressive Youth, 3rd Edition. Champaign, IL, Research Press, 2020

Glicken MD, Sechrest DK: The Role of the Helping Professions in Treating the Victims and Perpetrators of Violence. New York, Pearson Education, 2003

Goldstein RB, Chou SP, Saha TD, et al: The epidemiology of antisocial behavioral syndromes in adulthood: results from the National Epidemiological Survey on Alcohol and Related Conditions–III. J Clin Psychiatry 78(1):90–98, 2017 27035627

Gondolf EW, Bennett L, Mankowski E: Lessons in program evaluation: the ACTV Batterer program study and its claims. Violence Against Women 25(5):NP1–NP10, 2019 29361885

Gordon A, Wong SCP: Offence analogue behaviours as indicators of criminogenic need and treatment progress in custodial settings, in Offence Paralleling Behaviour: A Case Formulation Approach to Offender Assessment and Intervention. Edited by Daffern M, Jones L, Shine J. New York, Wiley, 2011, pp 171–184

Gottfredson M, Hirschi T: A General Theory of Crime. Stanford, CA, Stanford University Press, 1990

Groves Gillespie L, Seibel LL: Self-regulation: a cornerstone of early child development. Beyond the Journal: Young Children on the Web, July 2006. Available at: https://childhealthanddevelopment.files.wordpress.com/2011/06/self-regulation.pdf. Accessed August 1, 2020.

Gunderson JG (with Links P): Handbook of Good Psychiatric Management for Borderline Personality Disorder. Washington, DC, American Psychiatric Publishing, 2014

Gunderson JG, Links P: Managing suicidality and nonsuicidal self-harm, in Handbook of Good Psychiatric Management for Borderline Personality Disorder. Washington, DC, American Psychiatric Publishing, 2014, pp 37–45

Gunderson JG, Stout RL, Shea MT, et al: Interactions of borderline personality disorder and mood disorders over 10 years. J Clin Psychiatry 75(8):829–834, 2014 25007118

Gunderson J, Masland S, Choi-Kain L: Good psychiatric management: a review. Curr Opin Psychol 21:127–131, 2018 29547739

Hare RD: Hare Psychopathy Checklist—Revised, 2nd Edition. Pearson, 2020. Available at: www.pearsonassessments.com/store/usassessments/en/Store/Professional-Assessments/Personality-%26-Biopsychosocial/Hare-Psychopathy-Checklist-Revised-%7C-Second-Edition/p/100000336.html. Accessed August 7, 2020.

Harris GA: Overcoming Resistance: Success in Counseling Men. Lanham, MD, American Correctional Association, 1995

Hellerstein DJ, Aviram R, Kotov K: Beyond "handholding": supportive therapy for patients with BPD and self-injurious behavior. Psychiatric Times, July 1, 2004. Available at: www.psychiatrictimes.com/view/beyond-handholding-supportive-therapy-patients-bpd-and-self-injurious-behavior. Accessed September 16, 2020.

Hemphill JF, Hart SD: Motivating the unmotivated: psychopathy, treatment, and change, in Motivating Offenders to Change: A Guide to Engagement in Therapy. Edited by McMurran M. Chichester, West Sussex, UK, Wiley, 2002, pp 193–219

Hirstein W: What is a psychopath? The neuroscience of psychopathy reports some intriguing findings (blog). Psychology Today, January 30, 2013. Available at: www.psychologytoday.com/us/blog/mindmelding/201301/what-is-psychopath-0?page=1. Accessed September 20, 2020.

Holmes J: Attachment theory in clinical practice: a personal account. Br J Psychother 31(2):208–222, 2015

Hong V: Emergency departments, in Applications of Good Psychiatric Management for Borderline Personality Disorder: A Practical Guide. Edited by Choi-Kain LW, Gunderson JG. Washington, DC, American Psychiatric Association Publishing, 2019, pp 37–56

Hornsveld RHJ: Kraaimaat FW, Gijs LACL, Palmer E (eds): Assessment and Treatment of Violent and Sexually Violent Offenders: Integrating Theory and Practice. Cham, Switzerland, Springer Nature, 2019

Howard R, Duggan C: Mentally disordered offenders: personality disorders, in Forensic Psychology. Edited by Towl GJ, Crighton DA. Malden, MA, BPS Blackwell, 2010, pp 309–328

Howard R, Howells K: Afterthoughts on personality disorder and risk: tasks for the future, in Using Time, Not Doing Time: Practitioner Perspectives on Personality Disorder and Risk. Edited by Tennant A, Howells K. Chichester, West Sussex, UK, Wiley, 2010, pp 195–204

Human Rights Watch: Ill-Equipped: U.S. Prisons and Offenders With Mental Illness. New York, Human Rights Watch, 2003. Available at: www.hrw.org/sites/default/files/reports/usa1003.pdf. Accessed October 2, 2020.

Internet Movie Database: Star Trek: The Original Series (1966–1969): The Menagerie, Part 1. 2021. Available at: www.imdb.com/title/tt0394904. Accessed February 19, 2021.

Iowa State University: New intervention program reduces domestic violence recidivism rates, July 5, 2017. Available at www.news.iastate.edu/news/2017/07/05/actv. Accessed August 8, 2020.

Jackson S, Feder L, Forde DR, et al: Batterer Intervention Programs: Where Do We Go From Here? NCJ 195079. Washington, DC, National Institute of Justice, Office of Justice Programs, 2003. Edited by Jackson S, Feder L, Forde DR, et al. 2003. Available at: www.ncjrs.gov/pdffiles1/nij/195079.pdf. Accessed August 8, 2020.

Junewicz A, Billick SB: Preempting the development of antisocial behavior and psychopathic traits. J Am Acad Psychiatry Law 49(1):66–76, 2021 33408155

Kagan J: Personality and temperament, in Depression and Personality: Conceptual and Clinical Challenges. Edited by Rosenbluth M, Kennedy SH, Bagby RM. Washington, DC, American Psychiatric Publishing, 2005, pp 3–18

Kellerman J: Bad Love. New York, Bantam Books, 1994

Laumer K: Retief! Emissary to the Stars. Edited and compiled by Flint E. Riverdale, NY, Baen Publishing Enterprises, 2001

Lee R: Mistrustful and misunderstood: a review of paranoid personality disorder (abstract). Curr Behav Neurosci Rep 4(2):151–165, 2017 29399432

Little GL, Robinson KD: How to Escape Your Prison. Memphis, TN, Eagle Wing Books, 1989

Livesley WJ: Practical Management of Personality Disorder. New York, Guilford, 2013

Livesley WJ, Dimaggio G, Carkin JF (eds): Integrated Treatment for Personality Disorder: A Modular Approach. New York, Guilford, 2018

Logan C: Narcissism, in Personality, Personality Disorder and Violence. Edited by McMurran M, Howard RC. New York, Wiley, 2008, pp 85–112

Martens WHJ: The hidden suffering of the psychopath. Psychiatric Times, October 7, 2014 (originally published in 2006). Available at: www.psychiatrictimes.com/view/hidden-suffering-psychopath. Accessed August 7, 2020.

McLean Hospital: John Gunderson: borderline personality disorder trailblazer. January 29, 2019. Available at: www.mcleanhospital.org/news/john-gunderson-borderline-personality-disorder-trailblazer. Accessed September 23, 2020.

McMain SF, Links PS, Gnam WH et al: A randomized trial of dialectical behavior therapy versus general psychiatric management for borderline personality disorder. Am J Psychiatry 166(12):1365–1374, 2009 19755574 (erratum in Am J Psychiatry 167[10]:1283, 2010)

McMurtry J: Good love and bad love: a way of evaluation. Journal of Speculative Philosophy New Series 6(3):226–241, 1992. Available at: www.jstor.org/stable/25670036. Accessed July 9, 2021.

Meloy JR: Pathologies of attachment, violence, and criminology, in Handbook of Psychology, Vol 11. Edited by Goldstein A. New York, Wiley, 2003, pp 509–526

Miller NA, Najavits LM: Creating trauma-informed correctional care: a balance of goals and environment. Eur J Psychotraumatol 3:17246, 2012 22893828

Mizock L, Harkins D: Diagnostic bias and conduct disorder: improving culturally sensitive diagnosis. Child Youth Serv 32:243–253, 2011

Moody M: From under-diagnosis to over-representation: Black children, ADHD, and the school-to-prison pipeline. J Afr Am Stud 20:152–163, 2016

Moore J, Renn T, Veeh C, Pettus-Davis C: Associations of Childhood and Adult Trauma on Substance Misuse and Mental Health Among Incarcerated Men. Florida State University College of Social Work, Institute for Justice Research and Development Working Paper, July 2020. Available at: https://ijrd.csw.fsu.edu/sites/g/files/upcbnu1766/files/Publications/Workingpaper_Childhood_and_Adult_Trauma_Incarcerated_Men.pdf. Accessed November 28, 2020.

Moore KE, Gobin RL, McCauley HL, et al: The relation of borderline personality disorder to aggression, victimization, and institutional misconduct among prisoners. Compr Psychiatry 84:15–21, 2018 29660674

Myers WC, Burket RC, Husted DS: Sadistic personality disorder and comorbid mental illness in adolescent psychiatric inpatients. J Am Acad Psychiatry Law 34(1):61–71, 2006 16585236

National Institute for Health and Clinical Excellence: Antisocial Personality Disorder: Treatment, Management, and Prevention. NICE Clinical Guideline 77. London, National Institute for Health and Clinical Excellence, January 28, 2009. Last updated March 27, 2013. Available at: www.nice.org.uk/guidance/CG77. Accessed October 30, 2019.

Norcross JC: Toward the delineation of empirically based principles in psychotherapy: Commentary on Beutler. Prev Treat 3(1):1–5, 2000

Novalis PN, Singer V, Peele R: Clinical Manual of Supportive Psychotherapy, 2nd Edition. Washington, DC, American Psychiatric Association Publishing, 2020

Ocklenburg S: The dark side of boredom: new study shows that boredom can motivate harming others for pleasure (blog). Psychology Today, September 13, 2020. Available at: www.psychologytoday.com/us/blog/the-asymmetric-brain/202009/the-dark-side-boredom. Accessed June 20, 2021.

Olver ME, Stockdale KC: Assessing and treating violent offenders, in The Practice of Correctional Psychology. Edited by Ternes M, Magaletta PR, Patry MW. Cham, Switzerland, Springer, 2018, pp 143–172

Patrick CJ, Brislin SJ: Theoretical perspectives on psychopathy and antisocial personality disorder, in Handbook of Personality Disorders: Theory, Research, and Treatment, 2nd Edition. Edited by Livesley WJ, Larstone R. New York, Guilford, 2018, pp 436–443

Patterson M: As I Live and Breathe: A Perspective From a Prison Psychologist. Asheville, SC, Moonshine Cove Publishing, 2019

Perry JC, Banon E, Ianni F: Effectiveness of psychotherapy for personality disorders. Am J Psychiatry 156(9):1312–1321, 1999

Polaschek DL: Interventions to reduce recidivism in adult violent offenders, in The Wiley Handbook of Correctional Psychology. Edited by Polaschek DLL, Day A, Hollin CR. Hoboken, NJ, Wiley, 2019, pp 501–514

Polaschek DLL, Daly TE: Treatment and Psychopathy in Forensic Settings. Wellington, New Zealand, School of Psychology, Victoria University of Wellington, 2018. Available at: www.researchgate.net/publication/259158339_Treatment_and_psychopathy_in_forensic_settings. Accessed August 7, 2020.

Polaschek DLL, Kilgour TG: New Zealand's special treatment units: the development and implementation of intensive treatment for high-risk male prisoners. Psychology, Crime & Law 19(5–6):511–526, 2013

Reilly PM, Shopshire MS: Anger Management for Substance Use Disorder and Mental Health Clients: A Cognitive–Behavioral Therapy Manual. SAMHSA Publ No PEP19-02-01-001. Rockville, MD. Substance Abuse and Mental Health Services Administration, 2019

Reilly PM, Shopshire MS, Durazzo TC, Campbell TA: Anger Management for Substance Use Disorder and Mental Health Clients: Participant Workbook. SAMHSA Publ No PEP19-02-01-002. Rockville, MD. Substance Abuse and Mental Health Services Administration, Updated 2019

Rendell R: An Unkindness of Ravens. New York, Ballantine Books, 1985

Rendell R: Harm Done: An Inspector Wexford Mystery. New York, Vintage Books, 1999

Rendell R: The Babes in the Woods: A New Chief Inspector Wexford Mystery. New York, Vintage Books, 2002

Ritter S, Platt LM: What's new in treating inpatients with personality disorders? Dialectical behavior therapy and old-fashioned, good communication. J Psychosoc Nurs Ment Health Serv 54(1):38–45, 2016 26760134

Ross RR, Fabiano EA: Time to Think: A Cognitive Model of Delinquency Prevention and Offender Rehabilitation. Johnson City, TN, Institute of Social Sciences and Arts, 1985

Safren SA, Sprich S, Perlman CA, Otto M: Mastering Your Adult ADHD: A Cognitive-Behavior Treatment Program. Client Workbook. New York, Oxford University Press, 2005

Salters-Pedneault K: History of the term "Borderline" in borderline personality disorder. Updated April 10, 2020. Available at: www.verywellmind.com/borderline-personality-disorder-meaning-425191. Accessed September 30, 2020.

Sampson RJ, Laub JH: Crime in the Making: Pathways and Turning Points Through Life. Boston, MA, Harvard University Press, 1993

Schouten R, Silver J: Almost a Psychopath: Do I (or Does Someone I Know) Have a Problem With Manipulation and Lack of Empathy (The Almost Effect). Center City, MN, Hazelden Publishing, 2012

Shonkoff J, Phillips D (eds): From Neurons to Neighborhoods: The Science of Early Childhood Development. A Report of the National Research Council. Washington, DC, National Academies Press, 2000

Skodol AE, Bender DS, Gunderson JG, Oldham JM: Personality disorders, in The American Psychiatric Publishing Textbook of Psychiatry, 6th Edition. Edited by Hales RE, Yudofsky SC, Roberts LW. Washington, DC, American Psychiatric Publishing, 2014, pp 851–894

Stone MH: The personalities of murderers: the importance of psychopathy and sadism, in Psychopathology and Violent Crime. Edited by Skodol AE. Washington, DC, American Psychiatric Press, 1998, pp 29–52

Stone MH: Gradations of antisociality and responsivity to psychosocial therapies, in Psychotherapy for Personality Disorders. (Review of Psychiatry Vol 19, No 3). Edited by Gunderson JG, Gabbard GO. Washington, DC, American Psychiatric Press, 2000, pp 95–130

Stone MH: Personality-Disordered Patients: Treatable and Untreatable. Washington, DC, American Psychiatric Publishing, 2006

Stone MH, Brucato G: The New Evil: Understanding the Emergence of Modern Violent Crime. Amherst, NY, Prometheus Books, 2019

Tafrate RC, Kassinove H: The Practitioner's Guide to Anger Management: Customizable Interventions, Treatments, and Tools for Clients With Problem Anger. Oakland, CA, Impact Publishers, 2019

TB Alliance: TB is a global pandemic. 2020. Available at: www.tballiance.org/why-new-tb-drugs/global-pandemic. Accessed October 22, 2020.

Tobin J: The Honey Moon: A Comedy, in Five Acts. London, Longman Hurst, Rees & Orme, 1805

Trestman RL: Behind bars: personality disorders. J Am Acad Psychiatry Law 28(2):232–235, 2000 10888193

Trestman RL, Ford J, Zhang W, Wiesbrock V: Current and lifetime psychiatric illness among inmates not identified as acutely mentally ill at intake in Connecticut's jails. J Am Acad Psychiatry Law 35(4):490–500, 2007 18086741

Tye CS, Mullen PE: Mental disorders in female prisoners. Aust N Z J Psychiatry 40(3):266–271, 2006 16476155

Tyrka AR, Wyche MC, Kelly MM, et al: Childhood maltreatment and adult personality disorder symptoms: influence of maltreatment type. Psychiatry Res 165(3):281–287, 2009 19162332

Virdi S, Trestman RL: Personality disorders. In Oxford Textbook of Correctional Psychiatry. Edited by Trestman RL, Applebaum KL, Metzner JL. New York, Oxford University Press, 2015, pp 195–199

Walters G: The lifestyle approach to substance abuse and crime, in Antisocial Personality Disorder: A Practitioner's Guide to Comparative Treatments. Edited by Rotgers F, Maniacci M. New York, Springer, 2006, pp 91–114

Walters GD: Modeling the Criminal Lifestyle. Cham, Switzerland, Palgrave Macmillan (Springer Nature), 2017

Weinberg I, Finch EF, Choi-Kain LW: Implementation of Good Psychiatric Management for narcissistic personality disorder: good enough or not good enough? in Applications of Good Psychiatric Management for Borderline Personality Disorder. Edited by Choi-Kain LW, Gunderson JG. Washington, DC, American Psychiatric Association Publishing, 2019, pp 253–280

Widiger TA, McCabe GA: The alternative model of personality disorders (AMPD) from the perspective of the Five-Factor Model. Psychopathology 53(3–4):149–156, 2020 32526758

Winston A, Rosenthal RN, Roberts LW: Learning Supportive Psychotherapy: An Illustrated Guide, 2nd Edition. Washington, DC, American Psychiatric Association Publishing, 2020

Wolfe M: Can you cure a domestic abuser? The Atlantic, January 17, 2020

Wolff N, Shi J: Childhood and adult trauma experiences of incarcerated persons and their relationship to adult behavioral health problems and treatment. Int J Environ Res Public Health 9(5):1908–1926, 2012 22754481

Wong SCP: Treatment of psychopathy in correctional settings, in Correctional Psychiatry: Practice Guidelines and Strategies, Vol II. Edited by Thienhaus OJ, Piasecki M. Kingston, NJ, Civic Research Institute, 2013, pp 6-1–6-28

Wong SCP: A treatment framework for violent offenders with psychopathic traits, in Handbook of Personality Disorders: Theory, Research, and Treatment, 2nd Edition. Edited by Livesley WJ, Larstone R. New York, Guilford, 2018, pp 629–644

Wong SCP, Gordon A: The Violence Reduction Programme: a treatment programme for violence-prone forensic clients. Psychol Crime Law 19:461–475, 2013

Zeier JD, Baskin-Sommers AR, Hiatt Racer KD, Newman JP: Cognitive control deficits associated with antisocial personality disorder and psychopathy. Pers Disord 3(3):283–293, 2012 22452754

Zwirn I, Owens H: Commentary: boundary violations in the correctional versus therapeutic setting—are the standards the same? J Am Acad Psychiatry Law 39(2):164–165, 2011 21653257

PART IV

Important Considerations

11

Women in Prison

As we began to write this book, the Netflix series
Orange Is the New Black (Netflix Original Series 2013–2019) was entering its final season. "OITNB" was inspired by the true story of Piper Kerman, who was sentenced and lived in federal prison some years after the fact for moving drug money (Kerman 2011). In the series, she goes to a corruptly run private prison and suffers through abuse from correctional officers, a riot, and several murders. Although Piper Kerman's case (referring to the person, not her fictionalized version) is not typical, it draws attention to the fact that some female prisoners do not seem to need rehabilitation, since the circumstances related to their crime are a "one-off" and not repeatable. Or they themselves (like Ms. Kerman) have "moved past" the period of their lives in which they were committing crimes or spending time with co-offenders. There are also low-level offenders whose recidivism theoretically will not change appreciably in response to treatments. Therapy in such cases may have goals similar to those for a patient in the community but can also address the special needs of people in prison (e.g., the "serious psychological distress" measured by the Bureau of Justice Statistics that we introduced when we started this book).

There is great interest in the experience of women in prison, and in the drama that directors can find in either real or fictional relationships between women in prison. Some of it relates to concerns that women are punished disproportionately for minor, nonviolent, and/or victimless drug crimes, and to the likelihood that women with traumatic histories will be further traumatized by their experiences in prison. Other issues relate to the belief (probably true) that women invest more in personal relationships than men, which makes their prison lives more interesting and also (through involvement in criminal behavior for the sake of family or in a dependent relationship with a significant other) may account for their being in prison.

According to many reviewers, the fundamental message of OITNB is that women's prisons are about female bonding. Whether or not this is a trend or the reverse of a trend is hard to tell. Some researchers (e.g., Chesney-Lind and Pasko 2012) say that women are less likely to bond long-term than they used to and are more likely to remain isolated, possibly because the level of threat is lower than it used to be or because the prisoner population is less trustworthy than it used to be. OITNB also shows the influence of a significant other—Kerman's marginal "friend" Nora (a pseudonym, but her real name is known)—on her own decisions, the peer group influence of her loosely knit group of drug runners and money movers, her decision to engage in a "victimless" crime, and her use of rationalizations like "just this one time" to do the crime.

Not everyone runs their own website to record their life in prison, but there are many websites describing the social inequities and injustices that have put generally nonviolent women in prison. It should be noted, however, that OITNB has also been accused of sensationalizing racist and sexist stereotypes for the sake of its audience and has been discussed in college courses and the feminist literature (Householder and Trier-Bieniek 2016). More on feminism later. But in any case, OITNB is over. Many people would say that "Black Is the New Black," not a title we invented, since it has been used in the media already. "Black Is the New Black" does not mean that it is merely fashionable to talk about Black women, but that the time has come to address their issues. It has been recognized that Black Lives Matter, and it is certainly true that Black Women Prisoners Matter. Black women (and also Hispanic women) are disproportionately arrested, tried, convicted, and incarcerated compared with white persons of the same sex. To be sure, this is also true of Black (and Hispanic) men. However, Black women have special problems as they are caught between socioeconomic factors causing crime and loyalties to significant others, and have issues in relation to families, child-rearing, and violence in their communities (Ritchie 1996). Their involvement even starts as schoolchildren (Morris 2018). Do a search on "school to prison pipeline" and you will find numerous items including at least 10 books and videos.

Statistics and Comparisons

The number of women in prison is much less proportionately to the population than the number of men. Women represent about 7% of the prison population, but the percentage continues to grow. There are tremendous differences within the prison population itself, as elaborated in Table 11–1. This table is not meant to give you a lot of numbers; rather, we've included it to help you appreciate the differences between the populations. We then, in Table 11–2, provide guidelines to follow when treating women. Many of these will be discussed later.

Why is it that women in prison have such high rates of mental illness or distress? First, as with men, the criminal justice system tends to target mentally ill persons and has become the successor to the mental hospital for those with serious mental illness (see Chapter 8). Second, the high prevalence of mental problems in women is a result of their past life stressors and experiences. Third, which is related to the second, is the issue of trauma that we discussed in Chapter 6. But we thought to share (in addition to the numbers in the table) a few from a survey of women in Illinois prisons (Reichert and Bostwick 2010, p. 1):

- 83% were bothered by at least one symptom of PTSD in the past month.
- 71% were bothered by repeated, disturbing memories, thoughts, or images of a stressful experience and avoided thinking or talking about a stressful experience.

TABLE 11–1.   **Just the stats, Ma'am**

Part 1: Typically, women in prison

Are unmarried, unemployed, or underemployed prior to incarceration[1, p. 189]

In most cases, are never married and are in the reproductive age group[3]

Have minor children (average 2.4)[3]

Are likely to be the custodial parent of at least one child[1, p. 189]

Are socioeconomically disadvantaged and vulnerable and have major physical and mental health needs[3]

Are more likely to be white (but this reverses a previous minority predominance)[1, p. 201]

Do not have an extensive criminal background[2, p.11]

Are in prison for a drug-related offense (70%–80%)[5, p. 15-3]

Commit crimes such as drug-related crimes, larceny, or prostitution[3]

Are arrested for prostitution or fraud, especially fraud involving acting or artifice[2, p. 11]

Report childhood sexual abuse[5, p. 15-6]

Are in traditional feminine (i.e., not masculine) roles[7, p. 213]

Have comorbid substance use disorders and personality disorders (often more than one)[3]

Have histories of diverse and multiple traumas[6]

Are different (less well off) than the offender group as a whole (who get diverted before sentencing)

Part 2: More often than men or compared with men, women in prison

Have diagnosed mental health issues, with 60% requiring mental health services[1, p. 210]

Previously took psychotropic medication (24.3% vs. 11.4%)[7, p. 214]

Require more medical services[1, p. 208]

Come from extremely dysfunctional families[1, p. 204]

Have children

Are prone to self-despair resulting in self-injury[1, p. 211]

Are more likely to be employed (60% vs. 40% for men)[1, p. 201]

Are slightly more educated[1, p. 201]

Are more likely to be serving time for a drug-related offense[1, p. 200]

Are less likely to have been sentenced for a violent crime[1, p. 200]

But if violent, are more likely to have victimized a relative[1, p. 200]

Have shorter criminal records[1, p. 200]

Have shorter maximum sentences[1, p. 200]

Use more drugs[1, p. 200]

Tend to use drugs to self-medicate (but men use drugs for social reasons)[1, p. 207]

Are more likely to have committed their crime under the influence of drugs or alcohol[1, p. 200]

Are more likely to report having been physically or sexually abused as a child (three times more likely) or physically abused as an adult (six times more likely)[1, p. 200]

Are twice as likely to have grown up in a single-parent household[1, p. 202]

Are slightly older[1, p. 189]

Have serious psychological distress (see Bronson and Berzofsky 2017) or another measure of mental illness, with PTSD the most common diagnosis other than substance use disorder[3]

Are more likely to use hard drugs and use a greater number of drugs[4]

Have a short sentence

Are more likely to have murdered an infant

TABLE 11–1.   **Just the stats, Ma'am** *(continued)*

Part 2: More often than men or compared with men, women in prison *(continued)*

Are perceived as being harder to supervise[1, p. 189]

Receive institutional discipline[2, p. 35] 1.5–2.0 times the rate among men,[1, p. 224] possibly because they showboat (have altercations in front of officers) more than men[1, p. 224] and they are more heavily policed[1, p. 213]

Were a primary caretaker for their children[6]

Were head of a household[6]

Have a high school education[4]

Lived with their children prior to incarceration[6]

Committed a crime with a dominant decision-maker, usually male[2, p. 20]

Committed a crime with an opposite gender co-offender[6]

Were victimized by a person they know[6] in the context of an emotional relationship conflict[7, p. 213]

Have an income less than $600 a month or are at poverty level[3]

Are older (early 30s) than men (late 20s)[2, p. 8]

Are (better) educated[2, p. 8]

Are accused of child neglect or abuse

Have been convicted (and incarcerated) for the first time

Have a histrionic or borderline personality disorder

Have family members in prison (47% vs. 37%)[2, p. 10]

Have family with alcohol or drug abuse problems (33% vs. 25%)[2, p. 10]

If mentally ill, are more likely to commit a crime (either violent or nonviolent)[8]

Part 3: Less often than men or compared with men, women prisoners

Are less likely to engage in serious or lethal violence or large-scale riots[1, p. 213]

Are less likely to be violent toward officers or other prisoners[2, p. 28]

Are less likely to recidivate[1, p. 202]

Are less likely to be employed[3]

Are "[l]ess likely to follow the 'do your own time' mandate of the male prisoner subculture and are more involved in each other's lives"[1, p. 213]

Commit crimes of any sort, with the exception of prostitution, running away, or embezzlement[3]

Have one or no prior offense (51/39) or two or fewer (66/55)[2, p. 11]

Have a long sentence

If committing a homicide, less likely to kill an acquaintance or stranger (versus an intimate or relative)[3]

Commit a violent crime[2, p. 13]

If violent, are less likely to have committed the crime against a woman[5, p. 15-3]

If violent, are less likely to have committed a crime of which the consequences are severe[5, p. 15-3]

Are a serial murderer[2, p. 14]

Have antisocial personality disorder

Are a sex offender (much rarer in women)

Have a juvenile history

Commit suicide in jail or prison[3]

Source. [1]Pollock 2014; [2]Pollock 1998; [3]Lewis 2010; [4]Lewis 2015; [5]Piasecki 2007; [6]Scott et al. 2019; [7]Loper and Levitt 2011; [8]Hodgins and Klein 2019.
As above, but if not otherwise cited are widely reported or general knowledge.

TABLE 11–2.   **Guidelines for treating women in prison**

Use gender-specific assessment instruments whenever possible or, if not possible, instruments that have not been proven to have a gender bias.

Recognize that comorbidity involves substance use, personality disorders (often more than one), and mental illnesses, including major mental illness.

Recognize that psychopathy, while rarer than in men, occurs in women and that psychopathic women can victimize other women.

Create and maintain a safe environment for patient and therapists working together.

Employ trauma-informed services (see Table 11–4).

As with all patients, continuously assess for suicidal thinking and plans to prevent suicide and provide postattempt crisis response safety plans.

Assess for comorbidity of substance use disorder and personality disorder; treat mental illnesses along with these disorders.

Provide gender-specific substance use disorder programs based on the differences between male and female patterns of use (i.e., programs designed for men do not work for women because their reasons and patterns of use are different from men's) (Baird 2003, p. 9-8).

Find therapeutic communities for substance use disorder or mental illness.

Assign to efficient group programs for specific issues such as PTSD.

Provide services that address criminogenic factors if applicable to the individual patient.

Practice multiculturally sensitive therapy that reflects the contributions of feminist or intersectional psychotherapy, or relational-cultural therapy, with awareness of LGBTQ+ needs.

Provide supportive psychotherapy, which is strengths-based rather than deficit-based.

Consider mental/physical health goals rather than merely elimination of mental/physical illness.

Address family dysfunction prior to, during, and after (to extent practicable) release.

Provide training in job skills, parenting skills, and other skills that will be needed in the community.

Address the criminogenic environment faced upon release.

Serve as a positive role model throughout therapy.

Address dangerous behaviors through hospitalization or special mental units and specialized programs to prevent nonsuicidal self-injury.

Try to find case managers or social workers to help with linkage to other services.

Be very cautious in self-disclosures in therapy; avoid countertransference carelessness arising from the apparently less threatening nature of women's disorders or their projected vulnerability.

Coordinate discharge planning with an assigned case manager and arrange for housing.

- About one-fourth of the sample experienced trauma-related symptoms in childhood, 41% as teenagers and 84% in adulthood.
- 61% could potentially (according to the authors of the study) be diagnosed as having PTSD.

As suggested in Chapter 7, substance use is present in offenders in high numbers, probably 70%. Statistics show a group of "pure" substance abusers, of whom 92% do not have a mental illness diagnosis. But there is also much comorbidity (80%) of substance abuse in mentally ill female prisoners (Loper and Levitt 2011). So if you did nothing else but treat substance use disorders, you would be doing a good deed, since most of the people you see in prison have a substance use disorder, and about a third of women attribute their imprisonment to actions related to substance abuse, such as needing to get money for their drugs (Loper and Levitt 2011).

Programs for female substance abusers should be gender-based, since women's patterns of substance abuse are quite different from men's. It is thought that historically, many of the get-tough-on-drugs programs directed toward women were ill-thought out and victimized them further, lowering their self-esteem. We hope this time has passed, but you should vet your institution's substance use treatment program to be sure it is gender sensitive, not just *written* for women, but addressing *women's needs*.

As we discuss supportive psychotherapy with women, we remind you of the multiple other prison programs, not just for substance use, that you may interface with. Some are excellent and some are not. Some prison therapeutic communities, for example, are controversial because of poor outcomes and confrontational (i.e., nonsupportive) methods, punitive procedures (e.g., writing up offenders for small rule violations), and susceptibility to abuse and retribution from other prisoners (as sometimes happens with Prison Rape Elimination Act [PREA] allegations).

When beginning treatment with a woman in prison, you will, of course, know some things about her sentence and recidivism. You should also become familiar with the issues that have arisen in her therapy. An interesting question concerning what the differences are between short-timer and long-term prisoners is addressed in a much-cited study that looked at newly entered prisoners with short vs. long sentences, and a third group with long sentences who had been there a long time. The study found that

> [t]he inmate groups did appear to experience different problems and to cope with their experiences in different manners. The newly entered inmates were more apt to be members of "play" families and they were more concerned about safety. The newly entered short termers reported less control of events in the environment. Those who had served long terms in prison reported more situational problems such as boredom, missing luxuries, and lack of opportunities. (MacKenzie et al. 1989, p. 223)

Fortunately, the study showed that long-termers were generally realistic about the limitations of their environment and retained their ability to cope.

Feminism

Fast forward once more to the future, when one of the doctors expounds on the unfairness that a majority member of the human race has to (in certain circumstances) give up a most precious possession, her name (White 2001, pp. 462–463). To him this smacks of second-class citizenship or just plain stupidity, and to us of course a certain parochialism and prefeminist stance of James White's time, since there were and are cultures, countries, and individuals to which this does apply.

It would make sense that when treating women, practitioners should develop an understanding and an appreciation of, or at least a position with respect to, feminism. *Feminism* is the social philosophy or movement that promotes equal rights between the sexes. As with supportive psychotherapy, one can find a historical basis for feminism in Ancient Greece, since in his *Republic* Plato proposed a society with equality between for men and women except for occupations requiring strength. Somewhat later, a fascinating, elusive, and prolific playwright, Aphra Behn (1640–1689), said to be the first woman to support herself through writing, has been called a protofeminist, LGBTQ+ icon, and possibly a protoabolitionist as well. However, contemporary feminism is not one thing but a group of related social philosophies and—for our purposes—inclusive of theories of psychotherapy. The movement has evolved from more radical positions (we mean radical to mainstream thought) regarding the oppression of women in patriarchal European-American society to a social philosophy that attempts to embrace a multicultural prescription for the enlightened behavior of everybody, including men. There is a part of feminism that is rooted in anti-establishment and antimale sentiments, even if it has evolved far from that stance. Therefore, some feel that the name "feminism" has come to detract from the more general content of modern feminism. Many sites and sources now ask: "Why can't we all be feminists?" We mentioned our own philosophy of "enlightened multiculturalism" in Chapter 1 and made it an ethical principle of psychotherapy. Another term, *intersectionality*, was coined by law professor Kimberlé Crenshaw. We will discuss this shortly.

The history of modern feminism is parsed differently by different feminists. According to Laura Brown, it has evolved through the following stages (Brown 2018, p. 22):

- No-difference feminism (1960s–early 1980s)
  - Reformist feminist
  - Radical feminist
- Difference/cultural feminist (mid-1980s–mid-1990s)
- Difference with equal values feminism (mid-1990s–present)
- Multicultural, global, and postmodern feminisms (the early 21st century)
- Feminism of the globally connected world (2008–present)

Others describe feminism as occurring in waves. The first wave in the United States began in the mid-1800s, highlighted by the 1848 Seneca Falls Convention in New York, at which a "Declaration of Sentiments" and 12 resolutions were passed. Some 200 years after the birth of Aphra Behn, Sojourner Truth delivered her famous "Ain't I a Woman?" speech in 1851 in Akron, Ohio. However, it would be a long time before feminism represented the positions of minority race and economically marginalized women. The second wave began in the 1960s, reflecting a movement for civil rights and prisoner rights. The third wave developed from the 1980s into the 1990s with the birth of Generation X and attempts to accommodate difference, diversity, and change (Schram and Tibbetts 2014, pp. 285–287). A fourth wave started in 2012 and included the growth of the Me Too movement (founded in 2006 but becoming most prominent in 2017) and attempts to address sexual harassment, body shaming, and rape culture (Brunell 2020).

Finally, we mention that some feminists are concerned that what is now called the "carceral state" may actually have been aided by the feminist movement insofar as it promulgated incarceration for violence against women and has had unforeseen and adverse consequences (Gruber 2020). Intersectionality is an outgrowth of the second wave of feminism. It asserts that that people's experiences occur at and express the intersection of their various social and political identities, including gender, race, class, sexuality, and disability. The purpose of this approach is to better account for the wide-ranging experiences of all women, not just white women, and in particular to account for the power relationships that affect people's development. The term *intersectionality* was coined by Black feminist scholar Kimberlé Williams Crenshaw in 1989 (Wikipedia 2019a).

It is said that "[i]ntersectionality as an analytic tool gives people better access to the complexities of the world and of themselves" (Collins and Bilge 2016, p. 2). Since intersectionality has the potential to be a social philosophy that can be expressed by both men and women and all therapists, it does have great applicability to therapeutic situations. However, some of the doctrines of intersectionality are more controversial, and the qualifications and caveats in Wikipedia make that clear as well. It has also been criticized as being an untested ideology rather than a progressive social philosophy. Whether these criticisms are valid or not, we feel obliged to mention them and ask you to learn more about feminism and intersectionality on your own.

In culturally competent assessments, in fact, it may be appropriate to ask the patient about her attitude toward feminist philosophy. However, these are not likely to be issues you would ask about in a first interview or even at all. See the examples in Table 11–3.

There Is Nothing Like a Dame

(but most mainstream criminologists still don't know that)

Theories of crime reflect sensitivity to the biological and cultural differences, and this is especially true of feminist theories of crime. Back in Table 1–1 in Chapter 1, we summarized criminological theories, which included some feminist theories of crime. For example, the feminist pathways theory of crimes (attributed to many, including the already quoted Chesney-Lind and Pasko [2012] and obviously much earlier theorists) shows that women's paths often follow trajectories of escape from abuse and victimization. They may escape from these circumstances by running away from home, abusing drugs, and engaging in what are called survival crimes including prostitution. However, criminologists going back to the classical also had theories of female crime, for example, Cesare Lombroso's *The Female Offender* (Lombroso and Ferrero 1895). Biological theorists such as Otto Pollak (*The Criminality of Women*) in 1950 posited biological and psychological differences as the explanation of women's criminality but neglected the effect of social, political, and economic factors (Pollak 1950). Crimes by women are also addressed in so-called gender-neutral theories of crime, including social learning theory (Burgess and Akers 1966 and subsequently developed by Akers), and hybrid theories such as general strain theory (Agnew 1992). The power-control theory of John Hagan considered the effects of conflict and social control on delinquency in women (Hagan et al. 1985). Finally, the risk-need-responsivity (RNR) theorists hold a general personality and cognitive social learning theory of crime that combines psychological and social learning theories. However, even with this brief survey that shows growing recognition of the need to modify or develop entirely new criminological theories about women (but not of the sort that patronize or objectify them as "dames"—you can have a theory about women but it can be a bad theory), there is still a long way to go, as lamented in one article from a few years ago that urges criminologists to realize "that a more inclusive criminology has far more to of-

TABLE 11–3. **Examples of culturally competent assessment of gender issues**

Personal history item	Sample questions	Comments
Developmental cultural influence	How were you raised as a girl? What are the cultural expectations for a woman such as yourself from your parents? From your community? What do you see as a future for yourself? How does going to prison affect your view of your future?	Gender identity is shaped by family and cultural influences from birth onward (e.g., cultural meaning of names, dress, choice of toys and gifts, activities, schooling, allowable behaviors such as being encouraged to speak or play in a certain way).
Rites of passage	Have you ever participated in rites of passage in your culture?	Examples: bat mitzvah (Jewish coming of age ceremony for women); quinceañara (celebration of fifteenth birthday in the Hispanic community). Inquiries might have to be made (or gathered from records) of female genital mutilation in immigrants from African and Middle Eastern countries.
Identification with women's movement	What do you think about the feminist movement? Where do you see yourself relative to the movement? How does this affect your life choices? What would it mean to you to be a feminist in prison?	You should be prepared to justify such questions and explain the different types of feminist philosophies as they affect prison life.
Significant others and marital arrangement	What partners have you had in the past? Do you have a current partner? What role did your family play (if any) in selection of a partner?	Answers will vary considerably depending on culture of origin, life history, and desired choices.
Sexual orientation	Are you familiar with the designations LGBTQ+? How do you identify yourself (whether or not you use labels, what is it that you feel)? Are you attracted to men, women, both, are you unsure, or would you describe your relationships in another way?	This may lead to gender identity issues, gender dysphoria, and so forth.

Source. Primarily based on Andermann and Fung 2015, pp. 312–313, with additional correctional items.

fer in the future than was possible in the relatively gender-blind criminological past" (Cook 2016, p. 349).

An underlying premise when working with women is worth thinking about. Are women in general *less culpable* than men? We already know that they are, for example, less violent. How do we determine culpability? A syllogism is an old form of deductive logic that you may remember from that Philosophy 101 course you were required to take. The standard form of a syllogism is this:

> All men are mortal.
>
> Socrates is a man.
>
> Therefore, Socrates is mortal.

In thinking about culpability in women, are we reasoning like this?

> A person who commits a crime is culpable to the extent that she rationally chooses to break the law.
>
> Because of social oppression and life pathways, women more than men are constrained and oppressed in the choices they make to commit crimes.
>
> Therefore, women are less culpable than men.

In other words, how should we think of women: as offenders or as victims? Referring to what is now called the "blurred boundaries" theory of victimization and criminalization, it is argued that: "This false categorization of women as either offenders or victims does not provide an enhanced understanding about women who commit crime" (Schram and Tibbetts 2014, p. 307). We shall even reprise our traveling Galactic master chef, Gurronsevas, from Chapter 1. Gurronsevas has gotten himself into a spot of trouble and destroyed some cargo. In his defense, he argues that he cannot be held entirely responsible for the outcome because he did not have complete control over the situation, and in fact his level of responsibility should be much reduced because he had little control over his particular situation (White 1996, pp. 100–101). This would describe the situation in which many women in prison find themselves, and probably many other persons both within and outside of prison. (We should note that our point does not just suggest the legal term of *diminished responsibility* in many jurisdictions; it also alludes to the responsibility that people can reasonably be expected to exercise over their actions given their particular circumstances.)

What's Good for the Gander May Not Be Good for the Goose

Feminism is obviously relevant to psychotherapy with women. As far as proponents of feminism and intersectionality are concerned, there are serious issues of power imbalance when conducting therapy in coercive settings. Some feminist therapists believe that males ought not provide therapy because in those settings women will be passive, the male is not an accessible role model, the male plays the role of an expert, and the male will espouse supposedly liberated ideas that neither of them believe (Baird 2003, citing Ackerman 1987, pp. 27–28). Ackerman (1987) recommends that the goals of feminist therapy should be

- Providing reinforcement for actively seeking empowering solutions to problems.
- Changing the oppressive system.

- Getting women out of the victim role.
- Helping women to pay attention to their self-esteem in their daily interactions.
- Encouraging women to trust their own feelings and perceptions.
- Encouraging personal growth skills.

These goals sound reasonable, but one might wonder if the requisites of an egalitarian and consented psychotherapy can be met in a prison. Perhaps we can suggest that a therapist in prison is like a teacher or tour guide whom one can agree to follow or emulate as a role model, at least temporarily. Consider the tour guide analogy. As a therapist, liken yourself to being a tour guide "hired" by the prison. There are many possible sights, but following your guidance, your "tourists" are not allowed to wander off into the backwaters of an unknown country. They should go, trustingly, where you lead them. In addition, there are criticisms of a totally egalitarian psychotherapy. If a therapist is an equal, how can she be the expert? Also, authoritarianism in the transference can lead to more effective psychological change, provided that the transference is kept positive.

Some feminist therapists eschew structured assessment instruments, yet these are the heart and soul of the RNR methodology. There is also still debate about the need for gender-responsive risk assessment instruments. Some feminist therapists have objections to the use of standard DSM-5 diagnostic categories, preferring to use the terminology of distress and injury rather than disorders and diseases (Bloom and Covington 2008). It has been claimed that DSM-5 lacked evidence-based practices and that psychopathology is attributed to persons whose lives reflect reactions to sexism (e.g., racism, homophobia). We want you to be aware of these concerns, but they are still associated with controversy, and it does appear that DSM-5-TR has made some progress in addressing such concerns. So has the increased emphasis on social justice issues as they affect psychiatric diagnoses.

Many therapists oppose the labeling of victimized, distressed, and emotional women as having borderline or histrionic personalities, since it appears that emotional men do not receive those labels. In this regard, they urge us to seek alternative ways to describe behaviors that one might be accustomed to label in what might be a derogatory manner. For example, a person who is said to have a borderline personality disorder might better be said (using the language of Seeking Safety) as having intense emotional experiences. Of a person who is said to be attention-seeking, perhaps it is better to say that she finds it difficult to share the time with others. Other example of labels that have better descriptions include "manipulative," "immature," "uncooperative," or simply "untreatable" (for more items, see Williams et al. 2010, p. 38). Whether or not you can find more descriptive phrases, it is good advice when charting to use detailed behavioral language rather than simplified labels of a patient's behavior. For example, instead of writing "patient was aggressive today," give the behavioral details (e.g., "Patient yelled at the culinary worker for not getting an extra portion and pushed her neighbor away on the line"). If you say that the patient is delusional, give examples, or if you say she is hallucinating, explain how you know, what she said about her hallucinations, and how she interacted with them.

Speaking of disagreements with DSM-5, it has been argued that PTSD should be replaced by PTSI (posttraumatic stress injury), although that change was not accepted by the American Psychiatric Association in 2012 when DSM-5 was being finalized.

There are also the legal implications of diagnosing a woman with battered woman's syndrome and premenstrual dysphoric disorder when used as explanations for crimes. There is a type of psychotherapy, relational-cultural therapy (Jordan 2019a, 2019b), that recognizes the importance of relationships in women's lives and has developed on a parallel track to feminism. It recognizes the negative effects of isolation in women's lives and the need for satisfying connections with others.

Feminism can be used to provide what are called "genetic" (really, developmental) explanations in psychotherapy. A woman who was victimized and/or abused, or whose opportunities were limited due to sexism, can be educated about how this took place, not as an excuse for illegal future behavior, but as a way to help her reach an understanding of how she came to be where she was. Feminism can empower women in prison to change their personal circumstances as well as bring about change in the prison, although we would not use some of the terms we see, such as "revolution" and "resistance." As prisoners, they may wish to associate with such movements, but as therapists we do not feel that we can endorse wholesale resistance to the institution as opposed to advocacy for change (which we do endorse).

Despite the challenges that both male and female therapists face when working in a women's prison, we do agree with Baird (2003), who states that while it is a challenge to provide appropriate and empowering therapy to incarcerated women, it can provide "endless rewards" when they can make changes in their circumstances of unequal status and invisibility.

Feminism also can inform therapy in uncovering what are now believed to be legitimate biological (e.g., brain structure) and cultural differences between men and women. Women are said to value relationships more than men and define themselves more relationally. This helps us to understand their desires to establish relationships in prison and to function as family groups. When the PREA regulations were being developed, which took many years, it was suggested that women should be cut more slack in the area of touching, hand holding, and kissing. This was eventually rejected in the interest of equal treatment for the sexes. Yet, as we mentioned, prison management routinely allows differences, such as allowing women to use knitting needles. Then there are the sex-based (and often sexist) differences when the men's prison teaches sheet metal work and the women's prison processes the returns to department stores.

Supportive psychotherapy, being advisory or directive, must address issues of the inherent disparity of power and domination in the prison setting. We still believe that there is a place for *some* male role models in prison, yet at the same time we wonder: How can a male therapist *not* replay the male domination of an abused woman's past? Some would hold that it is undesirable to be treated by either a benevolent male despot or a malevolent one. Despite these risks and the risks of PREA allegations, we still think that male therapists should be available, although an attempt should be made to allow vulnerable women to opt out and see a female therapist. Consider this (based on Lewis 2015, p. 296): Women who have had trauma do not necessarily require treatment only by women. Gender-responsive programming does not require that they can demand only female treatment providers, which would be disruptive and limit their access to providers. There is no strong proof in the literature that they have better outcomes with female providers, and they should have the opportunity to work with qualified male providers.

Psychotherapy in prison, regardless of the gender or sexual orientation of the therapist, remains highly unequal in power. In giving direction of any sort, you risk expressing your biases. When a woman declares that she wants to become a high-rise steelworker, do you gently discourage it as unrealistic? Do you suggest she neglect her bruises and go into marital counseling rather than divorce for the sake of the children? Women will come to you with requests for advice. Do you withhold all advice to avoid the imposition of bias?

Feminist psychotherapy and intersectionality are approaches that are usually accompanied by gender-informed programming. Examples are Seeking Safety (addressing PTSD and substance abuse) (Najavits 2002; see also Seeking Safety 2020) and STEPPS (Systems Training for Emotional Predictability and Problem Solving 2021), which addresses what we have called borderline personality disorder (BPD) as a problem of emotional intensity. We do like STEPPS, an inexpensive program with a lot of support materials. For additional information see the websites for these programs and Chapters 6 and 12 of this book, as well as publications by Taylor et al. (2018, p. 117), Khilnani (2016), and Black and Blum (2017). Dialectical behavior therapy, of course, is probably the best-known program originally developed for the problems related to BPD.

Although RNR proponents claim it to be equally applicable to women and men, it has been adapted by others to a gender-specific model (Blanchette and Brown 2006). Since RNR generally discounts programs for low-risk offenders, it has also been questioned whether there is an obligation to treat them (Scott et al. 2019, discussing Van Voorhis 2012). One notable omission in the needs group as it applies to women has been parental needs. Gender-specific programming also follows a strengths-based model that is amenable to supportive therapy techniques. Strengths-based treatment "shifts the focus from targeting problems to identifying the multiple issues a woman must contend with and the strategies she has adopted to cope" (Bloom and Covington 2008, p. 173). Based on research on the comparative moral development of men and women, "an understanding of female biopsychosocial development, mutual caring and empowering relationships serve as useful tools to integrate in a gender-specific treatment approach. These differences should be viewed as strengths instead of weaknesses" (Khilnani 2016, p. 9).

We started our discussion of feminism with a literary allusion, so referring back to Ruth Rendell again, when discussing Freud's well-known question "What do women want?" her character (the daughter of her chief inspector Wexford) answers that they just want to be people like anyone else (Rendell 1978, p. 104). That makes sense, doesn't it?

At all phases of therapy, you will be hearing about and providing therapy regarding sexual behaviors, both within and outside prison. For years it has been known that interpersonal sexual activity is widespread in men's and women's prisons. Most interpersonal sexual activity is homosexual, although as dramatized in the media and statistics of PREA allegations, there is both heterosexual and homosexual activity between staff and prisoners. Those are serious crimes. All interpersonal sexual activity is a violation of rules, but the nature of the enforcement and PREA involvement depends on the parties involved and the level of coercion.

Most women who enter prison were heterosexual prior to incarceration, but many enter into same-sex relationships while in prison. Most will return to heterosexual relationships and exclusivity after release, but some may recognize in themselves bisexuality or gay interests in the future. Heterosexual women may experience distress in engaging in homosexual activity. Not only is it a rule violation, but there is an element of coercion and a certain amount of secrecy either overt or covert in much activity, even though there is considerably less violence associated with women's compared to men's sexual relationships in prison. The thought of developing or the actual development of a sexual relationship may create concerns and questions in a prisoner about her sexual orientation. Is she thinking of coming out or just being "gay for the stay" or "gate gay"? These questions are not limited to prisons, but occur in colleges, the military, and summer camps. Although you can take the official position that sexual activity is forbidden anyway, you may be issuing a lot of nonverbal cues of which you are unaware.

Sexual relationships in prison are not just a pairing off of temporary or stable couples. Relationships—whether they be of the parent-child type, of a type marked by a nonromantic friendship style, or intimate partner relationships—are important to both men and women in prison. Because of the general unavailability of opposite-sex relationships in women's prison, women may become involved with other women at any of the levels mentioned. This has been recognized for more than a century (see Wikipedia 2019b). Women, much more so than men, form "pseudo-families" or "fantasy families," often around a central couple and creation of mothers, fathers, sisters, children, and so forth. There is a prison word for every possible role. Gay, masculine, or "butch" women are cast in masculine rules and are referred to as "he" or "him" or addressed as "Mister." Prisoners who are used by others are called "tricks" and those who engage in sex for commissary items are called "commissary hustlers." Prisoners may experience jealousy, breakups, domestic abuse, and violence. They may attempt to change cells to be with each other or get away from each other. One person may state she is suicidal so she gets sent to the infirmary, and then another will do the same to be placed next door where they can talk to each other.

An example: Bursick (2018) describes the experiences of Angela, a woman who was in a heterosexual relationship with a man she considered to be her fiancé, but he soon ghosted her. She formed a relationship with Cam, a woman 6 years younger whom she described as somewhat unfeminine, but this relationship fell apart after a few months. Reporting data we have seen elsewhere, Burdick states that 30%–60% of women engage in lesbian relationships in prison, and once released 25% continue to be with women. People in the LGBTQ+ group are highly overrepresented in prison (surveys say they are six times as likely to be incarcerated as are heterosexuals), and they have their own issues of adjustment. Gay women may find it easier to continue being gay but are subject to harassment from officers and other prisoners.

Pseudofantasies as well as homosexual fantasies have been discussed in research, but some of the research may be flawed or out of date. You will find what is real in your own facility. We have certainly seen patients repeat the pattern of their past in reproducing the domestic violence of their families of origin in a prison family. Prisoners interviewed in Cuen (2016) discuss widespread, if not universal, sexual activity, ranging from handholding to brutality and violence. Opinions (and data) vary somewhat, but the general impression is that although many women remain celibate without being coerced into sexual behavior, others participate in homosexual relationships with one or more partners.

What is the role of a therapist when discussing these make-believe families? It is suggested that female prisoners turn to their therapists for support in understanding their use of these adaptations to prison life (Arrigo and Shipley 2005, p. 481). This includes helping correctional staff to understand why female prisoners develop these relationships.

When you talk to women about these relationships, you will no doubt find the workarounds of not referring to the sexual behavior. PREA forbids sexual behavior and requires you to report it. But you can talk about previous incidents that were reported and dealt with, and you can talk about romance and love. Most patients are aware of the difference between love and situational relationships. We find it is helpful to deal with the issues of falling in love, overcommitments, manipulation, and outright domestic abuse. Angela, mentioned above, had probably become overinvested and in love with Cam. Her therapist (if she had one) would need to help her through two major breakups in just the first year!

Having lived through the process ourselves, we think there has been much change in attitude since the implementation of PREA. There has been increased awareness and acceptance of female homosexual relationships in prison at the same time as even the mildest public expressions of affection in prisons have been forbidden. A journalist who has visited prisons throughout the world documented the frustration that prisoners experienced (before PREA): "Barbed prison walls and armed guards are everyday reminders of the fact that women can't kiss their girlfriends or walk together holding hands" (Talvi 2007, p. 107). These restrictions have to be balanced with her own observations: Mentioning a Reuters report that said that 20% of female prisoners had been coerced into a sexual relationship, she still feels that "[a]necdotally speaking, same-sex relationships in women's prisons rarely seem to be a matter of coercion or sexual violence, although intimidation and physical violence certainly do exist" (Talvi 2007, p. 200). We discuss these things with patients when they bemoan the fact that they can't hold hands in public. Women may be less violent than men, but they can still be sexually coercive, and we explain why PREA does not believe that prisoner-to-prisoner relationships can be consensual.

Trauma-Informed Services

Based on the predominance of trauma in history and of stressor-related disorders in women prisoners, there are established guidelines for providing trauma-informed services. We have discussed these in several previous chapters, especially Chapters 3 and 6. Elliott et al. (2005) set forth 10 principles of trauma-informed services for women (Table 11–4).

While taking into account the existence of trauma and victimization in the history of your patients, you cannot allow it to be used as an excuse for future criminal behavior. An example is given by Elliott and Verdeyen (2002, p. 112). Erika says she was sexually abused by her father and stepfather, ran away from home, started using drugs, and then sold them. She says "I didn't care about anything or anyone. Why should I? No one cares about me. Yeah, I sold drugs. I had to support my habit. That's why I'm here." Her past behavior is understandable: she was a victim of her father, stepfather, and the War on Drugs. However, she uses her life history to preempt criticism or commitment to developing a drug-free and crime-free lifestyle. Elliott and Verdeyen identify

---

TABLE 11–4.   Principles of trauma-informed services

---

1. Trauma-informed services recognize the impact of violence and victimization on development and coping strategies
2. They identify recovery from trauma as a primary goal
3. They employ an empowerment model
4. They strive to maximize a woman's choices and control over her recovery
5. They are based on a relational collaboration
6. They create an atmosphere that is respectful of survivors' need for safety, respect, and acceptance
7. They emphasize women's strengths, highlighting adaptations over symptoms and resilience over pathology
8. The goal of trauma-informed services is to minimize the possibilities of retraumatization
9. They strive to be culturally competent and to understand each woman in the context of her life experiences and cultural background
10. Trauma-informed agencies solicit consumer input and involve consumers in designing and evaluating services

---

Source.   Elliott et al. 2005, pp. 465–469.

at least two criminal thinking patterns in Erika's attitude: mollification and playing the victim. Citing Najavits (2002, mentioned above), they recommend trying to achieve a balance between praise and accountability. While it is important to listen to Erika as she relates her history, the staff need to generate an expectation that her deprivations do not absolve her of future responsibility for her actions.

Borderline Personality Disorder

More women than men are diagnosed with BPD, but men with borderline personalities, who are less common in the community, are overrepresented in prison populations and often violent and bizarre in their self-destruction and self-cutting. We remember one man who managed to swallow a tin of snuff (Hint: Anything bigger than a quarter gets stuck in the stomach). Another bypassed that oral route by stabbing himself in the stomach so much that he had created an opening (medically called a fistula) from the outside of his stomach to the inside. So from our personal experiences in both male and female settings, we have come to "appreciate" (to use the best word we can find) that there are many advantages to working with such self-destructive women in prison, since you actually have some means for improving their safety. Or, to put it somewhat sadly, you can sometimes make the same mistake *twice* when dealing with women's self-cutting behaviors and you do not always have that option with men. There may be times you wish you were back in a private office, but not when you get called by a borderline patient who says she is suicidal and hangs up. There's no hiding in the prison.

We discussed some relationships between borderline personality and criminality in the previous chapter. As for data specific to women, a study of incarcerated women in maximum security in Virginia found that 43% had antisocial personality disorder (ASPD), 24% had BPD, and 10% had narcissistic personality disorder. Comorbidity is high: of the 43% with ASPD, the same percentage (43%) also had BPD (Warren et al. 2002). However, surveys vary considerably. In the Trestman survey mentioned in Chapter 10, 12.9% of the sample had both (Trestman et al. 2007). But surprisingly, it appears that narcissistic personality actually has a stronger association with aggression than does borderline personality. The reason for this is hypothesized to be psychological defensive maneuvers due to the low self-esteem in women (Kalemi et al. 2019).

With women with BPD, we:

- Describe it as in STEPPS as an emotional sensitivity problem.
- As in the previous chapter, tell them that the historical meaning of "borderline personality" was that it meant the borderline of psychosis and that persons with borderline personalities can lose touch with reality and have micropsychotic episodes even though they do not have schizophrenia (unless they have both disorders).
- Cowrite a crisis response safety plan (see Chapters 5 and 6) and review it periodically.
- Automatically review any crises or meltdowns they have had between sessions (because they will often avoid telling you about them).
- Provide "a little bit" of the flexibility and availability of dialectical behavior therapy therapists by having some time to deal with crises.
- Reinforce good behavior by giving more therapy time when they are well than when they are in crisis. (This may sound paradoxical, but we do not wish to reinforce the use of crises to obtain therapy; when they are in a genuine crisis, they do not benefit from a long therapy session.)

Specialized programs and workbooks can also help. For example, *Beyond Anger and Violence* (Covington 2014) and *Beyond Violence* (Covington 2013), two of many books by Stephanie Covington, discuss adverse childhood experiences and trauma and their role in creating anger and violent behavior.

Alcohol and Substance Use Disorders

Because of the high percentage of alcohol and substance use disorders, either alone or with mental illness, most of your patients should be in concomitant substance use treatment as discussed in Chapter 7. Be familiar with the particular programs and periodically discuss their issues in therapy. Make sure that the interventions *you* use (e.g., relapse prevention) are compatible with the programs the patients attend. You can use techniques of motivational interviewing, but keep in mind that we find those techniques to be less effective than the ones we use for addressing criminal lifestyles and severe mental illness. The major advantage of working with substance users in prison is that for the most part patients are clean and sober and in a somewhat underfunded long-term residential treatment program. The main sentiment you must counter is the attitude that "I'm through with drugs. I'll never use them again and I don't need a drug treatment program when I get out." Why, you ask, don't they make arrangements for one in the "rare" instance that they need one? This is one of the issues in preventing recidivism.

Benefits and Risks of Working in Women's Prisons

There are many possible benefits of working in a women's prison. The environment and the therapy setting are less violent. Prisoner violence and ASPD are less prevalent, as are sex offenses. Manipulation schemes are probably less prevalent. There is more opportunity to talk about family matters and children. Group therapies and relationship issues are more interesting.

Risks can consist of losing caution, being too friendly, or giving out too much personal information. All therapists, but probably more often male than female, can end up in an eroticized transference or with eroticized countertransference. We do urge male therapists to have someone watching the therapy even if it is outside of the room. We would like to believe that all unjustified PREA allegations against staff members are dismissed, but they can be made vindictively and create stress while investigated.

Earlier, we did not rule out the use of a male therapist but discussed a prisoner's rights to change therapists. Staff being limited, that always slows down a request for change. Many women have had abusive or absent male parental or authority figures but still benefit or even thrive with male role models. A therapist can be a positive role model, although there are some women who have been so badly traumatized by men that they cannot work with a male therapist. Sometimes they will eroticize them, and of course they may also eroticize the relationship with a female therapist. If it is merely a matter of a little flirting or liking, there may be enough of what we call a positive transference to leave the situation alone. Women may also flirt with a therapist, perhaps in the belief (conscious or habitual) that this is the only way to get favors or the only way to be liked. If this is a safe but positive transference in supportive therapy, we may leave it alone or wait until it can be interpreted in a positive light (e.g., at the point where they know they do *not* need to flirt to be what they count as being "liked"). But when positive transference takes the form of romantic blandishments or love letters, it must be addressed immediately. Also, there is the possibility of a negative transference from a previously traumatized woman to a male therapist. This can become violent, and it also needs to be addressed or the therapist changed.

Consider a *New York Times* blog from a prison psychologist, Dr. Gross, who states that he has stopped reading the charts of his patients and just listens to what they have to say in their sessions. He says that the reason for this (other than joking about his laziness!) is the risk of being overwhelmed by the sad life stories of his patients. But to look at the patient's side of the encounter, she tells him that she has long ago given up telling people her life story because it overwhelms them and she gets too much false sympathy from it. She found her mother's body in the laundry room (dead by suicide) when she was 14, to just start it off. Dr. Gross muses that: "Inmates get clothes and food and shelter, maybe a G.E.D. But they don't get the kind of warmth, comfort and understanding that can help them truly change, prepare them for a better life outside" (Gross 2015, p. 4). We do hope that you can do this for female prisoners without becoming overwhelmed yourself. (But you should still read the chart!)

Common Gender-Predominant Issues

By gender-predominant issues, we mean those that are more likely to be found in women, but these do not have to be exclusive to women. The point of mentioning them is to improve your ability to do therapy when you encounter them. The lifelong perception of being a victim is found in many women prisoners, although it is not exclusively found in women. One researcher, Jessica Williams Saunders, kept a beat-up rag doll in her office and found that patients frequently made comments about their identification with it (Williams Saunders 2001, p. 15).

Women and men are different, and women's and men's prisons are different. Some of the differences are due to the vastly greater number of men than women in prison. As a result, women's prisons may have all security levels in one building. This can lead to security and movement issues, and also to inadvertent mistakes or presumptions on the therapist's part of "treating all patients alike" (e.g., both violent and nonviolent offenders). One moment you may be seeing a nonviolent embezzler and the next a murderer. You may see a meek and reserved drug user followed by a cunning and violent gang-involved drug distributor. Do you react to them in the same way or take different precautions based on the known differences in their risk classification? Even if the person won't tell you (and we have already urged you to find out from the file, and we will discuss this issue of how much to ask), there is usually a presentence report, separate from the medical records. Do you know to change gears both for safety and for therapeutic effect? Stopping drug use may be a goal in the treatment plan for the drug user and for the gang member, but will the interventions be the same? For example, the gang member ought to change her criminogenic thinking or codependent attachment to a male gang member (itself a controversial issue) and move away from her criminal associates. The drug user may have self-esteem and mental health issues.

Some therapists begin to slip or ease up in relating personal details to female patients. This happens to both male and female therapists. In women's prisons, despite the differences in security levels, you can be certain that every little detail of your life that you let slip in a therapy session with a prosocial schoolteacher eventually finds its way into the personal memory bank of the antisocial criminal: those HIPAA rules don't apply to your confidences to patients.

We do assume that everything we say will be shared. Sometimes we even use it (somewhat deliberately) to our advantage. For example, we are meeting one-on-one with a member of the therapeutic community and debating a change in policy. "You know, that's a great idea…I'll think about that [limiting statements strictly to 3 minutes on the clock] and we can talk about it tomorrow." By the next morning, the entire therapeutic community is buzzing about it. The patient feels special in being the first to spread the rumor, and so forth. Such "tricks" can backfire on you, or they can work several agendas (your relationship to the patient and the group). Use them wisely, but we think you will be using them on some occasions.

Psychodynamically trained therapists point out that women reenact scenes from their early lives involving having been victimized by close family members. They warn that although women are less violent than men with strangers, they are often violent with family members or substitute family members such as therapists. Thus, therapists may underestimate the violence risk when treating women and even become complacent because they are "being treated like family."

Displaced anger is seen in women's reactions to staff and therapists. Anger at a correctional officer may reflect displaced anger at parents. The therapist may have countertransference feelings or feel anger at the patient "for behaving like a child."

Fear of independence is a common theme in the therapy of women who have lacked it. Many have never been independent of a controlling or abusive partner or have had a succession of relationships with drug users. Some have no work skills and have never worked.

When women commit a violent crime (much less often than men), it is likely to be against someone they know in the context of an emotional relationship conflict. Processing the event and preventing similar future events therefore involves understanding the woman's skills or lack of them in handling intense or highly invested emotional relationships. Given the tendency to victimization, the finding is likely to be that violence in the context of an unhappy relationship is seen as the only option or is just an expression of anger and hopelessnessness without a thought to the consequences.

Splitting is a much-mentioned phenomenon attributed to persons with borderline personality disorder. "Prison staff may find themselves becoming favored by some women and rejected by others, often leading to splits in staff teams and inconsistent responses to women's needs" (Short and Barber 2010, p. 59). Meeting regularly with custody (within HIPAA limits) to share stories (be they horror or happy) can help to avoid the divisions between custody and clinicians. Finding out that staff have become split is sometimes the first recognition that a patient has borderline personality features. However, splitting frequently occurs as part of staff manipulations and can drag staff members into conflicts with each other that reflect staff members' desires to be super-good therapists who are going the extra mile for their patient.

Case Vignette

Ms. Sanchez, a 40-year-old woman, asks for an immediate appointment and is seen as a walk-in by her psychiatrist. "You have to move me to unit C [from unit B where she currently resides]." The psychiatrist is puzzled, because B is a quiet unit upstairs and most people prefer to live there. Ms. Sanchez says "No, it is terrible, it is noisy, and I am bored to death. I have asked the officers to move me and they refuse. Why are they punishing me?" The psychiatrist calls the lieutenant, who joins them in the office. "It's nothing personal," says the lieutenant, "but due to the COVID-19 restrictions, we aren't moving anyone to unit C right now. She can ask us again when the pandemic is over." After the lieutenant leaves, Ms. Sanchez angrily continues: "That's not true. If I broke the rules, they would move me out." [True, but she would be moved to a disciplinary unit.] The psychiatrist asks if there is some hidden reason, such as a friend in unit C that she wants to be closer to, but she angrily denies it. Finally, the psychiatrist says he can do nothing more but he says he will ask her therapist to look into it further.

Ms. Sanchez reiterates her concerns to the therapist and is still very emotional about it. In fact, Ms. Sanchez now "hints" that she "might become suicidal" if she does not get moved soon. The therapist does not think it would be productive to move Ms. Sanchez to the infirmary, but she still cannot get to the real reason (if there is one) for the request. The therapist promises to investigate it further and this requires going up to the associate warden level. The incident is discussed in the weekly mental health meeting. The associate warden does wonder why they are bothering him when his lieutenant already gave the correct answer and they are not going to make an exception for her.

Ms. Sanchez finally quiets down, and she eventually does get moved to unit C. That week, the therapist meets with another patient, 20-year-old Ms. Rivera. "Oh, Dr. Jones, thank you so much for moving Ms. Sanchez. We have been trying to get together ever since we got separated last month due to the COVID-19 cohorts! Oh, it's not what you think, Dr. Jones. It's perfectly respectable. We are doing all sorts of cooking together and she is teaching me how to raise my children! I do love her, but not in a romantic way. She is like the mother I didn't have at all."

"Aha," thinks the therapist. "Finally, we have the explanation of that whole episode. But if Ms. Sanchez' motives for moving were so pure, why didn't she just say so? Why did she have to lie to us, and repeatedly so?" The therapist reflects this back onto Ms. Sanchez. "Why did you lie to us?" she asks. "Why didn't you just tell us your reason?" Ms. Sanchez is silent for a minute and says, "I figured I could get what I wanted by lying to you guys. I lie all the time. That's what I do." The therapist goes through an abbreviated version of the Roy Horn story (see Chapter 4), and asks, "Do you just lie to us because we are the authority figures or do you lie to everybody?" The answer: "Oh, yes, to everybody. That's how I get what I want." The therapist asks: "Do you lie to Ms. Rivera?" Answer: "Sure, I said *everybody*, didn't I?" The therapist says, "We've got some work to do here!" The therapist thinks: "Do lying liars ever stop lying? Can a tiger shed its stripes?"

Ms. Sanchez' behavior may be an example of what we called the "spin the therapist" technique back in Chapter 4. Ms. Sanchez is not a psychopath but seems to have a psychopathic trait of lying repeatedly and without feelings about doing so. There is also another possibility—that she and Ms. Rivera do have a romantic relationship and that they are *both* lying about it!

Another (related) thing we have noticed is that sometimes it is not clear 1) who is really "treating" whom and 2) who is really getting better. This occurs in the therapy of severely ill and violent women. A treatment plan is developed with the behavioral goal of "fewer violent outbursts" and indeed, as time goes by, there are fewer violent outbursts. The treatment team is pleased that the patient is making progress. Then there is a change in the treatment team either temporary or permanent, for example, the therapist goes on vacation or is replaced, and the patient has another one or a series of outbursts. The team now begins to think that the patient has not changed very much at all. Is it just that the treatment team has become better at treating the patient (e.g., noticing the onset of violent thoughts and preventing a major break; anticipating problems in the patient's life, such as an upcoming parole board; and talking to them through these stressors to forestall the violent outbursts)? Maybe the patient has not changed at all, but the treatment team has learned to better control the patient's violence. This is a sobering thought in the treatment of severely ill and violent patients but can apply when treating any patient. Ask yourself for the proof that any improvements in behavior come from the patient, rather than from your ability to manage them. As therapists, we like to think we have aided permanent, beneficial changes in our patients. But there can be some wishful thinking involved.

It is true and not a cultural stereotype that women are less violent than men. Many male prisoners have ASPD, but it is thought that it is less common in women, although we presented some data in the previous chapter that suggested it is more common in women than generally believed. The differences in the two populations generate differences in the therapeutic approach. Or at least it ought to. Thus, we explained in the previous chapter what it means to have an ASPD, its relationship to psychopathy, and the differences of treatability in the two groups.

It is also important to note that there is a wealth of difference (and diagnostic detail) between ASPD and "adult antisocial behavior." We do find that even seasoned clinicians tend to refer to their patients as having ASPD even if the official diagnoses do not include ASPD. Another point we made when talking about severe mental illness was that the onset of ASPD is typically earlier than the onset of the mental illness that brings the patient into treatment. This is certainly true of schizophrenia and bipolar disorder, where onset is typically in the early and late 20s. But it is also often true of other disorders such an anxiety and unipolar depression. So keep in mind that your patient was probably antisocial before she developed mental illness. (Admittedly, though, histories of trauma can go back to infancy.)

More women than men have families to worry about and *that* they worry about. More women than men get into prison because of a co-offender (not necessarily male), and there is often a dominant partner in the decision to plan and undertake the crime. Crime is more of a solitary pursuit for men. In our first table, we mentioned the well-known fact that more women than men are in prison for killing their child. We have seen some women who were in prison for abuse or neglect (often in conjunction with the conviction of a codefendant) resulting in the death of a child. The codefendant may have been an abusive man, and there was often an "unindicted co-conspirator" of methamphetamine. We have followed some ambitious (a year of weekly therapy) accounts of therapists who worked with women with poor parenting skills imprisoned for child abuse and how they can eventually process their guilt at what they did (Franciosi 2001).

But as much as we like case studies and the successes we can recall in our personal experiences, we think that the generalizability of these therapies is uncertain, and these patients may not be shown to have recovery or parenting skills after that. Many women who kill their children have abject psychosis as did Andrea Yates, who drowned her five children in a bathtub while she was briefly alone in her house in 2001. In fact, the nature and quality of the psychosis were a serious matter of debate. The forensic experts argued about the case, one side saying that Ms. Yates' deliberate attempts to avoid detection showed that she was culpable for the crime. She was convicted, but the conviction was later overturned because of an error of the forensic psychiatrist on the prosecutor's side. She was then sent to a mental hospital and as of our publication remains in a low-security hospital. She continues to grieve for her children (Adams 2016). This case was widely reported. (For another account, see History Channel 2020.)

If you take on such cases in a regular prison, you should read the forensic reports carefully. If you work in a forensic setting, that observation is unnecessary because you will probably be inundated with documents. As in the Yates case, you may find mental health experts on both sides as they argue whether delusions were the dominant feature rather than knowledge that the action was morally or legally forbidden. What you say in psychotherapy might depend on your considered and expert decision of whether mental illness was involved in the act, or as in the first case, poor parenting skills and (not mentioned in the first case) substance abuse and neglect. The ethical issues are interesting. Such cases may have a singularity, because the parent may never be in a parenting or child-rearing situation again even if released after a long sentence. So the mission is to assess for guilt but not necessarily create it. The agenda might be to help her come to grips with what she did and get on with her life and family relationships—what is left of them.

Starting Work With a New Patient

As discussed in Chapter 3, entering prison is fraught with problems, but it is gratifying to find that some women put themselves in a drug/abuse/violence/family-free space that gives them a chance to think clearly, perhaps for the first time in their lives. "Possibly the most frequent comment made to probation staff by women in prison is that 'this is the first time I have ever had space to think about myself'" (Carless 2006, p. 153). You have the opportunity to (gently) step into this space, build an understanding of their previous behaviors, and help them plan for the future. Of course, this includes the good (family and children) with the bad (abusive partners and drugs). Also, as previous authors point out, that "space" may fill with flashbacks of past trauma and guilt. Anger at oneself may express itself in self-injury, acting out, aggression toward others, and destruction of personal and prison property.

We have cited some opposing opinions on groups for women (for substance use). However, we do think that in general women "tend to be more disclosing and cooperative [than men] in the group process" (Pollock 1998, p. 135). So don't forget to refer them, and do expect to talk to them about what happens in their groups. Keep in mind, however, that in all reasonable models, such as RNR, for preventing recidivism, advice and direction are required. RNR advocates unload their wrath on nondirective therapies. A correctional culture of "supportive direction" is recommended to reduce recidivism. It would be nice if people learned to be law-abiding on their own just by observing your good character. But that is not enough.

Of Day Residue, Shoes and Ships, and Sealing Wax

> "The time has come," the Walrus said, "To talk of many things: Of shoes—and ships—and sealing-wax— Of cabbages—and kings— And why the sea is boiling hot— And whether pigs have wings."
>
> "The Walrus and the Carpenter," Lewis Carroll (1872)

Freud used the term "day residue" to refer to the pieces of information collected during the day (and sometimes the previous day or two) that are worked on or reassembled in the dreams that follow at night. We appropriate the term to refer to the collection of recent events and things that come to mind before your patient goes to sleep for the night—and earlier than that—that is, what's been happening that they bring to the therapy room. Sometimes it may just be the stuff we have called "Happy Talk" (i.e., things to mention such as the fact that there was a fight on the yard or the hot water was out for a whole day). But pay attention: Often these supposedly random mentions have value. For example, the fight on the yard might be relevant to your patient's gang affiliations or create fears of retaliation. The lack of hot water may lead to a tirade about the deficiencies in prison care.

A frequent, often hot topic, as hot as the hot water is not, is the theme of mistreatment. Of course, this occurs with angry and paranoid men, but it has particular relevance to the women, as we shall see in a moment. Consider (based on Amiga 2019, p. 130): Jenny always claimed the staff were against her and she would assume the worst about their intentions, but as her therapy progressed she began to examine alternative possibilities such as that an officer might have actually been trying to calm her down rather than make her worse, or that a nurse's apparent rudeness to her might have been due to the nurse's personal problems.

The therapist teaches Jenny the skill of mentalization, which is the ability to grasp what is going on in other people's minds. We mentioned mentalization in Chapter 1 as one of several integrative psychotherapies. It was developed initially to treat women with borderline personality disorder. Jenny's therapist also teaches her mentalization "as a means of protection against interpersonal violence" (Amiga 2019, p. 130). That is, misreading the thoughts and intentions of others and reacting impulsively is a source of violent personal responses to staff or interactions with other prisoners. Often, it is seemingly innocent remarks or behaviors that set off these fights. Learning to delay responses and "think first" is another skill, used in anger management, to avoid an instant fight scene. The mention of an "automatic belief" above also brings to mind the automatic beliefs of cognitive-behavioral therapy.

However, the above scenario with Jenny has probably been enacted (without linking it to a theory of psychotherapy) with therapists going back a hundred years, and certainly before mentalization or cognitive therapy was invented. We supportive psychotherapists are happy to claim it also as a supportive intervention. The intervention with Jenny involves two aspects of supportive therapy. First, it reflects our recognition of her psychological defense of projection in which Jenny's own anger at the system and its staff is projected back onto the staff. She hates all of them and she thinks all of them hate her. Second, it reflects an aspect of the criminogenic thinking involving the externalization of blame: "Everybody always mistreats me! It's other people who are responsible for my unhappiness!" And if she really believes that everybody always mistreats her, we can pass the talking stick back to the cognitive therapists who will point out that it is the thinking error called "overgeneralization."

In other words, you can work on Jenny's belief from a number of angles, all with the common goal of helping her to find alternative explanations of the motives and actions of other people. You can point out that her remark is part of a pattern you have seen in which every remark from staff members is malevolent. Or that she seems to find particular fault with the male officers and this relates to the way she was treated by her father and subsequent male relationships. She expects all men to mistreat her, doesn't she? And this may be a fairly reasonable expectation based on her past experience, is it not? And so forth.

This is a way that we use the so-called day residue in psychotherapy, but in particular we use it to process those daily reports of prison maltreatment, which are extremely common. To review, we can think of at least seven angles of discussion, and perhaps you can find more:

- Mentalizing
- Learning to develop alternative explanations of others' behavior rather than jumping to conclusions

- Externalizing blame
- Projecting anger onto others
- Learning to delay angry responses
- Counteracting overgeneralizations about other people
- Relating these discussion points to past experiences with family members

Issues When Giving Advice

While someone is on the inside, the world goes on outside. Mothers remain mothers even in the physical absence of their children, and motherhood is a major topic of conversation. It may be difficult for children to visit their mothers, and institutions will set limits on visitation. Women may be ambivalent about having their children see them as prisoners or may have told the children they were in a hospital or somewhere else. They may have difficulty facing the separation that occurs at the end of a visit. They may have a grandiose recollection of how good their mothering was prior to prison, and unrealistic expectations of what their motherhood will be like when they leave. They may be overinvested in talking about their role of motherhood to the neglect of other needs (Morton 2004, pp. 212 ff.). In some such cases, you may need to choose your constructive criticisms wisely and in a timely manner. Laws (supposedly for the best interests of the child) limit the amount of time that children can spend in custodial agencies. Women are frequently presented with divorce and custody papers and ask for advice. They may feel pressured by outside sources, not always unbiased, including family and attorneys, to "do the right thing" for children (i.e., to relinquish custody). They have often given in to the pressure to "just sign this and I won't bother you again." Usually that means they *will* be bothered by the memory of having done it. They may sign and regret it or regret that they haven't signed it. They may ask you for direct advice, but you may have to give balanced and qualified advice that is appropriate for the situation. They struggle over issues of raising their children vicariously through custodial relatives or social workers. Pregnant patients will also ask for advice about custody. Parents and prospective parents have a lot of questions. Family issues include custody issues and disputes and conflict when a family member has custody. Therapists as mandated abuse reporters are also picking up the phone when the patient reports that they think their child is being abused (e.g., by their custodial ex-husband).

It is easy to be conflicted as to what, if any, advice to give. If you sit back and do absolutely nothing ("I can't give any advice about such an important matter"), what good are you? Are you only supposed to give advice about unimportant matters? Consider you should recommend they get legal advice before signing any legal papers, and social work advice for questions about custody or foster care type issues on the outside. You can also give them some expert opinions and take on a mediator type of role (between the two sides of the question!). Give them the resource materials from the parenting classes. If you would rather not tell them what you think (e.g., "Your ex-husband is a hateful, controlling person. Why would you even think for a minute that he should have your children?"), divide the issues into pros and cons and let them work it out.

In Chapter 4, we discussed the work of Walters (2002) in basing therapy on the observation that many criminals naturally stop ("desist" from) criminality at some point in their lives. This was supported by a study by Sommers et al. (1994) of how 30 women decided to change their criminal lifestyles. These women had a sense of despair that inspired them to question their criminal identity and world view. When you pick up on these feelings in your patients, that is the time to support them in this change.

Case Vignette

A 40-year-old woman emigrated here from Syria with her husband and children 20 years ago. They have been arguing for many years, often ending up with mutual pushing matches. On one occasion he actually did hit her in the face and broke her orbital bone, but in the emergency department she claimed she had "walked into a door." However, the last instance ended up with *her* in jail for domestic violence. As usual, her husband had pushed her, but she hit him with a coffee cup, which broke and resulted in multiple cuts requiring sutures. Although he did not wish to file charges, the DA did, and she got 3 months in jail (why she was not diverted to domestic violence classes is another story). She wants to know what she should do. How should you advise her?

Should you advise her and her husband to go to counseling? You do, but you hear that he rejects that option. He says, "In our country, marriage is a private affair. The police should never have gotten involved." Should she leave him? She points out that 100% of their income comes from his business. What do the children think? They are all grown, and their loyalties are divided. And so on. Should you even give advice? Then what other goals should you seek in your psychotherapy? If you advise her to leave, could he sue you for alienation of affection? Could *she* sue you for the same thing? But is a little pushing back and forth a reason for a divorce? A lot of couples (from different backgrounds) do the same thing. What do you need to know about Middle Eastern culture to properly advise her? What do you need to know about Syrian culture? Does it matter? Did you ask her if she loves him (yes)? Is love the same in all cultures (no)?

Of course, this is the other side of the issue that we introduced in Chapter 3 when we talked about a Latino patient who abuses his wife.

"Get Out and Stay Out!"

Please think about these women and beg the American public to ask for reforms in sentencing guidelines such as length of incarceration for first time nonviolent offenders and drug users. Those women would be much better off in rehabilitation programs than in prison, which gives them no real help and does not prepare them for life on the outside, where they will find themselves without the skills to live. (Our paraphrase of the words of a federal prisoner serving her sentence in 2004, quoted by Talvi 2007, p. 22)

There is a study of women released from prison in Massachusetts that found that "[o]ver the course of the five years,… not all of the women were re-incarcerated, but virtually none of the women moved into a safe and stable lifestyle with independent secure housing and employment" (Norton-Hawk and Sered 2018, p. 261). The women were captives of what the study authors call an "institutional circuit" made up of the numerous facilities that women are sent to from prison (p. 266). Many of them came from families that were already in the institutional circuit and could be described as "convicted at birth." Nearly all the women qualified for mental disability income, but that does not mean that they had severe mental illness as defined in Chapter 8. The authors recommend that women have a single case manager and primary care physician (called a "medical home," although we would add that mental health should be included).

As noted, prisoners doing well on the outside continue to do well on the inside and when released, but even they are touched by the conditions they see afflicting their co-prisoners, and even in a fairly "cushy" minimum security federal facility. So although the words above might have come from Piper Kerman, who was in federal prison in 2004, they actually came from celebrity Martha Stewart, who served 5 months in a federal prison for insider stock trading.

Same Old World

For newly released prisoners, "It's a whole new world" often does not apply. Rather, it is usually the same old world with problems in employment, housing, and family relationships. According to a Bureau of Justice Statistics 9-year study, 84% of, or 5 out of 6, released prisoners were rearrested within 9 years. For women, the rates are lower. The 9-year recidivism is 77%, and more than a third (35%) were rearrested in the first year versus 44% of the men (Alper et al. 2018).

Factors that protect against recidivism include completion of high school education and stable mental health. Lack of stable housing or employment increases recidivism. So do lack of access to drug treatment services and lack of car ownership, as many DUI offenders have lost their licenses and many others cannot afford a car. In fact, car ownership is a better predictor of obtaining or keeping work than is education or previous work experience. Some women have special needs. Women who were sex workers have been found to benefit from a diversion program. More money helps. An increase from $100 in salary up to $500 more is associated with a 24% reduction of recidivism (the findings in this paragraph are reported by Dehart and Lynch 2021). Also noted is that there are 20,000 statutes limiting the employability of people with criminal histories, such as prohibitions against licenses covering 350 occupations.

Attachment theory, discussed in the previous chapter, has also been researched as a factor in improving women's return to the community. A premise of such research is that women do value relationships more than men, and hence the reestablishment of weakened relationships is particularly important to women. A study evaluated women's earlier attachment difficulties and found an expected level of neglect and abuse in their relationships with one or both parents. It resonated closely with our own experience that "despite negative experiences with their parents a number of the women interviewed are either actively seeking to restore their relationships with their mothers and to a lesser extent, fathers, now they are adults…or expressed a wish to do so… a classic sign of ambivalence" (Plechowicz 2009, p. 27). This is an ambivalence both sides of which should be explored in your prerelease counseling in order to prepare for the possible outcomes including rejection and failure to reestablish a relationship. As the saying goes, "Hope for the best but prepare for the worst." Of course, the risks must be explored in linking up with a violent partner or a family system that is involved in criminal activity. More productively, the study showed the relative positivity of relationships with grandparents, a resource that should be explored in advance if possible in your therapy before discharge. The insecure attachment histories of the prisoners made it difficult for them to trust their counselors both before and after release. This is another issue worth exploring, but with the proviso that the trust required in the professional relationship may not reach the level of a good parent or grandparent. It should go a long way to have a "go-to person or confidant" on a crisis response safety plan when they are released. As one woman put it: "Someone I could just pick up the phone and talk to, somebody who could come and see me and talk to me if I've got problems, just talking to them" (p. 32).

There are various model programs to help facilities plan for reentry on both sides of the line between prison or jail and community. The Substance Abuse and Mental Health Services Administration APIC (Assessing, Planning, Identifying, and Coordinating) model is used, but facilities also have available one for mentally ill prisoners call FACT (Forensic Assertive Community Treatment), an elaboration of the well-known Assertive Community Treatment model (Substance Abuse and Mental Health Services Administration 2019). Coordination between programs starts as early as one year before discharge.

The Women's Prison Association has put the issues of transition into a matrix showing the tasks and developments at each stage of reentry (Table 11–5). We will discuss reentry for both men and women in Chapter 14.

Key Points

- While experts differ on the details, it is widely acknowledged that there are major differences between the women in jail and prison and the men. For example, women are much less violent and have a lower rate of antisocial personality disorder (ASPD).

- The differences in therapy needs between men and women are significant.

- It is thought that women have a more relational lifestyle than men, and this expresses itself in a variety of sexual and family-like relationships in prison.

- Feminism is not just one social philosophy but an evolving set of viewpoints about the nature of women in society and the implications for psychotherapy, such as the avoidance of diagnoses that stigmatize women more than men.

- There are still competing theories to explain why and how women become involved with crime. Feminist theories such as the pathways theory of crime posit that victimization is one of the major factors that leads women into criminal activity through running away and turning to survival crimes.

- Therapists incur risks when working in women's prisons, including the tendency to share too much personal information and the issues of allegations of PREA violations.

- The phenomenon of splitting can divide mental health teams from custody and among themselves, even when looking out for it.

- Therapists should not confuse signs of real progress with better management by the mental health team.

- ASPD differs from psychopathy and is a lot different from simple adult antisocial behavior.

TABLE 11–5.   Success in the community

Phase	Livelihood	Residence	Family	Health and sobriety	Criminal justice compliance	Social/civic connections
Survival	Gate money, money from prison accounts, general assistance, soup kitchens, religious charities	Shelter, family or friend, street	Locate or contact family members, arrange to visit or meet	Gate meds, crisis response safety plan (with individual and in multiple places)	Report to court and parole officer, comply with community supervision (e.g., if federal)	Receive peer support
Stabilization	General assistance, workfare employment, school, training program, clothes for interviews	Halfway houses, religious-based homes, home of family or friend	Shared custody, supervised visitation; start legal action to change custody arrangements, get refamiliarized with family	Community health and mental health clinics, public drug treatment programs; linkage to counselor and case manager established prior to discharge	Earn reduced supervision	Join support group or nurturing community Do volunteer work
Self-Sufficiency	Job that pays a living wage and provides benefits	One's own apartment with public subsidy or not	Reunify; receive family counseling, care for others	Regular health visits paid by health insurance; ongoing support: 12 step, therapy, community activities	Satisfy conditions of parole, probation, or community supervision	Help others Contribute to community life
Goal	Adequate money for food, clothing, transportation, and personal and family expenses	Safe, clean, affordable home that accommodates household comfortably	Reunify with children, parents, grandparents, other family; reconcile with family members	Physically and mentally healthy, or receiving affordable quality care including needed prescriptions	Expiration (end of supervision); become law-abiding citizen without return to prison	Form and maintain healthy friendships, network of supportive adults Pursue volunteer or paid opportunities to give back Participate in civic activities (voting if allowed by law)

Source.   Our modifications from Women's Prison Association 2020.

- Therapists can face difficulties in giving specific advice to women who ask for it, and we suggest some ways to make it easier, such as by having them list the pros and cons of a decision or providing research based on expert opinions.

- One of the most important things (in addition to resources) for a woman newly released from prison is to have one case manager and primary care physician or medical "home."

References

Ackerman HP: Therapy With Women in Jail: A Manual for the Mental Health Worker. Plantation, FL, National Institute of Corrections Information Center, 1987

Adams C: Andrea Yates now: hospitalized mom still "grieves for her children" 15 years after drowning them. People, Sept 1, 2016. Available at: https://people.com/crime/andrea-yates-now-she-grieves-for-her-children-15-years-after-drownings. Accessed June 30, 2021.

Agnew R: Foundation for a general strain theory of crime and delinquency. Criminology 30(1):47–88, 1992

Alper M, Durose MR, Markman J: 2018 Update on Prisoner Recidivism: A 9-Year Follow-up Period (2005–2014). NCJ 250975. Washington, DC, Bureau of Justice Statistics, May 2018. Available at: www.bjs.gov/index.cfm?ty=pbdetail&iid=6266. Accessed January 22, 2021.

Amiga S: "'I will never get out of here": therapeutic work with an Imprisonment for Public Protection prisoner caught up in the criminal justice system, in The End of the Sentence: Psychotherapy with Female Offenders. Edited by Stewart PW, Collier C. New York, Routledge, 2019, pp 123–136

Andermann L, Fung KP: Clinical Manual of Cultural Psychiatry, 2nd Edition. Edited by Lim RF. Washington DC, American Psychiatric Publishing, 2015, pp 287–338

Arrigo BA, Shipley SL: Introduction to Forensic Psychology: Issues and Controversies in Crime and Justice, 2nd Edition. San Diego, CA, Elsevier Academic Press, 2005

Baird S: Treating female offenders, in Correctional Psychology: Practice, Programming, and Administration. Edited by Schwartz BK. Kingston, NJ, Civic Research Institute, 2003, pp 9-1–9-22

Black DW, Blum BN (eds): Systems Training for Emotional Predictability and Problem Solving for Borderline Personality Disorder: Implementing STEPPS Around the Globe. New York, Oxford University Press, 2017

Blanchette K, Brown SL: The Assessment and Treatment of Women Offenders: An Integrated Perspective. Chichester, UK, Wiley, 2006

Bloom BE, Covington S: Addressing the mental health needs of women offenders, in Women's Mental Health Issues Across the Criminal Justice System. Edited by Gido RL, Dalley LP. Upper Saddle River, NJ, Pearson Prentice-Hall, 2008, pp 160–176

Bronson J, Berzofsky M: Indicators of Mental Health Problems Reported by Prisoners and Jail Inmates, 2011–2012. NCJ 250612. Washington, DC, Bureau of Justice Statistics, June 2017. Available at: https://bjs.ojp.gov/content/pub/pdf/imhprpji1112.pdf. Accessed June 14, 2019.

Brown LS: Feminist Therapy, 2nd Edition. Washington, DC, American Psychological Association, 2018

Brunell L, The Editors of Encyclopedia Britannica: The fourth wave of feminism. Updated August 27, 2020. Available at: www.britannica.com/topic/feminism/The-fourth-wave-of-feminism. Accessed September 18, 2020.

Burgess RL, Akers RL: A differential association-reinforcement theory of criminal behavior. Soc Probl 14(2):128–147, 1966

Bursick L: A former inmate talks lesbian relationships in prison. Outfront, February 16, 2018. Available at: www.outfrontmagazine.com/inthemag/former-inmate-talks-lesbian-relationships-prison. Accessed May 3, 2020.

Carless S: Constructive work with women offenders: a probation in prison perspective, in Constructive Work With Offenders. Edited by Gorman K, Gregory M, Hayles M, Paton N. Philadelphia, PA, Jessica Kingsley Publishers, 2006, pp 141–157

Carroll L: Through the Looking Glass. London, Macmillan, 1872

Chesney-Lind M, Pasko L: The Female Offender: Girls, Women and Crime, 3rd Edition. Thousand Oaks, CA, Sage, 2012

Collins PH, Bilge S: Intersectionality. Cambridge, UK, Polity Press 2016

Cook KJ: Has criminology awakened from its "androcentric slumber"? Fem Criminol 11(4):334–353, 2016

Covington SS: Beyond Violence: A Prevention Program for Criminal Justice–Involved Women. Workbook. Hoboken, NJ, Wiley, 2013

Covington SS: Beyond Anger and Violence: A Program for Women. Hoboken, NJ, Wiley, 2014

Cuen L: Here's what relationships are really like inside a women's prison. June 16, 2016. Available at: www.mic.com/articles/146276/here-s-what-relationships-are-really-like-inside-a-women-s-prison. Accessed July 3, 2020.

Dehart D, Lynch S: Women's and Girls Pathways Through the Criminal Legal System: Addressing Trauma, Mental Health, and Marginalization. San Diego, CA, Cognella, 2021

Elliott BE, Verdeyen V: Game Over! Strategies for Redirecting Inmate Deception. Alexandria, VA, American Correctional Association, 2002

Elliott DE, Bjelajac P, Fallot RD, et al: Trauma-informed or trauma-denied: Principles and implementation of trauma-informed services for women. J Community Psychol 33(4):461–477, 2005

Franciosi P: The struggle to work with locked-up pain, in Life Within Hidden Worlds: Psychotherapy in Prisons. Edited by Williams Saunders J. New York, Routledge, 2001, pp 69–88

Gross S: Prison psychotherapy (Opinionator). New York Times, December 22, 2015. Available at: https://opinionator.blogs.nytimes.com/2015/12/22/prison-psychotherapy. Accessed November 12, 2019.

Gruber A: The carceral state will not be feminist. The Gender Policy Report. August 4, 2020. Available at: https://genderpolicyreport.umn.edu/the-carceral-state-will-not-be-feminist. Accessed July 9, 2021.

Hagan J, Gillis AR, Simpson J: The class structure of gender and delinquency: Toward a power-control theory of common delinquent behavior. Am J Sociol 90(6):1151–1178, 1985

History Channel: The Defense Rests: This Day in History, March 7, 2002. Updated March 4, 2020. Available at: www.history.com/this-day-in-history/defense-rests-in-andrea-yates-trial. Accessed July 3, 2020.

Hodgins S, Klein S: Severe mental illness: crime, antisocial and aggressive behavior, in The Wiley International Handbook of Correctional Psychology, First Edition. Edited by Polaschek DLL, Day A, Hollin CR. Hoboken, NJ, Wiley, 2019, pp 251–264

Householder AK, Trier-Bieniek A (eds): Feminist Perspectives on Orange Is the New Black: Thirteen Critical Essays. Jefferson, NC, McFarland & Company, 2016

Jeffcote N, Watson T: Working Therapeutically With Women in Secure Mental Health Settings. New York, Jessica Kingsley Publishers, 2010

Jordan J: Relational-Cultural Therapy, 2nd Edition. Washington, DC, American Psychological Association, 2019a

Jordan J: What is relational-cultural therapy? 2019b. Available at: https://wholeperson.com/blog/what-is-relational-cultural-theory. Accessed November 11, 2019.

Kalemi G, Michopoulos I, Efstathiou V, et al: Narcissism but not criminality is associated with aggression in women: a study among female prisoners and women without a criminal record. Front Psychiatry 10(21):21, 2019 30792668

Kerman P: Orange Is the New Black: My Year in a Women's Prison. New York, Random House, 2011

Khilnani S: Gender-specific programming targets females' unique needs. Correctcare 30:7–11, 2016

Lewis CF: Female offenders in correctional settings, in Handbook of Correctional Mental Health, 2nd Edition. Edited by Scott CL. Washington, DC, American Psychiatric Publishing, 2010, pp 477–514

Lewis CF: Gender-specific treatment, in Oxford Textbook of Correctional Psychiatry, Edited by Trestman RL, Appelbaum KL, Metzner JL. New York, Oxford University Press, 2015, pp 293–308

Lombroso C, Ferrero W: The Female Offender. New York, D. Appleton & Company, 1895

Loper AB, Levitt L: Mental health needs of female offenders, in Correctional Mental Health: From Theory to Practice. Edited by Fagan TJ, Ax RK. Los Angeles, CA, Sage, 2011, pp 213–234

MacKenzie DL, Robinson JW, Campbell CS: Long-term incarceration of female offenders: prison adjustment and coping. Crim Justice Behav 16(2):223–238, 1989

Morris MM: Pushout: The Criminalization of Black Girls in Schools. New York, The New Press, 2018

Morton JB: Working With Women Offenders in Correctional Institutions. Lanham, MD, American Correctional Association, 2004

Najavits LM: Seeking Safety: A Treatment Manual for PTSD and Substance Abuse. New York, Guilford, 2002

Netflix Original Series: Orange Is the New Black. Lionsgate Television (created by Kohan J). Santa Monica, CA, Lions Gate Entertainment, 2013–2019

Norton-Hawk M, Sered S: Institutional captives: U.S. women trapped in the medical/correctional/welfare circuit, in Mental Health in Prisons: Critical Perspectives on Treatment and Confinement. Edited by Mills A, Kendall K. Cham, Switzerland, Palgrave Macmillan, 2018, pp 259–284

Piasecki M: Psychiatric care of incarcerated women, in Correctional Psychiatry: Practice Guidelines and Strategies. Edited by Thienhaus OJ, Piasecki M. Kingston, NJ, Civic Research Institute, 2007, pp 15-1–15-23

Plechowicz L: Is attachment theory and the concept of a "secure base" relevant to supporting women during the process of resettlement? Observations from The Women's Turnaround Project, Cardiff. The Griffins Society New Thinking About Women and Criminal Justice Research Paper, February 2009. Available at: www.thegriffinssociety.org/system/files/papers/fullreport/research_paper_2009_02_plechowicz.pdf. Accessed October 23, 2020.

Pollak O: The Criminality of Women. Philadelphia, University of Pennsylvania Press, 1950

Pollock JM: Counseling Women in Prison. Thousand Oaks, CA, Sage, 1998.

Pollock JM: Women's Crimes, Criminology, and Corrections. Long Grove, IL, Waveland Press, 2014

Reichert J, Bostwick L: Post-traumatic Stress Disorder and Victimization Among Female Prisoners in Illinois. Chicago, IL, Illinois Criminal Justice Information Authority, 2010. Available at: www.icjia.state.il.us/assets/pdf/ResearchReports/PTSD_Female_Prisoners_Report_1110.pdf. Accessed September 20, 2020.

Rendell R: A Sleeping Life. Garden City, NY, Doubleday, 1978

Ritchie BE: Compelled to Crime: The Gender Entrapment of Battered Black Women. New York, Routledge, 1996

Schram PJ, Tibbetts SG: Introduction to Criminology: Why Do They Do It? Thousand Oaks, CA, Sage, 2014

Scott T, Brown SL, Wanamaker KA: Female offenders: trends, effective practices, and ongoing debates, in The Wiley International Handbook of Correctional Psychology. Edited by Polaschek DLL, Day A, Hollin CR. Hoboken, NJ, Wiley, 2019, pp 297–314

Seeking Safety: The model Seeking Safety. 2020. Treatment Innovations. Available at: www.treatment-innovations.org/seeking-safety.html. Accessed July 23, 2020.

Short J, Barber M: Troubled inside: vulnerability in prison, in Working Therapeutically With Women in Secure Mental Health Settings. Edited by Jeffcote N, Watson T. New York, Jessica Kingsley Publishers, 2010, pp 57–65

Sommers I, Baskin DR, Fagan J: Getting out of the life: desistance by female street offenders. Deviant Behav 15:125–149, 1994

STEPPS (Systems Training for Emotional Predictability and Problem Solving): 2021. Available at: https://steppsforbpd.com. Accessed January 21, 2021.

Substance Abuse and Mental Health Services Administration: Principles of Community-Based Behavioral Health Services for Justice-involved Individuals: A Research-Based Guide—A Bridge to the Possible. HHS Publication No SMA19-5097. Rockville, MD, Office of Policy, Planning, and Innovation, Substance Abuse and Mental Health Services Administration, Available at: https://store.samhsa.gov/product/Principles-of-Community-based-Behavioral-Health-Services-for-Justice-involved-Individuals-A-Research-based-Guide/SMA19-5097. Accessed October 30, 2020.

Talvi SJA: Women Behind Bars: The Crisis of Women in the U.S. Prison System. Emeryville, CA, Seal Press, 2007

Taylor K, McDonagh D, Blanchette K: Assessing and treating women offenders, in The Practice of Correctional Psychology, Edited by Ternes M, Magaletta PR, Patry MW. Cham, Switzerland, Springer Nature, 2018, pp 103–126

Trestman RL, Ford J, Zhang W, Wiesbrock V: Current and lifetime psychiatric illness among inmates not identified as acutely mentally ill at intake in Connecticut's jails. J Am Acad Psychiatry Law 35(4):490–500, 2007 18086741

Van Voorhis P: On behalf of women offenders: women's place in the science of evidence-based practice. Criminol Public Policy 11(2):111–145, 2012

Walters GD: Maintaining motivation for change using resources available in an offender's natural environment, in Motivating Offenders to Change: A Guide to Enhancing Engagement in Therapy. Edited by McMurran M. Chichester, West Sussex, UK, Wiley, 2002, pp 122–135

Warren JI, Burnette M, South SC, et al: Personality disorders and violence among female prison inmates. J Am Acad Psychiatry Law 30(4):502–509, 2002 12539904

White J: The Galactic Gourmet: A Sector General Novel. New York, Tor Books, 1996

White J: Beginning Operations. New York, Tor Books, 2001

Wikipedia: Intersectionality. 2019a. Available at: https://en.wikipedia.org/wiki/Intersectionality. Accessed November 4, 2019.

Wikipedia: Prison Sexuality. 2019b. Available at: https://en.wikipedia.org/wiki/Prison_sexuality. Accessed November 15, 2019.

Williams J, Scott S, Bressington C: Dangerous journeys: women's pathways into and through secure mental health services, in Working Therapeutically With Women in Secure Mental Health Settings. Edited by Jeffcote N, Watson T. New York, Jessica Kingsley Publishers, 2010, pp 31–43

Williams Saunders J: An introduction to psychotherapy in prisons: issues, themes and dynamics, in Life Within Hidden Worlds: Psychotherapy in Prisons. Edited by Williams Saunders J. New York, Routledge, 2001, pp 1–36

Women's Prison Association: Success in the community: a matrix for thinking about the needs of criminal justice involved women. Plantation, FL, FedCURE, 2020. Available at: www.fedcure.org/information/USSC-Symposium-0708/dir_08/Lerner_WPASuccess_in_the_Community_Matrix.pdf. Accessed January 21, 2021.

12

Deception and Disruption

In this chapter we examine behaviors that include the elements of deception or disruption. We start with deceptive requests, downright malingering, and disruptive and dangerous behaviors that do not seem to serve a rational purpose.

Toxicity Leads to Duplicity

If you are a man, and interested in being or feeling masculine, there are many ways you could express your masculinity. For example, you could join the Navy and try out to become a Navy SEAL (U.S. Navy 2020). Their training is so grueling that only 20% graduate. More Navy SEALs are killed in training than in combat (Locker 2016). They don't make a huge amount of money compared with professional athletes or prestigious Harvard MBAs, but they get by, and with retention bonuses, yearly increases, and military retirement pensions they can live quite well and with the knowledge that they are universally revered as patriotic, self-assured, and supermasculine role models. (By the way, women are eligible for the program.)

Or…you could go to prison.

> Masculinity is arguably the central tenet underpinning and shaping the adult male prison experience. Masculinity can be seen woven into nearly every account [of prison experience] in some manner, through the notions of control, ownership, dominance, or dependence. (Sloan 2016, p. 157)

One theory of understanding masculine behavior is the concept of ideological scripts that are socially rather than genetically inherited basically by finding oneself in one's particular part of society at a certain time. The inherited ideological script is transformed into the script of a male by reinterpreting aspects of his experiences:

> Although the ideological script of macho is inherited within a macho culture by virtue of being a male, the macho male is socialized by his family in specific ways that can be summarized as transformations of feminine affects to masculine ones. Distress is trans-

formed into anger, fear is transformed into excitement, and shame is transformed into masculine pride. The macho ideology expresses contempt for the inferior, feminine affects. (Zaitchik and Mosher 1993, p. 231)

The terminology would be different today, as at the time the authors above wrote this passage there was emphasis on men getting into touch with so-called feminine characteristics. What has not changed much since 1993 is the still-present macho culture in many parts of society and a "souped up" version of it in prisons.

Prisons are an expression of *toxic masculinity*, which is in turn the incarcerated version of *hegemonic masculinity*, a term promulgated by Connell (1987). Hegemonic masculinity is the stereotypical and dominant form of masculinity or being "a real man" in Europe and the United States, which expresses itself in ruthless competition and hierarchical dominance between men, in anger as the only acceptable emotion, refusal to admit weakness or dependency, the devaluation of women and of feminine attributes in men, and homophobia (Kupers 2005). There are many forms of masculinity, and of course not all are toxic. There are loving, gentle, and sensitive fathers, brothers, husbands, and both gay and straight ones. There are sensitive artists and geeks without muscles who bulk up multi-billion-dollar corporations. But many young men are influenced by hegemonic masculinity. They prove themselves by joining gangs, stealing cars, or abusing women. Ironically, they then end up in a homophobic environment where homosexual behavior predominates, and where dominant men demean their male sex objects with femininized insults seemingly to perpetuate the oxymoronic myth that they are homophobic heterosexuals engaging in homosexual behavior. Or, as another one of Michael Connelly's characters tells us (a man who was gay before incarceration), guys do what they need to do in prison and say they love gays and then change their tune when they get out, in a classic case of self-denial (Connelly 2020, p. 156).

Despite the apparent contradictions, many male prisoners who consider themselves heterosexual engage in so-called consensual same-sex activities. The range from low to high security levels in one study was 12% to 30%, respectively (at the U.S. Penitentiary in Lewisburg, Pennsylvania, described in Hensley et al. 2013, p. 241). Rates for women also vary widely, from 32% to over 50% depending on whether the woman is part of a so-called pseudofamily. Other studies found even higher rates. It would seem reasonable that the rates of consensual same-sex activity are higher between women than between men, consistent with theories of male and female sexuality and relationships.

Rates of reported male-on-male rape vary widely, from 1% to 21% (usually reported per incarceration or per year) (Hensley et al. 2013, p. 247). LGBTQ individuals are at higher risk than are heterosexual individuals (for additional comments see below). Placing them in protective custody, however, effectively punishes them. In a regular housing unit, they are at a risk for victimization, something that can be lessened by caring and proactive correctional officers rather than prejudiced or abusive ones; however, prison systems differ in their approaches, which should always consider safety and dignity. A supportive therapist should try to sensitively uncover instances of coercion or victimization and address remedies.

The world outside has a long way to go, but the world inside is way behind the world outside. Inside the prison, means to assert masculinity are much more limited than they are outside, and the repertory of assertions includes violent and defensive maneuvers that are a caricature of those on the outside. It is not possible to have a real, trusting friendship, merely associates or acquaintances. Here is how two prisoners describe it: "Xavier used violence to survive prison by adopting predatory behavior as way to protect himself and not be sexually violated. 'I had two choices—I can be a predator or the prey—and I ain't no faggot.' Tyrone simplified the choice: 'When you go in, you can be an easy mark or do the marking'" (Middlemass 2017, p. 61).

We mentioned in Chapter 4 that the Convict Code, gang membership, and toxic masculinity cause treatment resistance. Prison culture is so damaging and destructive that it threatens to defeat not just psychotherapy but any programming that seeks to change men's attitudes. For example, when interviewed, one prisoner says he would just love to spill his feelings to and get support from a therapist, but he can't allow himself to be seen as weak (Sloan 2016, p. 38).

The Convict Code described by American criminologist Gresham Sykes states (Wikipedia 2020b):

1. Never rat on another prisoner, don't interfere with others' interests, don't be nosy, don't have loose lips, and never put another on the spot.
2. Don't fight with other prisoners, don't lose your head, and do your own time.
3. Don't exploit others. If you make a promise, keep it, don't steal from other prisoners, don't sell favors, and don't go back on bets.
4. Maintain yourself. Don't weaken, whine, or cop out. Be a man and be tough.
5. Don't trust guards or the things they stand for. Don't be a sucker, the officials are wrong, and the prisoners are right.

A central concept in both toxic masculinity and the Convict Code is *respect*. Prisoners hold respect to be sacrosanct. They will demand it. They will fight for it, they will kill others for it, and they will sometimes kill themselves due to lack of it. By showing respect for prisoners, although not for their criminality, we can encourage openness and truth in psychotherapy. Of course, when we think of the amount of fighting and exploitation that goes on in prisons, we must assume the code is more adhered to in the breach than in practice! (Or do you think that all those fights are in *defense* of the Convict Code?)

The Convict Code makes prisoners wary of relating anything that could be considered a confidence. This makes it impossible to talk about sexual relationships, since talking about it results in reporting it, and that is a form of ratting out. There is no panacea for overcoming the toxicity, but we do suggest some things you can do. As mentioned above, show respect, which can lead to more openness. Educate and explain about psychotherapy. "Men who go to prison are neither a population that typically resorts to psychotherapy when faced with emotional or relational difficulties nor are they men who are familiar with the ground rules and uses of psychotherapy. These men must keep their cards close to their chests and must refuse to disclose their needs and pains" (Kupers 2005, p. 720). So don't expect the men to break down emotionally in therapy. Kupers concludes with a few related strategies:

- Honor the resistances (i.e., respect a prisoner's reticence to talk about certain subjects), as he may know better than you why he cannot speak of them.
- Show concern for the prisoner's plight and the reasons that he does not feel able to speak freely; this may improve trust and open up communication.
- Discuss confidentiality and what we already noted must be reported.
- Negotiate what can actually be accomplished given the limits on confidentiality.

- Be willing to do some advocacy, even for matters that do not concern the individual prisoner.
- Show recognition of the things that cause disrespect to the prisoner and empathize with the feelings that accompany perceived disrespect.

Try to recognize their anger and consider asking them if they agree with James Baldwin's remark: "I imagine one of the reasons people cling to their hates so stubbornly is because they sense, once hate is gone, they will be forced to deal with pain" (Brainy Quote 2020).

Prisons create pressure on prisoners to defend themselves and put on public performances of their masculinity. If their manhood is threatened, they will fight over a bag of chips. Failure to do so may result in them being branded as weak and subject to future sexual and physical abuse (Phillips 2001). If you interact with prisoners in public space, as opposed to the private space of your office, keep in mind that your patient may feel obliged to put on a public show for the sake of his "other audience." Even in your office, pay attention to the changes in his behavior with coming and going, and if "the show" can be observed from outside. Of course, all this applies to the much-maligned practice of cell-side psychotherapy. It's not that the neighbors can hear the words. You may be able to ensure privacy at that level by talking softly. It's that the neighbors can hear how loud the show is and pick up the emotional tone of your patient's obligatory masculine displays.

Programs are being run to help prisoners redefine their masculinity in less toxic ways, such as the ManKind project (Karp 2010). A small program in California emphasizes self-acceptance rather than self-improvement and demonstrates its usefulness by reducing recidivism (Sterling 2019). Yet individual psychotherapy is still an important treatment in the toxically masculine environment we have depicted. In a private environment with some level of confidentiality, men express a variety of opinions regarding the effect of supermasculinity on their incarceration. For example:

> If you're not gonna be able to open up, you're never gonna get help. If you have a bunch of idiots tellin' you that you shouldn't open up, you're never gonna get to the root of the problem. Talking about things helps 'cause not everybody's able to have that self talk within themselves. (Morse and Wright 2019, p. 14)

Kupers (2001), in another article, assures us that "Great Gains Are Possible" even in this toxic environment if we recognize a few factors.

- Prisoners are in a position to admit that they made mistakes earlier in their life, and this can lead to a good therapeutic relationship. Our comment: (Does this really apply to all patients, including career criminals?)
- You can agree with most of your patients that domination by race, the rich, and social class, and inequality in education and workforce are central to their problems—that is, they do not bear total responsibility for their situation. But this is not an excuse for future criminality.
- Some men who abuse women have simply not learned the right way to express their feelings and needs.
- Substance abuse can often be looked at historically as a reaction to childhood abuse and the need to develop a "tough guy" persona.

- Even some violent prisoners can appreciate that there is pain and sadness behind their past angry and violent reactions.

Returning to the terminology of masculine-feminine, it is recommended that "intervention should proceed incrementally as the macho man is able to acknowledge and accept gradual doses of his so-called feminine aspects" (Zaitchik and Mosher 1993, p. 237). However, we do *not* describe what we are doing as a way of feminizing men. For one thing, there are numerous traditionally masculine activities that are not toxic, such as fatherhood, brotherhood, mentoring, patriotism, and protecting families and friends and community. For another, there are many supposedly or traditionally feminine activities that are just as amenable to male interpretation, including caring for children, creative arts, writing, and cooking.

The Substance Abuse and Mental Health Services Administration (SAMHSA) recommends that clinicians develop these issues of relationships within masculinity. In Table 12–1 we excerpt some of their advice in a compact form. In addition, there are a number of issues that can be addressed with specific interventions. We will summarize them here briefly, but more can be found in SAMHSA Treatment Improvement Protocol (TIP) 56 (Substance Abuse and Mental Health Services Administration 2013).

- Men who have difficulty accessing or expressing emotions

  - Teach them words to apply to emotions or interior physical experience.
  - Start with more readily available or comfortable emotions.
  - Address fears of losing control when emotional.
  - Develop self-grounding techniques to deal with strong emotions created by others.

- Men who need to learn to nurture and avoid violence

  - Use programs for anger management and violent behavior.
  - Teach affirming, caring, nurturing, forgiving, and patience.
  - Achieve bonding via sports and service activities.

- Men who need to learn to cope with rejection and loss

  - Teach that merely being denied does not demean self-worth.
  - Teach that women have reasons to say "no" and should be respected (both the reason and the woman as a person).
  - Note that rituals, especially in 12-step programs, can help them deal with rejection.

- Men who feel excessive shame (and who disrupt groups for that reason)

  - Assign to individual counseling rather than group.
  - Use psychoeducation about shame.
  - Use strong therapeutic alliance to make it easier for them to talk about shame issues.

- Men with sexual issues

  - Address child sexual abuse issues individually, not in group.
  - Consider possibility of a pattern of disrespect due to abuse in childhood.
  - Address use of substances to counteract shame associated with unresolved sexual identity issues.

TABLE 12–1.   **Advice from Substance Abuse and Mental Health Services Administration about masculinity issues**

Male offenders often are very concerned about the welfare of their children, although socially defined gender roles still put more pressure on women to be good parents.

It is particularly difficult for male offenders to admit that they failed as fathers. Being a good father is not, as some might expect, looked down on in prisons as a sign of "weakness," but rather is generally perceived as an important and valuable activity. However, an individual perhaps feels a conflict between his role as a caring parent and the role of a "hardened criminal" that he presents within the prison.

Many male offenders feel inadequate when dealing with their children and have never had any instruction or assistance in how to be a good father. Their own fathers often were poor role models, and some were (and may still be) incarcerated themselves, even in the same prison.

Few criminal justice clients want their children to wind up in prison. Discussions of parenting and the welfare of one's children often promote strong emotional explorations and counseling opportunities. Offenders are sometimes more receptive to treatment, and more willing to accept prosocial values, when the appeal is made for the sake of their children.

Learning how to relate to people and build relationships (including how to be a friend) takes a lot of work for men. In many cases, this is not a matter of rehabilitation but rather habilitation; some male offenders do not understand how to be a friend, family member, or significant other. They often experience great difficulty even talking about this issue, in spite of the fact that they want to learn these skills.

One of the attractions of gang participation is that it gives members a sense of belonging and a certainty about their relationships with one another that they do not have outside the gang. Thus, treatment should encourage men to form relationships based on a shared experience with recovery.

Relationship training also is important for job success. Learning how to communicate with peers and supervisors is necessary for maintaining employment and advancement.

Source.   Excerpted from Substance Abuse and Mental Health Services Administration 2005, pp. 100–101.

A three-part classification is made by a therapist, Tony Evans, who has practiced in these environments. One type of man has grown up to embrace the doctrines of hegemonic masculinity because of an abusive or absent father. A second type also learned hegemonic masculinity but has had some event in his life that has led him to question it, such as having children, being in a romantic relationship, undergoing substance abuse treatment, or taking classes in prison. A third actually grew up with a father who fostered an individual form of masculinity but has to go along with the group at least when in public (Sommers 2015). If you can find out which kind your patient is, you may be able to reach him faster or more easily.

Finally, one factor that seems to make hypermasculine prisoners more amenable to psychotherapy is *age*. Toch (citing the work of Mosher and Tompkins 1988) tells us that "hypermasculine men who approach maturity may be ripe for psychotherapy" (Toch 1997, p. 176). This is because "in corrections hypermasculinity is a recipe for bankruptcy and no-win stalemates" (p. 177). Prisoners get punished for that hypermasculine acting out, and the isolation of no human contact wears thin as a consequence of their hypermasculine scripts. Still, Toch and others note that programmatic changes are needed (including with corrections staff), not just individual psychotherapy, to change the hypermasculine culture. And another writer holds that programs and institutions will fail to extinguish masculine violence if they focus only on a single factor because the causes are multisystemic (Bowker 1998).

It's Reigning Men

(the gang's all here and why you should care)

Gangs exert a pernicious influence both within and outside prisons. Gangs attract members both in the community and in prison by their ability to provide social purposes and group cohesion. They provide protection among the various racial, ethnic, and political groups. Units and yards are run by "shot-callers." Prisoners have to "put in work" to prove their allegiance to the gang. They can also incur unpayable debts to the gang and seek mental health services because of genuine stress or to get away from gang members. Distinguishing genuine mental illness from malingering can be difficult (Jenesky 2013), and we'll mention this again later. To help gang members without letting them prey on vulnerable mentally ill persons after placement on a mental health unit, you must work with your institution's designated experts on security threat groups. Helping persons to achieve a coercion-free goal of prosocial behaviors in life may mean helping a gang member to leave the gang, or at least envision leaving it. Try to determine if your patient can be motivated to go through your institution's gang exit strategy or think about it. Once back in the community, it is actually easier than one might imagine to slowly drift away from a gang. Suggestions to gang members from a gang intervention project include the following (Young and Gonzalez 2013, p. 3):

- Avoid direct confrontations and making statements about leaving the gang.
- Spend less time with the gang or its individual members.
- Focus instead on your family, school, work, or court responsibilities.
- Practice refusal skills and excuses.
- Notify interventionalist or law enforcement specialist if you have concerns about your safety.

A brief but excellent account provides guidelines that we have summarized and augmented in Table 12–2 (Hanson 2015). It helps to assist gang wannabes to avoid being recruited (actually, this means being coerced) into joining and to prevent gang influences in prison units (i.e., what they call "playing politics," that is, gang politics, on units). The gang leaders or shot-callers recruit vulnerable or susceptible prisoners to do their business in the prison, carry contraband, attack officers, create disturbances, and so forth. In your therapy, consent and confidentiality must be addressed. Except in the normal areas where consent is not required (e.g., institutional disruptions, riot, future crimes), the gang member should participate in the overall strategy to leave, stay, ease his way out, or whatever. Another issue that you can provide input on is whether the prisoner is really a gang member or on the periphery or cusp of joining. If the latter, it will help to avoid having him placed in gang-associated housing, which would cement his participation in the gang and make him a full-fledged member. On the optimistic side, a surprising number of prisoners are able to resist joining gangs or are able to begin the disengagement process while in prison. A major factor that we suggest can be optimized while a gang member is engaged in therapy is the item of disillusionment, which was found in a large gang study project to be a major predictor of gang exit (Pyrooz and Decker 2019, pp. 231, 259).

LGBTQ Issues

The social inequality and injustice that brings many people to prison are especially significant in bringing LGBTQ persons into prison. For example, transgendered persons are subject to discrimination in housing and services and are more likely than other groups to be arrested for poverty-related offenses (Law 2012, p. 202). Violence against transgendered persons in prison is higher than that in the general population, and (although there are many recent changes) they continue to face questions of what is medically necessary in their treatment (Glezer et al. 2013). In the homophobic but toxically masculine environment of the prison, males in the LGBTQ group have additional problems. They have a higher risk of sexual assault than heterosexual men. They may have conflicts about coming out in certain prison environments, and this may depend on the housing arrangements for LGBTQ persons (if they decide to be uncloseted in that particular institution). LGBTQ persons, presumably because of the stresses they encounter, have higher rates of mental illness than the general population. They also have a higher risk of suicide (Balsamo 2016). Also keep in mind that LGBTQ communities in prisons are not monolithic and have different attitudes toward various subgroups, especially bisexual men, who may not be as well accepted as gay men (Hensley et al. 2013).

Lies

In Ruth Rendell's *Not in the Flesh*, Inspector Wexford, packing a little more wisdom than he did when talking about intimate partner violence, muses how it amazes him how their suspects lie constantly and even when successfully confronted about their lying, show no shame or guilt and basically pass it off as nothing unusual (Rendell 2007, p. 241). Lying is a way of life among prisoners and especially within prison culture—especially lying to staff. The behavior that constantly surprises therapists in corrections is not *that* patients lie. It is *how often* they lie, even when they know their lies will be discovered. Talking about another character (who is about to meet his demise, but that's not a spoiler alert, because his fate is given on the back cover), Rendell observes that being basically honest, he resents people who are deceitful with him—a quality that actual liars don't have themselves (Rendell 1981, p. 9). Like any good mystery writer, Rendell has a fascination with bold-faced (or bald-faced, or barefaced) liars. In her mind (and we agree) they seem to have total self-confidence in their ability to get away with it even when somebody is staring them in the face (Rendell 1995, p. 114)! This is a feature supported by research. When confronted about their lies, deceitful patients do not exhibit the normal reactions of guilt or remorse. Many of them have antisocial personalities, a group of people who do lie a lot, but not all criminals have antisocial personalities. As we took pains to show in Chapter 10, they are not necessarily hopeless therapy clients, although it is true that they often do not want or need psychotherapy. Moreover, distinguishing between antisocial personalities and

TABLE 12–2. Combating gang influences

Come on people now, get together: Meet with your department, other departments, custody, the warden, and the security threat group (STG) experts to understand and implement your policies and work as a coordinated group to get people out of gangs.

Explore the patient's history of gang membership: why they joined, what their role is in the gang now; what they're doing now (such as carrying contraband for the shot-callers).

Explore with nongang members: what the politics on the unit are, what the shot-caller wants them to do, how they can resist being recruited.

Describe to them the gang exit strategies of your institution, e.g., moving to protective custody

Acquire consent and confidentiality (as discussed in text)

Thus, with permission and their participations: Get the names and details

Determine coercion: Are they being coerced, is their family being threatened?

What will happen if they leave the gang? Often you will hear that they will be "greenlighted" (e.g., an order will be issued to have them killed) but this is not universally so.

What would happen if they change institutions? (e.g., is this gang's influence local only)?

Do they want to talk to the STG expert? If so, when and how to ensure confidentiality?

What is their mental health need? (e.g., anxiety, depression from their situation)

And some bad news:

Other than trusted members of antigang professionals, do not trust the "ordinary CO," who might be a (past or present) gang member or sympathizer or compromised by gangs.

Be aware of gang manipulations, such as sending supposedly suicidal people to the infirmary to communicate; feigning illnesses to obtain psychotropics, which are then sold; obtaining pill line passes so they can do gang business in the hallways; and so forth.

persons who have performed antisocial acts will often open up therapeutic possibilities for patients who can make changes in their present and future lives.

Detection of deception is difficult and most people (including clinicians) think they are better at it than they really are. There is a vast literature on lie detection, written for both popular and research use. In the former category we have encountered several popular books that present easily accessible advice (e.g., Gorman 2013; Houston et al. 2012, 2015; Walters 2000), although you may find a few inconsistencies depending on the research or experiential basis for them (e.g., the reports of a CIA profiler may differ from those of a corrections researcher). Helpful advice culled from such sources includes the following:

- Recognize the limitations of most "tells" of deception—that they are signs of stress in general and not necessarily lies.
- Get to know the baseline behavior (e.g., gestures and ways of expression) of the person being evaluated when they are not being evaluated for truthfulness.
- Suspect deception when (compared with the baseline) a patient stalls, repeats your question, or seems to show a brief smile when telling you about something (called "duper's delight")—and keep in mind that some criminals just lie for amusement.
- Be suspicious of unnecessary (for a truthful person) "denial flags" such as "To tell the truth," "Honestly," or "Why would I lie?"
- In order to avoid getting a reputation for an easy mark for deception, you can express general skepticism about someone's answers but try not to let them know

which behavioral "tells" led you to conclude they are lying because they may learn from their mistakes and improve their future performance.

- And of course, be suspicious when someone answers your questions irrelevantly. In "The Speckled Band" (1894), when the angry stepfather of his client bursts into 221B Baker Street demanding to know what his daughter is up to, Sherlock Holmes calmly replies "It is a little cold for the time of the year" and to a second demand answers, "I have heard that the crocuses promise well."

A respected researcher who also successfully popularized his findings, Paul Ekman, introduced us to microexpressions, or very brief expressions of emotions. These would generally be more fleeting than the somewhat obvious "duper's delight," and not everyone can catch them, but you can check out your own recognition skills and even take training to improve them (Ekman 2022).

Of course, if you are working with your patients by video or even audio only, something that was greatly increased during the pandemic, it can be more difficult to determine truthfulness based on visual cues or even from observation of the patient's body language. Fortunately, some of the research being reported shows that it is still possible to determine issues of truthfulness even in telephone forensic determinations (Yang et al. 2021). Despite the known disadvantages of telemedicine interviews (and there are many reports about that), one advantage you may find is that it is more difficult for an antisocial patient to intimidate you verbally or physically in the (often inadequate) interview setting. These are factors you may not be consciously aware of but can affect your diagnoses and documentation.

A quick summary of a top researcher's work covers the areas of nonverbal and verbal cues to deception. Indicators of deception include (Vrij 2008, pp. 57, 124):

- Pupil dilation
- High-pitched voice, increased latency of response, longer pause durations, shorter responses
- Vocal tension, discrepant/ambivalent statements, verbal and vocal uncertainty
- Raised chin, lip-pressing
- Word and phrase repetitions, interrupted and repeated words
- Appearing unconcerned or indifferent, seeming planned or lacking spontaneity
- Changes in foot movements
- Lack of facial pleasantness, verbal and vocal involvement, direct orientation, or intensity of facial expression
- Lack of a genuine smile (a genuine smile involves the muscles of both the lips and around the eyes; a social smile is just made with the lips)
- Fewer illustrators (the gestures people use to accompany conversations), hand/finger and leg/foot movements
- Fewer immediate answers, plausible answers

Some findings are counterintuitive and go against popular beliefs. For example, Vrij (2008) says that liars do *not* blink more often or have more grooming gestures than normal.

Counselors who work with difficult patients develop their own personal styles of dealing with lies. You already know about reframing, so here is one called "The Reframe Refrain." (We are not the only writers who use cute titles.) When the patient challenges you with "Are you calling me a liar?" you reply with variations (based on Stanchfield 2001):

- "I'm not calling you a liar. I'm telling you, I don't believe you."
- It is not believable.
- It defies logic.
- It is ludicrous.

Patients also tend to shoot these challenges back at you (also based on Stanchfield 2001):

- "Don't you trust me?" The response is that trust is not all inclusive, but if they want to know if you trust them all-inclusively, you absolutely do not. You can tell them in which areas you trust them and which you do not, and why.
- "Are you accusing me of something?" You can respond that prisoners often behave differently depending on whether staff are present and that you understand that observation may apply to them because you want to understand why that is so. (They are presumably saying things or doing things to please or impress you.)
- And finally, there is the patient who says (or even pouts), "You can't prove it." This is reflected back on him because he is the one who has to *do something* to meet his treatment goals, not you. However, you say that you will make your decisions based on what you believe to be true about him and what you think is in his best interest. This kind of challenge frequently comes up when the therapist has to give input into discipline, or drop a patient from a group because of allegations from others and so forth. We may respond, "This is prison, but it is not a court of law, and we make decisions based on reasonable certainty, so there doesn't have to be video of everything we believe."

Requests for Privileges

Case Vignette

"I can't be locked in my room because I have claustrophobia."

A prisoner tells his therapist that he has severe claustrophobia as shown by the fact that he hears bells ringing when the door is locked in his dormitory room during count. He claims that the dormitory officer is temporarily allowing him to get out of the room so he can walk around during count but that the officer says he needs to get a dispensation from mental health to be able to do this permanently. The therapist is relatively new to the institution and is surprised, if not incredulous, that anyone could make such a request. Why, the next resident might demand to be released entirely from the institution under the provisions of the Americans with Disabilities Act! However, the therapist does take this up with his supervisor, who runs it by the warden, who sends it back down the chain of command with a few choice words like "Are you kidding?" or something that we prefer not to print. But the gist of it is as expected: "This is a correctional institution and counts are integral to its operation, so the prisoner can't be excused from being counted."

Not entirely satisfied with this answer, the therapist does some digging (this being more like a dormitory than a metal barred prison) to see if the resident's initial claim about his dorm officer was accurate, and to his surprise he finds that it was true. Some dorm officers were letting this resident walk around while they counted the others in the room. Possibly, this was because the prisoner had lied to the dorm officers and claimed that there was a dispensation to do so, which he did not have. So the whole thing was based on a circular lie.

The therapist got back to his patient and told him that the dorm officers have considerable discretion in the way they run their dorms, but there is no special dispensation from mental health to be let out of the room during count. However, the therapist also expressed doubt as to whether a person would hallucinate during the stress of being locked in. He noted that according to the patient's history, he had been in the county jail for 3 years prior to transfer to the new facility. What did he do there about his claustrophobia? The therapist also noticed that the prisoner did not mention claustrophobia in his intake, nor was it mentioned in his mental health history.

The therapist offered therapy for the reported claustrophobia and offered to refer the patient to the psychiatrist for treatment of the hallucinations if they were that frequent or disabling. The patient declined the referral and did not raise the issue again. The therapist concluded that the request for a dispensation was a form of malingering, perhaps as a way of walking around the dorm and finding something to steal. Or maybe the prisoner wanted that extra freedom or "perk" during count.

Note that this prisoner's distress was limited to the 30 minutes of count time while he was in a room with his usual three roommates. So this is not a case of long-term social isolation. You might also think that the matter of special privileges for claims of claustrophobia would have been laid to rest by the therapist's interventions with the above patient, but in fact the mental health department continued to receive similar requests for newly arriving prisoners over the next 2 years, suggesting that attempts were still being made to "sound out" the therapists in the hope of getting some accommodation.

More Special Requests

You often field other special requests. We take on a stronger advocacy role for patients with severe mental illness, but not for the typical patient with minor problems. You will hear "Please refer me to medical for my headaches." You will point out that there is a standard procedure to ask for medical care that involves seeing the nurse or filling out a medical request form. Then you will hear "They were supposed to see me, but they never did" or "They never give me anything that helps." Or "I just got this headache, and I can't wait to fill out the form." There is a protocol for immediate referrals for chest pain, shortness of breath, severe dizziness, and so forth. You can check and see when they have an appointment. You can assure your patients that if there is some egregious omission in their care, you will advocate for them in the usual manner or even as an emergency. These interactions are also useful in working at the level of confrontations. Point out that your patient "forgot" to tell you he had just left the nurse's office or that he saw the medical provider yesterday and got a prescription. As for your own credibility, determine how often you feel comfortable stepping out of your office and asking for a nurse to check out a complaint. We have done that, but we also get some feedback implying that we are coddling our patients. Still, we do sometimes go to bat for certain patients when they appear to have a genuine problem that needs immediate attention. If it becomes a pattern, however, we explain it to them—as in "Why am I always asking for a nurse when I see you for therapy?" Their ventilation about poor medical care takes up time and leaves less time to discuss psychological problems. It may be a form of what we called "spinning the therapist" (i.e., patient just finding out if they can get you to run around and do something for them). Explain this to them. (And do not leave them unsupervised in your office if you step out.)

As with other complaints, special requests can present an opportunity to interpret various aspects of your relationship including the transference. "Are you uncomfortable talking about your mental headaches rather than the physical ones?" The answer may elucidate some aspect of the transference. For example, "My mother never helped me when I was a child. As you probably know by now, she neglected me totally except when she needed me to do housework." In keeping with our supportive therapy techniques, we reinforce the positive transference but address the negative transference. You can joke, "Well, I hope I am being a better mother to you than that!" The answer will be "Of course you are!" Reply "But I don't want to be better at dealing just with the bodily cuts and bruises. I want to be better at dealing with the mental cuts and bruises, and when you talk about your headaches instead of the mental problems, we lose time in the session."

Food and Hunger Strikes

The cheapness of prison food has always puzzled us. After all, what are the fundamentals of life? A prisoner loses his job, friends, family, fresh air, soft bed, and of course his freedom. What is left to savor, if at all? The food. But prisons like to save money on food, and in our opinion the consequential costs are greater than any savings. Be your own judge of this, but the average cost of a meal in a Maryland prison is $1.36 (Koola 2020), and many prisons spend less than $3 per person per day (Brown 2021). Food issues are now being looked at as human rights issues (Impact Justice 2020).

An aphorism, often attributed to the Russian writer Dostoevsky, says: "You can judge a society by the way it treats its prisoners." We repurpose this with one small change: "You can judge a society by the way it *feeds* its prisoners." Or "The quality of a society's mercy is directly proportional to the quality of its *prison food*." It is also said that "an Army marches on its stomach," which means that it is a good idea to feed your soldiers well. But prisoners might also be more productive and better behaved if their food and food choices were better, and the negatives about prison food unequally afflict the indigent who cannot afford the commissary. Complaints about food are, to mangle the Freudian term from Chapter 11, like "day residue on a plate" which is more printable than the Army's version of it. Prisoners frequently complain about prison food and request special accommodations or diets. Dietary requests that are not self-selected can normally be directed to medical or religious staff. However, since many such requests actually come from overweight or actually obese patients, we take the opportunity to use these requests to discuss lifestyle issues. For example, you can educate them about the meaning of their BMI (body mass index). Are they concerned that they are gaining weight? Are they exercising rather than buying snacks in the commissary? A good time for lifestyle interventions is when you notice that they have been to a provider for a medical problem such as hypertension. That is a good time to point out that they apparently care about their physical health and ask about their general lifestyle, "Despite being locked up, are you doing all you can to stay healthy both mentally and physically?"

Are complaints about food just complaints about food? (Didn't Freud once say, "Sometimes a hot dog is just a hot dog?") But why complain to you? Perhaps there are some therapeutic opportunities there:

- Complaining may serve the purpose of ventilation and simply to listen and empathize may be therapeutic. This is a good time for those "simple empathic statements" from Chapter 3. "The hot dog was so dried out you could use it as a hammer." "Uh-huh, I understand, that sounds awful."
- Complaining may express a transferential disappointment in you or your failure to fix the food or to fix them. If the complaining is repetitive and angry, it should be explored as a negative transference.
- Complaining may be simply an avoidance of more important issues. "It seems that every time I see you, you complain about the food. What is *really* on your mind?"
- Complaining can be a way of just annoying you and enjoying it. Reflect it back that way: "It seems that your complaining is meant to make me feel as uncomfortable as you feel. If so, why? Let's talk about your expectations here."
- Everyone has memories of food and family, of nurturing families and poisonous families. Talk about these and go where it leads you. "What were meals like when you were growing up? Who nurtured you, not just at mealtime but in other areas of your life?"
- Is food the only thing they enjoy? Do some positive psychology. "What are the good things you can pursue in prison? Read a book, do a journal, exercise. Work on something you can change. Remember the Serenity Prayer?"

Complaining, grieving, and suing constitute a way of life for some prisoners. If you can work with the anger behind these complaints, you can add that to your anger management interventions. "Anger can accomplish a of things, but the anger I see in you is not accomplishing things. Your grievances are always turned around and found unsubstantiated. You have grieved so many officers, it is no wonder that none of them will hold a conversation with you. How has that helped your day-to-day life here?" You may find or create with them a list of things that make them angry. And is the prisoner to blame for anything? And is everything someone else's fault? The serious complainers may also have psychosis and personality disorders (or both) and need a treatment plan. You can work with them supportively by agreeing with the reasonable items (the food is sometimes unpalatable) but (using the therapeutic relationship) explore alternative explanations of why they are the target of the slings and arrows of outrageous fortune.

Hunger strikes, as individual or group political actions, have been recorded since the beginning of historical time (e.g., see the chronology in Wikipedia 2021). There are various definitions of what constitutes a hunger strike, based on the time frame or items or meals missed, but they do involve the concept of voluntary or competent failure to eat or drink. Your institution has its definitions.

Hunger strikers may be politically motivated, advocating for a specific change in treatment, or recognition of a problem. They may be misguided, misinformed, personality disordered, or psychotic. When a prisoner goes on a hunger strike, we assume that he usually wants something. He may have suffered the loss of a previously granted privilege, which creates strong feelings of disrespect which he wants to showcase. He may feel that he is being singled out or unjustly punished. Or he may just be trying to exercise power over a powerless situation and see what he can accomplish, even if he has no real grounds for his demand.

Management of hunger strikers is multidisciplinary. However, psychotherapy for hunger strikers is at its essence supportive. It is an opportunity to provide education and supportive work for people who are profoundly angry, confused or divided in their motives or loyalties, suffering physically, or losing their capacity to think clearly. Research actually shows that in 80% of cases, the reason a person stops a hunger strike is unknown, but that the most productive action appears to be working with custody relating to the conditions of restrictive housing where most hunger strikes occur (Reeves et al. 2017).

Table 12–3 is a checklist to consider when you are seeing a hunger striker. Refer to your department and institutional rules for guidance. Hunger strikes spread as more and more prisoners join for social cohesion to obtain whatever benefits they think can be achieved. Decisions to join or continue with the strike may seem rational or may result from coercion or mental incapacity.

There remain differences of opinion between authorities. To the extent that a hunger strike is a political action, you may want to stay out of the prisoner's value decisions and stick with his psychological needs. Hunger strikes create ethical dilemmas because a clinician is aware of dangerous medical consequences from an intentional act and not by itself a medical condition (Xenakis 2017). One way to approach this is to say, "I respect your right to advocate for your goals, but it is my duty as a mental health professional to prevent suicide and self-injury. If you don't know a lot about the effects of a hunger strike let me give this handout and we can discuss it or I will send you to the medical people."

Group hunger strikers may be highly motivated and unshakable, as, for example, when they banded together to oppose solitary confinement and other practices at the Pelican Bay Prison in California (Wikipedia 2020a). One of the other practices, for example, was "debriefing," an attempt by authorities to obtain the names of gang members, which would contravene the Convict Code. Or some individuals may have a risk-involved goal of being sent to the medical hospital for a while, or of being transferred out of or released from the particular facility they are in. Some hunger strikers have severe or malignant narcissistic personality disorder and go on to a hunger strike after being "narcissistically wounded." For example, one of our patients felt he had been unjustly accused of instigating a fight and, rather than suffer the 30-day sanction, went on a 30-day hunger strike. To complicate matters, he had diabetes and stopped all medications, including his insulin. He was eventually convinced that he had put his life in danger (how imminently no one knew because he refused to have his blood sugar checked).

Most experts state that it is not the therapist's job to argue a hunger striker into eating. Most also advise therapists to avoid trying to argue political or religious points. However, mental health clinicians may be asked to do a competency evaluation in case an institution wants to consider forced feeding. The World Health Organization does not want competent hunger strikers to be force-fed. The American Medical Association does not want physicians to participate in forced feeding. However, practice in the United States has been to force feed some hunger strikers. Competency to do such evaluations is definitely beyond our scope here.

TABLE 12–3.   Checklist for approaching hunger strikers

❏ Who is on the hunger strike: individual, a few, small group, large group?

❏ How far along is the hunger strike? Days, meals, etc.

❏ What exactly is being eaten or refused? Everything? Water? ("Dry hunger strike" cannot last.) Medications? Just solid foods? Does the hunger striker take liquid supplements?

❏ What mental and physical conditions did the hunger striker start with? Does his age create additional risks?

❏ What is his physical status (including laboratory values if you follow these or have these explained to you) and the general assessment according to the medical providers?

❏ What was his baseline weight and body mass index, and how much has he lost so far?

❏ What is the stated purpose of the strike? What change is requested or demanded?

❏ Is the demand within the realm of reason or so outrageous as to question the rationality of the hunger striker? Is this just a public demand, when he is really planning to compromise for something less, such as transfer to another institution?

❏ Does the hunger striker have a history of mental illness, not only psychosis but also a mood or personality disorder?

❏ Can you do a baseline evaluation of his cognitive capacity that can be updated as time passes?

❏ Can you meet individually with the hunger striker? (An individual meeting allows you to assess the element of coercion as in the next item.)

❏ Is the individual being coerced by a group? Does he want to find a "way out" to start eating without deserting his cohorts or being physically injured in retaliation? Can you figure out an exit strategy for him?

❏ What is the effect of the individual's social milieu in prison on the decisions to start the hunger strike?

❏ Who initiated the decision to go on the hunger strike? Is he the leader? If not, is there a defined leader to the hunger strike? Or was the decision made collectively without a defined leader?

❏ Are spouse, parents, children, other family, or significant other aware, involved, agreeable to, or opposed to the decision? Is he in daily contact with them and able to revise his strategy?

❏ What would happen if he stopped the hunger strike now?

❏ Is the individual competent? (A competent hunger striker is one who is making a rational decision based on his personal values and applying knowledge using accepted principles of reasoning and consideration of facts, even though personally you might not come to the same conclusion as he does. It requires some understanding of cause and effect and how his actions may influence the actions of the prison officials. Competency is a forensic concept. It is relevant to the task at hand. There is no such thing as general competency. If you do not have training in assessing competency, you should decline to do such an evaluation. Even if you are "competent to assess competency," you will need to follow your institution's protocol or that of the legal department if the competency is going to be used to make a treatment decision such as forced feeding.)

❏ What knowledge does the hunger striker actually have or lack about the physical process of hunger striking? How long does he think he will live if he does not drink or eat or take his diabetes/blood pressure/asthma/chronic obstructive pulmonary disease/thyroid/antibiotics or other medicines for life-threatening conditions? If he does not know, can you educate him? What does he think will happen if or when he starts to eat again after a planned starvation (e.g., refeeding risks or syndrome)?

We think it is appropriate to evaluate the individual's mental health status. For example, is the hunger striker delusional and in need of treatment? Has the hunger striker stopped psychotropic medication along with stopping food? And so on. If qualified, the therapist can also discuss the hunger striker's medical condition (e.g., that of the diabetic we mentioned above). Urging hunger strikers to keep hydrated may also save them a trip to the emergency room. If consistent with policy, one thing you need to determine is if the hunger striker can designate a substitute decision-maker in case he becomes incompetent (Annas 2017).

Some hunger strikers are obstinate to the point of not caring whether they live or die—to clarify, that is, in the absence of any political agenda. They may have a lot of anger against the institution but have reflected it upon themselves. They sometimes have, or overtly express, a fantasy of how badly people will feel when they die, or of their family suing the institution. As difficult as it is to work with such patients, there is usually some issue to expand upon. Proposing to them that they appear to be deliberately suicidal—for what else could they be by risking death?—often stirs a healthy denial that can be discussed.

You will probably try to identify any mental health conditions that need treatment and discuss these with the patient. According to the previous authors (Reeves et al. 2017), about 45% of hunger strikers have mental conditions, most frequently personality disorders. Some situations (Daines 2007) include:

- Depressed people may wish to die and engage in the hunger strike out of suicidal thinking as a way of opposing the prison system or a wish to attach themselves to a meaningful political cause to defend against hopelessness or meaninglessness.
- Overtly psychotic patients are easy to recognize, but that is less true for people just becoming psychotic or just stopping their medications.
- Eating disorders can interact with food refusals (although we have read that the interaction with anorexia is not common).
- Persons with antisocial personality disorder go on hunger strikes for specific gains, but as with narcissistic personality disorder, the reasons can be vindictive, retributive, or punitive to others.
- Persons with borderline personality may have shifting allegiances to the political reason for the hunger strike but also be depressed and suicidal at times.

You should use your chain of command to discuss and resolve differences of opinion, and you can coordinate with other staff, including corrections regarding behaviors and risks that should be shared. Fortunately, most strikes end long before there is a major decision point such as when there is unconsciousness, severe deterioration of physical health or behavior, or loss of mental competency.

Rule Violations and Illegal Acts

Compromised staff members have been known to put money in a prisoner's accounts, open P.O. boxes to receive their love letters, give them cell phones, aid in their escape, or merely get fired and marry the prisoner afterward. One therapist held his patient's hand during tender moments. He did not last long, not because his colleagues noticed or reported it, but because the other patients got jealous. You may think that some of the stories you hear are apocryphal, but in general they are not. If it is possible for a therapist to be compromised in a certain way, it has probably happened more than once in more than one institution.

Borderline patients may declare, "You're the best therapist I have ever had" or "You're the best person in the world" or "I really love you!" However, manipulations leading to compromise are typically cumulative, insidious, and subtle enough to deceive even therapists. Even the gradual growth of feeling, respect, and enjoyment of the presence of a particular patient can lead to blind spots in judgment, special privileges the patient doesn't objectively deserve, and other deviations from appropriate therapy. Prisoners know that compromise falls on a slippery slope, starting with "ambivalent" comments that might be compliments or have a sexual content—maybe. If there is a doubt, warn them. If there is no doubt, write them up.

Is It a Privilege or a Protection?

It is reasonable that most prisoners want to avoid the isolation, embarrassment, loss of privileges, and punishment of being put in disciplinary housing, which is why you frequently hear comments like "You can't put me in solitary (special housing, restrictive housing, segregation are other names) because I have mental illness…because I will become suicidal even though I am not suicidal now…because I will bang my head and you will have to take me back."

Many prisoners are blatantly honest that they are simply trying to avoid discipline, such as the one who threatens to bang his head. A possible solution is the ability to impose a suicide watch in restrictive housing (e.g., with a suicide vest and a sitter). This does not answer the question of whether restrictive housing should be abolished, but at least it makes it safer.

However, despite the opposition to restrictive housing, single cells (not necessarily with the social isolation) are a "perk" in most institutions and prisoners will try get into single cells for multiple reasons. One of them would simply strip off his clothes and walk around naked any time he was double-celled. Lower bunk requirements are another perk, and the reasons are often medical, but sometimes they are requested due to a claimed fear of heights. Sometimes the complaint is claustrophobia as in "I don't like to be near the ceiling" or a complaint of migraines such as "I can't be near a bright light." It helps to have a history, and a confirmation that a relevant diagnosis was obtained in the initial evaluation.

Malingering Mental Illness

Prisoners frequently malinger symptoms of mental illness. Malingering is defined in DSM-5-TR as "the intentional production of false or grossly exaggerated physical or psychological symptoms, motivated by external incentives such as avoiding military duty, avoiding work, obtaining financial compensation, evading criminal prosecution, or obtaining drugs" (p. 835). This includes feigning the symptoms of a mental illness when one does not have the illness, motivated by an external purpose, known to the prisoner, other than the illness itself (e.g., privileges, therapy, or programming, or some other palpable advantage, often the avoidance of punishment). Malingering is one of those "other conditions that may be a focus of clinical attention." There are two other conditions, factitious disorder and somatization disorder, in which patients report symptoms of illness that, in the opinion of objective observers, they do not have. There is also a disorder of giving approximate answers to simple questions, popularly known as Ganser syndrome, which is currently considered a dissociative disorder, but it has in the past been called a "prison psychosis" because it was thought to be a form of malingering in prisoners. DSM-5-TR lists four situations in which malingering should be "strongly considered" (p. 835), and we will discuss them in Table 12–4 below because each one is subject to criticism (Vitacco and Rogers 2010).

Malingering, therefore, is not an illness, but its effect is to make a diagnosis of illness less certain. Malingering can be conceptualized as an adaptation to being in a difficult situation. It can be viewed as a way that a goal-directed prisoner who is unconcerned about the social value of being honest goes about getting what he wants. However rational it is from the perspective of someone who doesn't care about truth, it still perplexes and annoys people, including therapists, who do care about truth. It wastes resources and takes them away from people who really need services. In criminal proceedings, the stakes are high. Malingering can get a guilty person set free or at least diverted into a mental health system. For sentenced prisoners, it can be used to build a mental health history so that they can receive Social Security disability income when they are released. Malingering can also result in dangerous people and predators being placed in programs where they don't belong and prey on others. One of our sources cited earlier (Jenesky 2013) reprints a detailed set of instructions shared by gang members to malinger mental illness and get prescribed psych meds. The instructions recommend making threats of lawsuits if they don't get medications, and some advice is more subtle: Tell them you've been mentally ill half your life, that you hear voices constantly and "I can't take it anymore. My cellie prevented me from hanging myself" (Jenesky 2013). One of us also had a patient who followed a prepared scenario explaining how his infant son had died. Unfortunately (for him), his corrections officer also had a copy of it. When confronted, the patient just begged to be released from suicide watch so he wouldn't get a write-up.

But the rest of the story is just as concerning. According to the experts (Vitacco and Rogers 2010), when traditional criteria for malingering are used, too many people are classified as malingerers (high false positives), and there is a huge underclassification of those with actual mental disease (low true negatives). Therefore, an overly zealous or overly enthusiastic endorsement of malingering, possibly fueled by countertransference dislike of antisocial patients, may result in not treating genuinely ill patients. For it should not be assumed that habitual liars always malinger in such instances (Gerson and Fox 2006). Finally, for your consideration is the reality that there can be legal liability when diagnosing malingering (Weiss and Dell 2017).

There are many detailed articles, several major books, and training courses on detecting malingered mental illness. We will just cover minimally the psychotherapist's role in having to deal with it, not just in detecting malingering but in working with such patients in the long term (e.g., dealing with the long-term effects their malingering has on the relationship in supportive psychotherapy). So what this section is not is a guide to forensic detection of malingering. Forensic examinations typically require multiple lengthy interviews and a review of all available collateral evidence. A forensic report might cover 50 pages and take weeks to prepare. A final decision about malingering with serious consequences should not be made after a 20-minute interview. Even for certified forensic examiners employed by a court, who usually have a judicial immunity from lawsuit from the malingering defendant, declaring malingering can be difficult, uncertain, and stressful. Researchers know this because it is easy to get test subjects to malinger various symptoms, and then find out what percentage of malingerers are discovered by the researchers! Experts have usually studied the standard guides to malingering such as Rogers and Bender (2018). In addition to the multiple interviews and comprehensive background reviews, experts also use one or more objective tests of malingered psychological symptoms. Such tests have their own criticisms, but they add to the database.

However, although we have just reminded you that as a psychotherapist you are usually not a forensic examiner, it is helpful to be reminded of advice that the experts give to forensic examiners: As summarized by Blau (1998, p. 279), this includes:

- Do not rely on previous attorney reports claiming malingering.
- Do not speculate on motives based on your observations.
- Use an appropriate standardized manner to conduct your examination.
- Base your opinion on the majority of measures.
- Consider and report reasonable alternative explanations.
- Render an expert opinion in a conservative manner.

According to Vitacco and Rogers (2010), the most reliable strategies for detecting malingering are the recognition of rare, quasi-rare, or improbable symptoms, unlikely symptom combinations, reporting of all symptoms being severe or extreme, indiscriminate endorsement of symptoms from almost every diagnostic category, overreporting of both obvious and subtle symptoms, a discrepancy between reported versus observed symptoms, erroneous stereotypes, and spurious patterns of psychopathology (this last strategy only available through testing with the Personality Assessment Inventory; Morey 1991). We shall not discuss each item separately, but we note that these may be sorted into two general strategies of looking for *unlikely presentations* and *amplified presentations* (Walczyk et al. 2018). Eliciting these through interviewing requires skill and ability to work the relevant questions into a seemingly routine interview so that they do not seem unrealistic. For example, you can work in a question asking if your patient has ever thought that automobiles are members of an organized religion (Resnick 2007, p. 228).

We have taken items from several sources and our own experience—"yellow flags" (cautions) on the road to diagnosis—and presented them in Table 12–4. We have also included the criticized items from DSM-5. Most of these apply to malingering psychotic illness—that is, hallucinations or delusions—and are well known in the literature and are discussed in many places, although they may not be items that you have thought of prior to working in a correctional institution. Unfortunately, there does not seem to be a lot of research in determining the validity of complaints of depression (McDermott 2012, p. 869), and as we mentioned in Chapter 9, the popular PHQ-9 tends to overestimate the severity of depression. However, in the correctional setting, you have the opportunity to gather collateral information and not rely solely on self-reports.

We call our cautions yellow flags and not red flags, however, because they are usually not conclusive, except in the few instances of really bizarre and ridiculous behaviors. In fact, there are possible situations that would involve one or more yellow flags

TABLE 12–4. **"Yellow flags" (cautions) on the road to diagnosing mental illness (mostly applicable to severe mental illnesses)**

Objective testing

Patient scores high on one or more objective psychological tests for malingering (exceptions: see Knoll 2015)—people with intellectual disability may be confused by those tests; the tests are good but their specificity is still too low to be definitive (Pierre 2019).

Patient responds affirmatively or gives unusual answers to test questions for malingering such as "Do your visions appear upside down and vibrating?" (Knoll 2015); or says the words of the hallucinations are spelled out as they are spoken (e.g., patient answers "yes" to a series of questions with absurd assertions of that nature because he or she assumes "yes" answers are expected).

Raising possibilities of nonpsychotic hallucinations

Patient reports hallucinations but has no delusions or thought disorder (discussed in Chapter 8): the existence of isolated auditory hallucinations without other symptoms and possible nonpsychotic conditions has been increasingly recognized in the last 10–15 years, especially by European researchers, and is the basis of a "hearing voices" community; some persons report having heard hallucinations since an early age rather than the typical age at onset of schizophrenia.

Presentations that are rare or quasi-rare, report amplified symptoms, or are not credible

Patient reports primarily visual, tactile, or olfactory hallucinations (many persons with schizophrenia do have some visual hallucinations, but these are usually concurrent with auditory ones); or patient reports all three at the same time (not a typical presentation).

Patient reports multiple severe symptoms from different diseases (psychosis, PTSD, bulimia, all at the same time).

Patient reports symptoms that are always severe and unbearable (Resnick and Knoll 2018).

Patient is reciting symptoms verbatim that are found in a textbook list such as those of DSM-5.

Several patients present with detailed complaints that are exactly the same.

Patient reports seeing little persons or even little green men (micropsia is rare; medical causes and hallucinogenic drugs are typically the source of definite bright and colored hallucinations).

Patient reports seeing shadows (see previous item); we have encountered this item frequently in persons with histories of methamphetamine use, but these do not seem to suggest psychosis but a persistent perceptual illusion.

Patient reports hallucinations all the time (usually hallucinations are intermittent and occur in quiet situations such as nighttime).

Patient reports very sudden onset of major symptoms without a premorbid period in the absence of known stressors (not typical of psychosis, and this condition is not schizophrenia, which requires a premorbid period); there is a condition of brief reactive psychosis that should be distinguished clinically from this; exception (Knoll 2015): persons placed in solitary confinement may develop serious symptoms fairly rapidly.

Patient does not have the negative symptoms usually associated with schizophrenia.

Patient reports depression but has silly or happy delusions (patients with psychotic depression usually have mood-congruent delusions).

Patient reports hallucinations but cannot hear what is said or it is just mumbling or just hears noise (but exceptions are now being recognized [Pierre 2019] in persons with hallucinations who are not psychotic, as we discussed above).

Patient is evasive in answers or says he doesn't know simple things.

Patient says he doesn't remember things and then tells you what it is he does not remember in detail.

TABLE 12–4.   **"Yellow flags" (cautions) on the road to diagnosing mental illness (mostly applicable to severe mental illnesses)** *(continued)*

Presentations that are rare or quasi-rare, report amplified symptoms, or are not credible *(continued)*

Patient reports solely hearing music (musical hallucinations are rare).

Patient reports isolated command hallucinations but nothing else (Knoll 2015) (usually patients have a mixture of hallucinations).

Patient says he has no control over the hallucinations; patient reports "nothing" when asked how he copes with the hallucinations (people normally develop coping mechanisms such as listening to music, talking, and exercising).

Patient behaves normally socially or when out of the interview (e.g., he says he is hallucinating but does not show any odd behaviors such as talking to the walls at night).

Patient reports having heard voices for years but says he has never told anybody about it (exception: patient who was in another prison and states it was too stigmatizing to admit his illness; such cases need a more detailed history, including, for example, questions about the symptoms and onset).

Patient reports having heard voices "constantly since childhood" but has a normal history otherwise. (Childhood psychosis is rare and serious, and—with some exceptions as discussed above—hallucinations are not heard constantly for years with no consequences on function; as above, an exception might be nonpsychotic hallucinations.)

Patient reports having been treated previously, but records do not show treatment.

Patient reports having been treated but refuses to sign a release for records. (*Note:* records can still be obtained under a HIPAA exception for correctional institutions).

Patient reports having been treated, but a records request to that institution comes back as "no records found" (exceptions: yes, this happens, but is a caution, especially if from more than one place).

Symptoms are bizarre and definitely not typical of the purported illness or any known illness ("There's a 50-foot-tall angel sitting on your shoulder, Doc" or "That crazy chicken is talking to me all the time"—El Pollo Loco is a restaurant chain).

Patient reports hallucinations (as of the chicken) that are not people or are robotic; patient says he never hears the same voice twice, or only hears women or children; patient states the hallucinatory voice changes gender midsentence or addresses patient as "Mr." or "Mrs" (Resnick and Knoll 2018).

Patient reports black-and-white hallucinations (they are usually in color).

Patient reports hallucinations as if they are real people in all modalities (seen, heard, felt, smelled).

Other suspicious presentations (not so much the symptoms but the patient's behavior)

Patient accuses you of implying that he is faking a symptom—genuinely ill patients rarely do so (Resnick and Knoll 2018).

The gain is readily admitted by the patient, often in a jocular matter ("Oh yes, I know it would be good to get out of the discipline, but I really am ill").

Patient asks it as a special favor for him ("Doc, can't you just do me this favor; I really need it").

Patient admits to having fooled others in the past with similar claims.

Patient admits (to others) that he is deceiving you in this instance, playing you for a fool, etc.

Patient has a recorded history of pathological lying or known malingering.

Patient reports instant response to a low dose of medication (it can take weeks for resolution of psychosis). (Most patients with hallucinations report a partial response to medication; however we note that if the goal is medication [usually for sleep], the patient frequently writes a new request a few days later and says the medicine "does nothing" for him or is absolutely worthless.)

TABLE 12–4. **"Yellow flags" (cautions) on the road to diagnosing mental illness (mostly applicable to severe mental illnesses)** *(continued)*

Other suspicious presentations (not so much the symptoms but the patient's behavior) *(continued)*

Patient is a predator, and the mental illness diagnosis would gain admission to a program with potential victims (the history of being a predator should be made exclusionary).

Patient slowly repeats your questions (to give herself time to figure out answers).

There has been a dynamic change in external motivators (e.g., a new mental health program or unit just opened up, and the patient has expressed desire to get into the program or unit, or was just disciplined and the mental illness would exempt or mitigate discipline; the most common so-called malingering behavior in prison is probably the feigning of suicidal intent to avoid or delay punishment).

The hallucinations resolve as soon as the patient receives transfer into the program desired.

Patient does appear to have a psychotic disorder (e.g., has a well-established history) but is presenting in an unusual way or with an obvious motive (e.g., to be hospitalized).

Not so reliable? (the first four items from the DSM-5 discussion of malingering)

History of antisocial personality disorder (ASPD); typically the patient has a long criminal history and ASPD but no history of mental illness—until now; this DSM-5 comment was meant to apply to community populations, but ASPD predominates in prison, so that characteristic is too common to be useful; Vitacco and Rogers (2010) also think it creates distrust and hatefulness in the countertransference.

Discrepancy between observations of disability and reported symptoms; although there is some objective evidence that this is a good predictor of malingering (see Singh et al. 2007), Vitacco and Rogers (2010) say this is too vague to be useful.

Occurrence in medicolegal context; another DSM-5 comment, but basically all prisoners are in a medicolegal context, so this is not helpful.

Lack of cooperation in the diagnostic evaluation and noncompliance with the treatment program: Also criticized by Vitacco and Rogers (2010). Our comments: We agree that many seriously ill patients are uncooperative, inconsistent, and unreliable, Therefore, lack of cooperation per se is probably not enough to raise a caution. However, the way in which the patient fails to cooperate is often quite helpful (e.g., if the patient is clearly manipulating the interview, bullying or threatening the interviewer into making the diagnosis quickly). In other words, note behaviors other than the lack of cooperation itself that suggest deliberate attempts to get a diagnosis over and done with quickly.

And: No mental health history. See text.

And finally:

Don't overreact to the presence of *static* external motivators to malinger. Of course, the presence of an external motivator is a necessary condition for malingering as defined here, as opposed to malingering for the sake of the illness itself, which is diagnostic of factitious disorder. But in prisons this is extremely common, and often there is an external motivator of which the evaluator is unaware.

Source Correia 2009; Knoll 2015; Pierre 2019; Resnick and Knoll 2018; Rogers and Bender 2018; Vitacco and Rogers 2010.

but in which the patients still have psychotic illness. However, the patients may not have active symptoms at the time of the interview. Patients with known mental health histories, for example, may say that they are hearing hallucinations at times when they are not, perhaps in order to be moved to the infirmary or a psychiatric hospital, or to receive a higher dose of a sedating medicine.

But what about the *lack of* a history of mental illness. Is this a yellow flag or not? Prison engenders depression, insomnia, anxiety, and sometimes psychosis, although (contrary to some popular conceptions) it does not seem able to create schizophrenia or bipolar disorder. However, it is certainly possible that a prisoner could experience the onset of these illnesses while in prison. Segregation units may create disorders that are stressor-related, but it does not appear that the nontraumatic components of incarceration create PTSD. In addition to the sources we quoted in Chapter 8, a study by Zamble and Porporino (1988) followed prisoners in Ontario, Canada, and concluded that contrary to popular conceptions, the prisoners did not deteriorate psychologically (Maier and Fulton 1998, p. 160). However, prison puts prisoners in a psychological deep freeze and arrests psychological development by continuing immature modes of coping that can lead to criminal activity later in life.

Along with yellow caution flags there are also green "clear to proceed" flags. Like yellow flags, green flags are not conclusive indicators that a person has real illness, but somewhat more favorable indicators that the diagnosis is more likely. One instance is when the person involved is intellectually disabled, for then his descriptions of symptoms may suggest malingering when it is really his way of describing the world (see Table 12–5).

How should psychotherapists act if they are fairly convinced that a patient is malingering mental illness? First, do as thorough an evaluation as you can, given the circumstances. Try to refuse to do any forensic type of determination that is outside your professional scope or that should ethically be done by a non-treating clinician. Your job is to diagnose and treat. Refer for objective testing, which is often quite simple and inexpensive. As recommended by experts, give patients an opportunity re-interview and retest and tell them that "test data were not valid, and we recommend you take it again." Refer to another clinician for an additional opinion, and go to a committee or treatment planners for a group opinion.

At some time, you will probably have to document your encounter. Some clinicians will still use the term "malingering" outright, but practically we think this is unwise. The pendulum of "political correctness" seems to have swung strongly in the other direction. Some experts even recommend you avoid the disparaging use of the term "secondary gain." For one thing, from what we have been saying, there is a likelihood that you are wrongfully labeling an ill person as a malingerer. In addition, there will often be a difference of opinion when a patient who is a good malingerer is malingering. Some other clinicians, often a clinician in an outside hospital to which you have sent him, will give him a "genuine" diagnosis. For example, we sent a mute antisocial patient to the psychiatric hospital, and although he gave out no useful information while he was there, he came back with a diagnosis of paranoid schizophrenia. From another 2 years of working with that patient, we knew that diagnosis to be inaccurate.

Of course, if malingering were just a behavior to be diagnosed, it wouldn't matter, but it is an attempt to get something. If the "something" is psychotropic medication, the prescriber will ultimately deal with it, so it is not a therapy issue per se, although you may have to make the referral. We suggest you do that in any reasonable situation. In those circumstances, the prescriber can read about what you found and conduct a separate, confirming interview for the purpose of prescribing medication. This may sound unkind to the prescriber, but we view this as a competency issue. If you are not a prescriber, you are certainly competent to refer to a prescriber for potential use of medication, but only a prescriber can consider the risks and benefits of prescribing or not

---

TABLE 12–5.   **"Green flags," or factors that may suggest that symptoms are real**

Has history of extensive psychiatric treatment

Has history of traumatic brain injury

Has intellectual disability

Has no incentive to malinger

Is referred by someone else

Has high number of objective suicide risk factors

Does well or benefits from being on a mental health unit

Shows improvement on psychiatric medications.[a]

---

[a]We are not sure of this one. It is true that many persons who malinger claim that "nothing works" and escalate their doses of psychiatric medicine. On the other hand, we have seen patients who cease their claims of hallucinations a few days after they start a low dose of medicine (i.e., under circumstances in which it is unlikely that a person with hallucinations would report being completely better).
Source.   Knoll 2015.

to a person who might be malingering. We do have one (nonprescribing) colleague, however, who gives potential malingerers the (factually correct) litany of possible side effects, including diabetic ketoacidosis, extrapyramidal syndrome (twisted up muscles), neuroleptic malignant syndrome (sometimes fatal high temperature and muscular rigidity), and tardive dyskinesia (wormlike movements that can be permanent).

In our nonforensic roles of documenting possible malingering, we descriptively report the findings with the conclusions about rare, unusual, or bizarre presentations. We point out that certain items (e.g., a report of lifetime unvarying hallucinations) are not found in schizophrenia or whatever other illnesses are being considered. We report test data objectively with the standard explanations of the scores. We tell patients that objectively their presentation or test data are unusual but do not take the further step of telling them we believe they are lying outright. We do discuss the importance of telling their therapist the truth, even if we mention that in a general way rather than making a specific accusation. We tell supposed stories of other patients who seemingly malingered to get into programs they did not need. We remind patients that they are functioning rather well despite their complaints of bizarre hallucinations and that they do not need the special privileges that they asked for. As we now do for all patients with mental illness, we often "normalize" the hallucinations and do not automatically refer for medication unless there are dangerous commands and delusions that create risk. Of course, this takes judgment. The "benignly hallucinating" patient could get worse, either because of genuine illness or spite at not getting the medicine he wanted.

Some persons will malinger their way into programs that they do not need. Predatory and antisocial behaviors should be exclusionary for certain programs, anyway. Predators will malinger mental illness to be admitted to mental health units or the infirmary. But the reactions of others who feel threatened by them provide relevant data. Why do they feel threatened? If it is just because the group member is a little manic and loud, then this can be explained to the group, and they can be asked to show a little tolerance to the mental illness that was the hallmark of admission to their group anyway.

Malingering suicidal behavior is, of course, not forgettable since 1) there is always the possibility that the so-called malingerer is genuinely suicidal; 2) even malingerers, especially those with borderline personality disorder, may escalate their behaviors if they don't get the response they want initially; 3) persons with non-lethal "parasuicidal" behaviors can become suicidal; and 4) situations change, even as a real wolf once showed up to the boy who cried "Wolf!" We don't have all the answers here, but there was more information in Chapter 6. Issues also arise when dealing with disruptive patients, as we'll discuss later in this chapter.

We think you can tell by now that, in general, our advice is that when there is doubt, the patient should get the benefit of it, since it would be a harm to withhold needed treatment from a genuinely ill or suicidal person. As mentioned, we have to recognize that countertransference feelings can play a role. We may find it hard or simply galling to "allow" an antisocial criminal to get the better of us, even if it is just for a little sleeping pill, but every time we withhold treatment from somebody, we could be withholding treatment from someone who needs it.

Case Vignette

Mr. Barton, a 19-year-old man, enters the institution with a 3-year sentence for assault. He has been homeless and has no family support and no prior history. He is a small and vulnerable person and is placed by mutual agreement in protective custody. About a month after admission, he is found with a sheet wrapped around his neck. He says the voices tell him to kill himself. He is sent to the infirmary and the mental health doctors place him on an antidepressant and an antipsychotic medication. He reports resolution of suicidal ideation and is released back to PC. Two days later, he is back again after putting a sheet around his neck again.

During the next 2 years, Mr. Barton is sent to the infirmary and also hospitalized many times after the same "sheet around the neck" scenario. No one really believes he is suicidal, and soon no one really believes he hears voices. But with a year to go, Mr. Barton tells his therapist. "I don't really hear voices, you know. When I got here, this older guy in the cell next door told me that it would help my case to be suicidal a lot, so I tried it. It got me to the hospital a few times, and it was sort of fun. But now they are saying that I have to go into mental health housing when I get out, and I don't want that. So I am going to stop being suicidal."

The therapist was not terribly surprised at this revelation but brought it up to the mental health team. Someone actually decided to re-read the initial mental health evaluation that was done the day Mr. Barton was admitted. In it, Mr. Barton said, "I hear voices most days, and they tell me to kill myself, but I don't listen to them." Somehow or other, the initial assessment had been forgotten.

The team concluded that Mr. Barton really did have a psychotic illness and that his story about the helpful neighbor may not have been entirely truthful. What had changed, however, was his agenda, from getting attention by being suicidal to being left alone when he left prison. It was theorized that Mr. Barton was developing a psychotic illness at the time of his admission to prison but was probably exacerbating his symptoms for some type of gain. His medicines were reduced but not stopped during his remaining year, and he was transferred to a mental health clinic with the diagnosis of schizophrenia.

Did the team make any mistakes in their treatment of Mr. Barton? We think so. It was apparent that no one ever really confronted Mr. Barton about his somewhat overplayed suicide attempts. Mr. Barton was not and never had been an antisocial, litigious criminal with a "send me out" strategy as frequently occurs when outside psychiatric hospitals are used. He was a young, vulnerable, impressionable, but streetwise man who was doing what he could to make his prison stay more palatable. There was no real "downside" to confronting him about his behaviors and finding other ways to make his stay more comfortable. Education about his mental illness may have overcome his fear of being sent to a mental health clinic. Persons with mental illness can overrepresent their wellness as well as their illnesses. The availability and positive benefits of community services to avoid homelessness could have been addressed.

Never really knowing the ultimate truth, and certainly not being able to predict the future, we have to act on suicidal threats. However, in the long term, psychotherapy needs to address the issues outside of the suicide cell—that is, when the suicidal crises have been averted. There is plenty of opportunity for supportive work even if it involves confronting people who overuse mental health services by stating they are suicidal. It will be predictable that an antisocial prisoner will bristle and threaten at the mere suggestion that he is not really suicidal when he says he is. But others will be more amenable to discussion.

Violent, Aggressive, and/or Disruptive Prisoners

There are many violent and aggressive people in prison, and they often stir up spirited thinking about whether their behavior is "mad" (due to mental illness) or "bad" (due to deliberate maleficence or wish to harm and disrupt the prison). And when suicidal behavior is noted, staff may add the category of "sad" to denote suicidal thinking that arises from clinical depression. Persons within this group are often considered to have psychopathy or severe single or mixed personality disorders. In editions prior to DSM-5 with two axes of diagnosis, clinicians often debated whether a patient was an "Axis I or an Axis II." This distinction ended with a better understanding of the personality disorders that we have discussed already. However, our goal here is to provide guidance for psychotherapists in dealing with these difficult patients.

In Chapter 10, we mentioned that violence is distinguished as either *impulsive* or *premeditated* violence, because the difference may point the way toward treatment. The "good" thing about impulsive violence, at least according to the experts, is that it is often treatable with medication, even if the violence is performed by an antisocial or psychopathic person (Felthous 2013). Anger is kind of a chemical thing, and people do have some chemicals in them, and treatment may be as simple as an antidepressant and does not necessarily require heavy-duty medication regimens.

Having dispatched some of these violent patients to the prescribers, we are still left with people who are deliberately violent in some manner or other. This includes many patients who seem impulsive but can "turn on" and "turn off" their anger and violence. When there is disruptive behavior, the poor judgment found in severe mental illnesses must be considered, since severely mentally ill persons have more episodes of physical and verbal assault. Suicidal and self-injurious behaviors, while technically an assault on oneself rather than others, have been viewed as part of a continuum of disruptive behaviors (Helfand et al. 2010). Those authors provide evidence that both types of behaviors are example of impulse control disorders and hence can be managed with similar methods. However, for various reasons, including the focus on suicidal behaviors as a problem that requires a discrete set of responses to prevent self-injury, we addressed suicide as well as the personality disorders in separate chapters. For example, someone who floods their cell may end up in discipline or restraint but does not undergo a series of suicide risk evaluations.

When something can be done about violent behavior, it usually requires a multidisciplinary commitment. Some experts on prison violence summarize the best strategies as follows (no surprises, but notice that it is important to collaborate with custody staff) (Edgar et al. 2011, pp. 208–209):

- Focus on individuals' interests, values, and needs.
- Prevent prisoners from using the usual insults, threats, and accusations as their tactics.
- Improve communication between the prisoners and custody.
- Try to create win-win outcomes.
- Try to create a culture that favors negotiation.

Another disruptive behavior is exhibitionism. This can have several causes:

- Antisocial or deliberate hostility or revenge. Such behaviors call for appropriate management, since many institutions have reached the point of laughing them off, which only increases their frequency. Example: the institution placed a sitter next to the patient with a stack of "General Incident Reports." Every time the person exhibited himself, the sitter completed a report and held it up to him. The behavior stopped after three reports.
- Cognitive distortions that the behavior is sexually arousing to the viewer. These distortions may occur, for example, in some intellectually disadvantaged or poorly educated individuals. Such persons can be educated that their cognitions are off base; RNs see naked people all the time and are not impressed but might think that the perpetrator is just ignorant.
- True sex offending. Address with group therapy and a treatment program such as the Good Lives Model (see Chapter 13).

Consider this description of a prisoner from a Bureau of Prisons Management Plan (paraphrased from Nicholas and Bryant 2013, p. 197): The person has had multiple incidents of extremely disruptive and dangerous behaviors. He has also made suicidal threats in order to get out of the Special Housing Unit to be placed on a suicide watch. Other than his suicidal threats, he does not have a mental health history and specifically denied such a history in several interviews done since his admission to the facility. Once placed in a suicide watch cell, he was seen to be smiling, laughing, and joking with staff. Moreover, he told staff directly that he was never suicidal and made those threats to be removed from the Special Housing Unit.

This prisoner would seem to be manipulating or malingering. Helfand et al. (2010) and many others also warn us that manipulative suicide attempts can often turn into genuinely dangerous ones. However, there are many prisoners who engage in disruptive behavior that seems to have no obvious purpose and worsens their situation in the prison. Toch and Adams have worked with such persons and called them "disturbed disruptive" (Toch 2004; Toch and Adams 2002). They advise us not to be blinded to preconceptions or attachments created by the previous diagnostic labels that have been attached to such patients. Maladaptive behavior, unlike malingering, does not serve external goals such as avoiding punishment or getting a cell change. It is "pathologically tinged," meaning it does have some aspects of psychopathology, but it does not fall within the conventional parameters we used to described maladaptive behavior (Toch and Adams 2002, p. 5).

Case Vignette

Mr. Able is a 50-year-old man sentenced for assault. He was a heavy drinker and went through a prolonged detoxification upon arrival. Even after that, with the usual vitamins to prevent neurological impairment, he was delusional about nurses trying to kill him, and he also had some mild cognitive impairments. Because of his delusions, thought to be due to a persistent alcoholic disorder, he takes low dose of an antipsychotic medication. Lately, he has been slightly depressed about family issues, and the psychiatrist has prescribed an antidepressant. However, Mr. Able has never (in life or in jail) been suicidal or self-harming.

One day, however, things change. Mr. Able asks to see a therapist. He tells the therapist that there has been a death in the family. He says he is more depressed than usual. The therapist asks him if he is suicidal. He replies, "If I had a razor I would cut myself, but I don't have a razor right now." Considering that it is fairly easy to get a razor, the therapist puts Mr. Able on a suicide watch and asks the psychiatrist to see him to consider an increase in the antidepressant. The psychiatrist asks the suicide question and Mr. Able says angrily: "I am not suicidal. I never said I was. Dr. Jones misunderstood me. You can't do this to me. I am not crazy! I am not an animal! I want to go back to my unit and be with my friends and make telephone calls."

What's going on here? Is Mr. Able playing the "spin the therapist" game? The staff decided that Mr. Able's impaired cognition and judgment, combined with his paranoia, had indeed created a misunderstanding as his "hypothetical" about suicide was his way of explaining his depression, but that he never intended to hurt himself. If he had been given a razor at that moment, he would not have hurt himself. He was just making a point, somewhat ineptly. Clearly, he did not intend to be locked up, but he did seek out someone to whom he could ventilate. The solution? He was kept overnight on a suicide watch, after a stern talking to that he had to take responsibility for the suicide watch and that people were genuinely worried about him because he was a human being and not an animal. He was not pleased, but he finally calmed down. He was allowed to make his phone calls under supervision. His medications for depression and paranoia were increased. He was followed up as an outpatient the next day and he handled the bereavement well.

We think this case would be one of Toch and Adam's "pathologically tinged" examples. They say it is understandable to think that disruptive individuals are acting rationally, but in reality it is just not so. Such behaviors are purposive, from a perspective that incorporates the person's distorted world view, but their maladaptation shows ineffective coping. Such individuals can change and develop better coping skills. Based on a large study in the New York prison system, Toch and Adams (2002) sorted maladaptive behaviors into five types with many subtypes:

- Gratifying impulses—rule-violating conduct, predatory aggression, frustration to aggression, stress to aggression, Russian roulette (taking unreasonable risks and not caring about the outcome), "jailing" (accumulating illicit amenities), and games that turn sour
- Enhancing esteem—advertising toughness, conforming to a violent peer group, gladiating (displaying the violence), preempting unpopularity (self-fulfilling cre-

ation of rejection and hostility from the peer group), countering aspersions (reacting violently when offended or slighted), and standing fast
- Pursuing autonomy—dependence, conditional dependence (alternating between
dependence and rebellion), defying authority, and rejecting constraints
- Seeking refuge—searching for sanctuary (protective settings), catch-22 (seeking
and rejecting protective settings at the same time), sheep's clothing (once in a safe
setting, becoming assertive or predatory), bluff called (asking for protection after
an act of defiance), turned tables (similar, asking for help once their acting out back-
fires), earned rejection (seeking sanctuary to get away from others ostracizing him),
and stress avoidance
- Maintaining sanity—escape from reality, flight-fight, paranoid aggression, tinged
rebelliousness, cryptic outbursts (unmotivated attacks for reasons the clinicians
cannot access), and oscillating (between normal and disturbed behaviors)

It's uncanny how many of our difficult patients fit into the above categories, but what
to do about them? Many incidents in the first category have identified stressors. According to Helfand et al. (2010), stressful relationships with officers are a major cause
of misbehavior. Others have suffered negative events such as "Dear John" letters, legal
setbacks, and other losses, such as placements within the prison. Some moves are
done to avoid gambling debts. We saw many behaviors, sad to say, due to effects of the
COVID-19 pandemic on family members.

Table 12–6 is a strategy for therapists to lessen disruptive behaviors. It is a challenge
to teach a person to behave appropriately, even when it is in his own interest. Despite
all these efforts, which are successful sometimes, the "solution" (if you want to call it
that) may require a behavior management program, which involves identification of
the problematic behaviors; reinforcement of appropriate behavior by gradually restoring privileges, such as commissary; and a fallback to the use of physical restraint.
Schmidt and Ivanoff (2015) describe a management plan called the "egregious behavior protocol" that involves detailing and targeting undesirable behaviors and analysis
of behavioral incidents and doable responses of patient to re-earn privileges. This is
a complex team effort. You may be involved (along with correctional officers) in de-
escalating a patient. Give them practice in anger management in individual sessions.
Keep in mind that most of these prisoners have long had antisocial lifestyles and have
emotional habits that have actually reinforced their aggressive and dysfunctional behaviors (Schmidt and Ivanoff 2015, p. 287). You can help the patient to unlearn these
behaviors and substitute prosocial coping skills.

Key Points

- *Hegemonic masculinity*, and the closely related concept *toxic masculinity*, are
cultural expressions of masculinity that hich are exacerbated by imprisonment.
They involve concepts of supermasculinity as well as misogyny and may represent adaptations to a homosocial environment in which the primary available sexual activity is homosexual.

TABLE 12–6. **Tough customers: therapeutic strategies to lessen disruptive behaviors**

Remember that therapeutic groups and therapeutic communities are effective with antisocial behaviors.

Use a multidisciplinary treatment team to treat the patient with disruptive behaviors.

Coordinate with custody; determine which behaviors need referral (i.e., Do you want a mental health referral every time one prisoner slaps another prisoner? Or what if the person doing the slapping is already your patient?).

Consistent with the previous item, discuss all behavior incidents in therapy session.

Review all disciplinary violations with the patient, identifying the maladaptive nature of the behavior and how it fails to meet the supposed needs that it addresses and usually just worsens the situation.

Chip away at psychological defenses. "Much change literature has to do with ways of dealing with defenses. The prevailing wisdom is that defenses should not be attacked head-on but that they must be surfaced and redundantly highlighted and discussed" (Toch and Adams 2002, p. 351).

Teach social skills and behavioral self-control so that the patient can achieve his goals without the destructive behaviors he has become accustomed to.

Address the toxic masculinity of many of the behaviors by relabeling caring and prosocial behaviors as more masculine than exploitation.

Find alternative behaviors that enhance self-esteem (one patient was "saved" when it was discovered that he had a real aptitude for art and the institution nurtured it).

Attempt to develop a nurturing and caring relationship with a staff member, thus compensating for the lack of appropriate parental figures in the prisoner's childhood.

Determine goals, motives, and intent (if any), or whether it is random-type outburst.

Consider a problem with impulsivity (with or without any other diagnosis).

Treat mental illness.

Negotiate an outcome that is unique to the patient.

Use anger management techniques when appropriate.

Require the patient to take ownership and responsibility of his impulsive behaviors.

Require "buy in" to your treatment plan.

"SOC it to 'em!" By which we mean, a "Sitter Outside the Cell" keeps the patient in the original location of the suicide attempt (e.g., with common attempts such as wrapping a blanket around the neck). This prevents their intended move and access to the benefits of moving to the infirmary. We have COVID-19 to thank for this (and we certainly did not think we would be thanking COVID-19 for anything). Management did not allow this until they became overwhelmed with patients in various stages of isolation for the virus; they allowed it, and it worked, and lessened the types of suicidal behaviors we have mentioned.

Use behavior management plans as a last resort but in a graded fashion with control of privileges, rewards, time out of cell, and so forth, leading ultimately to walking restraints and finally five-point restraints.

- Prisoners live by a Convict Code, the main tenet of which is to not rat out another prisoner. Components of the Convict Code interfere with the ability to have open therapeutic relationships, so they need to be countered in therapy. The therapist should be aware that the patient may need to appear strong and untouchable outside therapy sessions while opening up to more sensitive issues within the therapy session.

- Lying is common in prisoners and must be countered by constructive rebuttals and verification of all claims.

- Gang "politics" affects the behavior of many prisoners, and therapists can be prosocial in assisting gang members who wish to separate from their gang safely either now or in the future. This involves coordinating with the institution's security threat group supervisor.

- Hunger strikes have many possible causes. Although some hunger strikes are undertaken for political purposes, many are not. The supportive therapist has a role in educating the patient about available choices and assessing for coercion and impairment.

- Malingering, or the reporting of symptoms that one does not really have, may be exhibited by patients who seek gain for external purposes. It is not a diagnosis, but it makes diagnosis more difficult. The 10 criteria of experts (Vitacco and Rogers 2010) can be summarized as referring to unusual, rare, or amplified symptoms.

- There are many yellow flags (cautions) in diagnosing genuine mental illness as opposed to malingering, and even some green flags that support the veracity of mental health claims, but it may not be possible to be definitive in either ruling in or ruling out malingering. In general, a diagnosis is made less certain by the possibility of malingering, and we give the patient the benefit of the doubt so as to avoid causing harm to a genuinely ill person.

- Disturbed disruptive prisoners can destroy property, require cell extractions, and threaten suicide repeatedly. They may not fit into any one diagnostic category. Management may require a multidisciplinary treatment team and, if necessary, a behavior management plan.

References

Annas GD: Hunger strikes by inmates, in Principles and Practice of Forensic Psychiatry, 3rd Edition. Edited by Rosner R, Scott CL. New York, CRC Press, 2017, pp 603–610

Balsamo DN: Suicide risk in transgender inmates. AAPL Newsletter (American Academy of Psychiatry and the Law) 41(1):12–13, 15, 2016

Blau TH: The Psychologist as Expert Witness, 2nd Edition. New York, Wiley, 1998

Bowker LH: On the difficulty of eradicating masculine violence: multisystem overdetermination, in Masculinities and Violence. Edited by Bowker LH. Thousand Oaks, CA, Sage, 1998, pp 1–14

Brainy Quote. James Baldwin Quotes. 2020. Available at: www.brainyquote.com/quotes/james_baldwin_105629. Accessed January 15, 2021.

Brown PL: The "hidden punishment" of prison food: In Maine, the inmates are growing vegetables and making meals from scratch to replace the deadly diets they have long been served. New York Times, March 2, 2021. Available at: www.nytimes.com/2021/03/02/opinion/prison-food-farming-health.html. Accessed August 26, 2021.

Connell RW: Gender and Power: Society, the Person and Sexual Politics. Stanford, CA, Stanford University Press, 1987

Connelly M: The Night Fire. New York, Grand Central Publishing, 2020

Correia K: Handbook for Correctional Psychologists: Guidance for the Prison Practitioner, 2nd Edition. Springfield, IL, Charles C Thomas, 2009

Daines MK: Hunger strikes in correctional facilities, in Correctional Psychiatry: Practice Guidelines and Strategies. Edited by Thienhaus OJ, Piasecki M. Kingston, NJ, Civic Research Institute, 2007, pp. 8-1–8-13

Edgar K, O'Donnell I, Martin C: Prison Violence: The Dynamics of Conflict, Fear and Power. New York, Routledge, 2011

Ekman P: Deception. Available at: www.paulekman.com/deception. Accessed February 12, 2022.

Felthous AR: The treatment of clinical aggression in prison, in Correctional Psychiatry: Practice Guidelines and Strategies, Vol II. Edited by Thienhaus OJ, Piasecki M. Kingston, NJ, Civic Research Institute, 2013, pp. 4-1–4-34

Gerson A, Fox D: Malingering, in Practitioner's Guide to Evidence-Based Psychotherapy. Edited by Fisher JE, O'Donohue WT. New York, Springer, 2006, pp 386–395

Glezer A, McNiel DE, Binder RL: Transgendered and incarcerated: a review of the literature, current policies and laws, and ethics. J Am Acad Psychiatry Law 41(4):551–559, 2013 24335329

Gorman CK: The Truth About Lies in the Workplace: How to Spot Liars and What to Do About Them. San Francisco, CA, Berrett-Koehler Publishers, 2013

Hanson AL: Clinical and legal implications of gangs, in Oxford Textbook of Correctional Psychiatry. Edited by Trestman RL, Applebaum KL, Metzner JL. New York, Oxford University Press, 2015, pp 331–335

Helfand SJ, Sampl S, Trestman RL: Managing the disruptive or aggressive inmate, in Handbook of Correctional Mental Health, 2nd edition. Edited by Scott CL. Washington, DC, American Psychiatric Publishing, 2010, pp 197–230

Hensley C, Eigenberg H, Gibson L: Gay and lesbian inmates: sexuality and sexual coercion behind bars, in Special Needs Offenders in Correctional Institutions. Edited by Gideon L. Los Angeles, CA, Sage Publications, 2013, pp 233–257

Houston P, Floyd M, Carnicero S: Spy the Lie: Former CIA Officers Teach You How to Detect Deception. New York, St Martin's Griffin, 2012

Houston P, Floyd M, Carnicero S: Get the Truth: Former CIA Officers Teach You How to Persuade Anyone to Tell All. New York, St Martin's Press, 2015

Impact Justice: Eating Behind Bars: Ending the Hidden Punishment of Food in Prison, Dec. 2, 2020. Available at: https://impactjustice.org/wp-content/uploads/IJ-Eating-Behind-Bars-Release1.pdf. Accessed August 26, 2021.

Jenesky E: Prison gangs, in Correctional Psychiatry: Practice Guidelines and Strategies, Vol II. Edited by Thienhaus OJ, Piasecki M. Kingston, NJ, Civic Research Institute, 2013, pp 8-1–8-13

Karp DR: Unlocking men, unlocking masculinities: doing men's work in prison. J Men's Stud 18(1):63–83, 2010

Knoll JL 4th: Evaluation of malingering in corrections, in Oxford Textbook of Correctional Psychiatry. Edited by Trestman L, Appelbaum KL, Metzner JL. New York, Oxford University Press, 2015, pp 117–122

Koola MM: Are umatched residency graduates a solution for "shrinking shrinks"? Clinical Psychiatry News 48(2):12–14, 2020

Kupers TA: Psychotherapy with men in prison, in The New Handbook of Psychotherapy and Counseling with Men: A Comprehensive Guide to Settings, Problems, and Treatment Approaches, Vol 1. Edited by Brooks GR, Good GE. San Francisco, CA, Jossey-Bass, 2001, pp 170–184

Kupers TA: Toxic masculinity as a barrier to mental health treatment in prison. J Clin Psychol 61(6):713–724, 2005 15732090

Law V: Resistance Behind Bars: The Struggles of Incarcerated Women, 2nd Edition. Oakland, CA, PM Press, 2012

Locker R: Since 2013 more SEALs have died in training than in combat, records show. USA Today, May 13, 2016. Available at: www.usatoday.com/story/news/politics/2016/05/13/since-2013-more-seals-have-died-training-than-combat-records-show/84347974. Accessed February 20, 2021.

Maier GJ, Fulton L: Inpatient treatment of offenders with mental disorders, in Treatment of Offenders With Mental Disorders. Edited by Wettstein RM. New York, Guilford, 1998, pp 126–167

McDermott BE: Psychological testing and the assessment of malingering. Psychiatr Clin North Am 35(4):855–876, 2012 23107567

Middlemass KM: Convicted and Condemned: The Politics and Policies of Prisoner Reentry. New York, New York University Press, 2017

Morey LC: Personality Assessment Inventory. Tampa, FL. Psychological Assessment Resources, 1991

Morse SJ, Wright KA: Imprisoned men: masculinity variability and implications for correctional programming. Corrections 1694854:1–23, 2019

Mosher DL, Tompkins SS: Scripting the macho man: hypermasculine socialization and enculturation. J Sex Res 25(1):60–84, 1988

Nicholas LAL, Bryant G: Mentally ill inmates, in Special Needs Offenders in Correctional Institutions. Edited by Gideon L. Thousand Oaks, CA, Sage, 2013, pp 155–201

Phillips J: Cultural construction of manhood in prison. Psychol Men Masc 2(1):13–23, 2001 Available at: http://citeseerx.ist.psu.edu/viewdoc/download;jsessionid=5A70F53A43320A09149EAAD024D66B33?doi=10.1.1.631.1180&rep=rep1&type=pdf. Accessed July 12, 2020.

Pierre JM: Assessing malingered auditory verbal hallucinations in forensic and clinical settings. J Am Acad Psychiatry Law 47(4):448–456, 2019 31519734

Pyrooz DC, Decker SH: Competing for Control: Gangs and the Social Order of Prisons. New York, Cambridge University Press, 2019

Reeves R, Tamburello AC, Platt J, et al: Characteristics of inmates who initiate hunger strikes. J Am Acad Psychiatry Law 45(3):302–310, 2017 28939727

Rendell R: Death Notes. New York, Ballantine Books, 1981

Rendell R: Simisola. New York, Crown Publishers, 1995

Rendell R: Not in the Flesh: A Wexford Novel. New York, Crown Publishers, 2007

Resnick PJ: My favorite tips for detecting malingering and violence risk. Psychiatr Clin North Am 30(2):227–232, 2007 17643838

Resnick P, Knoll JL 4th: Malingered psychosis, in Clinical Assessment of Malingering and Deception, 4th Edition. Edited by Rogers R, Bender SD. New York, Guilford, 2018, pp 98–121

Rogers R, Bender SD (eds): Clinical Assessment of Malingering and Deception, 4th Edition. New York, Guilford, 2018

Schmidt H 3rd, Ivanoff AM: Behavior management plans, in Oxford Textbook of Correctional Psychiatry. Edited by Trestman L, Appelbaum KL, Metzner JL. New York, Oxford University Press, 2015, pp 286–290

Singh J, Avasti A, Grover S: Malingering of psychiatric disorders: a review. Ger J Psychiatry 10:126–132, 2007

Sloan JA: Masculinities and the Adult Male Prison Experience. London, Palgrave Macmillan, 2016

Sommers J: Masculinity in prison: the "mask" men have to wear behind bars. Huffington Post UK, November 22, 2015, pp 1–9. Available at: www.huffingtonpost.co.uk/2015/11/21/masculinity-in-prison_n_8472628.html. Accessed July 1, 2021.

Stanchfield P: Clarifying the therapist's role in the treatment of the resistant sex offender, in Tough Customers: Counseling Unwilling Clients, 2nd Edition. Lanham, MD, American Correctional Association, 2001, pp 49–62

Sterling AL: Prisoners unlearn the toxic masculinity that led to their incarceration. Huffington Post, July 31, 2019. Available at: www.huffpost.com/entry/incarcerated-men-gender-roles-recidivism_n_5d378544e4b004b6adb78912. Accessed October 11, 2010.

Substance Abuse and Mental Health Services Administration: Substance Abuse Treatment for Adults in the Criminal Justice System. Treatment Improvement Protocol (TIP) Series 44. DHHS Publ No (SMA) 13-4056. Rockville, MD, Substance Abuse and Mental Health Services Administration, 2005

Substance Abuse and Mental Health Services Administration: Addressing the Specific Behavioral Health Needs of Men. Treatment Improvement Protocol (TIP) Series 56. DHHS Publication No (SMA) 13-4736. Rockville, MD, Substance Abuse and Mental Health Services Administration, 2013

Toch H: Hypermasculinity and prison violence, in Masculinities and Violence. Edited by Bowker LH. Thousand Oaks, CA, Sage, 1997, pp 168–178

Toch H: The disturbed disruptive, in Working With Dangerous People: The Psychotherapy of Violence. Edited by Jones D. Abingdon, Oxon, UK, Medical Press, 2004, pp 9–14

Toch H, Adams K: Acting Out: Maladaptive Behavior in Confinement. Washington, DC, American Psychological Association, 2002

U.S. Navy: SEALS. Available at: www.navy.com/seals. Accessed July 18, 2020.

Vitacco MJ, Rogers R: Assessment of malingering in correctional settings, in Handbook of Correctional Mental Health, 2nd Edition. Edited by Scott CL. Arlington, VA, American Psychiatric Publishing, 2010, pp 255–276

Vrij A: Detecting Lies and Deceit: Pitfalls and Opportunities, 2nd Edition. Chichester, West Sussex, UK, Wiley, 2008

Walczyk JJ, Sewell N, DiBenedetto MB: A review of approaches to detecting malingering in forensic contexts and promising cognitive load-inducing lie detection techniques. Front Psychiatry 9:700, 2018 30622488

Walters SB: The Truth About Lying: How to Spot a Lie and Protect Yourself From Deception. Napierville, IL, Sourcebooks, 2000

Weiss KJ, Dell LV: Liability for diagnosing malingering. J Am Acad Psychiatry Law 45(2):339–347, 2017 28939732

Wikipedia: 2013 California prisoner hunger strike. 2020a. Available at: https://en.wikipedia.org/wiki/2013_California_prisoner_hunger_strike#. Accessed November 28, 2020.

Wikipedia: Inmate code. 2020b. Available at: https://en.wikipedia.org/wiki/Inmate_Code#cite_note-Clear-1. Accessed July 12, 2021.

Wikipedia: Hunger strike. 2021. Available at: https://en.wikipedia.org/wiki/Hunger_strike. Accessed February 19, 2021.

Xenakis SN: Ethics dilemmas in managing hunger strikers. J Am Acad Psychiatry Law 45(3):311–315, 2017 28939728

Yang S, Baronia R, Ibrahim Y: Validity of psychiatric evaluation of asylum seekers through telephone. Case Rep Psychiatry 2021:8856352, February 10, 2021 33628562

Young MA, Gonzalez V: Getting out of gangs, staying out of gangs: gang intervention and desistance strategies. National Gang Center Bulletin (Bureau of Justice Assistance), No 8, January 2013, pp 1–10. Available at: www.nationalgangcenter.gov/Content/Documents/Getting-Out-Staying-Out.pdf. Accessed September 13, 2020.

Zaitchik MC, Mosher DL: Criminal justice implications of the macho personality constellation. Crim Justice Behav 20(3):227–239, 1993

Zamble E, Porporino FJ: Coping, Behavior, and Adaptation in Prison Inmates. New York, Springer, 1988

13

Special Topics

In this chapter we discuss a number of issues that affect supportive psychotherapists working in correctional settings—issues that may apply to special populations of prisoners or are particularly relevant to doing supportive work.

There but for Culture

In a world that has many books about culture and psychotherapy, we can only make some brief observations (cultured pearls?) about some facets of culture that we think relevant.

In the 2020 presidential campaign, then-candidate Joe Biden received a lot of flak when he said that the Latino community was more diverse than the Black community (Epstein 2020). So, if anything we say here, which is based on references to credentialed experts or persons speaking from within their own community, gives an impression of a stereotype or misapprehension that all persons in a culture are like the instance described, then consider it to be qualified by this observation. So-called American culture, Black culture, Latino culture, and so forth are diverse. In approaching any patient with a culture-tinted lens in our glasses, we are already bringing certain assumptions to the table. The only point in doing that is to make it easier and faster to understand him or her as an individual.

The word "culture" can mean different things. According to a famous (mis)quote, Hermann Göring said, "Every time I hear the word 'culture,' I reach for my gun" (for discussion, see Quote/Counterquote 2019). Expressing the American gun culture, Americans reached for guns and ammunition in record numbers in the spring of 2020, affected by coronavirus fears and outrages over racial injustices (Levine and McKnight 2020) and backlash to cultural change. When we hear the word *culture*, we reach for our DSM-5-TR, which defines culture in a fairly narrow way and then a page later much more broadly and encompassingly. Initially, it says:

> *Culture* refers to systems of knowledge, concepts, values, norms, and practices that are learned and transmitted across generations. Culture includes language, religion and spirituality, family structures, life-cycle stages, ceremonial rituals, customs, and ways of understanding health and illness, as well as moral, political, economic, and legal systems. Cultures are open, dynamic systems that undergo continuous change over time;

in the contemporary world, most individuals and groups are exposed to multiple cultural contexts, which they use to fashion their own identities and make sense of experience. This process of meaning-making derives from developmental and everyday social experiences in specific contexts, including health care, which may vary for each individual. Much of culture involves background knowledge, values, and assumptions that remain implicit or presumed and so may be difficult for individuals to describe. These features of culture make it crucial not to overgeneralize cultural information or stereotype groups in terms of fixed cultural traits. In relation to diagnosis, it is essential to recognize that all forms of illness and distress, including the DSM disorders, are shaped by cultural contexts. Culture influences how individuals fashion their identities, as well as how they interpret and respond to symptoms and illness. (p. 860)

This definition of culture informs the DSM-5-TR outline for cultural formulation, which briefly has the following parts:

1. Cultural identity of the individual
2. Cultural conceptualizations of distress
3. Psychosocial stressors and cultural features of vulnerability and resilience
4. Cultural features of the relationship between the individual and the clinician, treatment team, and institution
5. Overall cultural assessment

It is certainly worth reading the details of these items, and item 4 in particular if a patient is of a different culture from the therapist.

DSM-5-TR casts the definition of culture over nearly every influence in human development. The American gun culture does seem to fall under the DSM-5-TR cultural umbrella and is probably responsible for the incarceration of many of your patients, even if they may be forbidden to own firearms when they leave.

> In the CFI [Cultural Formulation Interview], the term *culture* includes:
>
> - The processes through which individuals assign meaning to experience, drawing from the values, orientations, knowledge, and practices of the diverse social groups (e.g., ethnic groups, faith groups, occupational groups, veterans' groups) and communities in which they participate.
> - Aspects of individuals' background, developmental experiences, and current social contexts and position that affect their perspective, such as age, gender, social class, geographic origin, migration, language, religion, sexual orientation, disability, or ethnic or racialized background.
> - The influence of family, friends, and other community members (particularly, the individual's *social network*) on the individual's illness experience.
> - The cultural background of the health care providers and the values and assumptions embedded in the organization and practices of health care systems and institutions that may affect the clinical interaction. (p. 862)

We similarly take a broad view of the term and include in our thinking issues such as socioeconomic status and the aforementioned American gun culture, and we would include a concept of "criminal culture" as applying to many prisoners. So using the broad concept, it should already be obvious to anyone who read the first page of Chapter 1 that there is something troubling about American culture. For example, the United States imprisons African Americans and other persons of color at rates much higher than it imprisons white persons. Of course, it could be supposed that

African Americans simply grow up in cultures (e.g., low socioeconomic status urban areas) where there is more crime. And if there is more crime in a family and community, the children of that family and community might commit more crime, and the system perpetuates itself, right? Maybe so, but there are many stronger forces at work, forces that most objective observers call *structural and systemic racism.*

We are talking about culture in treatment here, and space doesn't permit us to detail the many influences of racism. In Chapter 1, we alluded to the U.S. criminal justice system as a juggernaut that sweeps up enormous numbers of people of color, but here is more: It also, as Alexandra Natapoff (2018, p. 149) points out, marks people of color as criminals by piling on them fines and other punishments, all the while perpetuating the historical stereotypes that link them with criminality.

That's just a fraction of what that author found. But her voice is not one crying in the wilderness; it is one in a chorus of the voices from our cities. For example, Victor Rios, a gang member turned sociologist in Oakland, California, investigated the way that Black and Latino boys acquired their "negative credentials" as they are caught up in the American culture of punishment (Rios 2012). And as Jeffrey Reiman says in the title of his book, *The Rich Get Richer and the Poor Get Prison* (Reiman 2020).

In the past, many other policies, such as the differences between powder and crack cocaine penalties and stop-and-frisk laws, led to the differential incarceration of minority groups, and many other policies continue to do so today. As Kapoor and Griffith (2015) note, "The end result is that in many communities of color, incarceration is viewed not as a personal failure or source of shame but as the most recent battle in the ongoing struggle for civil rights" (p. 343). And, adding in the attitude of gang members who view prison time as an initiation, "Bravado, even pride, in incarceration is not uncommon" (Kapoor and Griffith 2015, p. 343, referencing Morris 2012).

So when you treat patients, you may become aware of a great deal of rage at racism and other unfairness in our society. This rage may be difficult to disentangle from your patients' attitudes toward criminal behavior and their concepts of themselves. To quote once more from Kapoor and Griffith (2015, p. 343), "Clinicians from a middle-class, white background may interpret an inmate's statements about the unfairness of the criminal justice system as evidence of callousness or lack of responsibility for actions. Clinicians may also view discussions about growing up fatherless or without positive role models as excuses for bad behavior." Your patients' attitudes, and your attitudes *toward* their attitudes, are part of the complexity of cultures interacting with theirs. We have learned a lot from our patients and how they got into prison, and even (for those to whom it applies) how they got to be career criminals. People come from many different houses, but they often end up in that "Big House." It helps to understand how our culture got them there.

Since Black men do constitute a large group of prisoners, a few more observations are worth considering, starting with a brief vignette slightly different from our usual ones.

Vignette: The Staff Break Room

Staff are watching the news on TV.

> STAFF PERSON #1: Did you hear that? They say that Reverend Al Sharpton is planning another one of his marches on Washington at the end of the month!
> STAFF PERSON #2: Oh, really, wow! I'd like to see that: Ten thousand angry Black men marching on the White House!

Comment: Who might be saying these things, correctional officers or professional mental health staff? Do these remarks, the first or the second, reflect a racial stereotype, outright racism, or merely sarcasm?

Reverend Al Sharpton actually led marches on Washington on August 28, 2020 and 2021 to commemorate the anniversaries of Martin Luther King, Jr.'s "I Have a Dream" speech, and they were large and peaceful protests, full of committed but not violent men and women of different races, ages, and sexual orientations. But stereotypes of "angry Black people" permeated and polarized American society as many people protested multiple instances of social injustice starting in the spring and summer of 2020. The anger and division in our society were still simmering at the time of the Reverend's second march.

Events in the outside world do affect relationships in psychotherapy in prisons, connecting in part to the toxic masculinity that afflicts all races there. An account of this is given by a Black therapist of an angry Black patient (Wade 2006). White staff feel threatened by the patient's expressions of anger, but the Black therapist does not perceive the threat, just the anger. The therapist also notices that when he gets expressive about a therapy issue in staff meetings, the other (white) staff start asking him if he feels okay, because they perceive his emotion as excessive. Are his colleagues stereotyping him as an "angry Black man"?

Kevin M. Simon, who is an uncommon person indeed—a psychiatrist who is Black—asks us to consider the following factors (Simon 2020, p. 8):

- *A comfortable environment.* The Black person may not be familiar with what happens in psychological evaluations.
- *Storytelling.* Doctors typically interrupt their patients too much. Let your patient tell his story.
- *Confidentiality.* It will be especially important to describe the limits of confidentiality in the prison setting, since Black men are used to violations of their trust and rights in society.
- *Nonverbal language.* Black men are used to being regarded as threats and will read the nonverbal reactions of a therapist closely.
- *Respect.* This gives the patient the space and time to make the appropriate decisions in treatment.

When we talked about women in Chapter 11, we introduced the social philosophy of intersectionality that draws attention to the multiple groups to which a person may belong and that could be called cultural in nature or thought of as identity markers. For example, prisoners are controlled by the official prison establishment. In the community, previously incarcerated persons are subject to discrimination in job employment and social status. And in addition to being a prisoner, a person might be Black, lesbian, disabled, and poor, all of which play a role in her identity. Her lack of opportunities and her individual family circumstances play a role in her behavior and have played a strong role in where she is now: Prison.

Some patients may be fully aware of their cultural histories and even blame many of their identity markers for their criminal behavior. Others, not so much. Patients may be aware that they come from a disadvantaged background but not that they are expressing the values of a criminal culture. So while your patient is a unique individual with a unique upbringing, he or she also shares a number of common elements with other prisoners. However, people are the product of multiple influences and many individual choices. The fact that multiple causes, including their own choices, led them to commit crimes does not excuse their future behaviors, but it does help them to understand their past. All poor people do not commit crimes, and few become career criminals. Explanations are not justifications.

As a therapist, however, you should try to understand your patient's culture. What do you say to the patient who says, "Doc, you're not Black and poor and you probably didn't grow up without a father, did you? So how could you possibly understand me or why I did what I did? So let's just forget about you trying to understand me."

You could respond with:

> We'll try to get you to see our one Black therapist, but he is inundated with similar requests and too busy to see you for a few months anyway, and he is probably not poor because he has a nice job here in the prison, although he might have grown up in a poor neighborhood and maybe he did grow up without a father—I've never asked him that question, but I did ask you that question because I was interested in how you grew up. So you may never find anyone who is enough like you to satisfy you. However, unlike you, I know about the backgrounds of hundreds of prisoners I've worked with and I've tried the best I can to understand prisoners of all races with all kinds of backgrounds and different family situations. So when I don't seem to understand a certain point, I hope you will help me out. And for the things that I can't convince you of, we are going to put you in group therapy with your peers and let *them* do some convincing that you won't be able to talk your way out of. But the fact that I am not 100% like you should not be an excuse for staying the same or refusing to make any progress here. Unless, of course, you're looking for such an excuse. Are you?

Cultural biases affect the way you do treatment. One, just mentioned, may be the way you react differently to emotions in Black men versus men of other races. In Chapter 8, we also noted that African Americans are overdiagnosed with psychotic disorders and underdiagnosed with mood and anxiety disorders. This can result in relative overuse of antipsychotic medications and undertreatment of depressive disorders (Courtney 2013).

Other suggestions from a practitioner experienced with Black and Latino men are (Wexler 2009, pp. 225–233):

- Interrogate yourself about your diversity self-awareness with questions like

  - What were my first experiences with people of this group?
  - Am I aware of my own biases and assumptions regarding persons of this group?

- Understand that the Latino concepts of masculinity connected to *machismo* also parallel concepts of *caballerismo*, a more positive concept of the male role involving nurturing of others. Reframe *machismo* rather than trying to directly counter it. Three concepts of the culture, certainly emphasized in supportive psychotherapy, have been found to enhance the connection with patients. These are *respeto* (recognizing and respecting their life experiences), *personalismo* (having an ability to chat, which includes some of the friendliness we called "Happy Talk") and *simpatía* (not identical to but similar to empathy).

- Even if you do not wish to respond at the time, listen to your patients' experiences with discrimination, disenfranchisement, and hate crimes. Try to understand the "invisibility" experience of Black men (history of being slighted and discounted).

Cultural sensitivity is sometimes equated with cultural relativism, but this leads into controversy. Cultural relativism is often promoted as the doctrine that all cultures are equal. We have trouble with that claim, even though some proponents of cultural relativism say that any attempt to impose Western values on other cultures is a form of cultural colonialism. Cultural relativism should mean merely that people's actions are best understood within the context of the cultures they are in. For example, in Chapter 12, we described the concept of ideological scripts that are socially inherited and modified by individual upbringing. A man who enacts a macho script and is hurtful to women needs to be understood but not congratulated for his adherence to his cultural normal and family upbringing. Cultural relativism helps us understand why he enacts that script. But cultural relativism should not be equated with moral relativism, which is the doctrine that moral laws are all relative to culture and there is no one right set of moral laws. We do believe that there is a common morality. This is a concept that societies are evolving toward a set of common moral laws and universal human rights that arise from human nature and self-consciousness. Common morality is particularly relevant to our work because it has been paired with the set of medical ethics called *principlism* associated with the work of Beauchamp and Childress (2019). A set of "moral laws" proposed for common morality can be found in several places, such as Bernard Gert's *Common Morality* (Gert 2014). Here is one of them:

1. Do not kill.
2. Do not cause pain.
3. Do not disable.
4. Do not deprive of freedom.
5. Do not deprive of pleasure.
6. Do not deceive.
7. Keep your promises.
8. Do not cheat.
9. Obey the law.
10. Do your duty.

These laws are not absolute, and they may come into conflict with one another. The resolution of all this is probably why Prof. Gert had to write a book about it. For example, you may note that killing somebody in self-defense might justify violating the first law, and so forth. And perhaps you are wondering if prisons, including the death penalty, violate these supposed laws of common morality.

Consider when (suggestive of Mr. Lopez in Chapter 3) a patient says, "In my culture, women are just property. So my wife has no right to argue with me, and I have the right to hit her, and the police have no right to intervene in a private matter." You might say, "Mr. X, you are in our airspace now, and you should fly by our rules. You don't hit women. And if you do, you end up here. And…I think it is wrong in *any* culture to hit women, although I understand how you came to feel the way you did because you grew up in a patriarchal culture, but you are somewhere else now and need to change." Similar advice could be given to the Syrian woman in Chapter 11, that she has the inherent right to be equal to her husband in their marriage. Curiously, we ran into a parallel argument, in an account of what is called *energy psychology*, of a Middle Eastern woman who discovers her primordial self cannot be subservient to her husband.

She is said to uncover the self she had before she was acculturated, a self that has (what the author considers) a "primordial" right to be respected in direct opposition to what she was taught in her culture (Mayer 2009, p. xl). (For more about the discussion of common morality, see Veatch 2003 and related articles.)

Once more we will mention our galactic Master Chef Gurronsevas, whose adventures takes him into various culinary environments that are food cultures but not moral ones. In feeding the various species in Sector General, his huge hospital at the edge of the galaxy, he has to enact some rules. One of them is that no food can be sentient. Eventually it appears that all the foods have to be vegetarian, because many cultures eat meat that *resembles* the species of other cultures, even if it is not sentient itself. And sentience is, after all, a matter of degree. It would be objectionable to the humans under his care to see human-like beings fed to some other carnivorous species. So gradually, there evolves a set of rules that govern culinary decisions, which are of course cultural, subject to rules of a common morality that apply to all species of the galaxy. This is not to say that vegetarianism is part of the common morality, but it shows the process by which decisions are made in that sphere. Everything we do is not just a matter of taste. The cultural is not merely culinary. Culture is not like cuisine. All "menus" are not created equal. Some of them subjugate human beings; some do not, and so forth.

And indeed, in James White's galactic Sector General hospital, there is the assumption that all intelligent species evolve toward a common morality. Moreover, it is asserted (perhaps another element of science fiction) that there is no such thing as a completely evil alien race because any species that has technologically evolved to engage in space travel must be civilized (White 2002, p. 186).

One last admonition: Members of gangs or organized crime subcultures cannot use their subcultures as justifications for their crimes. They have an awareness that the subculture they join is illegal and immoral by the standards of the larger culture of their upbringing.

It's About Time

There is a group of prisoners who have problems with carceral time. Some of them may be lifers or elderly so that the only time they face is in prison. Time for those on death row is supposedly limited, but we know in practice that it takes years, and few persons are actually executed. People with really long sentences, or what has been called "durance vile," are in the minority but have their issues. Patients with serious terminal illness are also running out of time.

Sometimes in therapy we have something special to discuss and we casually or reflexively ask the patient if he has time for it. Often we hear, "Doc, you know I've got all the time in the world." James Knoll (2009), to whom we have referred, reminds us that lifers have a high rate of mental illness (1 in 4). Many of them have made a positive adjustment and have a maturity and leadership position with respect to younger prisoners. Some are career criminals who continue to function in organized crime, directing criminal enterprises, including murders both within and outside the prison. Putting that group aside, however, Knoll says that many prisoners and recidivists score lower than those in the community on tests for purpose in life such as the (aptly named) Purpose-in-Life Test (Crumbaugh and Maholick 1969). He interviews a lifer who has found meaning in his "lifer's group" and by mentoring others.

Case Vignette

Mr. Wilson is a 61-year-old white man who is midway through a long sentence for DUI causing death. He has not had mental health services before but puts in a request. We pick up after the usual preliminaries.

THERAPIST: Tell me some more about why you wrote your request.

MR. WILSON: Well, I'm getting depressed, I think. I found out that my dad is dying. He's 80 years old, and now they say he's only got a few months. I wanted to get out there and just be with him one more time.

THERAPIST: Where is he now?

MR. WILSON: He moved in with my sister [who is a few years younger than patient], or rather she moved in with *him*. They say he's got some sort of dementia, so he really can't be left alone, and he's got heart failure and a lot of other things. He barely gets out of bed.

THERAPIST: Oh, so there's no way he can come here?

MR. WILSON: Not a chance. He can't even stand up. That's why I wanted to get out and see him. And I began to think there was a chance, with the COVID-19 thing going on.

THERAPIST: You mean, to get a humanitarian release?

MR. WILSON: Yes. You see my chart. I've got diabetes, COPD, and high blood pressure.

THERAPIST: [Thinks—sure, but this man is only halfway through his sentence, and they are releasing people who have completed 75% of their sentences.] Yes, I see. [Don't dash hopes.]

MR. WILSON: Yeah, so I started thinking, what if I die before I get to see him again, and then I started getting depressed.

THERAPIST: And you've never been depressed before?

MR. WILSON: No, not really. I mean, I was devastated when I first came in. This is my first and only prison term. And what I did…I killed a guy because I was drunk and in a car, get it? It was so stupid. I mean, not just stupid, but bad. Of course, I've had 6 years to think about that.

THERAPIST: How long have you been feeling depressed?

MR. WILSON: I guess 3 or 4 weeks, but I thought it would pass. But my sister tells me that my dad is getting worse and worse.

THERAPIST: Have you had any thoughts of hurting yourself?

MR. WILSON: No, nothing like that at all. But sometimes I wish I could just go to sleep and, should I say, not have to think about getting up the next morning.

THERAPIST: Well, I'm glad you feel comfortable telling me that. When people get depressed, it's a warning sign that we should get to know you better and address the depression.

MR. WILSON (*not happy*): You're not going to put me in the infirmary for that, are you?

THERAPIST (*reassuringly*): I wasn't planning to, but I would like to know a little more about your depression. I've got a little questionnaire that should take about 5 minutes [The Geriatric Depression Scale, available at numerous sites, including Stanford University 2020].

The therapist assesses the depression and considers if a referral for medication is needed or if it can be delayed for a while as he gets to know the patient better, knowing that in older patients, "[p]sychotherapy is comparable with the effectiveness of antidepressants" (Kok and Reynolds 2017, p. 2119). He learns about the patient's younger sister, who is his main contact in the community, but discovers that the patient has two sons with whom he has had minimal contact since entering the prison. What is that all about? The sister talks to them frequently, but he doesn't. Why not?

Mr. Wilson has an issue with a common form of grief when dealing with aging parents: anticipatory grief. Grief counseling, as discussed in Chapter 5, is by no means required or useful for cases of ordinary grief (Campbell 2016), but such counseling may be helpful for prisoners with losses related to being in prison, especially those with long periods of prison time.

John J. Lennon is a prison journalist with a long list of bylines and a broad readership who is serving 28 years-to-life for second-degree murder. In a recent *Washington Post Magazine* issue (Lennon 2019) on prisoners and prison, he writes about the process he went through in trying to apologize to the family of the man he murdered in 2001 when he was involved in drug dealing and using. After joining a creative writing workshop, he began to be published and became quite well known in prison as well as in general circulation publications. Through counseling, being mentored, and through his own writing, Lennon began to come to terms with what an apology really is. Although clearly proud of his writing and its success, he deals with anxiety and depression, using his writing as therapy. But other than a kind of lip service to the idea of an apology that he would address in his articles by saying that he had committed the murder (and other crimes), his only real apology was a "tag line" in some of his articles that said "I'm sorry for killing him and taking all the life he could have had," while at the same time saying that he felt the murder was justified because his victim had beaten a murder rap and had "shaken down" one of his street dealers (Lennon 2019). Until recently, he had never apologized to the family of his victim.

There is a service in many states known as an apology bank that allows prisoners who are not permitted to contact victims or families directly to write and send a letter that will then be shared only if the victim requests it. However, Lennon was advised early on to try to apologize directly and ask for forgiveness as part of his therapy and addiction recovery, and he struggled with the notion that most prisoners wrote apologies to look good to the parole board without really internalizing the need to make amends. Finally, having been interviewed for a special on incarceration that was aired in 2018 on HLN, the family acknowledged that they had never received such a letter. Now, of course it seemed to him rather self-serving in that he now knew that the lack of a letter was public, but he went ahead and wrote it after several drafts. What he came up with was an acknowledgment of the hurt and trauma he had caused and an acknowledgment that going forward he would need to better represent his victim's memory in his work.

The conclusion Lennon makes in the process of writing his apology letter was that there is a need in prison, especially for long-termers, for therapy to address their remorse, like the one in Sing Sing called the Longtermers' Responsibility Project, which helps people realize the effects of their actions and come to terms with their responsibility for it.

Given what we have just said, we wish to refer once more to the morality of the next millennium in James White's Sector General Hospital. Here is one of the stories.

Lioren is a military surgeon who overzealously treats a newly discovered civilization called the Cromsaggar who are dying from a wasting disease. Through a misunderstanding of the illness, he creates a situation in which thousands of them on the planet die, leaving only the ones in Sector General Hospital alive. Lioren blames himself and thinks he should be put to death for his mistake. The administration sees it as a medical error and strips him of his rank and surgeon's license but allows him to become a trainee in the psychology department. (You would be wrong to think this reflects a negative opinion of psychology, because Sector General is in fact run by Dr. O'Mara, a psychologist, and O'Mara has chosen the assignment deliberately.) Lioren spends months talking to patients, including suicidal ones, who feel guilty about things they have done. Finally, he decides that the only way to deal with his guilt is to go to the remaining Cromsaggar and apologize, come what may—they can kill him on the spot if they want to.

But the Cromsaggar do not kill Lioren. They forgive him. And Lioren learns from this that there is benefit on both sides of the apology: a personal apology may be shameful for the person committing the offense, but forgiveness from the victim can have lasting benefits for both of them well beyond the knowledge that the offending person has received punishment (White 1991, p. 214). And by the way, Lioren is so moved and transformed by the forgiveness that he becomes—no, not the psychologist that O'Mara probably thought he would become, but—the hospital chaplain.

The concept raised here (published in 1991) would seem to refer to what is known as *restorative justice*, the foundational book of which was published in 1990 by Howard Zehr, although the concepts go back to biblical times. We do not know whether James White was familiar with restorative justice. However, it involves restoring the imbalance of society created by a crime by (usually) bringing together perpetrator and victim or members of the victim's community. It may involve restitution. It seems to lessen the recidivism in offenders. Many propose it as an alternative to punishment. It is now a major field of interest. Zehr's own delineation of it is well known in telling us what it is not. Restorative justice is not any particular program, is not about mediation, and is not designed to reduce recidivism. Restorative justice is not primarily about forgiveness or reconciliation, but it is not necessarily the oppositive of restitution. From the positive perspective, it involves the following five principles in victims, communities, and offenders (Zehr and Gohar 2003, p. 33):

1. Focuses on harms and consequent needs.
2. Addresses obligations resulting from those harms.
3. Uses an inclusive, collaborative process.
4. Involves the stakeholders in the process.
5. Seeks to put right the wrongs.

In concluding this section, it is clear that there is a lot of time to be spent with people who do have time, but we list a few therapy pointers in Table 13–1.

Sex Offenders: Throw Away the Keys or Give Them the Keys to a Good Life?

> SPIRIT: "My time with you, Ebenezer, is about done. Will you profit by what I have shown you of the good in most men's hearts?"
> SCROOGE: "I don't know. How can I promise?"
>
> *A Christmas Carol* (Desmond-Hurst 1951)

TABLE 13–1. **Agenda for treating time-challenged prisoners***

Remember that some of these prisoners may have a lot of carceral time to go but no time outside.

Consider that in the prison setting with typical prisoners' health conditions, a "geriatric" patient may be age 50 or older.

When in doubt, do formal simple and quick mental status testing, using, e.g., the MoCA (www.mocatest.org; Doerflinger 2012) or SLU Mental Status Exam (St. Louis University 2020), both of which have multiple versions and website support.

If patients do not test well, repeat tests and follow at least yearly, because in many cases there is a progression to dementia.

Find linkages to the outside world: persons and programs on the outside.

Link to or create a program on the inside (e.g., for lifers, over-50's).

Counter loneliness through programs and mentoring (must monitor for abuse or exploitation in either direction).

Give patients help in finding or creating meaning or purpose in life.

Offer education and personal growth activities.

Cultivate mindfulness.

Show an interest in patients (your relationship to them is part of their treatment).

If appropriate, develop past-looking activities (e.g., autobiographical or life narratives).

Write diaries, prison blogs, or books.

---

*Not for gangbangers, shot-callers, organized crime leaders, or incorrigible psychopaths—they can fend for themselves unless there is a genuine issue you can help them with.

There are prisoners who usually live in special units or attend programs tailored for their needs. They are often a reviled group of people who, like psychopaths (and some of them are psychopaths), are often considered untreatable and incorrigible, and it is true that some of them are. However, the risk-need-responsivity (RNR) theorists tell us that sex offenders can be treated using the same RNR principles as everyone else. In Chapter 1, we described a relationship between supportive psychotherapy, positive psychology, and the Good Lives Model (GLM), which has been applied to both sex offenders and, to a lesser extent, violent prisoners. Proof of the efficacy of treatment for sex offenders was fairly mixed until recently, although a recent government report reviewed numerous studies showing a positive effect favoring those with adherence to the RNR model (Przybylski 2017). While the GLM model is gaining adherents internationally, the efficacy research is still ongoing.

Treatment of sex offenders is specialized, and some places require additional certification above licensure. Treatment (or "management," as it is sometimes called) is often not referred to as psychotherapy because it is more proscriptive and has less than the usual limits on confidentiality (Saleh et al. 2015).

In your work, you will meet prisoners who at one time were in such programs. In fact, the recidivism studies show that 1) sex offenders actually have low recidivism for sex offenses per se but may continue to commit other criminal offenses, and 2) criminals who committed nonsexual offenses may include sex offenses in their repertory (discussed in Saleh et al. 2015). So we think it is reasonable to recommend that you become familiar with concepts such as GLM and consider using them in supportive therapy with such patients, as permitted of course in your institution, as well as violent individuals to whom the GLM concepts have also been applied. If you find these concepts interesting, you can certainly get one of the GLM workbooks (e.g., Yates and Prescott

2011) and use them with individual patients. Here are some ideas, based on supportive therapy and the Good Lives Model, that will enable you to understand these individuals and help them even if you lack the specialized expertise to treat sex offenders (see Table 13–2 for a summary).

The Good Lives Model is a method of offender rehabilitation that is complementary to the RNR model. Like supportive psychotherapy, it emphasizes and relies upon a strong therapeutic alliance with the patients—something their proponents say is lacking in the RNR approach. Proponents counter what they call the deficits-based RNR model with their own strengths-based approach. There is actually some disagreement between some RNR and some GLM proponents. To some, the attempt to graft GLM onto RNR is seen more like GLM trying to ride the coattails of the established, evidence-based (in reducing recidivism) RNR!

As our subtitle to this section suggested, GLM was developed primarily to treat sex offenders as an alternative to "throwing away the keys." It shares many of the underpinnings of positive psychology and offers people a set of attractive positive goals (rather than negative, demeaning treatment paradigms) that foster patients' "buy-in," which is vital to success. GLM assumes that individuals are goal-directed and that their behavior is aimed at seeking primary human goods. These goods are defined by each person representing their core values and priorities (Yates et al. 2010, pp. 65-66):

- Life
- Knowledge
- Excellence in play and work
- Excellence in agency
- Inner peace
- Friendship
- Community
- Spirituality
- Happiness
- Creativity

It is asserted that people strive for these primary goods by means of secondary or instrumental means that may be misguided or criminal. For example, a sex offender could strive for happiness by manipulating or coercing others in relationships, or a person could strive for excellence in work by embezzling money.

GLM asserts that sex offenders are similar to other people in that they strive for these goals, but they do so in inappropriate ways. They can do this indirectly or directly. Indirect maladaptive behavior occurs when a legitimate goal (e.g., getting respect) is approached with inappropriate means (e.g., hitting the spouse who appears disrespectful). Such a person needs to learn that hitting his wife is not going to create respect in the relationship, and furthermore that such behavior reflects attitudes that are destructive to a genuine relationship. He is offered training in emotional management (a GLM version of anger management or the packaged program called *Cage Your Rage*; Cullen 2013). The latter is consistent with a feature of GLM concerning self-regulation. "In other words, crime and psychological problems are hypothesized to be a direct consequence of maladaptive attempts to meet human needs" (Ward and Maruna 2007, p. 111). Our view of this is that offenders need to be taught to regulate themselves. Or as Thomas Gray (1747) wrote:

TABLE 13–2.   **Supportive psychotherapy interventions for sex offenders***

Familiarize yourself with your institution's own programs and the one(s) your patient is enrolled in.

Know the cognitive strengths and weaknesses of your patient and educate accordingly.

A good beginning is to ask patients who are sex offenders how they are doing in their treatment program; ask them what they are learning or if they are having problems with any lessons; you do not have to ask about their current offense.

Discuss the patient's life goals and kinds of things he is willing to work for (which the Good Lives Model believes are common to most people).

Show respect and interest in their investment in legal, common goods.

Address social support for the isolated, lonely offender.

Assess the role of high or low self-esteem related to the offense; if the offense was related to low self-esteem, it is good therapy to use self-esteem raising methods; if the offense was related to high self-esteem, explain how the defense of grandiosity can be comforting at times but leads to dire consequences.

For the relevant group of male offenders, review attitudes toward women and discuss realistic and respectful characterizations of women.

For most coercive and violent offenders, address antecedents and triggers for coercive violence.

Show respect and interest in the patient's investment in common, legal goods.

*Not meant to be a program for treatment, but contains suggestions for individual psychotherapy compatible with programmatic treatment of sex offenders.

> And be with caution bold.
> Not all that tempts your wandering eyes
> And heedless hearts, is lawful prize;
> Nor all that glisters, gold.

Direct maladaptive behavior occurs when the behavior itself is illegal, such as when a pedophile feels attracted to a young boy and develops a sexual "relationship" with him. He only stops, because of his arrest, when the boy reports the relationship to his teacher. The direct offender is told that he desires a common good, a satisfying sexual relationship with another human being, but that he needs to redirect his impulses of attacking vulnerable children into socially acceptable impulses to relate to equals in a respectful dyadic relationship. The GLM analyst thinks that the pedophile has inadequate social skills and low self-esteem so that he is fearful of relating to person of his own generation. He is told that he is a worthwhile human being but one who needs to learn social skills and cultivate mature relationships.

There is a lot more structure to GLM, but it does give the (correct) impression that GLM, as well as positive psychology, holds the premise that people are basically good (Ward and Maruna 2007, p. 117). Those authors say, for example, that they are not sure if anyone is a pure psychopath because nearly everyone can be helped. They imply that just about everyone can be convinced through their own personal self-interest to become prosocial and law-abiding persons. We tend to think that such a sweeping and heavily value-laden assumption is a bridge too far. We believe that human beings do have some variety of free will and make decisions that can be wrong and can display or develop character that is morally evil. GLM, however, says that "[c]riminal behavior can be understood as the product of distortions in an individual's value/belief system. Yet the origins of these distorted self-narratives are always in the person's cultural environment" (Ward and Maruna 2007, p. 121). There we are again, back to culture as the overwhelming influence on a person's behavior. So although there is much in common between supportive psychotherapy and the Good Lives Model, we do part company on a number of issues, psychopathy being one of them.

Serving Those Who Served

Although the number is going down, veterans now constitute about 8% of prison populations. This group is overwhelmingly male (99%). Three reasons that veterans do end up in prison are:

- Use of alcohol and drugs that is in turn related to adjustment difficulties, trauma history, or difficulties with families.
- Adjustment difficulties related to lack of work or work that lacks the structure of military assignments.
- Economic difficulties leading to illegal actions (Rice-Missouri 2017).
- Behaviors related to PTSD.

There are some differences between the reasons for imprisonment. Income is a little higher in veterans, and homelessness a little less. Compared with nonveterans, veterans are more likely to have been incarcerated for violent and sex offenses, and in military prisons, one in three persons is there for a sex offense, often a sexual assault of a nonstranger. Veterans have less extensive criminal histories than nonveterans but receive longer sentences presumably because of the greater prevalence of violent offenses. Combat veterans are no more likely to be violent than noncombat veterans. Comparing veteran with nonveteran state offenders, veterans are more likely to have known their victims (69% vs. 51%) and much more likely to have victimized a relative (22% vs. 9%), but the victimization of intimates is about the same (11% vs. 9%). Combat veterans, when arrested, were less likely to have a criminal history and so were more likely to be first-time offenders.

Veterans have served their country, and the value system that leads to service and the service itself is more prosocial than that of many other social groups. The problems they get into upon return to civilian life can be related to their military services but certainly not their prosocial and service orientation. However, there will also be a portion of the population who have criminal orientations. In Vietnam veterans a distinction was found between criminality and so-called outlaw behavior that was illegal and related to impulsivity (Pentland and Dwyer 1985).

A felony conviction does not terminate a veteran's benefits. About 80% of veterans were honorably discharged and would be eligible for veterans' benefits (Mumola 2000), but there are some veterans who have no benefits. However, eligibility for medical benefits is wider than eligibility for disability benefits, so there are several situations in which a dishonorably discharged veteran may receive medical benefits.

Veterans may be reluctant to self-identify for fear of losing benefits while incarcerated (which is a law). Nongovernment veterans' groups are active in state prisons and provide a camaraderie that only veterans can give. There are legal restrictions on the services the Veterans Affairs (VA) can provide to prisoners, but the VA is involved in veterans' units and provides reentry services. The use of veterans' units has been associated with a lowered recidivism (9% in 4 years in a New York program reported by Rosenthal and McGuire [2013]).

Mental Illness and Substance Use Disorder in Veterans

Alcohol abuse is higher among prisoners who are veterans than among nonveteran prisoners; abuse of other drugs remains substantial. Rates of mental illness are higher in all settings (for veterans vs. nonveterans, it is 19.3% vs. 15.8% in state prisons, 24.6% vs. 15.2% in local jails, and (a big difference) 13.2% vs. 6.2% in federal prisons (Mumola 2000). It is reported that 9% of federal and 11% of those in state prison with mental illness have been told by a mental health professional that they have PTSD. Eleven percent of federal and 20% of state prison veteran prisoners report co-occurring mental illness (possibly including PTSD) and substance use disorder (including alcohol use disorder).

Suicide risk and traumatic brain injury (TBI) in veterans have received much attention. Fifteen percent of veterans in state prisons and 8% in state prisons report a previous suicide attempt. The Bureau of Justice Statistics did not address TBI, but the VA did actual screening of more than 100,000 veterans and confirmed TBI in 61% (Veterans Health Administration and Defense and Veterans Brain Injury Center 2015). This is much higher than the prevalence in the general community (8.5%), but as we learned in the previous section, TBI had a similarly high rate (60.25%) in one study (Shiroma et al. 2010) and a little lower rate (46%) in a meta-analysis of papers (mostly from the United States) (Durand et al. 2017). The VA has many resources, including a website devoted to PTSD and information about suicide (see Chapter 6).

The mix of TBI and disciplinary action will come up. Special programming for veterans will help. Understanding military culture is important—for example, that military training has to desensitize a soldier to killing (Rosenthal and McGuire 2013). Rosenthal and McGuire (2013) point us to a project of the Walter Reed Army Institute of Research that discussed the training program called "Battlemind," which creates strengths in combat. The program must change as veterans transition from combat to the community. The 10 areas of transition are as follows (Castro et al. 2006, p. 42-5):

- Buddies (cohesion) vs. Withdrawal
- Accountability vs. Controlling
- Targeted Aggression vs. Inappropriate Aggression
- Tactical Awareness vs. Hypervigilance
- Lethally Armed vs. "Locked and Loaded" at home
- Emotional Control vs. Anger/Detachment
- Mission Operational Security (OPSEC) vs. Secretiveness
- Individual Responsibility vs. Guilt
- Non-defensive (combat) Driving vs. Aggressive Driving
- Discipline and Ordering vs. Conflict

Each of these transitions may have created trouble with employers, family, or the law. Each of these represents an issue you can discuss. A veteran convicted of assault might say, "My training kicked in, so I defended myself." He may or may not appreciate, or he may appreciate but be unable to control, his aggression and anger. He may be unaware of or unable to control his secretiveness and personal defensiveness at home. An issue you might face is the use of what we have called "genetic" (e.g., historical) explanations for behavior—in this case, one's military training and experience—as providing an understanding of why your patient did what he did. Does that make him less responsible? Not necessarily. But it provides what most people seek: an understanding of why they acted the way they did and a chance to examine future similar situations that can prompt violent or illegal behavior.

Prisoners With Cognitive Impairment

A portion of incarcerated individuals have low educational attainment and have significant impairments in social and intellectual skills. Prisoners may be affected by poor education; intellectual and developmental disabilities; TBI; abuse, neglect, and poverty at a young age; and other trauma leading to developmental or cognitive impairments. Profoundly impaired individuals with IQs of less than 50 are most likely to be diverted into treatment programs rather than prison, but the low level of cognitive ability in a large portion of the prison community presents a challenge in treatment. The Bureau of Justice Statistics surveyed prisoners in jails and state and federal prisons and, on the basis of self-reporting by those surveyed, found that 4 in 10 jail prisoners and 3 in 10 of those in prison reported having at least one disability. The most common disability reported was cognitive impairment (2 in 10 of those in prison and 3 in 10 of those in jail). In addition, about half reported co-occurring chronic conditions. Prisoners were several times more likely to report psychological distress within the last 30 days, including more than one-third of those with cognitive disabilities (Bronson et al. 2015).

While the criminal offenses of people with cognitive disabilities are similar to those of the incarcerated population at large, the intellectual capabilities of these individuals may vary widely. Lower intelligence is a criminogenic risk, but those with IQ of less than 70 are less likely to offend than individuals with borderline levels of IQ (70–85), and it is also true that persons with borderline intellectual functioning are less likely to commit crimes than people of average intelligence (Mears and Cochran 2009). However, the rates of incarceration for people with intellectual disabilities appear to be higher than those for people of average intelligence, perhaps because this sector of the population also experiences greater deprivations than the population at large, including education, poverty, single parent homes, disadvantaged neighborhoods, and abuse, including bullying (Rice et al. 2020).

Intellectual and cognitive disabilities may be caused by:

- Genetic disorders: Down syndrome, autism spectrum disorders, fragile X syndrome, Prader-Willis syndrome, Smith-Magenis syndrome, Williams syndrome, XYY syndrome.
- Developmental disabilities stemming from physical and mental difficulties such as attachment disorders, ADHD, and comorbidity with other mental disorders.
- Educational disadvantages leading to poor reading and reasoning ability.
- Brain damage from illness, violence, birth defects such as fetal alcohol syndrome, or accident such as TBI.

In jails and prisons, the presence of cognitive impairments may lead to other disadvantages, including a lack of effective treatment, the inability to communicate needs, and the inability to understand correctional culture. Problems both before and during incarceration may include the following (Giamp and West 2003; Marshall-Tate 2019; Rice et al. 2020):

- Failure to diagnose specific disabilities
- Delayed access to treatment
- Difficulties in communication
- Emotional problems in coping with rules
- Abuse by staff and other prisoners
- Comprehension, sensory processing, social functioning, moral reasoning, impulse-control, and anger management
- Victimization and exploitation and injury within the institution
- Disciplinary actions
- Longer sentences with less opportunity for parole largely due to the disciplinary problems
- Lack of services that address their individual problems

Traumatic Brain Injury

Durand et al. (2017) studied research about TBIs in prisoners in several countries. The prevalence of TBI averaged about 46%. Causes included sports injuries, traffic accidents, violence, and explosions. Those with TBI as compared to those without the diagnosis reported more psychiatric disorders, especially anxiety; substance use; epilepsy; and hospital care. Those with TBI reported greater rates of cognitive, memory, and socializing difficulties.

Mood and motor ability problems such as anger, difficulty in processing information, or specific physical functions may result from brain injury as well (Magaletta et al. 2010).

Problems faced by those with TBI include hygiene/grooming, cell sanitation, problems completing work detail assignments, memory impairment, following directions, making decisions, agitation, aggression, and impulsivity.

Intellectual Disabilities

Intellectual disability (ID) is a permanent deficit in intellectual functioning, problem-solving, language limitations (both expressive and receptive), and impulse control, and persons with ID find it difficult to deal with change. Many need support to manage their lives in the community such as supportive housing. ID is also associated with psychiatric conditions, especially aggression and obsession, psychoses, and schizophrenia. Physical problems include seizures, sleep apnea, and hypothyroidism. People with IDs in prison are vulnerable to the social conditions and the physical environment of incarceration and may need staff to give them protection and attention. The stressors of prison, including the structure of prison life and the vulnerability of persons with IDs to bullying and exploitation by others, as well as lack of understanding by staff, can make the prison experience more difficult. In addition, prisoners with ID are more likely to receive disciplinary actions because of failure to follow rules and aggressive behavior, often because their communication skills are inadequate (Kalinowski 2007).

Autism Spectrum Disorder

While not all people with autism spectrum disorder have low cognitive functioning in terms of learning, they do present with a lack of social skills and understanding and are prone to obsessional behaviors that can lead to criminal offenses. Their deficits include social naivete leading to opportunities to be exploited, inability to process changes to routines, and poor understanding of social communications (Kalinowski 2007).

Fetal Alcohol Syndrome

Birth defects such as fetal alcohol syndrome, defects due to use of other substances, and defects due to illness or accident during pregnancy can cause behavioral and cognitive problems in children that persist into adulthood. These include problems with cognition, memory, language, executive functioning, motor functioning, attention deficits, social skill deficits, and sensory problems. These problems lead to disruption in school and with the law, with an estimated 50% facing some form of incarceration (Kalinowski 2007).

Down Syndrome and Other Genetic Syndromes

People born with genetic syndromes may present with emotional and physical problems as well. Disruptive behavior, psychiatric disorders, and social and executive problem-solving are often issues for them. Problems leading to incarceration can include naivete about right and wrong, the inability to follow directions, and poor problem-solving. Since genetic effects may be visible, as with Down syndrome, bullying, abuse, and neglect are common.

Low Educational Attainment

In addition to genetic and physical causes of ID, many prisoners have very low educational attainment due to problems in school or in the education system itself, neglect or abuse in childhood interfering with school achievement, homelessness leading to frequent schooling disruption, or high dropout rates. Prisoners with low literacy rates in both reading and math may also be deficient in reasoning and understanding skills. The Rand Corporation conducted a study for the Bureau of Justice Statistics on the value of education as part of prison programs and found that education reduces recidivism by as much as 40%, particularly GED and postsecondary and vocational education (see Chapter 14). However, many prisoners have very low education attainment compared with the general population. In 2004, 37% of prisoners had completed less than a high school degree compared with 19% of the population overall, and literacy levels were also much lower (Davis 2019). Education programs in prison have been improving since 2004, with an estimated 95% of prisons offering high school–level courses, but some prison programs are not available to all, and many individuals have a literacy level of less than 4th grade. Rampey et al. (2016) conducted a survey and assessment of literacy, reading comprehension, numeracy, and problem-solving in the context of use of technology among incarcerated adults. They found that compared with the population at large, those in prison faced many disadvantages, including the following:

- Education level. Only 4% of the prison population had an associate degree or higher, 64% completed high school, but 30% had not completed high school.
- Literacy level. Prisoners scored significantly lower than the general population on the literacy scale.
- Numeracy. Prisoners scored significantly lower than the general population on the numeracy scale.

Treatment and Interventions

With all cognitive disabilities, there is a need for staff awareness and training to identify the specific deficits that each individual experiences. Working with individuals with cognitive problems requires sensitivity to the limits of their understanding and, likely, considerable repetition, strategies for dealing with emotional and cognitive concreteness, and understanding of lack of both nuance and self-awareness on the part of patients. In particular, cognitive impairments that are not the result of inferior education or treatable mental disorders may not be treated so much as managed. That is, genetic and brain injury may in fact be a permanent condition for the patient, and therefore treatment strategies need to help the patient adapt and improve skills. For example, TBI patients may get worse in terms of aggression over time (Magaletta et al. 2010) but may learn to control impulses, and Down syndrome patients will not improve in IQ but may learn better ways of functioning. Specific areas to be addressed are impulse control, communication, decision-making, and social skills as discussed below.

Social problem-solving is a challenge for persons with IDs. Because these individuals have trouble with complex and nuanced communications, they may become confused and disruptive when presented with the need to follow directions, plan tasks, or face discipline for not being able to do these things. Verbal skills of patients with IDs are also limited, and their thinking tends to be concrete. Such patients are very aware of their disability and have had a lifetime of shame and embarrassment about their ID, including, in many cases, bullying and abuse. While those with significant impairments are most often diverted from the prison system, those with more moderate disabilities might find themselves angry at their circumstances but without the skills necessary to find a way forward. Many may have developed a "learned helplessness" that gives them an excuse not to behave (Novalis et al. 2020).

Patients with IDs may approach therapy with significant trepidation and distrust, so it helps to begin with emotional support, explaining the purpose of each session and your plans for proceeding with therapy and medication, if needed, should be clear and concise (Keller 2000). Approaches to treating people with intellectual disabilities in prison should begin with establishing a therapeutic alliance that takes into consideration the level of communication skills that the patent has. For example, if a patient is less verbal, acting out feelings or drawing might help. Your language should be simple, straightforward, and compassionate. You will need patience when communication stalls and progress is slower than "normal." Also, it may be difficult for some of these patients to complete homework assignments once the therapy session is over, so finding activities that can be done in short spurts with your guidance is important. Repetition will be important, and tools such as short lists of things to be remembered and perhaps worked on between sessions may assist the progress of therapy.

Prison environments are harsh and structured and can be quite hostile. Supportive psychotherapy techniques and education should be focused on helping the individual to recognize and improve the person's own strengths and overcome negative feelings of depression, anxiety, and the fears faced in the prison environment. Identifying activities that can alleviate some of the unpleasantness, such as art, entertainment, or improving skills and knowledge can help the individual develop a sense of self-efficacy, even in such an environment.

Morasky (2007) identified four components of therapy that you should use in planning the treatment of patients with IDs:

- Speed of thought. Patients may take longer to communicate problems and feelings.
- Number of problems. Starting with difficulty in understanding the world around them, patients face physical, mental, and emotional issues because of both their deficits and their history.
- Abstraction. Patients with IDs have difficulty in understanding abstract concepts.
- Complexity. Such patients may not be able to predict or understand consequences of actions and decisions.

Talking to Your Intellectually Disabled Patients

People with IDs have difficulty in communicating verbally because their reading and comprehension are limited, physically because they have not learned to read physical communications, and intuitively because they tend to be concrete in their thinking and lack ability to be abstract or nuanced in communication. They may not have learned to think about the consequences of their problems or their actions and tend to act impulsively as a result. Such patients also need frequent repetition and reminders of both the purpose of the therapy and the progress made. When you are treating people with cognitive disabilities, it is important to answer simple questions, repeat the questions and answers as necessary, and have the patient put the question in his own words to make sure that it is understood. You should also look at techniques such as role-playing, art, and nonverbal cues to communicate.

In prison, the challenges to this population begin in becoming acclimated to the institution, its rules, and its culture, especially where special programs for the ID population are not available. Therapy and education should focus initially on this adaptation, with habilitation for life after prison the goal of a complete program (Arrigo and Shipley 2005).

In counseling, several factors are important. Insight and behavior may not be closely related: your patient may be able to repeat your advice but be unable to actually follow through on a behavior. Therapy and discussions need to proceed in smaller steps with this group and repetition and review are necessary. He may not remember the advice, so you should consider making out a crisis response safety plan as in previous chapters. The wording should be simple, direct, and at the patient's reading and comprehension level. It may be helpful to develop this "card" into a "memory" book and add information from therapy sessions as needed. For individuals who have difficulty reading, having the patient make drawings about problems may make the solutions easier to understand. The cognitively impaired patient may find it difficult to apply things learned about one situation to another, so it may be helpful to teach methods of considering the consequences of behavior before acting. Be straightforward with your patient about behaviors when they are inappropriate. Other points to consider (Substance Abuse and Mental Health Services Administration 2012):

- Modify materials to make sure they are concise and to the point.
- Give several examples and present material is several ways.
- Encourage use of the memory book.
- Use the memory book to remind the patient of appointments, homework assignments, and specific lessons.
- Review main points before and after each session.
- Help with assignments and give a lot of feedback.
- Recognize that noncompliance may not be resistance, but may reflect attention deficits.

Key Points

- Using the concept of culture and the DSM-5 Cultural Formulation Interview, we see how culture profoundly affects the conduct of psychotherapy and the psychotherapist.

- Those whom we call "time-challenged" prisoners require special attention because their lives are dominated by prison time, which creates major limitations for them.

- Sex offenders have often been considered reprehensible and untreatable. The Good Lives Model, which is related to positive psychology and shares many of the assumptions of supportive psychotherapy, is an approach that shows promise in offering the goods and benefits that most people desire as a way for sex offenders to change their behavior in a prosocial manner.

- Incarcerated veterans are an important part of the prison population (about 8%) and have issues regarding violent crime and sex crimes, often with non-strangers, as well as suicide risk and traumatic brain injury.

- A significant number of inmates have intellectual disabilities, developmental problems, and poor educational attainment.

- Inmates with intellectual and educational limitations frequently have problems in abstraction and may have trouble verbalizing their problems.

References

Arrigo BA, Shipley SL: Introduction to Forensic Psychology: Issues and Controversies in Law, Law Enforcement, and Corrections, 2nd Edition. Burlington, MA, Academic Press/Elsevier, 2005

Beauchamp TL, Childress JL: Principles of Biomedical Ethics, 8th Edition. New York, Oxford University Press, 2019

Bronson J, Maruschak LM, Berzofsky M: Disabilities Among Prison and Jail Inmates, 2011–2012. NCJ 249141. Washington, DC, Bureau of Justice Statistics, December 14, 2015. Available at: www.bjs.gov/index.cfm?ty=pbdetail&iid=5500. Accessed December 26, 2020.

Campbell S: Can therapy make your loss worse? Psychology Today, August 2, 2002; last reviewed June 9, 2016

Castro CA, Hoge CW, Cox AL: Battlemind training: building soldier resiliency, in Human Dimensions in Military Operations—Military Leaders' Strategies for Addressing Stress and Psychological Support. Meeting Proceedings RTO-MP-HFM-134, Paper 42. Neuilly-sur-Seine, France, RTO, 2006, pp 42-1–42-6. Available at: https://apps.dtic.mil/dtic/tr/fulltext/u2/a472734.pdf. Accessed November 27, 2020.

Courtney K: Cultural aspects of correctional psychiatry, in Correctional Psychiatry: Practice Guidelines and Strategies, Vol II. Edited by Thienhaus OJ, Piasecki M. Kingston, NJ, Civic Research Institute, 2013, pp 3-1–3-23

Crumbaugh J, Maholick L: Manual for Instructions for the Purpose-in-Life Test. Munster, IN, Psychometric Affiliates, 1969

Cullen M: Cage Your Rage: An Inmate's Guide to Anger Control, Second Edition. Alexandria, VA, American Correctional Association, 2013

Davis LM: Higher education programs in prison: what we know now and what we should focus on going forward. Santa Monica, CA. RAND Corporation, August 28, 2019. Available at: www.rand.org/pubs/perspectives/PE342.html. Accessed February 20, 2021.

Desmond-Hurst B (dir): A Christmas Carol (Orig. title Scrooge). Starring Alistair Sim. Renown Pictures, George Minter Productions, 1951

Doerflinger DMC: Mental Status Assessment in Older Adults: Montreal Cognitive Assessment: MoCA Version 7.0 (Original Version). Try This: Best Nursing Practices in Nursing Care to Older Adults, Issue No. 3.2, Revised 2012. Available at: https://micmt-cares.org/system/files/mental%20status%20assessment%20in%20older%20adults%20moca_0.pdf. Accessed August 17, 2020.

Durand E, Chevignard M, Ruet A, et al: History of traumatic brain injury in prison populations: a systematic review. Ann Phys Rehabil Med 60(2):95–101, 2017 28359842

Epstein J: Biden apologizes for comments on racial diversity among blacks. Bloomberg, Aug. 2, 2020. Available at: www.bloomberg.com/news/articles/2020-08-07/biden-apologizes-for-comments-on-racial-diversity-among-blacks. Accessed December 6, 2020.

Gert B: Common Morality: Deciding What to Do. New York, Oxford University Press, 2014

Giamp JS, West ME: Delivering psychological service to incarcerated men with developmental disabilities, in Correctional Psychology: Practice, Programming, and Administration. Edited by Schwartz BK. Kingston, NJ, Civic Research Institute, 2003, pp 8-1–8-31

Gray T: Ode on the death of a favourite cat drowned in a tub of goldfishes (1747). Poetry Foundation. Available at: www.poetryfoundation.org/poems/44302/ode-on-the-death-of-a-favourite-cat-drowned-in-a-tub-of-goldfishes. Accessed August 1, 2020.

Kalinowski C: Working with individuals who have intellectual disabilities, in Correctional Psychiatry: Practice Guidelines and Strategies. Edited by Thienhaus OJ, Piasecki M. Kingston, NJ, Civic Research Institute, 2007, pp 14-1–14-21

Kapoor R, Griffith EEH: Cultural competence, in Oxford Textbook of Correctional Psychiatry. Edited by Trestman RL, Applebaum KL, Metzner JL. New York, Oxford University Press, 2015, pp 341–346

Keller E: Points of intervention: facilitating the process of psychotherapy with people who have developmental disabilities, in Therapy Approaches for Persons with Mental Retardation. Edited by Fletcher RJ. Kingston, NJ, NADD Press, 2000, pp 27–47

Knoll JL: Discussing the meaning of life with a "lifer." Psychiatric Times 26(9):1, 4, 5, 8, 2009. Available at: www.psychiatrictimes.com/view/discussing-meaning-life-lifer. Accessed August 7, 2020.

Kok RM, Reynolds CF 3rd: Management of depression in older adults: a review. JAMA 317(20):2114–2122, 2017 28535241

Lennon JJ: The apology letter. Washington Post Magazine, October 28, 2019. Available at: www.washingtonpost.com/magazine/2019/10/28/ive-built-career-prolific-prison-journalist-so-why-did-it-take-me-so-long-write-letter-family-man-i-killed/?arc404=true. Accessed January 1, 2021.

Levine PB, McKnight R: Three million more guns: the Spring 2020 spike in firearm sales. Brookings Up Front, July 13, 2020. Available at: www.brookings.edu/blog/up-front/2020/07/13/three-million-more-guns-the-spring-2020-spike-in-firearm-sales. Accessed October 18, 2020.

Magaletta PR, Diamond PM, McLearen AM, Denney RL: Traumatic brain injuries in correctional populations—understanding and responding to an important need, in Managing Special Populations in Jails and Prisons. Edited by Stojkovic J. Kingston, NJ, Civic Research Institute, 2010, pp 20-1–20-12

Marshall-Tate K: Learning disabilities: supporting people in the criminal justice system. Nursing Times June 17, 2019

Mayer M: Energy Psychology: Self-Healing Practices for Bodymind Health. Berkeley, CA, North Atlantic Books, 2009

Mears DP, Cochran JC: What is the effect of IQ on offending? Crim Justice Behav 40(11):1280–1300, 2009

Morasky RI: Making counseling/therapy intellectually available. NADD Bulletin X(3):3, 2007

Morris EJ: Respect, protection, faith, and love: major care constructs identified within the subculture of selected urban African American adolescent gang members. J Transcult Nurs 23(3):262–269, 2012 22477722

Mumola C: Veterans in Prison or Jail. NCJ 178888. Washington, DC, Bureau of Justice Statistics, March 2000. Available at: www.bjs.gov/content/pub/pdf/vpj.pdf. Accessed November 27, 2020.

Natapoff A: Punishment Without Crime: How Our Massive Misdemeanor System Traps the Innocent and Makes America More Unequal. New York, Basic Books, 2018

Novalis PN, Peele R, Singer VS: Clinical Manual of Supportive Psychotherapy, 2nd Edition. Washington, DC, American Psychiatric Association Publishing, 2020

Pentland B, Dwyer J: Incarcerated Viet Nam veterans, in The Trauma of War: Stress and Recovery in Viet Nam Veterans. Edited by Sonnenberg SM, Blank AS, Talbott JA. Washington, DC, American Psychiatric Press, 1985, pp 403–416

Przybylski R: The effectiveness of treatment for adult sex offenders, in Sex Offender Management Assessment AND Planning Initiative. NCJ 247059. Washington, DC, Office of Justice Programs, March 2017 (updated), pp 155–179. Available at: https://smart.ojp.gov/somapi/initiative-home#rfl4xq. Accessed August 1, 2020.

Quote/Counterquote: "Whenever I hear the word 'culture'…" April 30, 2019. Available at: www.quotecounterquote.com/2011/02/whenever-i-hear-word-culture.html?m=1. Accessed October 18, 2020.

Rampey BD, Mohadjer L, Xie H, et al: Highlight from the U.S. PIAAC Survey of Incarcerated Adults: Their Skills, Work Experience, Education, and Training. Washington, DC, National Center for Education Statistics, 2016

Reiman J: The Rich Get Richer and the Poor Get Prison: Thinking Critically about Class and Criminal Justice. New York, Routledge, 2020

Rice LJ, Einfeld SL, Howlin P: Behavioural and cognitive phenotypes in genetic disorders associated with offending, in The Wiley Handbook on What Works for Offenders With Intellectual and Developmental Disabilities. Edited by Lindsay WR, Craig LA, Griffiths D. Hoboken, NJ, Wiley, 2020, pp 69–98

Rice-Missouri S: 3 reasons U.S. veterans end up in prison. Futurity, September 6, 2017. Available at: www.futurity.org/military-veterans-prison-1535212. Accessed November 27, 2020.

Rios VM: Punished: Policing the Lives of Black and Latino boys. New York, New York University Press, 2012

Rosenthal J, McGuire J: Incarcerated veterans, in Special Needs Offenders in Correctional Institutions. Edited by Gideon L. Thousand Oaks, CA, Sage, 2013, pp 345–376

Saleh FM, Grudzinskas AJ, Malin HM: Treatment of incarcerated sex offenders, in Oxford Textbook of Correctional Psychiatry. Edited by Trestman RL, Applebaum KL, Metzner JL. New York, Oxford University Press, 2015, pp 336–340

Shiroma EJ, Ferguson PL, Pickelsimer EE: Prevalence of traumatic brain injury in an offender population: a meta-analysis. J Correct Health Care 16(2):147–159, 2010 20339132

Simon KM: How can we better engage black men as patients? Clinical Psychiatry News 48(7):8, June 20, 2020

Stanford University: Geriatric Depression Scale. 2020. Available at: https://web.stanford.edu/~yesavage/GDS.html. Accessed August 19, 2020.

St Louis University: SLU Mental Status Exam (SLUMS). Available at: www.slu.edu/medicine/internal-medicine/geriatric-medicine/aging-successfully/assessment-tools/mental-status-exam.php. Accessed August 17, 2020.

Substance Abuse and Mental Health Services Administration: Substance Use Disorder Treatment for People With Physical and Cognitive Disabilities. Treatment Protocol (TIP) 29. SMA12-4078. Rockville, MD, U.S. Department of Health and Human Services, July 2012. Available at: https://store.samhsa.gov/product/TIP-29-Substance-Use-Disorder-Treatment-for-People-With-Physical-and-Cognitive-Disabilities/SMA12-4078.

Veatch RM: Is there a common morality? Kennedy Institute of Ethics Journal 13(3):189–192, September 2003

Veterans Health Administration, Departments of Veterans Affairs, and Defense and Veterans Brain Injury Center, Department of Defense: VA Traumatic Brain Injury Veterans Health Registry Report (cumulative from 1st Qtr FY 2002 through 4th Qtr FY 2013, October 2001 through September 2013). Released May 2015. Available at: www.publichealth.va.gov/docs/epidemiology/TBI-report-fy2013-qtr4.pdf. Accessed November 27, 2020.

Wade JC: The case of the angry black man, in In the Room With Men: A Casebook of Therapeutic Change. Edited by Englar-Carlson M, Stevens MA. Washington, DC, American Psychological Association, 2006, pp 177–196

Ward T, Maruna S: Rehabilitation. New York, Routledge, 2007

Wexler DB: Men in Therapy: New Approaches for Effective Treatment. New York, WW Norton, 2009

White J: The Genocidal Healer. New York, Ballantine Books, 1991

White J: Alien Emergencies: A Sector General Omnibus. New York, Tor Books, 2002

Yates PM, Prescott DS: Building a Better Life: A Good Lives and Self-Regulation Workbook. Brandon, VT, Safer Society Press, 2011

Yates PM, Prescott DS, Ward T: Applying the Good Lives and Self-Regulation Models to Sex Offender Treatment: A Practical Guide for Clinicians. Brandon, VT, Safer Society Press, 2010

Zehr H: Changing Lenses: A New Focus for Crime and Justice. Scottsdale, PA, Herald Press, 1990

Zehr H, Gohar A: The Little Book of Restorative Justice. 2003. Available at: https://sites.unicef.org/tdad/littlebookrjpakaf.pdf. Accessed January 29, 2021.

14

Time to Say Goodbye

*More broadly, desistance from crime is intimately tied to social and eco-
nomic reintegration. (Harding et al. 2019, p. 8)*

Almost all people come from families, homes, and communities
where they have freedom: to move about, seek jobs and friendships, and make their
own decisions, however right or wrong. When people come into contact with the
criminal justice system, that changes. A person could certainly consider his entry into
a correctional facility as an alien experience—as described in the introduction to this
book, it might even be like a Close Encounter of the Fourth Kind. Or, using a word we
have heard repeatedly over the past few years, it has been described as similar to putting someone in quarantine—a behavior of a of a risk-averse society that fails to provide
the opportunities to pursue prosocial lifestyles to persons with criminal records (Ward
and Maruna 2007, p. 81).

Less obvious, perhaps, is that *leaving* the system might seem like leaving a spaceship
and visiting an Earth that looks and feels like an alien planet, and without a space suit
for protection! For one thing, one's drop-off point may be far from home; for another,
it is certainly another environment and culture, and the returnee's contact with her
last locale and the people in it (even the food, occupation, and activities) may be completely changed or even unfathomable.

Throughout this book, we have discussed the stresses of entering prison and how
the experience can be traumatic. Leaving prison might therefore seem to be a good
thing or a great relief, but for some people it can be as traumatic as entering prison in
the first place. Returning to society is especially challenging to individuals who have
problems with mental illness, substance use, low educational levels, or a history of
poverty, abuse, or trauma.

According to a Bureau of Justice Statistics report (Alper et al. 2018), over a 9-year
period, 83% of people who left prison were rearrested, with 44% rearrested in the first
year, 68% arrested within the first 3 years, and 79% within 6 years. Excluding parole and
probation arrests would have reduced the recidivism rate overall to 82%. Since American jails and prisons release between 600,000 and 800,000 people each year, the scope
of the problem is obvious (Nelson and Trone 2000). Clearly, programs that can address

this problem are necessary. Preparing individuals for the end of their sentences and helping them to be successful must be a goal of programs within prisons and in the community. This chapter explores the problems faced by released prisoners and the ways in which therapists can assist them in finding a way forward.

Challenges of Leaving

Ninety-eight percent of people in prison will return to society—some after many years, some after just a year or two—but all will face barriers to success and problems in adjusting, especially if the socioeconomic and educational resources available to them are limited. Leaving prison raises obstacles in obtaining housing, jobs, and health care; reestablishing (or leaving) pre-prison relationships; caring for oneself and family; and perhaps, most importantly, navigating the world while desisting from crime.

Anybody who works in a psychiatric hospital knows that treatment plans have a section for discharge planning that is part of the treatment from the moment of arrival. Similarly, Petersilia (2003) recommends that prisons build programs that from the very beginning of incarceration focus on preparing individuals for leaving. She suggests that prison environments change to more closely resemble society at large with work, education, recreation, and community activities that help individuals become accustomed to the rhythms and norms of society in a prosocial way. The scope of reentry research and program development over the past two decades has shown the success of targeted programs and intensive treatment in helping more successful reentry and reducing recidivism.

Harding et al. (2019) describe reentry as a process that proceeds unevenly; there will be progress and backslides, and there will be leaps toward success and frustrations. For some, the outcome of reentry will depend on the motivation of the individual and/or the practical challenges of finding and keeping housing and jobs or affording education. For others, it will depend on whether relationships with family can be reestablished. Requirements for reporting to authorities under parole and probation structures, or for participating in day programs, substance use disorder programs, and other activities, are designed to help, but adding another layer of responsibility for the individual can also hinder success.

It still seems early to see if large-scale reduction of jail and prison populations due to COVID-19 will affect recidivism statistics, but this event, which was of course not predicted, should encourage programs in prisons to focus sooner rather than later on preparing individuals for life after prison. While data are still preliminary, such states as New Jersey (Star-Ledger Editorial Board 2022) report that the recidivism rate for those released due to COVID-19 is low: only 9% of the first 2,500 persons released were reincarcerated over the next 14 months as compared with the historical figure of 14%. The year 2020 saw fluctuations in crime rates and led to, as of mid-2021, a concern about the increase in violence in the large cities. The movements against social injustice and systemic racism have led to examination and review of policies concerning incarceration rates and prison conditions and programs. An interesting study conducted by Kuziemko (2013) looked at recidivism in Georgia after changes to parole and sentencing guidelines resulted in early unplanned release of prisoners. Kuziemko draws two major conclusions. The first is that the length of prison sentences directly affects the rate of recidivism, with 1 month longer time in prison associated with more than 3% reduction in recidivism. The second is that providing incentives toward lessening sentences is effective. Recidivism was also reduced when prisoners had the ability, through education, work, and other goals, to directly affect the length of their sentences when compared to fixed sentences, by working to reduce their own recidivism.

Haney (2002) suggests comprehensive changes in the approach that institutions take in preparing individuals to reintegrate into society. These include:

- Prison systems should develop decompression programs to reacclimate people to the "free world" (p. 7).
- They should provide prisoners insight into the ways prison life has changed them.
- They should provide job training and job placement services.
- They should have specialized services for those with mental illness and/or developmental disabilities both before and after release.
- Services in the community for those returning must take the needs of the individuals into account, and coordination between the institution and the community service providers is vital. The primary goals of postrelease services must be gainful employment, family counseling, and support and housing.
- Parole and probation services need to be reoriented toward helping individuals to succeed in transitioning to home rather than controlling every detail of behavior, with return to prison a last resort (Haney 2002, p. 7; see also Haney 2020).

Petersilia (2003) has similar recommendations, with an emphasis on increasing the continuity of services and conditions from incarceration through successful reentry. One recommendation is to have reentry courts that function like drug and mental health courts. In the years since Haney and Petersilia began their work, in fact, orientation of prison programs has shifted toward these goals. The U.S. Department of Justice (2017) developed a Roadmap to Recovery that lays out five components to lessen recidivism:

1. Individualized plans for reentry that reduce risks of recidivism
2. Education, employment training, life skills, and substance use and mental health treatment
3. Resources and opportunity to maintain family relationships and strengthening of the support system that will help individuals succeed
4. During transition back to the community, halfway houses and supervised release services
5. During incarceration, comprehensive information and access to resources necessary for success

Mears and Cochran (2015) discuss the need for such programs to begin by preparing individuals for life in prison before or as they begin their sentences so that they learn how to best use their time in order to be successful in reentry.

Practical Aspects of Reentry

Obstacles faced by those returning to the community are practical, emotional, and physical. Underlying many of these problems can be structural racism as well as negative attitudes toward those who have been in prison.

Having a Place to Live

Many individuals returning to the community will move at least once within the first few months after leaving prison. An editorial in the *Los Angeles Times* about the needs of services for people in light of the effort to reduce incarcerated populations to prevent spread of the COVID-19 virus cited the need for housing as the most immediate need. Beyond temporary housing that was created to accommodate a large "outflux" from the jail, concern for stable placement beyond temporary housing was a key concern (Los Angeles Times Editorial Board 2020). Another factor in reentry is that families are in many cases without adequate resources and may find it difficult to help support the person in their homes because of cost, space, and restrictions on who might be eligible to live in the apartment, including the need for background checks (Mears and Cochran 2015).

Finding a Job

It is well established that the ability to find a job is essential to success in reentry (Tharshini et al. 2018). Barriers to finding work include low skill levels and experience, the requirements of parole/probation reporting, difficulties accessing transportation, and background checks that make many jobs unattainable. Also, many of the jobs that people get are low paying and physically demanding in terms of the work and the time and resources needed to manage life needs such as health care and child care. It is unclear at this writing how the changing employment needs of businesses after the COVID-19 pandemic will affect this. Meeting financial obligations of legal fees, treatment costs, and commuting as well as rent and food can be daunting. One approach might be transitional jobs programs that provide jobs that are subsidized, giving them an income and the opportunity to gain experience (Latessa et al. 2015).

Credit

With no immediate income other than public assistance, individuals returning to the community may not be able to afford the costs of job hunting and education. Moreover, many will have incurred such expenses as fees levied from the time of incarceration, including processing fees, court costs, and costs of electronic monitoring. Entry-level jobs may barely cover their living expenses, let alone let them acquire the resources to establish credit for such things as rent deposits, tuition for school, and other expenses.

Transportation

Many jobs (and certainly the job hunting), parole officer meetings, and prescribed treatment or community service locations often will not be close to where the newly released person is living. Costs of transportation and the inconvenience of public transit may hamper timeliness and attendance and, indeed, the willingness to persevere. As we said earlier, having a car was a significant factor in post-incarceration success.

Probation/Parole

Most former prisoners enter the probation/parole system (some individuals are in both because of multiple arrests). In 2018, there were about 878,000 people in the parole system in the United States (Kaeble and Alper 2020). Generally, about 80% of prisoners enter the parole system. The community justice system exerts considerable control over the lives of participants, including electronic monitoring, frequent reporting, unscheduled home visits, and prescribed courses of treatment. Parolees are subject to strict requirements as well as expected to be law abiding. Many feel that it is just another term of imprisonment. Indeed, they are held to a much more stringent set of behavioral standards than the general population is, with minor or technical violations sometimes a ticket back to the institution. Although the number of people reincarcerated for parole violations is small—about 1% of recidivism overall (Alper et al. 2018)—parole and probation services are costly, and merging them with other postrelease programs might result in better outcomes.

Voting

Some states still prohibit those previously incarcerated for felonies and parolees from voting. Lack of participation exacerbates a sense of detachment from society as a whole among this population.

Stigma and Discrimination

People who have served time find that that status may persist for many years if not their whole lives and in fact may feel ashamed of their history. Public assistance, housing, jobs, and social connections are very often adversely affected. Even simple identification may be difficult to obtain. This was evident in the spring of 2020 when many bureaucratic offices were shut down because of COVID-19. Many job and housing applications require background checks, and a criminal history limits opportunities.

An ex-prisoner faces social stigma because of his "record." He may also have a personal feeling of shame for having been in prison or having committed a crime that caused hurt to someone else. He may have an adjustment disorder as a result of his criminal history, a mental illness, and the incarceration. Many prisoners come from poor communities and are from minority groups who face racist attitudes in society, and having a history in the criminal justice system, a history of mental illness, and poor work experience all contribute to the stigma and barriers to success even if the person is able to avoid criminal behavior. People who have been in therapy in prison may need mental health services after leaving.

Personal Relationships

As people serve out their sentences, their families and friends live their lives, grow up, and change. This may be true of the people in prison as well, but the development is taking place in parallel universes, with phone calls, letters, and visits being rare, often expensive, and insufficient to maintaining relationships. The family situation of some former prisoners may sometimes, in fact, be one of the causes of the criminal behavior, because of a culture of illegal activities, negative and often traumatic history with members of the family, or simply poverty and lack of resources. Although maintaining personal relationships during incarceration is more difficult for all prisoners, it is especially difficult for parents hoping to reestablish their connection with children when they return home. Women in prison are especially affected since there are fewer facilities for women, most often only one in a given state. Increasing visitation, including video meetings, and making phone calls more accessible are practical actions that can help incarcerated individuals maintain relationships (Mears and Cochran 2015).

For parents, relationships with children may be adversely affected by the incarceration. Alternative custody arrangements may have been in place, and the children may have become emotionally estranged from the parent who has been gone. Prison life puts up many barriers to keeping up family relationships, from distance to the prison, limited visiting hours and opportunities, expensive telephone services, and limited email accessibility (Hairston 2003). Many correctional systems are beginning to offer parent education and training related to interpersonal relationships, family dynamics, and violence within families to assist individuals after they leave.

Cultural Changes

Some people have been incarcerated for a long time, even decades. With the availability of technology, interactions with the outside world are more accessible now than ever before, but the equipment and technology available within an institution are usually not the same as outside. Mores change as well: even something as simple as clothing styles can be disorienting. For example, before the turn of the century, clothing was much more formal, especially in work and church attendance. With COVID-19, as another example, many more people are working from home. Rideshare and food delivery services are only a few years old, and much of television is now streaming rather than broadcast. The COVID-19 pandemic also brought about such changes as mask-wearing and social distancing.

Mental and Physical Health

Inadequate education, low literacy, mental health issues and substance use, poverty, systemic racism, and extreme adversity in early childhood all contribute to the causes of crime and mental and physical health problems. As we have documented in many places, being in prison is also a time of adversity. Stressor-related disorders are common issues, as are any underlying medical and mental problems (see Chapter 6). A mitigating factor is that health care, and especially mental health care, if used by the individual, may be more accessible in prison, where it is free, although perhaps more limited than in the community. One aspect of reentry that we emphasize here is that continuity of care and coordination between in-prison services and the community to which the patient returns are critical to successful reentry.

Released prisoners will do better if they continue to take appropriately prescribed medications. For example, researchers evaluating the use of psychotropic medications among a cohort of violent offenders in Sweden found that postrelease violence was reduced when medications were used appropriately (Chang et al. 2016).

Since more than 60% of justice-involved individuals used substances prior to incarceration, many will resume these behaviors once back in the community. People who work with newly released prisoners are familiar with the Saturday night overdose phenomenon. Such individuals are often treated in hospitals for unintended overdoses of alcohol and drugs. Having been sober because of the lack of opportunity in prison, individuals are not always aware that they have lost their tolerance for substances used prior to incarceration. A study in North Carolina found that those who were newly released were 40 times more likely to die of an opioid overdose than were individuals in the community as a whole (Ranapurwala et al. 2018). Merrall et al. (2010) estimated that there was a three- to eightfold increased risk of drug-related deaths in the first few weeks after reentry compared with the subsequent 3 months. In fact, the leading cause of death after release is drug overdose, especially in the first few weeks (followed by cardiovascular disease, suicide, cancer, and motor vehicle accidents). This suggests that programs for substance use disorders may be of paramount importance in prison and in postrelease programming and that attention to health, and especially mental health, might improve outcomes (Binswanger et al. 2007). A review of a broad sample of studies found that prison programs addressing substance use can lead to a reduction of use once individuals return to the community. Opioid maintenance treatment is effective in treating opioid use disorder in prison and after, reducing substance use disorder and recidivism (de Andrade et al. 2018; Fox et al. 2015).

Leaving prison may exacerbate preexisting mental and physical problems, since health care is more accessible, if not ideal, within the institution and accessing services in the community may be more difficult. The abrupt change in conditions can also lead to further health problems. Dealing with disorientation; reestablishing relationships; getting reestablished in job, home, and community; finding needed services; and complying with parole requirements are major stressors that lead to health problems (Middlemass 2017; Wallace et al. 2015). A study conducted with the Washington State Department of Corrections from 1999 to 2003 found that the death rate for recently released prisoners was as much as 3.5 times that of the general public and 12.7 times that of the population at large in the first 2 weeks of reentry (Binswanger et al. 2007).

Health interventions, especially mental health services, have been shown to reduce reoffending of the seriously mentally ill, especially programs that help patients navigate return to the community through therapy and social services (Hopkin et al. 2018). Dual diagnosis patients should be directly enrolled in both substance use disorder treatment programs and psychiatric services for maintaining their mental health therapy and medications. Coordination between prison therapists and outside services, if allowed, should be a priority. In discussing barriers to mental health care among African Americans, Rostain et al. (2015) recommend increasing awareness of public programs and low-cost insurance, providing education about the nature of illnesses and the appropriate treatments, using remote access such as telemedicine to increase availability of services, and providing enhanced cultural training for professionals including recognizing biases and advocating for the patient. We would add that this is true for former prisoners in general, especially those in minority groups, low-income areas, and rural areas where services are few.

Paperwork

In almost all of the potential problems discussed above, an individual will encounter the need to fill out an application (e.g., for a job, housing, or health insurance). The paperwork can be intimidating and the questionnaires can be difficult to understand. The difficulty is magnified when the individual has limited education or is not fluent in English. Required information, such as birth certificates, credit history, and even photo identification, can be difficult to obtain and expensive to procure, especially before a person has a job.

Psychological and Emotional Challenges of Leaving Prison

Prison changes people. Some of these changes are easily reversed by many individuals. Others are more lasting and different individuals will react differently. The loss of personal control over even the most mundane details of life in prison can lead to disorientation when most or all of these decisions are now required. Some of the results are subtle as individuals adapt to the strictures of the prison environment and culture, but many are quite profound, even in some cases leading to adjustment disorders or PTSD (see Chapter 6). Haney (2002) does not believe that these changes are pathological or dysfunctional for most prisoners; rather he considers them to be adaptive responses to the circumstances.

Even a cursory review shows that there are many programs being run successfully by corrections departments and charitable organizations around the country. Criminal justice reform has become a major issue in American politics and the COVID-19 pandemic as well as the recent demonstrations protesting police use of excessive force have accelerated the discussion. In some cases, decarceration has been increased in order to protect the health of individuals. These programs include diversionary programs such as drug and mental health courts before imposing prison sentences; education, counseling, and training programs in the institutions, including internships and work release programs; and programs such as halfway houses, addiction treatment, day centers, and education and job training and placement services (Nelson and Trone 2000). In some states and in the federal prison system, the rate of incarceration increased steadily from the 1990s through 2010. In recent years, that rate has decreased slightly (Kaeble and Alper 2020). Additionally, because of COVID-19, there has been an increased rate of releases from prison and jails in 2020. Violent crime had previously decreased since the mid-1990s (Wikipedia 2020b), and there is increased activity in efforts to reduce prison populations. While many postrelease programs have not yet been subject to comprehensive and rigorous research, individual programs report some success.

Harvard University surveyed programs in various jurisdictions and found that assistance in health, housing, employment, and education were key to successful programs (Price-Tucker et al. 2019). The survey authors concluded that these programs should be part of in-prison programming as well as services in the community. They found that among the most important aspects of programs were training for interpersonal skills, such as anger management, parenting, and goal-setting. In addition, overcoming the negative influences of antisocial peer relationships and attitudes was essential. One of the most important factors is continuing such programs for a year or more. Successful mentorship pairs mentors who come from similar backgrounds (e.g., gender and ethnic) as the prisoner and who have been successful after leaving the justice system.

Programs and Approaches

There are many programs within institutions that focus on adjusting to life outside. These programs can be helpful, although it should be noted that participants may have a distrust of the programs offered and dropout rates may be high. Programs are structured around a curriculum and often have a group format. The approach is geared largely toward the practical considerations of release (finding the parole officer, getting a job, getting a place to live) and may gloss over the mental and emotional stressors the individual will face. Also, these programs are not necessarily focused on identifying, and achieving, the individual's own goals.

Such programs focus on education, counseling, and proactive coordination with the individuals. Identifying which programs will help which individuals is one of the more important, if difficult, tasks facing prison managers. In this book we have discussed two widely used ones. First was the risk-need-responsivity model (RNR). RNR assesses individuals for programs based on their 1) risk of reoffending, 2) need for skills, education, and counseling to counter those risks, and 3) estimated responsivity to such programs. Such assessments have been used since 1928 as formal tools in use in a variety of prison, jail, diversionary programs, juvenile, and postrelease programs (Latessa et al. 2015). RNR programs have as their primary goal to give individuals the skills and attitudes that lead to a productive life outside of the institution. The programs are structured, intensive, and comprehensive in providing skills needed for vocational and social interaction and approaches to avoid re-offending and participate in society and contribute to family and community. Unfortunately, as such programs become entrenched in the organizations presenting them, often a common program is offered to all participants, forgoing the role of assessment and individualization that is often key to success. While effective in reducing recidivism, RNR programs also have a high rate of participant dropout (Ward and Maruna 2007).

More recently, professionals working with incarcerated individuals have developed programs that extend the nature of training and counseling beyond attending RNR programs toward helping clients with figuring out what it is they want to do and how to get to a prosocial lifestyle. New programs begin with the positive psychology concepts of Seligman (1999), Peterson (2006), Seligman and Csikszentmihalyi (2000), and others to enhance self-efficacy and strength-building to help individuals discover their own goals and develop attitudes and skills that will help them plan for attaining those goals once they are back in the community. The theory behind this approach is that developing a prosocial and self-managed set of goals and learning how to achieve them will also address criminogenic needs and encourage desistance from criminal behaviors (Ward and Maruna 2007). Haney (2002, 2020) argues that without helping individuals to see their own potential outside the criminal history with which they entered prison, there will be no incentive for them to seek a noncriminal lifestyle.

The second program we have discussed (see Chapter 13), The Good Lives Model, has been widely used to treat sex offenders and has been broadened to other settings. It is based on the concept that in order to succeed, one must have a sense of place in society, attitudes that are pro-social, and goals for achieving success. GLM programs use RNR techniques to help individuals change criminogenic thinking and learn strategies for avoiding reoffending, but in addition, they work with people to identify their own strengths, goals, and aspirations and learn how to achieve success. In helping people to learn to desist from crime and helping them find prosocial ways of achieving their primary goods, GLM assumes that offending is the result of flaws in the person's life plan for obtaining those goods. Helping the individual to reimagine his or her approach is the goal of the programs (Willis and Ward 2013). In a related endeavor, Huynh et al. (2015) created a positive psychology program in Washington state and reported that participants felt that they had improved on several aspects of self-efficacy.

Education and Training

Since many incarcerated people have had low educational levels, literacy and high school programs are present in most American prisons as are job training opportunities. Programs such as those of the Vera Institute of Justice promote postsecondary education. Obtaining skills for success in society outside prison is a goal, and the program includes occupational training (Walsh and Delaney 2020). Programs for vocational and academic training may have the overt aim not of changing criminogenic thinking, but rather of giving them practical knowledge about specific careers or topics they wish to pursue. There are a variety of pre- and postrelease programs to help individuals with the practical and attitudinal skills and support they need to "make it" on the outside. Tables 14–1 and 14–2 present several of these and their attributes.

Prisoners are often undereducated as discussed in Chapter 13, and many have limited literacy both in reading and in math skills needed for effective employment. Literacy and math education provides them with skills that they lacked when detained—skills needed to be more successful on the "outside" and tools to manage practical aspects of their lives. Education, both pre- and post-reentry, provides individuals with skills and opportunities for engaging in society. Community college, which allows both academic and vocational paths, is well suited to this pathway because such institutions have social, academic, and mental health resources to assist students in their reintegration into life outside the prison (Feldman 2017). Many prisons in the United States now require high school equivalency programs and make vocational training available. One of the problems encountered in many facilities, however, is that enrollment is limited and there are significant waiting lists. Once beyond high school, tuition for postsecondary education may be a barrier to people in prison. For example, the Vera Institute of Justice (Walsh and Delaney 2020) works with prison administrators to implement Second Chance Pell grants. This program was initiated in 2015 by the U.S. Department of Education and has enrolled more than 17,000 prisoners. The Vera Institute estimates that recidivism for those who participate in college programs was reduced by 48% compared with those who did not enroll.

Supportive Psychotherapy

Many prisoners participate in psychotherapy because of underlying mental health issues. In light of the programs available, the practical and emotional tasks of reentry, and individual needs, supportive psychotherapy techniques can be of significant value in this process. In particular, individuals are looking for strategies to help them succeed after incarceration. Although the RNR programs discussed earlier focus primarily on the cognitive-behavioral models of treatment and have a wide acceptance in programming, and Good Lives Model–type programs look at individual goals and aspirations of individuals beyond addressing their criminogenic needs, there is still a need for individual psychotherapy that addresses prisoners' emotional and mental health needs. This is where supportive psychotherapy techniques come into play.

Listening

What are the individuals saying about their personal experience? It can make the dividing line between success and failure in reentry (Middlemass 2017). By actively listening, you can identify clues to that person's needs and make suggestions for meeting those needs. Just the respect shown in the listening process is an important aspect of this process. As therapy proceeds, by example and advice, active listening is a significant skill that will help the individuals to cope with relationships as they leave the institution and make their way in society.

TABLE 14–1. **Examples of prerelease reentry programs**

Program	Description
Shortimer (nationwide) Sponsor: Prison Fellowship	Comprehensive manual for soon-to-be released people with an agenda of tasks and information to help individuals navigate the reentry process, starting before release.
Connecting Access to Resources for Entering Society (Clark County, NV)	Program to assist people who are in jail and expecting to be released within 45 days to obtain ID cards, connect with social services, receive counseling, and navigate the DMV.
U.S. Department of Justice Prerelease Program	Reentry planning program that begins with initial intake interviews and reentry readiness is assessed at periodic reviews and at 30 months prior to release. It includes planning and training about health, employment, finance, availability of community resources, release requirements, and plans for personal growth and development. In addition, community correctional facilities, halfway houses, and supervised home confinement may be used.
Prerelease center (Montgomery County, MD)	Prerelease center that involves parole and probation officers in the process of helping individuals prepare to enter the community.
Thinking for a Change (T4C) (Alabama Department of Corrections)	Cognitive-behavioral change program that was implemented statewide with continuous assessment of the effectiveness.
Gender Responsive Opportunities for Women (GROW) (Santa Clara County, CA)	Comprehensive program of services by county agencies providing both pre- and postrelease assistance in transitional housing, service navigation, and employment assistance to women.

Source. Ellis and Henderson 2017; Grega 2020; National Institute of Corrections 2018; Nelson and Trone 2000; Prison Fellowship n.d.

TABLE 14–2. **Examples of postrelease reentry programs**

Program	Description
Oklahoma Partnership for Successful Reentry	Works to integrate community services with state resources to encourage locally oriented programs.
Tulsa Reentry One-Stop (Tulsa, OK)	Offers career reentry services, particularly in areas of high demand for labor and coordinates training and placement as well as follow-up services.
Citizen Potawatomi Nation and Oklahoma Inter-Tribal Reentry Alliance	Provides services that are specific to the community and tribal culture, including "talking circles" that involve reentering persons discussing issues and providing assistance to one another.
Safer Foundation (Chicago, IL)	Provides comprehensive services for education and employment as well as other social services.
Leap for Ladies (Florida)	Provides training prerelease and mentors to help women develop skills and resources and assistance upon release.

Source. LEAP Reentry Programs 2022; Price-Tucker et al. 2019.

Therapeutic Task of Promoting Personal Goods and Reducing Risk

Creating an alliance that does not view the patient as a moral stranger is key. Ward and Maruna (2007) note that it is rare for individuals to be completely evil. They point out that these individuals' criminal acts do not necessarily come from wanting to be criminals; rather, their goals and needs have led them to believe that these acts will fulfill some need. Establishing respect for an offender's ability to change and work toward a more prosocial set of goals is essential to helping him.

Narrative therapy helps patients develop healthier self-narratives and shift their understanding and perhaps their behavior (Ward and Maruna 2007, p. 86). Telling their individual stories helps provide visibility and value to their particular experience. Sharing stories with other people and interacting about both the shared and unique experiences can help the individual to better understand where they came from and where they are going, both experientially and psychologically.

Developing an alternative prosocial self-identity to justify change from criminal thinking and identity helps patients to identify strengths and goals beyond past actions and ideas to find the things that will lead to growth and positive action in the future.

Strategic Storytelling

Writing from the perspective of creating opportunities for minority populations who have begun the process of reentering, Feldman (2017) advocates for strategic storytelling within the community that these individuals find themselves. Such storytelling helps individuals to create their own narratives, sharing experiences and wisdom gained and "refuting the notion that their experiences are invisible" (p. 19). This allows them to frame their lives as moving forward, rather than as deficits. Indeed, learning the stories of people leads to powerful empathic understanding of their needs and ways in which they wish to be and can be helped.

Self-Efficacy

Providing job training, even early in incarceration, gives individuals a sense of and capability for self-efficacy by allowing them to develop a plan for reentry. Education and skills training are goals in and of themselves and should be available to all prisoners. You should assist patients in developing goals and finding methods to achieve them (Liem 2016). West (2017) recommends that reentry practitioners go through the training themselves to understand the holistic needs of reentering people.

Quality of Life and Enhanced Treatment Engagement

Willis and Ward (2013) begin with intensive assessments of risk and needs, intensively working with the individual to identify core commitments and the day-to-day activities and experiences to come to an understanding of the reasons the individual committed offenses. This enables the therapist to help the patient identify ways of achieving those goals and developing a comprehensive treatment plan for intervention and strategies. These include cognitive restructuring, victim impact and empathy training, social skills training, and techniques for avoiding reoffending, as well as developing practical skills for obtaining employment, finding recreational activities, and improving interpersonal relationships.

Therapists who work with incarcerated people have a lot of experience interacting with and listening to their life stories, but how many of them have had similar life experiences? After all, the overwhelming majority of prisoners come from disadvantaged communities and have low education levels, are often poor, and disproportionately come from minority backgrounds—almost like a different planet from the one people trying to help them inhabit. This can lead to unconscious biases and negative attitudes on the part of therapists and negative attitudes in the participants. To counter this, you should encourage some flexibility and allow participants to develop their own approach and narrative, rather than imposing every single facet of a packaged program.

Prerelease Jitters

If entering prison is stressful, leaving may be more so. Jail and prison give incarcerated individuals little control over day-to-day activities, diet, and even sleep/wake cycles. Returning to the society at large may leave individuals with a sense of disorientation and even fear of the unknown (Arehart-Treichel 2010). Prior to release there is a peak in prevalence of mild depression at about a month before leaving. From 1–4 weeks after release, the prevalence drops to 8%, but it increases to 20% by 3–4 months later. Even in tightly controlled halfway house circumstances, the changes from the mundane, such as the clothing one wears, to the profound, such as reestablishing family relationships, can be stressful (Middlemass 2017). Navigating probation, finding a job, finding housing, and reconnecting with family are obstacles to be overcome.

Therapists should be prepared for the stressors and anxieties that may affect patients as the end of their incarceration nears. It is duly suggested that "if prisoners were given the opportunity to discuss their feelings about leaving the prison environment before they reentered the community, it might decrease any depression or anxiety they have and increase their chances of a successful reintegration into the community" (Arehart-Treichel 2010, p. 3). In particular, patients with mental health issues need to be reassured that they can get the resources they need to navigate life after prison. You can help your patients understand some of the challenges ahead and work with them to develop plans for creating a path for success (Latessa et al. 2015). The planning process will help to allay some of the "jitters" as will your counseling.

A study by Bahr et al. (2010) explored the success of reentry and the impact that factors such as drug treatment, friends, work, family ties, and age contributed to success. The researchers, and we as well, were surprised to learn that family ties, being a parent, and education were not linked in this study with successful reentry. However, many other studies that we have cited here have shown that it is important to address these areas in therapy in prison to facilitate the transition and help individuals to develop social skills and job qualifications. The bonding with friends is beneficial to parolees because associating with law-abiding friends may help with discouraging the parolee when they are tempted to violate their parole. Parolees may also consider the likelihood of losing friends and/or employment should they become involved with the legal system again. Those individuals most likely to succeed had taken a class while in prison and spent time in enjoyable activities with friends. Additionally, those who worked a minimum of 40 hours a week were more likely to complete parole successfully. Working more than 40 hours enables the parolee to earn more money and to have less time to be involved with those who could contribute to his downfall, and to provide each person with opportunities for cultivating associations with law-abiding citizens.

Short Timer's Syndrome

In addition to the use of "short timer" as an objective description of someone who is leaving soon, prisoners often use the term "short timer's syndrome" to refer to someone who acts out or burns their bridges in a "don't care" frenzy as their term winds down. The term is used similarly in business forums, and prisoners warn each other about it (Prisontalk.com 2010). Prisoners can sabotage their release, incur discipline, and even anger family and friends. Some may plan to reoffend immediately when they go out. We are aware of one man who left the federal prison and immediately walked into a bank, robbed it, and waited around to be arrested.

Coordination of Programs Pre- and Postrelease

While many programs have been instituted in prisons nation- and worldwide that have been shown to succeed, it still remains in many states that programs and services in prisons and jails are not coordinated with services in the community. Individuals whose terms have expired may be left at a bus stop with little in the way of money, proper clothing, or orientation to services. Persons on parole may have a parole officer who is often overworked and with little time to help, or there may not be comprehensive services, including transitional housing, vocational services, and health care.

Petersilia (2003), Haney (2002), and many others have spearheaded research and development of programs to improve services in prison for reducing recidivism and have inspired many public and private providers to develop services for returning individuals to reinforce the skills needed for success. For example, medical and mental health services that are provided in the institutions are often handed off to outside providers with little more coordination than a 30-day supply of medications. This circumstance is changing as a result of the criminal justice reform movement with such groups as the Vera Institute, the Urban League, and many local government and nongovernment organizations. Successful reentry is predicated on the ability of the individual prisoner to develop necessary skills in social and employment circumstances, and the ability to access services such as employment, health, and family relationships. Improving coordination between prison and the community, the following should be included (Price-Tucker et al. 2019; Prison Fellowship n.d.):

- Seeking involvement of the family in working on reestablishing relationships and understanding the challenges the individual faces as well as finding resources for success.
- Exploring options for education and vocational training to provide skills for employment and managing postrelease life.

- Developing a network of resources, including assisting with financial planning, physical circumstances (e.g., housing), and necessary paperwork, and making contact with these resources.
- Developing relationships with people who can help: a mentor, professional helpers, family.
- Helping individuals to get Social Security (or other assistance), clear any legal issues such as outstanding warrants or charges, and sealing of any records that do not pertain to employment, driver's licenses, certificates of completion of programs, and voter registration, if available. Also identifying reporting requirements for parole or probation.
- Developing a plan for reentry, such as transportation home, living arrangements, and job opportunities (and applications).
- Obtaining medical records and identifying health services nearby.

One important factor, which is now becoming more common, is the coordination of treatment between caregivers on both sides of the person's experience. This is the focus of a set of guidelines for people with mental disorders or substance use disorders by the Substance Abuse and Mental Health Services Administration (SAMHSA) as reported by the National Commission on Correctional Heath Care (Fiscella 2017). As we have discussed, reentry planning actually begins on intake into a facility with screening and assessment for identifying problems and placing individuals in appropriate settings. This should lead to individualized treatment and service plans and collaboration between justice and behavioral health approaches for each person. From the first hours to several weeks after, it is critical to identify and coordinate and facilitate continuity of care and interventions that may be needed. Sharing of information, treatment plans, and approaches is important. SAMHSA also recommends that professionals in prison and the community cross-train so that the collaboration is strengthened.

Working With the Soon to Be Released Person

As a therapist, it is important to know the programs available to individuals in your facility and after they leave. Compounding the problems of reentry for your patients are the mental health issues for which you are treating them. Whether a personality disorder, substance use history, or stressor-related disorder, each patient will need an individualized plan. Working with your patients to develop an approach will give them specific goals and strategies for success. Involvement in the planning will provide the patient with a sense of control while facing an unknown future. Possible points of departure for these discussions include:

1. Do you know the terms of your release?
2. What plans have you made for where you are going? Are you going to a halfway house, or will you live with family? Do you know the transportation arrangements for your release?
3. What areas of support do you need? Monetary, job, health, living arrangements?

4. What emotional/mental health support will you need?
5. What are your medications? Do you plan to take them after you leave?
6. What people do you have that you can ask for social support, and are they ready to help? Have you contacted them? What information have they provided?
7. What will your professional contacts or support systems be (e.g., P&P, clinics, housing, social services)?
8. What will your personal supports be? Family? Friends? Peer (prisoner, mental health) support group?
9. Do you have children, and what are their living arrangements? Do you expect to have custody? How do you intend to reestablish your relationship with them?
10. Do you think you need to add family counseling to your therapies?
11. What are your goals for yourself? What work do you want to do, what are your qualifications, do you need further training, and do you have any job prospects?
12. What are your concerns about leaving? How do you feel about it?
13. Do you feel you will be successful in avoiding behaviors that will cause you to get involved with the police?
14. Where do you see yourself in 6 months? A year? 5 years?

In helping your patients prepare, you should also try to help them make the transition through the following:

- Discuss the use of long-acting injectable medications based on your knowledge of their motivation and adherence to their treatment recommendations.
- Link them to community services.
- Talk to the community providers yourself.
- Ask the case manager to come to the prison to meet them in advance.
- Build strengths for the community transition: anticipate opportunities for family interaction, school, work, and social development; many who cannot work can take a course in a local community college or work or study online.
- Discuss diet, exercise, and other lifestyle decisions, since many newer medications cause increased hunger and weight gain.
- Discuss how to deal with violence in the community. What is their community crisis response safety plan for suicide or violence? They can learn to back off from violent situations, go home, call their case worker, go to the emergency room, call the police, and so forth.
- Coordinate with the patient and community providers.

What Do You Say Before You Say "Goodbye"?

Directing the conversation toward practical and practicable plans for release can help patients look realistically at their prospects. With patients who have mental disorders or intellectual disabilities, helping develop a way to cope with feelings and behaviors while also creating concrete steps that can be taken will go a long way to reducing anxiety.

As these questions are discussed, a good idea would be for the patient to create a sheet of important information or a full crisis response safety plan as discussed below and shown in Figure 14–1. Based on the plans we have discussed throughout, we sug-

Warning signs I am getting suicidal or going to hurt myself [Side 1]

When I'm sleeping less or sleeping poorly

When I stop going to the yard

When I stay in my cell

When I stop eating

When I start to hear voices again

When I think of cutting my arm

When I think I should be dead

When I start to feel guilty about being in prison

When I think abut what my father did to me and I am so mad

When I pick up the razor and start playing with it

Warning signs of my PTSD

External triggers (things seen or heard or felt)

CO opens and slams door

Someone touches me unexpectedly

Someone yells at me or gets in my personal space

Seeing people in uniforms

Someone says or does something to me that makes me feel unsafe or threatened

Watching people argue and hit each other

Hearing a police siren or seeing squad car lights go by

Hearing a firecracker or real gunfire

Upsetting events on a movie, TV show, or news such as an accident

Anniversary of something that happened

Certain prisoners or staff who remind me of an abuser

Other things that are special to me _____

Internal triggers (thoughts, moods, or behaviors)

Becoming more irritable, angry, or depressed

Having more upsetting dreams or nightmares

Missing people and feeling lonely

Feeling different from my usual self

Feeling unsafe or vulnerable

A resurgence of my PTSD symptoms such as memories and flashbacks

An increase in my pain

Feeling tense and ready to "go off"

Warning signs that my reentry plan is at risk

Losing my job

Suicidal thoughts (see my warning signs of suicide)

Running with the old crowd

Urges to use or using

Running out of money

Lost my housing

Fight with my family

Abused by my S.O. or contacting previous abusers

Symptoms of my mental illness returning

FIGURE 14–1. Crisis Response Safety Plan—Trauma-Informed and Reentry Version (CRSP-TR)

How can I cope by myself when I start getting into trouble?   [Side 1, continued]

Coping with thoughts of hurting myself

Read a book

Put away any knives and razors

Do some of my drawings

Read the Bible with the passages I marked and mark some new passages

Do physical exercises

Just go to sleep

Do my deep breathing

My progressive relaxation that they taught me

My mindfulness exercises

Trauma: coping with my PTSD triggers

Do any of the above and more

Use my coping cards

Repeat my mantra

Put in my earplugs at night

Who can I contact? Personal

My significant other 202-×××-××××

*My best friend and primary contact
202-×××-××××*

My mother 202-×××-××××

My brother 202-×××-××××

Who can I contact? Professional

My counselor here in the group home

My sponsor 202-×××-××××

My PO 202-×××-××××

My rehab program 202-×××-××××

My case manager 202-×××-××××

My mental health therapist 202-×××-××××

My mental health clinic 202-×××-××××

My medical clinic 202-×××-××××

National Suicide Prevention Lifeline
1-800-273-8255

My reasons for living   [Side 2]

My family

My children

Suicide is a sin, and I don't want to do that

I am out of prison now, and I can do the things I wanted to do

I can get my A.A. degree

I like watching television

My resilience strategies

Do my problem-solving exercises

Do my resilience exercises (yoga or mindfulness)

Read my inspirational book

My medications

××××××× is for my depression

××××××× is for my anxiety

××××××× is for my hallucinations

FIGURE 14–1. Crisis Response Safety Plan—Trauma-Informed and Reentry Version
(CRSP-TR) *(continued)*

gest a further update to apply to community life. If relevant, it can include the enhancements for trauma as well. The reentry version of a crisis response safety plan should remind individuals of their goals and contacts that they will need in case of emergency or other developments. It may include inspirational messages to help keep them on track; a list of phone numbers and addresses of therapists, probation officers, family members, or friends who can be called in case of need; and a to-do list of actions that can help them navigate the "outside." It may be helpful to include their list of medications and a reminder to be sure to take the medications as prescribed.

Whatever form the crisis response safety plan takes, individuals should plan to keep it with them at all times. They might want to make several hard copies of it and carry a copy on their person, place a few where they can be retrieved, and give a copy to trusted individuals such as relatives, therapists, and/or their parole officer. A good idea is to keep a reduced-size copy of emergency contacts and list of medications in a shoe once in the community in case of some adverse event, such as a robbery or accident, where the person's phone is lost or stolen. Also, if possible, the person should memorize two or three names and phone numbers. Even if newly released persons have no access to a personal smart phone or computer, a free email account can be created at any public library and the information loaded into an email to themselves.

We summarize the therapist's agenda in Table 14–3.

Give Them a Chance

The year is 1942, the city Perth, Australia, and newly paired Malachi Stormes, decorated captain of the submarine *Firefish*, is having bit of dinner repartee with Kensie Richmond, decorative daughter of a prominent rancher and mine owner. Captain Stormes asks her if there is an Australian aristocracy similar to the English one. Not quite, she laughs, but they did have some robber barons as they did in the United States, and he should keep in mind that many Australian men are descendants of convicts who were sent there from England (Deutermann 2018, p. 80).

But to the facts (courtesy of Wikipedia). Great Britain and Ireland sent about 162,000 people called "convicts" to Australia between 1788 and 1868. That certainly strikes *us* as a huge number given the population of Australia in 1788 (uncertainly estimated between 300,000 and 1.25 million according to Wikipedia's "History of Indigenous Australians" [Wikipedia 2020c]), many of whom were Aboriginal people and who were soon killed by disease or other people. Most of the people were sent there for petty crimes because the more serious crimes carried the death penalty and those offenders were kept behind.

Kensie's comment is slightly misleading, though, as she refers only to men. In fact, about 1 in 7 were women, but the rest is correct. Most of the emancipated prisoners stayed in Australia, and many of them became prominent citizens. While descent from a so-called convict was initially stigmatized, "it is now considered by many Australians to be a cause for celebration to discover a convict in one's lineage. Almost 20% of modern Australians, in addition to 2 million Britons, are descended from transported prisoners. The 'convict era' has inspired famous novels, films, and other cultural works, and the extent to which it has shaped Australia's national character has been studied by many writers and historians" (Wikipedia 2020a).

TABLE 14–3.   **Therapist's agenda for the "nearly departed" person**

It is to be hoped you are not blindsided by the discharge plan, but plans do change. Ideally, the discharge plan should have been an ongoing part of the treatment plan.

Be aware of the type of discharge (e.g., expiration of sentence, parole, probation, community supervision) and site (e.g., halfway house, family, public substance use treatment, sober-living facility, adult foster care, mental health group home).

Remember that discharges to mental hospitals would probably just be considered transfers in most systems, but the therapist still has an agenda in assisting with the transition.

See if the person is living on a prerelease unit and attending the prerelease classes.

Make sure veterans are set up with their outpatient services.

Review the prerelease curriculum on the prerelease unit first by yourself and then periodically with your patient to make sure he or she is actually learning it and doing the tasks.

Make sure *you* have made any possible or allowable contacts with outside providers, mental health case managers, and therapists.

See if you can get the outside contact to visit the prison.

Review the individual's release version of the crisis response safety plan (see Figure 14–1).

Review the instructions to have multiple copies and memorize one or two phone numbers in case "everything" gets stolen on the outside.

Make sure the individual has made his or her calls to personal and professional contacts.

Review the medications; ask the individual whether he or she plans to take them; if not, why not? Question decisions that appear foolish. This could be your last chance to do so.

Review the substance use history and relapse prevention plans (unless the individual is going into a specific substance rehab program).

Make sure there is follow-up for medical problems (there is an increased suicide risk for these individuals).

Explore, as only you can, the patient's thoughts, feelings, apprehensions, hopes (e.g., false, pessimistic, realistic, overly optimistic) about reentry.

Explore, as only you can, the person's short- and long-term goals (same range as in previous item).

Address the problems to mitigate future issues now and plans to mitigate future problems.

Protect against the Saturday night drug overdose due to loss of tolerance to opioids.

Warn about the possibility of depression after a few months back in the community.

Consider how to terminate a last session before discharge.

If allowed, give the individual a chance to give you feedback from the community.

In other words, give them a chance. We can thank Great Britain and Ireland for populating an entire continent with prisoners and giving them the opportunities for personal success, if not nation-building.

But as the television commercials say, "Wait, there's more!" We said that the transport of persons convicted of crimes to Australia started in 1788. Why was that? The American Revolution happened. Prior to that: "It is estimated that some 50,000 British convicts were sent to colonial America and the majority landed in the Chesapeake Colonies of Maryland and Virginia, as well as in Georgia. Transported convicts represented perhaps one-quarter of all British emigrants during the 18th century" (Wikipedia 2020d). Did they make good? James Bell stole a book from a London bookstall in 1723 and was punished by being sent to the Colonies as an indentured servant. The story of these persons and the history of individuals are now documented (Vaver

2011). So suffice it to say merely that most of those immigrants and their descendants probably did succeed in life and make a contribution to their new country.

In other words, give them a chance (redux).

But wait, there's more (coda). We do not wish to leave you fuming about our remark about "decorative Kensie" above. That "decorative Kensie" was a *trauma surgeon*. Deutermann, whose military novels are meticulously researched, was aware that there was a history of Australian women surgeons dating back to the Great War. Unfortunately, "None of this valuable experience advanced their career prospects as military surgeons. It was another 20 years before the Australian Army commissioned its first female doctor (a medical administrator), and almost 70 years before it deployed a female surgeon on operations. In the amnesia that follows war, their achievements were simply forgotten" (Neuhaus 2013, p. 717).

So, as for any disadvantaged and discriminated-against group, be it women, persons of color, or previously incarcerated citizens, as a society we need to learn (as we have not yet learned):

Give them a chance.

Reentry Capsule

JACK: So what's new?

JILL: Well, it's certainly no comparison to being a real prisoner, but while self-isolating from the coronavirus I have been reading Daniel Defoe's *Journal of the Plague Year*.

JACK: Any good?

JILL: Not as good as his other book, *Robinson Crusoe*.

JACK: If you liked that one, you might like Sir Isaac Newton's *Calculus and other Rocks I picked up from Route 1666*.

JILL: Don't be snarky. Everyone knows that Newton invented calculus while hiding out from college during the London plague of 1665–66.

JACK: I thought we had discussed all the plague and pestilence books in our last dialogue. Except maybe Anthony Trollope's Doctor Omicron Pie. Is there nothing new, or does history just repeat itself?

JILL: I suppose so, as long as the world doesn't end entirely. That would be a "one-off."

JACK: Well, then, I have some questions about reentry.

JILL: OK. Since the SpaceX program finally got their astronauts up there and back, reentry is a breeze, at least figuratively, since there are no breezes in outer space.

JACK: Is "astronaut" another Sanskrit word like "juggernaut"?

JILL: No, silly, "astronaut" comes from the Greek words for "star" and "sailor."

JACK: Then tell me about prisoners, not astronauts. From what I've read, reentry is by no means a breeze for prisoners. They have to negotiate a maze of regulations, move around from one location to another, reestablish relationships with family members but avoid all persons convicted of felonies, and get a job or go back to school.

JILL: You think it's easy for astronauts? They have to plunge into the atmosphere, risk overheating, ending up in the wrong location, and open the doors of their space capsule while underwater.

JACK: I think that reentering prisoners have the same problems but a lot less money to do it. They have to enter a hostile atmosphere, risk overdosing rather than overheating, and financially they are almost always underwater.

JILL: I've read that it helps to have a centralized case manager for social issues and a so-called medical home or primary care provider for their medical and mental issues.

JACK: Sure, like a Mission Control for prisoner reentry.

JILL: Good idea. Reentering from carceral space is like reentering from outer space! Are you going to use that in the book?

JACK: I already have. Except I didn't use the word "cars-are-all" since I couldn't spell it.

JILL: Is there something wrong with the car?

JACK: No, except that the battery is probably dead because we haven't left the house in 3 weeks.

JILL: Well, then, to get back to the subject, I think we all hope that reentry from carceral space will be 100% successful as in the SpaceX program.

JACK: I wish.

JILL: But it's so good to hear that civilized nations have stopped the barbaric practice of sending their so-called criminals to other countries.

JACK: No, not really. The United States still does that.

JILL: No way! You're joking, of course.

JACK: Not at all. According to Pew Research, in fiscal 2018 the U.S. deported about 337,000 immigrants. Moreover: "Immigrants convicted of a crime made up less than half of deportations.....Of the 337,000 immigrants deported in 2018, some 44% had criminal convictions and 56% were not convicted of a crime. From 2001 to 2018, a majority (60%) of immigrants deported have not been convicted of a crime" (Budiman 2020).

JILL: Okay, okay. That sounds like a bad thing, but what does it have to do with the book?

JACK: How soon you forget! In the beginning of Chapter 1, we noted that 20,000 people were being held in immigration detention facilities, down from 50,000 before the COVID-19 crisis, but it will probably go up again when the crisis is over. These people have exceptional and unique mental health needs, similar in many ways to persons in jail, facing an uncertain "verdict" if you want to call it that, the verdict being "deport" or "let stay."

JILL: Well, hope their attorneys can get the best possible verdict for them.

JACK. Only if they have attorneys. Deportation is considered a civil action, and most immigrants are not entitled to a public defender.

JILL: That sounds unfair. Deportation is a serious thing, and certainly could deprive a person of "life, liberty and the pursuit of happiness." Did you catch the quotes?

JACK: I sure did. But whatever the outcome, and pending the development of a new immigration policy, we need to be mindful of the mental health needs of these immigrants while they are detained.

JILL: Maybe we need to think outside the box, if you get my drift.

JACK: Yes, and to get rid of pestilence that *is* the box. Camus said, "A pestilence isn't a thing made to man's measure; therefore we tell ourselves that pestilence is a mere bogy of the mind; a bad dream that will pass away. But it doesn't always pass away and, from one bad dream to another, it is men who pass away, and the humanists first of all, because they haven't taken their precautions" (Camus 1991, p. 37).

JILL: And your point is…

JACK: My point is that COVID-19 is not a bogy of our minds, but our "Plague of Prisons" *is* a creation of our minds. We created it, and we can cure it, especially we who think of ourselves as humanists.

JILL: Yes, we need to think outside of the box, while we fix what (or who?) is inside the box.

JACK: I agree. It's better than "Waiting on the World to Change."

Key Points

- Preparation for reentry should begin at entry to prison (if not before), especially for people with mental disorders and intellectual disabilities.

- A plan for activities and programs for reducing each person's risk of recidivism should be formulated as initial assessments are made and should be tailored to the person's level of education, social and economic conditions, and mental health needs.

- A number of programs and approaches are available. Your institution may have its own. It will be helpful to know about it so you can know best how to supplement it.

- Planning for release is the province of the prisoner. You should provide the kind of information and advice that will help the person make good decisions and take control of the process and the outcomes.

- Taking medicine after release should be a major recommendation and a commitment the patient makes in the plan.

- Each person needs access to resources in the community to which he or she is going and an understanding of how to obtain these once they are out. Preferably, these contacts will be made before the individual is released.

- A crisis response safety plan for reentry should be prepared by the prisoner that includes the name and phone number of people the prisoner has identified who can provide support in the community, a list of medicines if appropriate, and strategies to cope with stressors that he or she may encounter. The individual should memorize the phone numbers and establish a free online account such that it can be accessed from the phone or at a public library or other institution where access to a computer is possible.

- Many persons convicted of crimes were sent to Australia as well as Colonial America in the early years of their history. Most of these people stayed in their adopted countries and made good, and many Australians and Americans are their descendants. It helps to give disadvantaged people a chance. It's good for the individual, and it's good for the society as a whole.

References

Alper D, Durose M, Markiman J: Special Report: 2018 Update on Prisoner Recidivism: a 9-Year Follow-Up Period (2005–2014), NJC 250975. Washington, DC, Bureau of Justice Statistics, May 2018. Available at: https://bjs.ojp.gov/content/pub/pdf/18upr9yfup0514.pdf. Accessed September 13, 2020.

Arehart-Treichel J: Inmates' prerelease anxiety levels surprise researchers. Psychiatric News, August 20, 2010. Available at: https://psychnews.psychiatryonline.org/doi/full/10.1176/pn.45.16.psychnews_45_16_030. Accessed September 13, 2020.

Bahr SJ, Harris L, Fisher JK, Harker Armstrong A: Successful reentry: what differentiates successful and unsuccessful parolees? Int J Offender Ther Comp Criminol 54(5):667–692, 2010 19638473

Binswanger IA, Stern MF, Deyo RA, et al: Release from prison—a high risk of death for former inmates. N Engl J Med 356(2):157–165, 2007 17215533

Budiman A: Key findings about U.S. immigrants. Pew Research Center Numbers, Facts and Trends Shaping Your World, August 20, 2020. Available at: www.pewresearch.org/fact-tank/2020/08/20/key-findings-about-u-s-immigrants. Accessed November 28, 2020.

Camus A: The Plague. Translated by Stuart Gilbert. New York, Vintage Books, 1991

Chang Z, Lichtenstein P, Långström N, et al: Association between prescription of major psychotropic medication and violent reoffending after prison release. JAMA 316(17):1798–1807, 2016 27802545

de Andrade D, Ritchie J, Rowlands M, et al: Substance use and recidivism outcomes for prison-based drug and alcohol interventions. Epidemiol Rev 40(1):121–133, 2018 29733373

Deutermann PT: The Iceman. New York, St Martin's Press, 2018

Ellis A, Henderson JM: The U.S. Bureau of Prison's prelease program: getting out early. Crim Justice 21(4):20–22, 2017

Feldman C: Education outside of the box, in Race, Education and Reintegrating Formerly Incarcerated Citizens. Edited by Chaney JR, Schwartz J. Lanham, MD, Lexington Books, 2017, pp 15–26

Fiscella K: New guidelines aid in the reentry of those with mental/substance use disorders. Chicago, IL, National Commission on Correctional Health Care, 2017

Fox AD, Maradiaga J, Weiss L, et al: Release from incarceration, relapse to opioid use and the potential for buprenorphine maintenance treatment: a qualitative study of the perceptions of former inmates with opioid use disorder. Addict Sci Clin Pract 10(2):2, 2015 25592182

Grega K: Local inmates on verge of release find help to ease shift back into society. Las Vegas Sun, February 29, 2020. Available at: https://lasvegassun.com/news/2020/feb/29/inmates-verge-release-find-help-ease-shift-reenter. Accessed November 26, 2020.

Haney C: The psychological impact of incarceration: implications for post-prison adjustment, in From Prison to Home: The Effect of Incarceration and Reentry on Children, Families, and Communities. U.S. Department of Health and Human Services, Office of the Assistant Secretary for Planning and Evaluation, January 2002. Available at: https://aspe.hhs.gov/reports/prison-home-effect-incarceration-reentry-children-families-communities. Accessed February 20, 2020.

Haney C: Criminality in Context: The Psychological Foundations of Criminal Justice Reform. Washington, DC, American Psychological Association, 2020

Hairston CF: Families, prisoners, and community reentry: a look at issues and programs, in Heading Home: Offender Reintegration into the Family. Edited by Gadsden VL. Lanham, MD, American Correctional Association, 2003, pp 13–38

Harding DJ, Morenoff JD, Wyse JJB: On the Outside: Prisoner Reentry and Reintegration. Chicago, IL, University of Chicago Press, 2019

Hopkin G, Evans-Lacko S, Forrester A, et al: Interventions at the transition from prison to the community for prisoners with mental illness: a systematic review. Administration and Policy in Mental Health Services Research 45:623–634, 2018

Huynh KH, Hall B, Hurst MA, Bikos LH: Evaluation of the positive re-entry in corrections program: a positive psychology intervention with prison inmates. Int J Offender Ther Comp Criminol 59(9):1006–1023, 2015 24618877

Kaeble D, Alper M: Probation and Parole in the United States 2017–2018, NCJ 252071. Washington, DC, Bureau of Justice Statistics, August 4, 2020. Available at: www.bjs.gov/index.cfm?iid=6986&ty=pbdetail. Accessed November 26, 2020.

Kuziemko: How should inmates be released from prison? An assessment of parole versus fixed-sentence regimes. Q J Econ 128(1):371–424, 2013

Latessa EJ, Listwan SJ, Koetzle D: What Works (and Doesn't) in Reducing Recidivism. London, Routledge, 2015

LEAP Reentry Programs: Our program. 2022. Available at: https://leapforladies.org/program. Accessed March 6, 2022.

Liem M: After Life Imprisonment: Reentry in the Era of Mass Incarceration, New York, New York University Press, 2016

Los Angeles Times Editorial Board: Freed inmates face brutal lives of poverty and homelessness. Don't blame coronavirus. Los Angeles Times, May 28, 2020

Mears DP, Cochran JC: Prisoner Reentry in the Era of Mass Incarceration. Thousand Oaks, CA, Sage Publications, 2015

Merrall EL, Kariminia A, Binswanger IA, et al: Meta-analysis of drug-related deaths soon after release from prison. Addiction 105(9):1545–1554, 2010 20579009

Middlemass KM: Convicted and Condemned. New York, New York University Press, 2017

National Institute of Corrections: Report to the Nation, Fiscal Year 2018: Results and Innovations. Washington, DC, National Institute of Corrections, 2018. Available at: www.nicic.gov. Accessed October 20, 2020.

Nelson M, Trone J: Why Planning for Release Matters. New York, Vera Institute of Justice, 2000

Neuhaus SJ: Australia's female military surgeons of World War I. ANZ J Surg 83(10):713–718, 2013, 23924307

Petersilia J: When Prisoners Come Home. Oxford, UK, Oxford University Press, 2003

Peterson C: A Primer in Positive Psychology. Oxford, UK, Oxford University Press, 2006

Price-Tucker A, Zhou A, Charroux A, et al: Successful Reentry: A Community-Level Analysis. Boston MA, Harvard University Institute of Politics, 2019

Prison Fellowship: Shortimer Handbook: preparing for release. n.d. Available at: www.prisonfellowship.org/training-resources/reentry-ministry/ministry-tools-2. Accessed November 17, 2020.

Prisontalk.com: Short-timers syndrome. Cactus, November 19, 2010. Available at www.prisontalk.com/forums/showthread.php?t=514211. Accessed November 27, 2020.

Ranapurwala S, Shanahan M, Naumann R, Marshall S: Former inmates at high risk for opioid overdose following release. Gillings School of Global Public Health, July 19, 2018. Available at: https://sph.unc.edu/sph-news/former-inmates-at-high-risk-for-opioid-overdose-following-prison-release. Accessed November 26, 2020.

Rostain AL, Ramsay JR, Waite R: Cultural background and barriers to mental health care for African American adults. J Clin Psychiatry 76(3):279–283, 2015 25830447

Seligman MEP: Positive social science. Journal of Positive Behavior Interventions 1(3):181–182, 1999

Seligman ME, Csikszentmihalyi M: Positive psychology. An introduction. Am Psychol 55(1):5–14, 2000 11392865

Star-Ledger Editorial Board: Reducing the prison populations saved lives. Now let's invest in those lives. Updated January 19, 2022. Available at: www.nj.com/opinion/2022/01/reducing-the-prison-population-saved-lives-now-lets-invest-in-those-lives-editorial.html. Accessed February 3, 2022.

Tharshini NK, Ibrahim F, Mohamad MS, Zakaria E: Challenges in re-entry among former inmates. International Journal of Academic Research in Business and Social Sciences 8(4):970–979, April 2018

U.S. Department of Justice: Roadmap to recovery: reducing recidivism through reentry reforms at the Federal Bureau of Prisons. 2017. Available at: http://static.politico.com/1a/bb/8e265a0d4db9a6768ed5b967aa27/roadmap-to-reentry.pdf. Accessed November 26, 2020.

Vaver A: Bound with an Iron Chain: The Untold Story of How the British Transported 50,000 Convicts to Colonial America. Westborough, MA, Pickpocket Publishing, 2011

Wallace D, Eason JM, Lindsey AM: The influence of incarceration and re-entry on the availability of health care organizations in Arkansas. Health Justice 3(3): 2015

Walsh B, Delaney R: America ready to reinstitute Pell grants for students in prison. Vera Institute, November 20, 2020. Available from: www.vera.org/blog/america-is-ready-to-reinstate-pell-grants-for-students-in-prison. Accessed November 20, 2020.

Ward T, Maruna S: Rehabilitation. New York, Routledge, 2007

West RJ: Reexamining Reentry: The Policies, People and Programs of the United States Prisoner Reintegration Systems. Lanham, MD, Lexington Books, 2017

Wikipedia: Convicts in Australia, 2020a. Available at: https://en.wikipedia.org/wiki/Convicts_in_Australia. Accessed November 28, 2020.

Wikipedia: Crime in the United States, 2020b. Available at: https://en.wikipedia.org/wiki/Crime_in_the_United_States. Accessed November 18, 2020.

Wikipedia: History of Indigenous Australians, 2020c. Available at: https://en.wikipedia.org/wiki/History_of_Indigenous_Australians. Accessed November 27, 2020.

Wikipedia: Penal colony, 2020d. Available at: https://en.wikipedia.org/wiki/Penal_colony. Accessed November 27, 2020.

Willis GM, Ward T: The Good Lives Model: does it work? Preliminary evidence, in What Works in Offender Rehabilitation: An Evidence-Based Approach to Assessment and Treatment. Edited by Craig LA, Dixon L, Gannon TA. Malden, MA, Wiley-Blackwell, 2013, pp 305–318

15

Conclusion

By the time you read this book, we hope the world is pretty much finished with the COVID-19 virus, but there is still some uncertainty about that. In fiction, at least, if we look ahead a few hundred years to the Sector General Hospital, one of its doctors finds an old medical textbook that mentions a disease similar to what they are finding in their patients. It turns out that their patients are suffering from a variant of influenza that has resurfaced with severe symptoms because of the waning natural immunity over the centuries since it first appeared (White 2002, p. 97).

However, as far as this book is concerned, we're done. We really are. Like well-meaning teachers, we hope we've told you what we're going to tell you, actually told you that, and reminded you (in the Key Points for each chapter) what we told you.

Yes, we're done. But you're not. You still have to work in your jail or prison. There are a variety of resources (not terribly expensive, and your department can purchase or share) to assist in doing psychotherapy. These will include those texts you choose for other forms of psychotherapy such as cognitive or interpersonal treatments based on your own predilections and specialized programming for your patients. Also, you will want to get some workbooks with handouts for prisoners or compile your own set of handouts on major topics such as insomnia, anger management, grief, and trauma. Surf the internet and collect some stuff. Perhaps you will also want some pages for journaling or just activities to pass the time, especially for seriously mentally ill patients.

We hope you appreciated the parallels we drew between the pandemics of COVID-19, tuberculosis, and mass incarceration. We are winning the battles against the first two, and the battle against the third is a work in progress. We have not tried to overdo the parallels, but there could also have been comments about the global AIDS epidemic that claimed 32 million lives (Avert 2021) and the prevalence of now-curable hepatitis C, both of which disproportionately afflicted incarcerated persons.

But recognize that we are primarily responsible for psychotherapy for *mental health* problems. So why all the emphasis on pandemics? There is a worldwide pandemic that is underrecognized and undertreated, and as we have learned so painstakingly, it is greatly magnified in our jails and prisons. It is the pandemic of mental illness. By this we do *not* mean the claims that COVID-19 has itself created a pandemic of mental illness—it has created a lot of mental distress, but experts say that this distress does not reach the level of a pandemic (Kelly 2020), although the bereavement created by the dreadful losses is real. And there is growing concern about "long COVID" and the persistence of neurological and mental impairments.

The pandemic we mean is the pandemic of mental illness itself, a pandemic that arguably is responsible for most of the deaths in the world by suicide (since it is thought that the majority of suicides are the outcome of mental illness), and presumably for millions of what the medical researchers call "YPLL," or "years of potential life lost." For example, the average number of YPLL in a person with schizophrenia is 14.5 (Hjorthøj et al. 2017). The National Institute of Mental Health defines two general categories of mental illness: any mental illness (AMI) and serious mental illness (SMI). In 2019, 20.6% of adults in the United States (51.5 million) had AMI, of which only 44.8% (23 million) received services. Of adults, 5.2% (or 13.1 million) had SMI, and 65.5% (or 13.1 million) received mental health services (National Institute of Mental Health 2020). Of course, we've gone over the much higher numbers of mental illnesses in prison.

You'll want to pick your battles wisely, fix what you think you can fix, and not spend more time than required trying to fix anything that doesn't seem to warrant the effort. We are referring, of course, to those prisoners who may not benefit from any form of psychotherapy, group or individual. Unless you work in Shangri-La (which is unlikely, because it does not have any prisons), you should advocate for changes in your institution and society as a whole. And we certainly do wish that when the time comes for the next edition of our book, the publishers will say, "We don't need a book about therapy for prisoners, because we deal with crime in the community." Then we would really be in Shangri-La!

So network with your colleagues locally and nationally and even meet with them if the current viruses allow. Hopefully, since nearly all prisoners do leave, you will have the opportunity to prepare some of your patients to get out, help find them homes, and help them to lead productive lives—and not do their intakes again.

We know that the revolving door of admissions can often seem like the labor of Sisyphus. You roll up your patients, roll them out the door, and find them rolling back into intake a month or year later. You talk your patients out of suicide, only to have them attempt it again. You teach your patients about relapse prevention, only to have them relapse when they go home. Or you teach them to be prosocial, only to hear they have committed a violent crime that horrifies the community. Reprising Camus, he reminds us of the myth of Sisyphus, who was condemned by the Gods to roll a boulder to the top of a mountain and then watch it roll down again. There is nothing worse, says Camus, than being forced to do a futile and hopeless task (Camus 1942/2018, p. 119). By one account, Sisyphus was punished for putting Death in chains for a while and depriving Pluto of his usual foot traffic. Consider that you deal in life and death matters on a day-by-day basis, and perhaps it's not with iron links but with your concatenations of words that your therapy puts Death and Destruction in chains, at least for a little while, in your patients' lives. As the ancient Greeks would say, it takes a lot of hubris to do that, and you've got to expect some pushback from Death and Destruction for impinging on their territories! (Of course, those folks should really have no complaints for what they accomplished in 2020.)

Thank you for spending this time with us. Go forth and therapize—but supportively!

References

Avert: Global HIV and AIDS statistics. 2021. Available at: www.avert.org/global-hiv-and-aids-statistics#:~:text=Since%20the%20start%20of%20the%20epidemic%2C%20an%20estimated,in%202004%20and%201.4%20million%20in%202010.%202. Accessed June 4, 2021.

Camus A: The Myth of Sisyphus (1942). Translated by O'Brien J. New York, Vintage, 2018

Hjorthøj C, Stürup AE, McGrath JJ, Nordentoft M: Years of potential life lost and life expectancy in schizophrenia: a systematic review and meta-analysis. Lancet Psychiatry 4(4):295–301, 2017 28237639

Kelly BK: COVID-19: Real problems but no pandemic of mental illness: COVID-19 is stretching our resilience, but we are stronger than we think. Psychology Today, November 17, 2020. Available at: www.psychologytoday.com/us/blog/psychiatry-and-society/202011/covid-19-real-problems-no-pandemic-mental-illness. Accessed November 29, 2020.

National Institute of Mental Health: Mental illness, 2020. Available at: www.nimh.nih.gov/health/statistics/mental-illness.shtml#:~:text=Mental%20illnesses%20are%20common%20in%20the%20United%20States.,severity%2C%20ranging%20from%20mild%20to%20moderate%20to%20severe. Accessed November 20, 2020.

White J: Alien Emergencies: A Sector General Omnibus. New York, Tor Books, 2002

Index

Page numbers printed in **boldface** type refer to tables and figures.